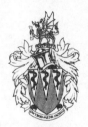

BENIGN DISORDERS AND DISEASES OF THE BREAST

Concepts and Clinical Management

Second Edition

Commissioning Editor   Sue Hodgson
Project Manager   Helen Sofio
Design Direction   Ian Spick/Deborah Gyan

BENIGN DISORDERS AND DISEASES OF THE BREAST

Concepts and Clinical Management

Second Edition

L.E. Hughes MB DS FRCS FRACS Emeritus Professor of Surgery

R.E. Mansel MB MS FRCS Professor and Chairman of Division of Surgery

D.J.T. Webster MD FRCS Senior Lecturer and Consultant Surgeon

University of Wales College of Medicine Heath Park Cardiff UK

With the collaboration of

K. Lyons MB BCh BAO FRCR Consultant Radiologist University Hospital of Wales and Breast Test Wales

D. M. Davies MS FRCS Consultant Plastic Surgeon Charing Cross Hospital London UK

S. J. Leinster MD FRCS Professor of Surgery University of Liverpool UK

With a Foreword by Kirby I. Bland

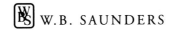

W.B. SAUNDERS

London Edinburgh New York Philadelphia St Louis Sydney Toronto 2000

WB Saunders
An imprint of Harcourt Publishers Limited

© Copyright Harcourt Publishers Limited 2000

W.B. SAUNDERS is a registered trademark of Harcourt Publishers Limited

The right of LE Hughes, RE Mansel and DTJ Webster to be identified as the authors of this work has been asserted by them in accordance with the Copyright, Designs and Patents Act, 1988.

First published 2000

ISBN 0 7020 20699

Cataloguing in Publication Data:
Catalogue records for this book are available from the British Library and the US Library of Congress.

Note
Medical knowledge is constantly changing. As new information becomes available, changes in treatment, procedures, equipment and the use of drugs become necessary. The editors, authors, contributors and the publishers have, as far as possible, taken care to ensure that the information given in this text is accurate and up to date. However, readers are strongly advised to confirm that the information, especially with regard to drug usage, complies with the latest legislation and standards of practice.

Printed and bound by Grafos, SA Arte Sobre papel, Barcelona, Spain

The
Publisher's
Policy is to use
**paper manufactured
from sustainable forests**

To quote the editors of Harrison's Principles of Internal Medicine, "No greater opportunity, responsibility or obligation can fall to the lot of a human being than to become a physician." Harrison's editors continue, "The physician should ask of his destiny no more than this; he should be content with no less." In the care of the suffering, a physician requires constant refinement of technical skills, scientific knowledge and human understanding. Those who follow these basic precepts with courage, humility and wisdom build an enduring edifice of character within themselves and provide the patient a unique service. The practice of medicine seeks to utilize scientific methods and principles in the solutions of its problems. As all those engaged in medical practice know, it is an art as much as it is a science.

With this book, Les Hughes, Robert Mansel and David Webster have raised the science of medicine in a particular discipline to an art. The thorough descriptions of the many benign conditions of the breast are enhanced by explanation of the etiologic and physiologic processes that initiate these benign states. Special attention is paid to understanding physiologic and anatomical reasons for treatment failures, illuminating for those of us who have failed, and who among us has not? Detailed, well-illustrated step-by-step descriptions of operative techniques ensure that surgical practitioners can achieve superior technical results.

The authors appropriately emphasize that past medical approaches to benign disease have focused attention solely on the exclusion of neoplastic disease and/or cancer risk; however, these authors elucidate the characteristics of these conditions in their own right. This reference, to my knowledge, delivers the most comprehensive coverage of benign breast disorders of any books in the current literature.

The authors point out the terminologic confusion that exists, because of the unwillingness of breast scholars to remove all imprecise, vague and fallacious jargon from the nomenclature. I strongly agree with the authors that the term 'fibrocystic disease' must be dismissed as antique, obfuscatory parlance. More precise pathological and clinically meaningful terminology should be promulgated by physician–scientists working with pathologists to provide more accurate descriptions of benign and malignant disorders.

Not content with the simple presentation of basic physiologic characteristics, these experts take great strides towards replacing confusing definitions with a better system. They argue for acceptance of new terminology derived from the 'aberrations of normal development and involution' (ANDI) – a comprehensive, meaningful and descriptive construct for nomenclature of benign disorders.

A new chapter in this edition deals with psychological implications of benign entities. Another new chapter surveys state-of-the-art cosmetic approaches. The varying claims of systemic disease induced by silicone implants are reviewed; the evidence convincingly documents that there is no causal relationship of silicone implants to cancer or other syndromes. The loss, perhaps temporary, of this valued method for rehabilitation after total mastectomy has created a major void in the physical–mental rehabilitation of these patients.

The content and concepts in this book reaffirm our fealty to the noble principles and the noble art of surgical practice. *Benign Disorders and Diseases of the Breast* provides the clinician with a thorough fundamental knowledge of aspects of benign breast diseases – valuable to all in the practices of internal medicine, family medicine, surgery and radiation oncology.

Kirby I. Bland, MD
Professor of Medical Sciences
J. Murray Beardsley Professor and Chairman
Brown University Department of Surgery
Surgeon-in-Chief, Rhode Island Hospital
Executive Surgeon-in-Chief, Brown University Affiliated Hospitals
USA

PREFACE TO THE SECOND EDITION

Our first edition was written to meet a need – the lack of a textbook dealing comprehensively with the benign conditions which constitute 90% or more of clinical problems related to the breast. Its aim was threefold.

The first aim was to provide a comprehensive account of all benign conditions affecting the breast, through a detailed review of the literature of the past 100 years, interpreted alongside the distillation of our own experience in a clinic started in 1972 to deal specifically with cyclical mastalgia and other benign conditions.

The second was to provide a pragmatic approach to diagnosis and management, again based primarily on our own experience from the many open studies and controlled clinical trials carried out over 17 years, and on an assessment of the somewhat disparate literature available.

Third, to discuss in greater detail the ANDI concept of pathogenesis and classification developed in this unit, based on the increasing recognition that many clinical presentations are based on minor abnormalities of normal physiological processes, with only a few being associated with sufficient morbidity or potential morbidity to justify the term disease. Hence BBD is better considered as mainly benign breast disorders, rather than benign breast disease.

The gratifying response to the book has confirmed a need, and 10 years on the need to update it with a second edition is just as great. There have been many developments in each of these three areas. Examples are new insights into aetiology, such as the influence of smoking on periductal mastitis: data on cancer risk has been refined; while developments in molecular biology are at last promising new insights into pathogenesis. Interest in benign breast disease has increased exponentially, with a parallel increase in the literature, much more geographically widespread than was the case 10 years ago. A comprehensive and critical review of the publications of the past 10 years has been rewarding.

The need for our dedicated clinic has not abated, so we continue to see even more patients after 27 years. Significant changes in management have occurred, such as acceptance of conservative management of fibroadenoma and percutaneous drainage of abscesses, but the greatest changes lie in diagnosis and assessment. The day of the multidisciplinary, one-stop clinic has arrived, so that diagnosis should be available at first attendance in most cases, much of this due to improvements in imaging modalities. These critically important developments are fully covered.

The ANDI classification and concepts have been increasingly accepted – not least by an international multidisciplinary working party – but the old concept and terminology of fibrocystic disease continues to fight a rearguard action in spite of almost universal recognition that it is falsely based and inaccurate. The past 10 years have seen many interesting developments supporting the ANDI concept, some from molecular biology.

New chapters have been added on cosmetic surgery, psychological aspects and geographical variations. The underlying pathology and disease processes are again covered fully for each condition, but histopathology has not been covered in a specialist chapter. It is felt that such a complex and detailed subject is best approached by interaction with pathology colleagues or through pathology textbooks, but a short chapter written from a clinician's viewpoint seeks to help clarify some of the terminology for the clinician who is unable to meet regularly with his pathologist colleague.

LH, RM, DW
October 1999

ACKNOWLEDGEMENTS

We owe a debt of gratitude to many people who have contributed to work on which this book is based. Foremost are those research fellows who have been responsible for the day-to-day conduct of many studies and clinical trials in this department over the last 27 years: Paul Preece, John Wisbey, Nigel Pashby, Jonathan Pye, Sandeep Kumar, Anurag Srivastava, Barney Harrison, Paul Maddox, Graham Pritchard, Stephen Courtney, Glyn Neades, Richard Cochrane, Eleri Lloyd-Davies, Chris Gateley and Anup Sharma.

We are much indebted to co-operation from the Departments of Radiology – especially Dr Huw Gravelle and Dr Kathleen Lyons, and of Pathology – especially Drs Winsor Fortt and Tony Douglas-Jones. This book could not have been produced without the exceptional service given by the Department of Medical Illustration under Professor R Marshall and now Professor R Morton.

The secretarial staff of the University Department of Surgery, both clinical and academic, have facilitated all aspects of the clinical and research work and documentation behind the book, and Mrs Edna Lewis has given many years of voluntary service to the Mastalgia Clinic.

Above all we are grateful to our wives and families who have foregone so much over many years in the cause of research and the writing of this book.

THIS BOOK IS DEDICATED TO

CD Haagensen
Surgeon Pathologist

JD Azzopardi
Surgical Pathologist

Whose meticulous studies have cast so much light on breast disorders, and
whose monographs are quoted so freely in this book.

Problems of concept and nomenclature of benign disorders of the breast

CONTENTS

KEY POINTS AND NEW DEVELOPMENTS

1. Only by taking a historical view of benign disorders of the breast can the confusion persisting until recent decades be understood.
2. In the past, benign conditions (and the patients carrying them) have been regarded as requiring exclusion of cancer or cancer risk, rather than entities requiring management in their own right.
3. Clinical conditions, such as painful nodularity, have been equated with and confused with histological conditions, such as fibrosis or hyperplasia.

4. Most accept that the concepts and terminology of 'fibrocystic disease' and 'fibroadenosis' cannot be justified, but this recognition has so far been matched by masterly inactivity.
5. Accurate and meaningful terminology will be achieved only if those in the field agree on one and use it and accept it. The aberrations of normal development and involution (ANDI) concept and terminology provides a means of achieving this.

THE SOURCE OF THE PROBLEM

The condition commonly called fibrocystic disease, or fibroadenosis of the breast, has been a clinical problem for centuries, as reflected in writings as early as those of Astley Cooper at the beginning of the nineteenth century. For patients it causes discomfort and anxiety which varies from nuisance value to serious interference with the quality of life. For clinicians, the condition causes a range of problems of diagnosis, assessment and management which are not always clearly recognized.

Although all clinicians have a concept of what fibrocystic disease represents, it is difficult to define, and none of its protagonists has given a meaningful differentiation between it and normality. One definition[1] is 'palpable lumps in the breast, usually associated with pain and tenderness that fluctuate with the menstrual cycle and become progressively worse until the menopause'. Despite giving a definition, this author, like many before him, states that the term fibrocystic disease has no real meaning and should probably be abandoned. Nevertheless, he also lists the histological features, fibroadenomas, macrocysts, fibrosis, duct dilatation and stasis, periductal round cell infiltrate, fat necrosis, papillomatosis, apocrine metaplasia, sclerosing adenosis and hyperplastic lesions of duct and lobule. This covers the whole range of benign conditions of the breast, and it is clearly inappropriate to equate this histological panorama with a mild, or even severe, degree of painful nodularity.

With such a loose equivalence between clinical and histological detail, it is not surprising that Foote and Stewart wrote in 1945: 'chronic cystic mastitis is so ingrained in the minds of some pathologists that this diagnosis of a locally excised portion of the breast almost amounts to a surgico-pathological reflex'.[2] What is surprising is that pathologists are still the most insistent single group to maintain the use of the term, despite this stinging remark from eminent members of their own discipline.

Greater interest in benign breast disorders in recent years has led to a more precise understanding of the clinical pictures associated with individual elements, and the histological changes of cyclical nodularity are increasingly recognized as lying within the range of histological appearance in the normal breast. Many authors have tried to determine and assess premalignant potential of fibrocystic disease but most attempts have resulted in confusion and frustration. Recent workers, especially Page and co-workers,[3,4] have shown that only a few specific histological patterns have an association with cancer and these show no consistent correlation with the clinical picture which in the past has been ascribed to fibrocystic disease. This poor correlation between histology and clinical symptoms led Love and her co-authors[5] to conclude that fibrocystic disease of the breast is a 'non-disease'. Their arguments are cogent in a histological context by denying the loosely defined cancer risk, but a concept of non-disease does little to help the many women who suffer from a variety of physical symptoms – sometimes of distressing severity. Disorder is a better term than disease because so many of the symptomatic conditions lie within the spectrum of normality. The magnitude of the problem is escalating with the wider concern of women about breast disease and the wider introduction of breast screening programmes.

Benign conditions of the breast have always been neglected in comparison to cancer, despite the fact that only one out of ten patients presenting to a breast clinic suffers from cancer. This is not surprising in view of the emotional implications of breast cancer and its treatment, but it has meant that the study of the benign breast has been undeservedly neglected. Until the 1970s reported studies were directed largely towards a possible relationship to cancer, rather than towards the basic processes underlying benign conditions.

There has been a noticeable and welcome correction to this neglect in recent years, but already the interest in benign disorders evident for two decades is again on the wane, at a time when advances in molecular biology give promise of understanding the basic physiology of human breast development, function and involution.

This neglect is most evident in standard textbooks (the most recent comprehensive texts on breast disease devote less than 5% of their material to benign conditions) because interest in benign processes can be found when studying historical reference material. Great names in surgery such as Hunter, Astley Cooper, Billroth, Cheatle, Semb, Bloodgood and Atkins appear in the literature. But whereas breast cancer has stimulated a continuous, on-going body of research – each new project building on the work preceding it – benign disease has been the subject of a relatively small number of isolated and unconnected projects, earlier related work having often been ignored. The sporadic nature of these investigations and the insularity of the resulting publications had led to much confusion which has had more serious consequences than neglect alone.

Consideration of benign breast disorders from a historical point of view provides a clearer understanding of how the present problems have arisen.

HISTORY

Sir Astley Cooper was an important early worker in this field. He described many aspects of benign breast disorders as well as malignant disease, in his monograph, *Illustrations of Diseases of the Breast*,[6] published in 1829. Among the conditions discussed are cystic disease, pain and fibroadenoma. He distinguished two main groups of patients with mastalgia – those with and those without a palpable tumour, which we might now better define as painful nodularity and noncyclical breast pain. He also laid much of the basis of the macroscopic anatomy of the breast in his book on the anatomy of diseases of the breast published in 1845. The French surgeon Reclus gave an excellent description of the clinical and pathological aspects of cystic disease in 1893, recognizing both the multiplicity and bilaterality of the cysts.[7]

Many of the current problems in terminology and understanding derive from the publications of German surgeons in the late nineteenth century. Koenig[8] called the disease 'chronic cystic mastitis', because he believed it had an inflammatory basis. At the same time, Schimmelbusch[9] described the same condition, compounding the problem by calling it 'cystadenoma'. Both authors gave the disease inexact names, and both gave incomplete descriptions of the pathology. Certainly they did not recognize the wide range of histological appearances found in these breasts, and they failed to recognize these as merely variants of normal processes within the breast.

There was an early reaction to this confusion. Cabot[10] questioned the inflammatory connotation of the term chronic cystic mastitis and urged more precise terminology, but unfortunately his pleas fell on stony ground. In the 1920s there were major studies by Semb in Norway[11] and Cheatle and Cutler in the UK[12] and their disease descriptions and data are still worth serious study. However, Cheatle and Cutler gave the name 'cystiphorous desquamative epithelial hyperplasia' to the clinical spectrum we have termed aberrations of normal development and involution in Chapter 3 and this can hardly be regarded as helpful. The tendency of the Scandinavians to use Semb's term 'fibroadenomatosis' also caused difficulty because of its confusion with the term fibroadenoma.[11] In spite of detailed investigations, Cheatle and Cutler confused changes of cyclical nodularity with both duct ectasia and fibroadenomas[12] and the term they finally chose – 'mazoplasia' – is hardly evocative in a descriptive sense.

While most workers concentrated on the clinical problems of fibrocystic disease, some gave accurate descriptions of other benign breast conditions. The paper on 'the varicocele tumour' by Bloodgood is a striking account of the clinical and macropathological aspects of duct ectasia and its clinical variants.[13] The accuracy and detail of the observations come as a surprise to those who believe advances in medical understanding are recent.

Special clinics for breast disease set up by Atkins in London and Geschickter in the USA concentrated experience and allowed adequate documentation and assessment of the results of treatment for the first time during the 1940s. Both authors made many contributions to benign breast disorders,[14,15] but suffered equally from the limited knowledge at that time of basic pathology and endocrinology of the breast. They both unfortunately continued the use of the term chronic mastitis. The 50 years since their contributions has seen an increasing momentum in investigation of benign breast conditions. Great benefit has derived from histological study of the normal breast and the development of hormonal estimations using radioimmunoassay. In particular, the autopsy study of Sandison[16] showed that most of the changes previously regarded as disease are so common as to be within the spectrum of normality and his work stimulated others to define the wide range of histological appearances of the normal breast. For example, Parks[17] studied both surgical and autopsy specimens and showed a gradation between normal lobules and fibroadenomas, and between involuting lobules and cyst formation. He also showed that papillary epithelial hyperplasia of the terminal ducts is so common in the premenopausal period as to be regarded as

normal, and that these lesions regress without treatment after the menopause. In 1961 Oberman and French[18] also stressed the concept of a continuum between normality and benign conditions: 'adenofibromas, fibrocystic disease and intraductal papillomas do not appear to represent distinct entities, but rather form a spectrum of conditions having their basis in an abnormality between hormonal stimulus to the breast, principally estrogen, and stromal and epithelial response'.

These writers have had a profound insight into the concepts discussed in this book, and it is salutary to go back even further. In 1922, McFarland[19] wrote: 'The so-called chronic mastitis is not inflammatory, and is not a pathological entity; it is nothing but a result – or at most a perversion – of involution. The only difficulty lies in clearly defining when the process of involution can be said to become abnormal, when it is so diversified.' The seed scattered by these workers has largely fallen on stony ground.

THE PRESENT AND THE FUTURE

In the past, each worker has tended to introduce their own terminology for a condition, either to stress a particular aspect they have noted, or through ignorance of work that has gone on perhaps many years before. As an illustration of this, Table 1.1 shows the large number of names that have been associated with just three conditions: so-called fibrocystic disease, duct ectasia and giant fibroadenomas.

Table 1.1 Some of the names used for common benign breast disorders
Cyclical nodularity
Fibrocystic disease
Fibroadenosis
Cystic hyperplasia
Hyperplastic cystic disease
Schimmelbusch's disease
Chronic cystic mastitis
Cystic mastopathy
Duct ectasia/periductal mastitis
Plasma cell mastitis
Varicocele tumour
Comedo mastitis
Mastitis obliterans
Secretory disease
Giant fibroadenomatous tumours
Giant fibroadenoma
Cystosarcoma phyllodes
Phyllodes tumour
Juvenile fibroadenoma
Serocystic disease of Brodie

This list is by no means comprehensive; some 40 names have been used to describe the variety of conditions covered by the old term, chronic fibrocystic disease, none of which can be considered satisfactory.

Because of their multiplicity and lack of specificity, past terms are better replaced by the use of clinical or histological terms which are specific and accurate in relation to the clinical and/or histological condition to which they refer. Examples of appropriate clinical terms are mastalgia and cyclical nodularity. Examples of appropriate histological terms that have evolved over recent years are sclerosing adenosis, atypical ductal hyperplasia, etc. Terms that accurately reflect both clinical and histological counterparts are fibroadenoma, duct papilloma and macrocyst, for example.

When it is desirable to cover the whole range of (unspecified) benign breast disorders, it is appropriate to use a term which, unlike fibrocystic disease, does not imply a disease state, but acknowledges the spectrum of change extending from normality and recognizes that most of the spectrum does not represent disease. We suggest that 'aberrations of normal development and involution' (ANDI) is a term which meets these criteria; it is comprehensive, and meaningful and descriptive in terms of pathogenesis.

Why has it taken so long to reach a reasonable understanding of the processes involved in benign breast conditions? The main stumbling block has been the failure to appreciate the range of basic physiological and structural changes within the normal breast – an organ dynamic throughout the reproductive period of life as it first develops, then undergoes repeated cyclical change and finally involutes. Because it is an organ under systemic hormonal influence, one would expect the breast to be uniform throughout in its appearance and behaviour, but this is not so. Like other endocrine target organs such as the thyroid, it varies greatly from one part to another, and end-organ response must be a factor in this variability. It has been usual practice to concentrate on the local findings as shown by biopsy, at one point in time when the patient presents with a clinical problem, assuming that the particular clinical condition at that time is directly associated with the local radiological and biopsy findings. It is tempting to ignore the findings of Parks and Sandison and others, that all these apparently specific findings are frequently found in asymptomatic breasts. So a particular clinical event that leads a patient to biopsy must be assessed against the background of this almost random variation in histological appearance which is a part of normality.

A further source of confusion has arisen from the association of radiological appearances with pathological descriptions, without adequate correlative studies to establish a relationship. An example of recent decades has been the description of radiological density as 'dysplasia' in relation to Wolfe patterns – when detailed study can show that density is unrelated to epithelial dysplasia.[20] The situation was then compounded by using the term 'dysplastic breast' for a radiological pattern, without histological correlation or confirmation. The welfare of the patient with benign breast problems will be best served by abandoning terminology that implies disease, and substituting terminology which reflects the normality of many of the underlying processes, reserving 'disease' for those conditions where clinical morbidity or histological significance warrants such a term. The terminology should come from consideration of the basic physiological and pathological processes that lead a patient to present to a breast clinic.

Perhaps the reason for persisting and increasing confusion is an unwillingness to be sufficiently radical in moving away from ideas that do not fit in with present knowledge. Not only must the concept of fibrocystic disease as a clinical concept or a histopathological entity be done away with, it must be replaced by an accurate terminology consistent with present knowledge. Many breast physicians accept the first half of this statement, but are unwilling to accept the corollary inherent in the second half.

These basic aspects of the non-malignant breast, and the arguments for the aberrations of normal development and involution terminology, are considered in Chapter 3.

REFERENCES

1. Scanlon EF. The early diagnosis of breast cancer. *Cancer* 1981; **48**: 523–526.

2. Foote FW & Stewart FW. Comparative study of cancerous versus noncancerous breast. II. The role of so-called chronic cystic mastitis in mammary carcinogenesis. *Annals of Surgery* 1945; **121**: 197–222.

3. Page DL, Vander-Zwag R, Rogers LW *et al*. Relationship between component parts of fibrocystic disease complex and breast cancer. *Journal of the National Cancer Institute* 1978; **61**: 1055–1063.

4. Page DL & Dupont WD. Anatomic indications (histologic and cytologic) of increased breast cancer risk. *Breast Cancer Research and Treatment* 1993; **28**: 157–162.

5. Love SM, Gelman RS & Silen W. Fibrocystic 'disease' of the breast. A non disease. *New England Journal of Medicine* 1982; **307**: 1010–1014.

6. Cooper A. *Illustrations of Diseases of the Breast*. London: Longmans, 1829.

7. Reclus P. Maladie Kystique De La Mammelle. *La Semaine Medicale* 1893; **13**: 353–354.

8. Koenig P. Mastitis chronica cystica. *Centralblatt für Chirurgie* 1893; **20**: 49–53.

9. Schimmelbusch C. Das Fibroadenom der Mamma. *Archiv für Klinische Chirurgie* 1892; **64**: 102–116.

10. Cabot RC. Irritable breasts, or chronic lobular mastitis. *Boston Medical and Surgical Journal* 1900; **CXLIII**: 555–557.

11. Semb C. Pathologico-anatomical and clinical investigations of fibroadenomatosis cystica mammae. *Acta Chirurgica Scandinavica Supplementum* 1928; **64**(10): 1–484.

12. Cheatle GL & Cutler M. *Tumours of the Breast*. London: Edward Arnold, 1931.

13. Bloodgood JC. The clinical picture of dilated ducts beneath the nipple frequently to be palpated as a doughy, worm-like mass – the varicocele tumour of the breast. *Surgery, Gynecology and Obstetrics* 1923; **26**: 486–495.

14. Atkins HJB. Chronic mastitis. *Lancet* 1938; i: 707–712.

15. Geschickter CF. *Diseases of the Breast*, 2nd edn. Philadelphia: JB Lippincott & Co., 1945.

16. Sandison AT. An autopsy study of the human breast. *National Cancer Institute Monograph No. 8*, US Dept Health, Education and Welfare, 1962.

17. Parks AG. The microanatomy of the breast. *Annals of the Royal College of Surgeons of England* 1959; **25**: 295–311.

18. Oberman HA & French AJ. Chronic fibrocystic disease of the breast. *Surgery, Gynecology and Obstetrics* 1961; **112**: 647–652.

19. McFarland J. Residual lactation acini in the female breasts. Their relationship to chronic cystic mastitis and malignant breasts. *Archives of Surgery* 1922; **5**: 1–64.

20. Mansel RE, Gravelle IH & Hughes LE. The interpretation of mammographic ductal enlargement in cancerous breasts. *British Journal of Surgery* 1979; **66**: 701–702.

Chapter 2

Breast anatomy and physiology

CONTENTS

KEY POINTS AND NEW DEVELOPMENTS

1. The key structures of the breast are the ductolobar segmental systems as the functional macro-unit and the terminal ductal lobular unit (TDLU) as the functional micro-unit.
2. The macroscopic ductolobar segmental units based on the excretory ducts at the nipple vary greatly in extent, shape and functional capability, and do not conform (as usually represented) to a regular pyramidal shape radiating from the nipple.
3. The microscopic TDLU is the site of origin of most ductal and lobular carcinoma-in-situ (DCIS and LCIS). The epithelium here consistently shows the highest mitotic rate of any breast epithelium.
4. Four types of lobules represent progressive phases of lobular development from menarche (type I) to the post-lactational state (type IV). Types I and II are more reactive to chemical carcinogens in-vitro and DCIS and LCIS may originate in them. Type III lobules are thought to be involved in involutional changes of aberrations of normal development and involution (ANDI).
5. The same four lobule types seen through 40 years of adult reproductive life are found in the lobules of infants compressed into the first 2 years of childhood.

6. The importance of the structure and activity of the basement membrane is increasingly recognized – a complex lattice-like structure lying between stroma and epithelium, with a complex paracrine pathway between stromal, myoepithelial and epithelial cells.
7. An increasingly complex role for oxytocin in breast function is now recognized.
8. The mechanisms of breast involution are related to ovarian function. While follicle-stimulating hormone levels rise progressively from the age of 30 to the menopause, oestradiol and luteinizing hormone levels remain relatively constant.
9. The differing relationships of mitosis to apoptosis during the menstrual cycle in different age groups may explain the onset of the involutional changes of ANDI.
10. The anthropomorphic measurements of the aesthetically 'ideal' breast have been defined. These are important in advising and assessing the results of reconstructive and cosmetic surgery.

DEVELOPMENT

The prepubertal breast is identical in both sexes and consists of a number of small ducts embedded in a collagenous stroma. The ducts develop *in utero* from an ectodermal mammary ridge which invades the epidermis at the seventh embryonic week and progresses to a budding stage at the twelfth week. The classical view has been that the mammary ridge extends from the base of the upper limb bud to the base of the lower limb bud (Figure 2.1).

This view arose from theories derived from comparative anatomy, and are not supported by studies of human embryos, which show that the mammary ridge extends only over the axillopectoral area. (Pathology in the groin mimicking mammary disease mostly arises from mammary-like anogenital glands (MLG), which are normal constituents of the vulva and perianal region. They are considered to be related to eccrine and apocrine glands, and to be the source of mammary-like pathology in this region, such as lactating glands, fibroadenoma, extramammary Paget's disease, etc.[1])

Already by the 12-mm stage the mammary ridge is shortening and migrating dorso-ventrally, so by the 14-mm stage it is found only as an elevated nipple primordium on the ventral wall of the thorax.[2] The epithelial bud then branches and canalizes between weeks 13 and 20 to form the 15–20 major ducts found in the adult breast. The major ducts at this stage only have small vesicles at the distal ends and no lobular development is visible. The increasing development of the fetal breast parenchyma induces considerable growth and specialization of the surrounding stroma. A comprehensive three-layer vascular network forms at the 9–10 week budding stage and eventually produces a cylindrical vascular envelope around each of the major ducts.[3] From the tenth week *in utero* to birth a series of developments occur. Ingrowth of connective tissue gives rise to partitions between each of the end-vesicles (primitive alveoli) and acts as a framework for the adult segmental pattern. Specialized fat cells also invade the matrices between the blood vessels and fibrous septae. Externally the nipple is small and flattened, although rudimentary sebaceous glands and Montgomery's tubercles are present. The circular interlacing smooth muscle fibres that give the nipple its erectile properties are already developed at this stage.

All the above changes are completed by the time of birth. At this time, transient secretory changes occur in the newborn breast which give rise to the clinical entities of 'witches' milk' or 'neonatal mastitis'. In late pregnancy the high levels of luteal and placental hormones in the mother's blood cross the placenta into the fetal circulation and cause stimulation of the fetal breast. This primes the primitive fetal end-vesicles for milk production in an analogous fashion to the adult female breast in late pregnancy. Birth inevitably causes separation of the maternal

and fetal circulations, resulting in a rapid fall in circulating sex steroids in the baby's blood, whereas prolactin secretion is maintained by the baby's pituitary. These conditions correspond once more to the maternal situation and result in secretion of colostrum which can be expressed from the nipple in 80–90% of newborn breasts of either sex. The newborn prolactin levels then decline and the secretion dries up over the next few weeks. Thus the secretion of colostrum and the swelling of the newborn breast are both normal physiological events and should not be considered as due to disease unless they become persistent.

A recent histological study has provided detailed information about the state of the breast during this neonatal period and the first 2 years of life.[4] The pattern is identical in males and females. Three morphological degrees of development are seen, varying from minimal blunt budding to fully developed lobules equivalent to the type 1 virginal lobule described in the adult by Russo and Russo (see below). Five functional stages are described which are seen as a continuum, proliferation

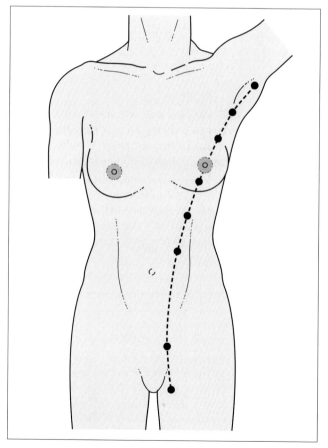

2.1 The classical view of the extent of the fetal mammary ridge. It is now accepted that the ridge does not normally extend as far as the abdomen in the human. Hence in practical terms accessory nipples or breasts are found only along the proximal half of this line (see Chapter 15).

proceeding to active secretory epithelium followed by apocrine metaplasia, formation of microcysts and involution. Embryonic fat is sometimes seen as well-defined islands surrounded by fibrous tissue. The morphology of the myoepithelial cells varies, apparently in tandem with the functional activity of the underlying epithelial cells. The intralobular stroma also shows changes, being very loose and vascular during the secretory stage, and more dense, less cellular and vascular during the involutional stage. All these changes are remarkably similar to those seen during adult reproductive life.

CHANGES AT PUBERTY

The next steps in development are activated at puberty in the female and follow the well-ordered sequence described by Marshall and Tanner[5] and Zacharias et al.[6] (Figure 2.2).

The first change (at about the age of 10 years) is growth of the mammary tissue beneath the areola with enlargement of the areolar area producing the characteristic swelling known as the breast bud or mound. This development is often asymmetrical. At 12 years the nipple begins to grow outwards and the breast elevation increases, but there is no distinct separation between nipple and areola. Between the ages of 14 and 15, increasing subareolar growth leads to elevation of the areola above the breast outline giving the 'secondary mound'. The familiar shape of the adult resting breast is then attained by a recession in the level of the areola to that of the surrounding breast, leaving the nipple projecting.

The exact physiological mechanisms that trigger and control the changes of puberty are not fully understood but the primary event in the initiation of puberty is the increasing secretion of follicle-stimulating hormone (FSH) and luteinizing hormone (LH) from the anterior pituitary in response to increasing stimulation by the hypothalamus. Detectable levels of FSH and LH are found in pre-pubertal children showing that some hypothalamic activity is present even in young children. As maturation proceeds,

this hypothalamic activity increases progressively between the ages of 8 and 18, and during these years sexual development can be shown to correlate with plasma oestradiol levels. This is probably due to a change in frequency of the pulsatile secretion of the gonadotrophin-releasing factors.[7] The increased FSH/LH causes activation of primordial ovarian follicles and secretion of oestrogen which is responsible for the first stages of breast development. Oestrogen, predominant during the anovulatory cycles typical of the first years, induces duct sprouting and branching but lobular development at this stage consists only of small buds. Adult levels of progesterone are required for further development of the lobular component at puberty as well as during the menstrual cycle and pregnancy.[8] Oestrogen also induces connective tissue and vascular growth which is required for the support of the new ducts; the connective tissue in turn stimulates fat deposition. When ovulating cycles begin, luteal function improves, the increased output of progesterone balances the oestrogen and results in differentiation of the terminal ductular buds to produce adult lobules. These differential growth patterns associated with the two major ovarian steroids have been studied principally in animals,[9,10] but appear to be true also for the human. While it is generally accepted that progesterone is important for lobulo-alveolar development at puberty, during menstrual cyclical changes and during pregnancy, details of the underlying mechanisms remain unclear. It is still uncertain whether the action on cell proliferation is direct via progesterone receptor, or by some other progesterone-related factor. Insulin, growth hormone, corticosteroids and prolactin are also required for optimal growth of the breast but only play minor roles.

ADULT ANATOMY

The adult female breasts lie on each side of the anterior thorax with their bases extending from about the second to the sixth ribs. Medially the breasts reach the sternal edge

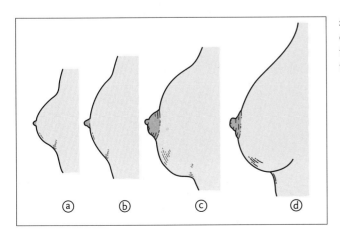

2.2 The stages of breast development at puberty. (**a**) Breast bud elevation; (**b**) growth and protrusion of the nipple; (**c**) elevation of the secondary areolar mound; (**d**) regression of the areolar mound to the level of the general breast contour.

and laterally the midaxillary line and extend up into the axilla via a pyramidal-shaped axillary tail (Figure 2.3).

The breast lies on a substantial layer of fascia overlying the pectoralis major muscle in the superomedial two-thirds and the serratus anterior muscle in the lower outer one-third. Duct injection under pressure to distend terminal ductules shows that duct-containing breast tissue often extends more widely than this – to the midline, and well up into the axilla.[11] Breast tissue extends below the costal margin in 15% of cases, and beyond the anterior border of latissimus dorsi in 2%. Ductal elements also extend very close to the skin. This wide extension explains the difficulty of removing all breast tissue by subcutaneous mastectomy and is important for matching the contralateral breasts in cosmetic and reconstructive surgery. Hicken's findings have been confirmed more recently in surgical studies.

Considerable asymmetry is frequently found among normal women, and the patient may not be aware of it, or may accept it as a normal variant. One half of women have a volume difference of 10% between left and right breasts, and a quarter have a 20% difference.[12] The left breast is usually the larger.

Westreich[13] has recently reviewed the anthropomorphic measurements of the 'aesthetically perfect' breast, important in assessing the need for and results of reconstructive and cosmetic surgery. This paper provides a simple protocol for measurement of the breast and its landmarks in relation to fixed skeletal points. The precise position of the nipple areolar complex varies widely with the fat content of the breast and the age of the woman. In the nulliparous breast, it lies between 19 and 21 cm from the suprasternal notch measured diagonally.

The amount of fat within the breast varies widely, as would be expected. The intimacy with which it is mixed with glandular tissue also varies, and is important in relation to the use of liposuction as an adjuvant to reduction mammaplasty. The question has recently been studied quantitatively in material removed during reduction procedures.[14] The proportion of the breast mass constituted by fat varied from 2% to 78%, with a mean in this group of patients of 48%. Breast fat increases with age, body mass and total breast volume, but this is not absolute; fat can predominate over glandular tissue in young women as well. The amount of fatty tissue in the breast is well imaged by MRI, but CT scanning is less accurate.

The nipple extends about 5–10 mm above the level of the areolar skin and is covered with rugose skin which is variably pigmented (Figure 2.4).

The surface of the areola shows a number of small protuberances. These are the openings of modified large sebaceous glands called Montgomery's glands, which lubricate the areolar skin during suckling. Montgomery originally described his tubercle as a combined sebaceous unit and mammary lactiferous gland, and this has recently been confirmed by Smith et al.[15] The sebaceous gland produces the palpable lump. The lactiferous duct opens into the sebaceous duct close to the areola, or occasionally directly onto

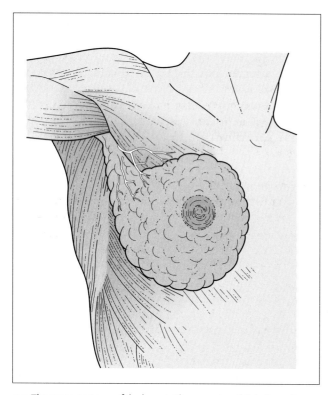

2.3 The gross anatomy of the breast. The upper two-thirds lie on the pectoralis major and the lower one-third on the serratus anterior. Note the prolongation of the upper outer quadrant into the axilla. Breast tissue extends much more widely than shown here in a significant minority of women.

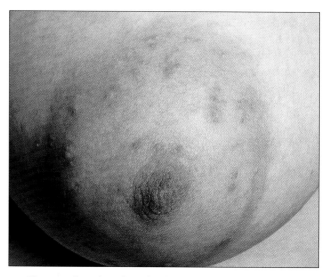

2.4 The normal nipple and areola. The pinker areolar skin is clearly demarcated from the surrounding breast skin and shows several small nodules which mark the openings of Montgomery's tubercles.

the areola alongside. The lactiferous gland lies deeper in the breast, can produce milk and is subject to the development of typical breast pathology (see Figure 14.11).

Apocrine sweat glands occur in the nipple and areola, but are not reported elsewhere in the skin of the breast. This is surprising, since hidradenitis suppurativa is rare in the areolar region (contrary to early reports which apparently confused periareolar fistula with hidradenitis) but not uncommonly affects peripheral skin of the breast, especially in the submammary region. This confusion is compounded by the imperfect correlation of hidradenitis with apocrine glands.

The nipple and areolar skin are rich in smooth muscle fibres which are responsible for nipple erection. While predominantly circumferential, some are radial and yet others are longitudinal, extending along the lactiferous ducts up into the nipple.

The adult ductolobar system

The breast consists of lobes separated from each other by fascial envelopes – usually stated to be 15–20 in number, but from a clinical point of view, more of the order of 7–8. The higher number comes from looking at transverse sections of the nipple, but is in conflict with the clinical experience that excision of a ductolobar unit appears to remove far more than one-twentieth of the breast. The reason for the difference is largely explained by two papers, one recent and the other old. Koenecke[16] in 1934 examined in detail the breast of a woman who died after childbirth. He showed that about half the ducts radiating from the nipple (and seen histologically in cross-section) are rudimentary, and do not drain a functional lobe. They extend only to 3–4 branchings, and do not form lobular structures. Koenecke believed that 95% of breast function is provided by about seven fully developed duct systems.

Recently Moffatt and Going[17] have used computer modelling software to reconstruct a three-dimensional model of the breast of a young woman from 2-mm slices examined in detail. The amount of work involved was such that only 10 duct territories, those in the centre of the breast, were covered. They showed that each duct drains its own territory, but the territories vary greatly in extent and shape; the volume of individual lobes varied by a factor of 20–30 times. Interlocked like a three-dimensional jigsaw, the transverse sectional outline of individual lobes was also variable, convex, concavo-convex, flattened or biconcave. Most lobes do not conform to the pear-shaped structure usually illustrated in operative diagrams of segmental excisions. The shapes suggest contact inhibition between adjacent ducts as they develop their individual territories. Some lobes have a long duct before branching, so that they have a deep territory close to the pectoral fascia, others branch very early, or have a series of lobules leaving the duct by short extralobular ducts. Taken in conjunction with Koenecke's work,

some of the smaller lobes may not function at all during pregnancy, perhaps overwhelmed by pressure from their larger neighbours.

Each lobe is drained by a ductal system from which a lactiferous sinus (5–8 mm in diameter when distended) opens on the nipple, and each lactiferous sinus receives a lobar duct 2 mm or less in diameter. Within the lobe are up to 40 (or more) lobules, the 'definitive' anatomical and functional entity. A lobule is 2–3 mm in diameter and may be visible to the naked eye. Each lobule contains 10–100 alveoli (or acini), the basic secretory unit. Some prefer to reserve the terms alveolus or acinus for the pregnant/lactating breast only, using the term ductule or ductulo-tubule for the non-pregnant state.

The lobar structure based on an individual duct system is more important than previously recognized, since it is the anatomic-pathological entity requiring excision of some multifocal papillary conditions, particularly in the elderly, and possibly the important macro-entity (in contrast to the micro-entity of the TDLU) in some cases of DCIS.

Vascular anatomy

The blood supply is from the axillary artery via its thoracoacromial, lateral thoracic and subscapular arteries, and from the subclavian artery via the internal thoracic (mammary) artery. The internal thoracic artery supplies three large anterior perforating branches through the second, third and fourth intercostal spaces. Perforating branches from the anterior intercostal arteries also come through these spaces more laterally. The veins form a rich subareolar plexus and drain to the intercostal and axillary veins and to the internal thoracic veins.

The detailed vascular anatomy of the breast[18] is important in more extensive procedures for benign conditions, particularly in relation to avoiding nipple and areolar necrosis.

Lymphatics of the breast

The lymphatic drainage of the breast is of great importance in the spread of malignant disease of the breast but of lesser importance in benign breast disease. Several lymphatic plexi issue from the parenchymal portion of the breast and the subareolar region and drain to the regional lymph nodes, the majority of which lie within the axilla. Most of the lymph from each breast passes into the ipsilateral axillary nodes along a chain which begins at the anterior axillary (pectoral) nodes and continues into the central axillary and apical node groups. Further drainage occurs into the subscapular and interpectoral node groups. A small amount of lymph drains across to the opposite breast and also downwards into the rectus sheath. Some of the medial part of the breast is drained by lymphatics which accompany the perforating internal thoracic vessels and drain into the internal thoracic group of nodes in the thorax and on into the mediastinal nodes. The older accounts of breast lymphatics derived from dissection studies have been clarified and superseded by dynamic studies *in vivo*,[19] and recently confirmed by sentinal node studies.

Nerve supply

The innervation of the breast is principally by somatic sensory nerves and autonomic nerves accompanying the blood vessels. In general, the areola and nipple are richly supplied by somatic sensory nerves while the breast parenchyma is mostly supplied by autonomic supply which appears to be solely sympathetic. No parasympathetic activity has been demonstrated in the breast.[20] Detailed histological examination has failed to show any direct neural end-terminal connections with breast ductular cells or myoepithelial cells, suggesting that the principal control mechanisms of secretion and milk ejection are humoral rather than nervous mechanisms. It is interesting that the areolar epidermis is relatively poorly innervated whereas the nipple and lactiferous ducts are richly innervated; these findings are supported by the clinical findings of poor appreciation of light touch and two-point discrimination over the areola. The rich nipple innervation is thought to be the basis of the well-known suckling reflex whereby a neural afferent pathway causes rapid release of both adenohypophyseal prolactin and neurohypophyseal oxytocin on suckling.

The somatic sensory nerve supply is via the supraclavicular nerves (C3, C4) superiorly and laterally from the lateral branches of the thoracic intercostal nerves (third to fourth). The medial aspects of the breast receive supply from the anterior branches of the thoracic intercostal nerves which penetrate the pectoralis major to reach the breast skin. A major supply of the upper outer quadrant of the breast is via the intercostobrachial nerve (C8, T1) which gives a large branch to the breast as it traverses the axilla.

The detailed nerve supply to the nipple is important in operations in this region, and has recently been reinvestigated.[21,22] The subareolar nerve plexus receives branches on the lateral side from the third to the fifth intercostal nerves, and on the medial side from the second to the fifth intercostal nerves. This supply is quite variable, and may differ on the two sides of the same patient, but the majority supply comes from the third and fourth nerves.

Fascia of the breast

The fascial framework of the breast is important in relation to clinical manifestations of disease and surgical technique. Because the breast develops as a skin appendage, it does so within the superficial fascia, such that the superficial part of the superficial fascia forms an anterior boundary and the deep layer of the superficial fascia forms a posterior boundary. In between, condensation of this interlobar fascia gives rise to the pyramidal-shaped ligaments of Cooper, called suspensory ligaments because they provide a supporting framework to the breast lobes. They are best developed in the upper part of the breast and are connected to both pectoral fascia and skin by fibrous extensions. In spite of these fibrous extensions, the superficial layer of superficial fascia gives a plane of dissection between the skin and breast. (The small subcutaneous fat lobules are readily differentiated from the much larger mammary fat lobules.) Likewise, the retromammary space provides a ready plane of dissection between the deep layer of superficial fascia and the deep fascia of pectoralis major and serratus anterior. This structural fascial support is so intimately connected to interlobular and intralobular fascia with their enclosed ductal units, that no ready plane of dissection exists within the breast substance and all surgery must be carried out by sharp dissection. The skin overlying the breast has been shown to vary in thickness from 0.8 mm to 3 mm on mammograms of normal breasts and tends to decrease with increasing breast size.[23]

MICROSCOPIC ANATOMY

The terminal ductal lobular unit (TDLU)

The adult resting breast has a branching major duct system leading to TDLUs (Figures 2.5 and 2.6).

The entity of the TDLU, described in detail by Wellings *et al.*[24] and comprising extra- and intralobular terminal ducts and the lobules arising from the intralobular terminal ductule (ITD), is an important entity in the origin of much breast disease, benign as well as malignant. The tree-like branching structure of breast ductules is very nicely shown by the technique of microradiography, which has been developed in Cardiff for small pieces of breast tissue (Figure 2.7).

Lobular development during reproductive life

Four types of lobules, representing progressive stages of lobular development from lobular bud to complete differentiation, have been recognized in the human breast.[25] Type I lobules are the most undifferentiated, bud-like structure; type II are more complex, with a higher number of ductules per lobule. Further progression to types III and IV is seen especially during pregnancy and lactation. Type I is seen at the menarche consisting of about 10 alveolar buds clustered around a terminal duct. Types II and III consist of increasing ductules around the duct, and type IV has fully developed acini.[26] The average number of components per lobule increases from type I to type IV with mean figures of 11, 47, 81 and 180, respectively. After weaning, there is an abundance of type III, which are more differentiated, have a low oestrogen receptor content and low proliferative activity. In nulliparous women, type I is the most frequent found at all ages, while type III is the most frequent found in parous women. Type I has a high content of oestrogen receptors and a high rate of cellular proliferation.

Type I is considered to be the site of development of ductal carcinoma-in-situ, and type II of lobular carcinoma. Type III is thought to originate adenomas, fibroadenomas sclerosing adenosis and cysts. Types I and II lobules have proved to be more reactive to chemical carcinogens-in-vitro than type III.

Changes in lobule number and structure with age have been studied in detail.[27] The largest number of lobular units occurs in the third decade, and decreases rapidly thereafter until the sixth decade, with a parallel decrease in size of the lobules. The greatest proportion is seen in the upper quadrants a decade earlier than in the lower quadrants, and the upper outer quadrant shows a surprising second peak in the fifth decade, in contrast with the steady decline in the others.

The epithelial cells

The ductal and alveolar epithelium are similar in structure and consist of two layers of cells, the basal cells being cuboidal and the surface cells being cylindrical with their long axes at right angles to the duct wall. Surrounding the ductal and alveolar walls is a discontinuous fenestrated layer of contractile myoepithelial cells. The myoepithelial cells contract in response to oxytocin stimulation and are responsible for the ejection of milk from the expanded TDLU of pregnancy into the larger ducts.

Light microscopy has shown some variation in the epithelial cells and two main cell types have been described by Bassler.[28] The more numerous basal cells have a light cytoplasm and were called clear basal B cells by Bassler, who thought they might function as stem cells for differentiation into myoepithelial cells or the second cell type (A cells). The darker A cells are luminal cells and have an eosinophilic cytoplasm packed with ribosomes which are responsible for the darker appearance under the microscope. Bassler postulated that the dark A cells develop from the clear B cells under the influence of oestrogen and migrate towards the luminal surface where they engage in secretory activity. A number of dark cells show regressive changes and are then shed as cellular debris into the lumen. Some dark A cells which have large membrane-bound vesicles containing lipid have been described as 'foam cells'; these may represent phagocytic histiocytes.[29]

Ultrastructural studies show that breast epithelial cells have well-developed luminal microvilli and complex interdigitating basal laminae with prominent desmosomes at intercellular boundaries. Cytoplasmic densities have been shown to vary in the same way as observed in light microscopy, in that a population of pale and dark cells can be identified.[30,31] As might be expected, myoepithelial cells

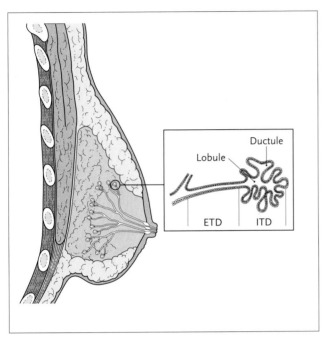

2.5 Cross-section of the breast to show the ductal and lobulo-alveolar structure. The expanded diagram shows the schematic structure of the TDLU. ETD, extralobular terminal ductule; ITD, intralobular terminal ductule.

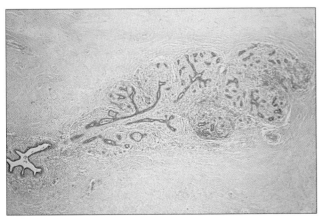

2.6 Histological section showing a TDLU adjacent to a major duct, the latter showing typical infolding. The pale and loose intralobular connective tissue contrasts with the denser collagenous interlobular stroma.

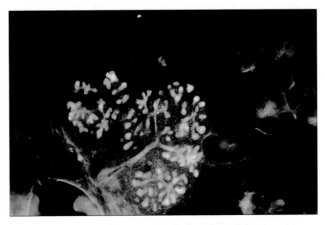

2.7 Microradiograph of breast tissue showing a small duct branching into ductules and lobules.

contain well-marked contractile myofilaments and cilia running parallel to the long axis of the cell. Myoepithelial cells are closely related to the basement membranes of the luminal epithelial cells and to the basal lamina, to which they are attached by numerous hemidesmosomes. Ultrastructural studies have revealed the unsuspected complexity of the epithelial stromal junction (ESJ), which is the crucial interface across which all nutrients must pass to reach the breast ductal cells.[30,32] The ESJ consists of a complex intertwining of fibroblasts, elastic fibres and endothelium and it is possible that the cause for some of the puzzling aspects of benign breast disease may lie in disorders of this region. It is also the area at which much of the paracrine and autocrine activity associated with growth factors occurs, as discussed below.

Recent work from Coombes' unit suggests that major advances in producing experimental models to understand lobular development and growth will soon be made with the human breast.[33] Having developed techniques for separating epithelial and myoepithelial cells from normal breast lobules, they have been able to identify some of their nutritional requirements and growth characteristics. This has allowed them to put the two cells together again and form typical two-cell-layer alveolar structures.

The basement membrane

The increasing knowledge of the activities of the basement membrane constitutes an exciting element of breast physiology and pathology. A complex, lattice-like structure lying between the epithelium and stroma, it clearly influences both. It is a dynamic structure, with both lysis and resynthesis going on to give constant remodelling. Principal constituents include collagens, fibronectins and proteoglycans. Enzymes capable of degrading the basement membrane may be found in stromal cells, myoepithelial cells and blood vessels. Contact with adjacent epithelial cells determines their polarity, contributes to their differentiation and helps control their secretory functions. At the same time, the epithelial cells are capable of stimulating the formation of a basement membrane.

The breast stroma

The importance of the stroma in general organ development was illustrated graphically by the mouse experiments of Kratochwil.[34] He showed that mouse mammary epithelium grown in organ culture grew normally when co-cultured with mammary stroma, but developed salivary morphology and invasive properties when co-cultured with salivary stroma. Much work in murine culture systems has defined aspects of this interaction. Macromolecules, such as collagen and proteoglycans produced by fibroblasts, influence many aspects of epithelial cell behaviour – from proliferation to cell division and motility. Conversely, epithelial cells have similar effects on fibroblasts, including deposition and resorption of matrix molecules and structures. While these experimental systems are far removed from the human breast *in vivo*, it is likely that the general principles will be

found to be similar as more sophisticated techniques are brought to bear on human studies, and in particular on the interaction of epithelium and stroma within the lobule. Indeed, Ferguson and co-workers have been able to demonstrate changes in the lobular extracellular matrix at different times of the menstrual cycle: interlobular fibroblasts showing characteristics of 'fetal' fibroblasts, intralobular fibroblasts showing the characteristics of 'adult' fibroblasts, and fetal fibroblasts showing enhanced migratory function compared to adult fibroblasts.[35]

Careful histological study by Parks has shown the heterogeneity of connective tissue in the breast.[36] The intralobular and periductal connective tissue is probably as important in physiological terms as the interlobular Cooper's ligaments in structural terms, although only recently is our knowledge of the physiology of the lobular stroma extending beyond the rudimentary. The segmental and interlobular fascia is dense and reticular, while the periductal and intralobular stroma is much looser – a contrast between loose and dense reminiscent of the papillary and reticular layers of the dermis, the tissue from which the breast arises.

The interlobular fascia often shows a large amount of fatty infiltration, especially in the larger breast. Further differences can be detected between periductal and lobular stroma. Periductal connective tissue is found as a cuff of loose stroma around the ducts in which the lymphatic vessels run. It is more cellular (fibrocytes) than the supporting fibrous tissue and contains a considerable amount of elastic tissue, which tends to increase with age and parity. The lobular stroma is even more loose, more vascular, more cellular and markedly mucoid – a structure which facilitates expansion of the developing acini in pregnancy. Recent biochemical studies[37] have shown that the distribution of a cell-surface enzyme called dipeptidyl peptidase IV provides a clear delineation of two functionally distinct populations of breast fibroblasts: those of the intralobular stroma and those of the interlobular stroma. This is a striking confirmation of the difference suspected from conventional histology.

Similarly, fetal antigen 2 (FA2) is present in the intralobular stroma as a broad band around acini, but is not found in the interlobular stroma.[38] The lobule contains no elastic tissue and this fact is helpful to the pathologist in differentiating lesions arising from the lobule from those arising from ducts. Lobular stroma, and probably periductal stroma, is under hormonal influence, but little is known about the detailed hormonal responsiveness of this tissue.

Durnberger et al.[39] have shown that the differentiation of the mammary epithelial bud in the male fetal rodent occurs in response to a transient increase in testosterone secretion which does not affect the mammary ductular epithelium directly but is mediated by the surrounding stromal fibroblasts. Work from our laboratories has shown that human breast fibroblasts are highly stimulatory to human breast cancer cells in an *in vivo* nude mouse xenograft model.[40] These experiments point to a major regulatory role for breast fibroblasts in epithelial cell growth, while other work points to a possibility that breast epithelial cells may influence the stroma, particularly intralobular stroma.

McCune et al.[41] have demonstrated three transforming growth factor (TGFβ) isotopes lying intracellularly in most active epithelial cells, but not within stromal cells. At the same time, a technique which demonstrates the same isotopes in extracellular conformation stained normal intralobular stroma, and particularly the stroma of active fibroadenomas, lesions believed to develop from lobules. This indicates a possible paracrine and autocrine interaction between TGFβ from epithelial cells and the surrounding intralobular stroma as a control mechanism in mammary development and the pathogenesis of disease. Similar findings relate to immunoreactive endothelin-1, which is found only in mammary epithelial cells, but with cell-surface receptors found only on fibroblasts – a possible mechanism by which epithelial cells may influence stromal cells, as discussed in Chapter 7.

The long-term administration of androgens to female-to-male transexuals has provided a clinical experimental system.[42] When administered to hormonally normal women, the main effect on the breast has been a marked hyalinization of both intralobular and extralobular stroma, with especially marked periductal fibrosis. This is accompanied by atrophy of ductal epithelium and marked decrease in ducts and lobules. A similar effect has been reported in mice.

The cellular changes in the stroma during progression from the benign breast to malignancy has recently been reviewed.[43]

BIOCHEMICAL CONTROL OF BREAST EPITHELIUM

The breast tissues are under a complex system of control by systemic factors, particularly hormones acting through their respective receptors, and a number of local factors. These include paracrine hormones, released by one type of cell to influence adjacent cells of similar or differing function; juxtacrine factors, situated on the surface of the producing cell to influence adjacent cells by direct contact; and autocrine hormones, which act on the same cell by intracellular or surface receptors. All interact, as the systemic hormones also act, by influencing the locally derived factors – cell adhesion-related proteins as well as autocrine and paracrine hormones – to produce signal pathways that finally result in cell regulation and stimulation.

Studies of the molecular mechanisms controlling breast epithelium have concentrated on cancer cells; only recently has the situation in the normal breast been studied. The growth factor receptor EGF-R and the oncogene product C-erbB-2 are involved in the control of proliferation and probably differentiation of breast epithelial cells, although their precise role in the normal breast is still unclear.[44] EGF-R is found mainly in the stroma (periductal and perilobular fibroblasts), myoepithelial cells and to

a lesser extent basal epithelial cells, whereas C-erbB-2 expression is exclusively epithelial, mainly on the inner layer of epithelial cells of duct and lobule. Some heterogeneity of staining from one lobule to another in the same biopsy was found in this study, although both were more strongly expressed in the luteal phase.[44]

C-erbB-2 appears to be negatively related to proliferation of mammary epithelium and positively related to differentiation. The predominant distribution of expression of EGF-R suggests a paracrine pathway between stromal, myoepithelial and basal epithelial cells, influencing the basal epithelial cells which are proliferating. Some of the more superficial cells which fail to express EGF-R could still be cells which produce, or are stimulated by, epithelial growth factor (EGF) or TGFα, since ligand binding can lead to a decrease in receptor levels by internalization or degradation. TGFα is a member of the EGF family which binds to EGF-R, and has been detected in normal breast cells.

Until recently the only function of oxytocin in the breast was thought to be related to lactation. The discovery that oxytocin receptors are widely distributed in the brain and that some are strongly influenced by steroids such as oestrogen, progesterone and testosterone has led to more detailed study of the breast. The mammary gland, and especially the nipple, is richly innervated with peptidergic nerve fibres with receptors to which oxytocin can bind. Oxytocin functions are thought to be very wide, perhaps even being responsible for the anxiolytic effect of breastfeeding, since oxytocin levels vary inversely with anxiety and aggression.[45]

There is increasing evidence in animals that oxytocin is related to differentiation of myoepithelial cells, and now a similar function has been demonstrated in humans. Oxytocin receptors (OT-R) can be found in myoepithelial cells of normal ductules, in benign hyperplastic lesions and some cancer cells, and are abundant in sclerosing adenosis.[46] OT-R-positive cells in hyperplasias are likely to be myoepithelial rather than classical epithelial cells, and there is evidence that this is so. Epithelial and myoepithelial cells differ markedly in the production and response to growth factors[47] in that myoepithelial cells produce basic fibroblast growth factor (FGF-2), which in turn affects the proliferation and survival of epithelial cells.

Much interest has also been shown recently in the fact that prostate-specific antigen (PSA) can be found in many breast conditions, such as in cyst fluid or nipple secretions. Yu et al.[48] have shown that it can often be demonstrated in normal breast tissues (33% of samples), benign breast disease (65%) and cancers (28%). The highest levels were found in fibroadenomas. Parathyroid-like peptide (PLP), structurally homologous to parathyroid hormone but of uncertain function, is another substance recognized in breast cancers, and now found with more sophisticated tests to be in the cytoplasm of normal and benign proliferative breast epithelial cells; it is increased in lactation and benign adenosis or ductal hyperplasia, and decreased in atrophic lobules. Its association with calcification in cancers suggests that it may play a local role in calcium metabolism in the normal breast.

Hepatocyte growth factor/scatter factor is present in benign, lactating and malignant breast epithelium, and an autocrine loop action in proliferating epithelium has been suggested.

Peptide growth factors such as EGF and TGFα can be obtained from breast fluid aspirated from the nipple. Individual women secrete consistent and individually distinct levels, which in some cases can be correlated with circulating hormone levels.[49]

CYCLICAL CHANGES IN BREAST EPITHELIUM

Physiological control of ovarian function

Ovarian function is increasingly recognized as much more complicated than earlier conventional concepts. Ovarian activity is under the control of the pituitary gonadotrophins – FSH and LH. The latter is secreted in pulsatile fashion under control of gonadotrophin-releasing hormone (GnRH), but modulated by a negative feedback effect of oestradiol and progesterone, and responding to a positive feedback in midcycle leading to the LH surge responsible for ovulation. FSH control is more complicated since it is partly under the control of GnRH, but partly independent of this. As well as the negative feedback from oestradiol and progesterone, there is a further negative feedback from inhibins and a positive stimulating effect of activins. Inhibins are dimeric glycoprotein hormones from the ovary suppressing FSH by a direct effect on the pituitary; activins are dimers which act mainly at a local level in paracrine or autocrine fashion. Activins are in turn activated by follistatin, an activin-binding third gonadal peptide.[50]

The breast during the menstrual cycle

Each breast cell has a finite lifespan before progressing to mitosis or apoptosis. The balance between mitosis and apoptosis is obviously of great importance in many aspects of breast functioning. Oestrogen tends to cause mitosis in ductular and alveolar cells, and during the follicular phase there is a modest increase in mitoses in the ductular cells, little in those of the alveoli.

Progestogens have a biphasic effect, at first stimulating mitosis with movement from G_1 phase to S phase, but then slowing down mitotic activity by arresting the cells in early G_1 phase. Progestogens also induce cytoplasmic changes conducive to lactation, with accumulation of fluid, protein and electrolyte. Hence administration of progesterone in clinically moderate dosage will give full tender breasts for a few weeks, but these symptoms will ease as apoptosis exceeds mitosis in the alveolar cells.

Anderson and co-workers[51] have quantified the incidence of mitosis and apoptosis morphologically in relation to the stage of the menstrual cycle. Both processes reach a peak incidence towards the end of the cycle and during men-

struation, but with a statistically significant difference of 3 days between the two peaks – day 25 for mitosis and day 28 for apoptosis. This is the mirror image of the changes in the endometrium, when maximal mitosis occurs in the first half of the cycle. The results did not vary with parity, history of contraceptive pill use or with the presence of a fibroadenoma, and the changes observed in the cells of the lobules were also seen in the cells of the adjacent ductules. The cyclical nature of the changes was most marked in younger women – indeed there was no cyclical pattern for apoptosis in the 35–45-year age group. This may reflect the involutional changes usually detectable throughout this age period. Likewise there is a trend towards a decreased incidence of mitosis, but a more significant decrease in apoptosis with increasing age, shown as a loss of the late cycle peak. This more marked decrease in apoptosis than mitosis in the 35–45 group could also be responsible for some of the involutional changes of ANDI.

There was a consistent finding of a higher rate of apoptosis in the right breast than the left. It is interesting to speculate that this lower level of natural cell death on the left may be related to the higher incidence of many disease conditions found in this breast.

Russo et al.[52] used DNA-labelling techniques to measure cell proliferation in normal breast tissue adjacent to biopsies. The DNA-labelling index and the growth fraction were always greatest in the terminal ductule of the TDLU, less in the alveolus and still less in the ducts (0.74 vs. 0.22 vs. 0.04). This decreased with age, but even in the older patients the index was greatest in the terminal ductule (0.33 vs. 0.08 vs. 0.04). There is increasing evidence that mitogenic factors other than the sex hormones influence these cells; EGF is one candidate.

These and similar studies have helped to clarify the previous conflicting evidence regarding cyclical changes in breast epithelium, while animal studies are also producing new insights. For instance, a fatty acid-binding protein, mammary-derived growth inhibitor, can be shown to act locally in the mouse to inhibit growth of ductal epithelioid cells, produce no effect on the stroma and stimulate the development of lobulo-alveolar structures.

In the human, Haagensen[53] emphatically stated that he was unable to confirm any cyclical variation in the number of acini per lobule – despite a search for the purported specific changes. A paper by Vogel et al.[54] suggested that specific changes were seen which correlated with the phase of the menstrual cycle, although an unspecified inter- and intraobserver variation was admitted.

Anderson et al. have summarized the situation at present.[55] Both epithelial and stromal cells show cyclical changes reflecting menstrual hormone fluctuations. Epithelial proliferation peaks in the midluteal phase and is followed by increased apoptosis. There is a dissociation between steroid receptor expression and cell proliferation. estrogen receptor (ER)-positive cells are distributed evenly throughout the lobule, and

96% of ER-positive cells are also progesterone receptor (PR)-positive. Since the proliferating cells are usually ER- and PR-negative, it is likely that oestrogen has its main proliferating effect via adjacent ER-positive cells acting in paracrine fashion. Oral contraceptives prolong the length but not the magnitude of cellular proliferation and the degree of fluctuation becomes much less in older women.

Despite the conflicting evidence of histological change, there is clearly documented evidence that breast volume measured by water displacement methods increases during the luteal phase of the cycle and falls at menstruation.[56] These changes are noticed by a large number of women and may be explained by vascular or lymphatic changes without requiring obvious changes in breast histology, although cellular proliferation in the lobules is believed to contribute to breast swelling. Mammary bloodflow shows a cyclical increase, an oestrogen effect, maximal for 3–4 days before menstruation, and this plays a part in the increased breast volume and discomfort typical of this period.

Matrix metalloproteinases play an important role in such basic functions as proliferation, differentiation and apoptosis[57] under the regulation of reproductive hormones.

Breast size correlates (in epidemiological terms) with height, weight and body mass index. However, current use of the oral contraceptive pill causes independently an increase in breast size which overrides this association.[58]

As a sexually responsive organ, the breast shows vascular engorgement and enlargement following sexual arousal, with nipple congestion and erection, followed by detumescence. In a similar manner to increased vascularity in the pelvic organs, these changes may be associated with discomfort that may become a cause for clinical presentation.

CHANGES DURING PREGNANCY AND LACTATION

Anatomy

The greatly increased levels of luteal and placental sex steroids, with the addition of placental lactogen and chorionic gonadotrophin in pregnancy, cause a remarkable increase in lobulo-alveolar growth. Prolactin levels also increase progressively throughout pregnancy but this hormone appears to be mainly concerned with milk production at the end of pregnancy after the preceding hormones have primed the breast by inducing marked proliferative changes. The chronological changes are shown in Table 2.1.

Histologically, the most remarkable features are the great predominance of dilated alveoli and the conversion of the resting two-layer epithelium to a monolayer within the alveoli (Figure 2.8).

The large ducts maintain their two-layer configuration.

Physiology

Basal prolactin levels increase from the non-pregnant level of 10 ng/mL to peak values of over 200 ng/mL at week 40,

postpartum prolactin levels fall over the next 4 weeks to around 20 ng/mL but are immediately elevated to about 10 times basal levels on suckling the infant. Although, as previously described, some colostral secretion is visible in the breast before term, the process of milk production proper begins 2–5 days after birth. The change from colostrum to milk is caused by high levels of prolactin maintained against a rapidly falling level of ovarian and placental sex steroids.

Prolactin is the primary stimulant for galactopoiesis and has been shown to have a variety of actions on breast tissue, which would contribute to milk production.[60] The increased mitosis required for alveolar growth and early

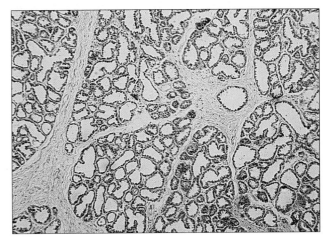

2.8 Histological section (H&E) of lactating breast showing grossly dilated acini lined by a low cuboidal epithelium. Note the high ratio of epithelium to stroma.

Table 2.1 Changes in the breast during pregnancy	
Week	**Change**
0	Resting breast approx. 200 g in weight
1–4	Ductular sprouting/lobular formation
5–8	Breast enlarges/vascular engorgement/areolar pigmentation/predominant lobular formation
>12	Large alveoli with single epithelial cell layer. Beginning of colostrum formation
>20	Alveolar dilatation/colostrum formation. New capillary formation/myoepithelial cell hypertrophy
Term	180% increase of mammary bloodflow Weight approx. 400 g Fat droplet accumulation in alveolar cells
After Vorherr.[59]	

colostrum production is stimulated primarily by ovarian and placental sex steroids, placental lactogen, cortisol and growth hormone, with the placenta supplying the bulk of the sex steroids and lactogenic factors. Although some milk protein and fat synthesis is seen from midpregnancy onwards, the full lactogenic stimulation of prolactin is inhibited by the high levels of circulating sex steroids. Birth and the consequent loss of the placenta reverses the inhibition and full milk production then begins. The predominant role of prolactin in lactopoiesis is illustrated by the fact that ovariectomized women and animals can successfully breastfeed.

Established lactation

Once established, lactation will continue almost indefinitely provided the milk is regularly removed from the breast. After 48 hours of milk stagnation, milk synthesis begins to fall rapidly.[3,61]

During milk secretion, alveolar cells change shape and histological appearance. During active lactation, the upper part of the cell breaks away or is extruded and the cell changes from a columnar shape to a low cuboidal shape. Thus milk secretion is an apocrine- and merocrine-type secretion as only part of the cell is lost. The fat globules in milk are surrounded by a membrane which is presumably derived from the luminal cell membrane of the alveolar cell. Following secretion, resynthesis of milk proteins such as lactalbumin and casein and milk fats occurs and the cell begins to elongate. Prolactin is the primary stimulant for lactose synthesis by stimulation of lactose synthetase and protein synthesis by stimulation of nuclear RNA polymerase. Lactose synthesis takes place in the Golgi apparatus and the cell becomes large and swollen with secretory products.[62,63] Secretion then takes place with fats and protein being excreted by apocrine secretion, lactose by merocrine secretion and inorganic ions by a combination of active transport and diffusion. The cycle of extrusion and resynthesis then restarts.

The active transport processes across the luminal cell (the blood–milk barrier) are of considerable interest as recent studies of cyst fluids suggest that different morphological types of epithelium may differ in the handling of ions.[64] Umemura and colleagues have carried out a histochemical study to define the cell kinetics and functional morphology of the lactating breast. They have defined four types of lobules: type I, prelactating; type II, lactating; type III, early regression; and type IV, advanced regression.[65]

Postlactational involution

Postlactational involution starts on weaning and is initiated by local mechanical factors causing alveolar distension and capillary obstruction. The one-layer secretory alveolar cells regress and reform the two-layered epithelium characteristic of the resting breast. This process is facilitated by cell death and phagocytosis performed by invasion of the alveoli by histiocytes. A lymphocytic infiltrate is also characteristic, but connective tissue regression

is limited. The branching alveolar structures become fewer in number but the ductular structure remains mostly intact. This is the fundamental difference between postlactational and postmenopausal involution; in the latter both lobules and ductules are reduced in number. The ducts become smaller although some secretion persists in the duct lumen in the postlactational breast and can be aspirated or expressed from the nipple in most parous women.[66] The fluid aspirated from 61% of women is of sufficient volume to study the cellularity and hormone content.[66]

Much work in rodents is currently in progress identifying the precise hormonal and biochemical substances and mechanisms responsible for this remarkable involution. In time, this will undoubtedly throw light on the human process.

POSTMENOPAUSAL INVOLUTION

Physiological control

FSH levels rise progressively from the age of 30 to the menopause, while levels of oestradiol and LH remain relatively constant during this period. This rise in FSH in the presence of a maintained oestradiol may be due to a fall in inhibins, produced by the granulosa cells of the ovary. With this change from the age of 30, it is not surprising that the involutional structural changes of ANDI may be seen in the breast long before the menopause. Oestradiol levels fluctuate widely in individuals at the time of the menopause, and very high levels in some women may be responsible for the breast tenderness that is sometimes seen at this time. Surprisingly, tissue steroid levels show little difference in premenopausal and postmenopausal women, despite the differences in circulating levels.

In the postmenopausal state, oestradiol levels are ten times lower, and FSH levels ten times higher than during reproductive life, and inhibins are generally undetectable.[50]

In postmenopausal women, continuous oestrogen administration may stimulate ductal cell proliferation, leading to breast fullness with discomfort and paraesthesiae of the nipple, but these changes do not persist. However, administration of combined oestrogen/progesterone supplementation may give more marked and persisting fullness and tenderness.

Histological changes

The process of postmenopausal involution can be divided into a preclimacteric phase starting at about the age of 35 and a postmenopausal phase starting at the time of the menopause. The predominant feature is regression of the glandular epithelium and adjacent connective tissue with gradual replacement by fat. In the preclimacteric phase there is a gradual loss of lobules and infiltration by round cells and the specialized loose connective tissue around the lobules changes into dense collagen. In the postmenopausal phase, the typical outline of a lobule is lost and is replaced by dense collagen containing a compressed epithelial remnant. Lobular involution may proceed to formation of microcysts which may be mistaken for cystic disease microscopically. The essential difference between the two conditions is the preservation of the specialized lobular stroma in the former.[67] Stromal changes dominate and fat deposition accelerates and connective tissue regression is marked. The end result is that the branching major duct system is visible, but very few lobules can be seen and these are embedded in dense fibrotic capsules unlike the loose stroma surrounding the lobules in the breasts of younger women. Some lobules may develop into microcysts by dilatation, possibly due to obstruction of the terminal ductule, and interlobular connective tissue is greatly reduced. Externally these changes produce the shrunken, pendulous breast of the old woman and, when mammography is performed, are responsible for the good contrast of parenchyma to fat obtained on mammograms of the older breast. Variations of this process are responsible for many of the clinical presentations and histological appearances of benign breast disease and are discussed fully in the next chapter.

REFERENCES

1. Van der Putte SC. Mammary-like glands of the vulva and their disorders. *International Journal of Gynecological Pathology* 1994; **13**: 150–160.

2. Hughes ESR. The development of the mammary gland. *Annals of the Royal College of Surgeons of England* 1950; **6**: 99–119.

3. Dabelow A. Die Milchdruse In: Bagman W (ed.) *Handbuch der mikroskopischen Anatomie des Merchen*, Vol 3, Part 3, *Haut und Sininesorgane*, pp 277–485. Berlin: Springer-Verlag, 1957.

4. Anbazhagan R, Bartek J, Monaghan P *et al*. Growth and development of the human breast. *American Journal of Anatomy* 1991; **192**: 407–417.

5. Marshall WA & Tanner JM. Variations in pattern of pubertal changes in girls. *Archives of Diseases of Childhood* 1969; **44**: 291–303.

6. Zacharias L, Wurtman RJ & Schatzoff M. Sexual maturation in contemporary American girls. *American Journal of Obstetrics and Gynecology* 1970; **108**: 833–846.

7. Wildt L, Marshall G & Knobil E. Experimental induction of puberty in the infantile female rhesus monkey. *Science* 1980; **207**: 1373–1375.

8. Graham JD & Clarke CL. The physiological action of progesterone in target tissues. *Endocrine Reviews* 1997; **18**: 502–519.

9. Topper YJ & Freeman CS. Multiple hormone interactions in the developmental biology of the mammary gland. *Physiological Reviews* 1980; **60**: 1049–1106.

10. Grahame DJ & Clarke CL. Physiological action of progesterone in target tissues. *Endocrine Reviews* 1997; **18**: 502–519.

11. Hicken NF. Mastectomy: A clinical pathologic study demonstrating why most mastectomies result in incomplete removal of the mammary gland. *Archives of Surgery* 1940; **40**: 6–12.

12. Loughry CW, Sheffer DB, Price TE *et al*. Breast volume measurement in 598 women using biostereometric analysis. *Annals of Plastic Surgery* 1989; **22**: 380–385.

13. Westreich M. Anthropomorphic breast measurement: protocol and results in 50 women with aesthetically perfect breasts and clinical application. *Plastic and Reconstructive Surgery* 1997; **100**: 468–479.

14. Lejour M. Evaluation of fat in the breast tissue removed by vertical mammaplasty. *Plastic and Reconstructive Surgery* 1997; **99**: 386–393.

15. Smith DM, Peters TE & Donegan WL. Montgomery's areolar tubercle. *Archives of Pathology and Laboratory Medicine* 1982; **106**: 60–63.

16. Koenecke IA. An anatomical study of the mammary gland twenty four hours postpartum. *American Journal of Obstetrics and Gynecology* 1934; **27**: 584–592.

17. Moffatt DF & Going JJ. Three dimensional anatomy of complete duct systems in human breast – pathological and developmental implications. *Journal of Clinical Pathology* 1996; **49**: 48–52.

18. Maliniac JW. Arterial blood supply of the breast. *Archives of Surgery* 1943, **47**: 329.

19. Turner-Warwick RT. The lymphatics of the breast. *British Journal of Surgery* 1959; **46**: 574–582.

20. Vorherr H. *The Breast: Morphology, Physiology and Lactation*. New York: Academic Press, 1974.

21. Sarhadi NS, Dunn JS, Lee FD *et al*. An anatomical study of the nerve supply of the breast, including the nipple and areola. *British Journal of Plastic Surgery* 1996; **49**: 156–164.

22. Jaspars JJP, Posma AN, Van Immerseel AAH *et al*. The cutaneous innervation of the female breast and nipple areola complex: Implications for surgery. *British Journal of Plastic Surgery* 1997; **50**: 49–59.

23. Wilkson SA, Adams EJ & Tucker AK. Patterns of breast skin thickness in normal mammograms. *Clinical Radiology* 1982; **33**: 691–693.

24. Wellings SR, Jensen HM & Marcum RG. An atlas of subgross pathology of the human breast with reference to possible pre-cancerous lesions. *Journal of National Cancer Institute* 1975; **55**: 231–273.

25. Russo J & Russo IH. Toward a physiological approach to breast cancer prevention. *Cancer Epidemiology, Biomarkers and Prevention* 1994; **3**: 353–364.

26. Russo J & Russo IH. Development of the human mammary gland. In: Neville MC & Daniel CW (eds) *The Mammary Gland* 1987. New York: Plenum.

27. Hutson SW, Cowen PN & Bird CC. Morphometric studies of age related changes in normal human breast and their significance for evolution of mammary cancer. *Journal of Clinical Patholoy* 1985; **38**: 281–287.

28. Bassler R. The morphology of hormone-induced structural changes in the female breast. *Current Topics in Pathology* 1970; **53**: 1–89.

29. Toker C. Observations on the ultrastructure of a mammary ductule. *Journal of Ultrastructure Research* 1967; **21**: 9–25.

30. Stirling JW & Chandler JA. The fine structure of the normal, resting terminal ductal-lobular unit of the female breast. *Virchows Archiv. A, Pathological Anatomy and Histopathology* 1976; **372**: 205–226.

31. Ahmed A. In: *Atlas of the Ultrastructure of Human Breast Diseases*, pp 1–26. Edinburgh: Churchill Livingstone, 1978.

32. Stirling JW & Chandler JA. The fine structure of ducts and subareolar ducts in the resting gland of the female breast. *Virchows Archiv. A, Pathological Anatomy and Histopathology* 1977; **373**: 119–132.

33. Gomm JJ, Coope RC, Browne PJ & Coombes RC. Separate breast epithelial and myo-epithelial cells have different

growth factor requirements in vitro but can reconstitute normal breast lobulo-alveolar structure. *Journal of Cellular Physiology* 1997; **171**: 11–19.

34. Kratochwil K. Organ specificity in mesenchymal induction demonstrated in the embryonic development of the mammary gland of the mouse. *Developmental Biology* 1969; **20**: 46–71.

35. Ferguson JE, Schor AM, Howell A & Ferguson MWJ. Changes in the extracellular matrix of the human breast during the menstrual cycle. *Cell Tissue Research* 1992; **268**: 167–177.

36. Parks AG. The micro-anatomy of the breast. *Annals of the Royal College of Surgeons* 1959; **25**: 295–311.

37. Atherton AJ, Monaghan P, Warburton MJ *et al.* Dipeptidyl peptidase IV expression identifies a functional sub-population of breast fibroblasts. *International Journal of Cancer* 1992; **50**: 15–19.

38. Rassmussen HB, Teisner B, Andersen J *et al.* Fetal antigen-2 in the stromal reaction induced by breast carcinoma. *APMIS* 1992; **100**: 39–47.

39. Durnberger H, Heuberger B, Schwartz P *et al.* Mesenchyme-mediated effects of testosterone on embryonic mammary epithelium. *Cancer Research* 1978; **38**: 4066–4070.

40. Horgan K, Jones DL & Mansel RE. Mitogenicity of human fibroblasts in vivo for human breast cancer cells. *British Journal of Surgery* 1987; **74**: 227–229.

41. McCune BK, Mullin BR, Flanders KC *et al.* Localisation of transforming growth factor-beta isotypes in lesions of the human breast. *Human Pathology* 1992; **23**: 13–20.42. Sapino A, Pietribiasi F, Godan A & Bussolati G. Effect of long-term administration of androgens on breast tissue of female to male transexuals. *Annals of the New York Academy of Sciences* 1990; **586**: 143–145.

43. Ronnov-Jessen L, Petersen OW & Bissell MJ. Cellular changes involved in conversion of normal to malignant breast: importance of the stromal reaction. *Physiological Reviews* 1996; **76**: 69–125.

44. Gompel A, Martin A, Simon P *et al.* Epidermal growth factor receptor and C-erb-2 expression in normal breast tissue during the menstrual cycle. *Breast Cancer Research and Treatment* 1996; **38**: 227–235.

45. Uvnas-Moberg K & Eriksson M. Breast feeding: physiological, endocrine and behavioural adaptations caused by oxytocin and local neurogenic activity in the nipple and mammary gland. *Acta Paediatrica* 1996; **85**: 525–530.

46. Bussolati G, Cassoni P, Ghisolfi G *et al.* Immunolocalisation and gene expression of oxytocin receptors in cancerous and non-neoplastic tissues of the breast. *American Journal of Pathology* 1996; **148**: 1895–1903.

47. Coombes RC, Bullweza L & Gomm JJ. The role of myo-epithelial derived growth factors in the human breast. *Endocrine-Related Cancer* 1997; **4**: 35–43.

48. Yu H, Diamandis EP & Levesque M *et al.* Prostate specific antigen in breast cancer, benign breast disease and normal breast tissue. *Breast Cancer Research and Treatment* 1996; **40**: 171–178.

49. Gann P, Chatterton R, Vogelsong K *et al.* Mitogenic growth factors in breast fluid obtained from healthy women. *Cancer Endocrinology, Biomarkers and Prevention* 1997; **6**: 421–428.

50. Burger HG. The menopausal transmission. *Baillière's Clinical Obstetrics and Gynaecology* 1996; **10**: 347–359.

51. Anderson TJ, Ferguson DJP & Raab GM. Cell turnover in the 'resting' human breast – influence of parity, contraceptive pill, age and laterality. *British Journal of Cancer* 1982; **46**: 376–382.

52. Russo J, Calaf G, Roi L & Russo IH. Influence of gland age and topography on cell kinetics of normal breast tissue. *Journal of the National Cancer Institute* 1987; **78**: 413–418.

53. Haagensen CD. *Diseases of the Breast*, 3rd edn, pp 50–54. Philadelphia:Saunders, 1986.

54. Vogel PM, Georgiade NG, Fetter BF *et al.* The correlation of histologic changes in the human breast with the menstrual cycle. *American Journal of Pathology* 1981; **104**: 23–34.

55. Anderson E, Clarke RB & Howell A. Change in the human breast throughout the menstrual cycle: relevance to breast carcinogenesis. *Endocrine-Related Cancer* 1997; **4**: 23–34.

56. Milligan D, Drife JO & Short RV. Changes in breast volume during normal menstrual cycle and after oral contraceptives. *British Medical Journal* 1975; **iv**: 494–496.

57. Hulboy DL, Rudolph LA & Matrisian LM. Matrix metalloproteinases as mediators of reproductive function. *Molecular Human Reproduction* 1997; **3**: 27–45.

58. Jernstrom H & Olsson H. Breast size in relation to hormone levels, body constitution and oral contraceptive use in healthy nulligravid women aged 19–25 years. *American Journal of Epidemiology* 1997; **145**: 571–580.

59. Vorherr H. Puerperium: Maternal involutional changes and lactation. In: Posinsky JJ (ed.) *Davis' Gynecology and Obstetrics*, Vol I, Chap 20, pp 1–46. New York: Harper, 1972.

60. Cowie AT. Induction and suppression of lactation in animals. *Proceedings of the Royal Society of Medicine* 1972; **65**: 1084–1085.

61. Zilliacus H. Physiologie und Pathologie des Wockenbettes. In: Kasero O *et al.* (eds) *Gynakologie und Geburtshilfe*, Vol II, pp 966–997. Stuttgart: Thième, 1967.

62. Turkington RW. Measurement of prolactin activity in human serum by the induction of specific milk proteins in mammary gland in vitro. *Journal of Clinical Endocrinology and Metabolism* 1971; **33**: 210–216.

63. Turkington RW, Brew K, Vanaman TC & Hill RC. The hormonal control of lactose synthetase in the developing mouse mammary gland. *Journal of Biological Chemistry* 1968; **243**: 3382–3387.

64. Dixon JM, Miller WR, Scott WN & Forrest APM. The morphological basis of human cyst populations. *British Journal of Surgery* 1983; **70**: 604–606.

65. Umemura S, Osamura RY & Tsutsumi Y. Cell renewal and functional morphology of the human lactating breast. *Pathology International* 1996; **46**: 105–121.

66. Petrakis NL. Physiologic, biochemical and cytologic aspects of nipple aspirate fluid. *Breast Cancer Research and Treatment* 1985; **8**: 7–19.

67. Azzopardi JG. In: Bennington JL (ed.) *Major Problems in Pathology*, Vol II, *Problems in Breast Pathology*, Chap 2, pp 8–22. London: WB Saunders, 1979.

Chapter 3

Aberrations of normal development and involution (ANDI): A concept of benign breast disorders based on pathogenesis

CONTENTS

KEY POINTS AND NEW DEVELOPMENTS

1. Terminology in benign breast disease has been confused by a multiplicity of terms which do not relate accurately to clinical or histological patterns, and which are not based on sound concepts of pathogenesis.
2. Most benign breast disorders derive from minor aberrations of the normal processes of development, cyclical activity and involution.
3. The ANDI classification allows precise definition of an individual patient problem in terms of pathogenesis, histology and clinical significance.
4. ANDI replaces the conventional view of 'normal' and 'disease' with a spectrum ranging from normal, through slight abnormality (aberration), to disease.
5. Recent developments in molecular biology give support to, and provide possible mechanisms for, the concept.

The ANDI classification of benign breast disorders[1] provides an overall framework for benign conditions of the breast, encompassing both pathogenesis and degree of abnormality. It was developed because the concepts used in teaching about, and managing, benign conditions of the breast (particularly 'fibrocystic disease') have been bedevilled by obscurities and inaccuracy. This is in marked contrast with breast cancer, where there is a clearly defined framework. A patient with cancer is investigated along two directions – a 'longitudinal' direction which will assess the tumour in temporal terms, *in situ* or invasive, size and extent of primary tumour, presence or absence of lymph node involvement and systemic spread; and a 'horizontal' direction assessing biology – histological type (e.g. lobular, ductal or other), grading, hormone receptor/growth factor status, etc. This will allow a patient to be placed within this well-recognized and well-defined framework, with a management policy appropriate to her individual status.

The situation with benign conditions has been different until recently. A large number of clinical and histological conditions, such as fibroadenoma, duct papilloma, subareolar abscess and nipple discharge right through to the ubiquitous fibrocystic disease have been seen as individual and unrelated entities in terms of pathogenesis and management. Alternatively, some workers equated the whole range of benign breast disease with fibrocystic disease and tried to push all its manifestations into this one ill-defined complex, with even greater confusion. There was no overall framework for benign disorders into which an individual condition could be placed for assessment and management. Thus, historically patients with breast cancer have been managed more logically, consistently, comprehensively and with more conviction than those with benign breast disease.

The ANDI classification, also a bidirectional framework, provides a means to reverse this disparity (Table 3.1), and

is based on the fact that most benign breast conditions arise from normal physiological processes.

The horizontal assessment defines the position along a spectrum from normality, through mild abnormality ('aberration') through to severe abnormality ('disease'). The vertical component defines the pathogenesis of the condition, for almost all conditions are related to the three different phases of activity in the breast during reproductive life. Together the two provide a comprehensive framework, into which can be fitted most aspects of benign breast disorders, in terms of concept, pathogenesis and severity (Table 3.2).

The basic principles underlying the ANDI classification are set out in Table 3.3.

Since the ANDI concept was first proposed in 1979, and published in 1987, a great deal of new information, relating both to physiology and to pathology, has come forward, providing a surprising degree of support to those elements of the concept which were speculative at that time. The ANDI classification was accepted and recommended by an international multidisciplinary working party in 1992.[2]

The ANDI framework is consonant with and builds on work of many earlier workers, extending back as far as 1922.[3] Yet its postulates are in total contrast to the widely accepted concepts of fibrocystic disease, and hence it is necessary to present the background, rationale and supporting material in some detail.

RECOGNITION OF THE NORMALITY OF MUCH BENIGN BREAST 'DISEASE'

In the 1950s, a number of seminal studies demonstrated that the histological changes of fibrocystic disease are widely distributed in patients who had not claimed to be symptomatic or demonstrated overt disease. Parks[4] showed, from studies of both surgical and autopsy specimens, a complete gradation between normal histology and disease; for example, between developing lobules and fibroadenomas, and between involuting lobules and macroscopic cysts. He also showed that epithelial hyperplasia is so common around the menopause as to be normal and that these lesions, so often in the past regarded as indicative of cancer risk, could regress without treatment.

Extensive autopsy studies over the past 50 years have shown that most of the benign changes previously considered as disease are so common that they must be regarded as lying within the spectrum of normality. Recently, such a study of 200 breasts at autopsy from 100 postmenopausal patients (mean age 62 years) without clinical breast disease confirmed earlier studies and showed changes of 'fibrocystic condition' (normal to aberration) in 54% of cases, with only 46% histologically normal. Hyperplasia with severe atypia (disease) was seen in only 3% of patients.[5]

Mastalgia provides an example of horizontal assessment. Studies in Cardiff over the past 20 years have shown the high incidence of painful nodularity: two-thirds of a population

Table 3.1 The basic bidirectional framework of the ANDI classification

Vertical – Pathogenesis based on reproductive period	Horizontal – Spectrum of severity		
	Normal	Aberration	Disease
Development (15–25 years)			
Cyclical activity (25–45 years)			
Involution (35–55 years)			

Table 3.2 Classification of the more important conditions of BBD into ANDI and non-ANDI

Stage	Main clinical presentations		
	Normal process	**Aberration**	**Disease**
Early reproductive (15–25 years)	Lobular development	Fibroadenoma	Giant fibroadenoma
	Stromal development	Adolescent hypertrophy	Gigantomastia
	Nipple eversion	Nipple inversion	Subareolar abscess/ Mammary duct fistula
Mature reproductive (25–40 years)	Cyclical changes of menstruation	Cyclical mastalgia Nodularity	Incapacitating mastalgia
	Epithelial hyperplasia of pregnancy	Bloody nipple discharge	
Involution (35–55 years)	Lobular involution	Macrocysts Sclerosing lesions	
	Duct involution – dilatation – sclerosis	Duct ectasia Nipple retraction	Periductal mastitis/abscess
	Epithelial turnover	Simple epithelial hyperplasia	With atypia
Non-ANDI	Conditions of well-defined aetiology, such as fat necrosis, lactational abscess etc, together with extrinsic precipitating factors such as smoking and oro-nipple contact in severe non-puerperal abscess.		

Table 3.3 The principles underlying the ANDI concept

1. Most benign disorders are related to normal processes of reproductive life.
2. There is a spectrum that ranges from normal to aberration, and occasionally to disease.
3. The definition of normal and abnormal is pragmatic.
4. The ANDI concept embraces all aspects – symptoms, signs, histology and physiology.

of working women will experience mastalgia. The clinical significance of mastalgia was quantified in the Cardiff Mastalgia Clinic through accurate classification and assessment of impact on patients' lives by visual linear analogue scales and breast pain charts. This has demonstrated that much breast pain can be considered as 'normal', some is sufficiently troublesome to warrant attention and can be regarded as a 'disorder', but in a minority pain is sufficiently severe as to be a major interference with quality of life and to be regarded as disease.

Individual conditions can also be put into a longitudinal grouping related to the three main phases of breast activity during reproductive life, since these conditions can be recognized as arising from aberrations of normal processes within the breast.

While the changes of ANDI, both clinical (painful nodularity) and histological ('fibroadenosis'), are now recognized as part of a spectrum extending from normality and probably arising from minor hormonal abnormalities, no specific aetiological factors have been identified, except for those of altered prolactin secretion and possibly changes in fatty acid intake. Nor is there any good evidence as to whether the condition has always occurred with the same frequency. A recent study of women of all age groups showed less histological changes of ANDI than were reported in the 1950s and 1960s.[6] While microcysts were seen in most breasts and duct ectasia in one-third, both conditions showed a uniform age spread. In contrast, epithelial hyperplasia and sclerosed lobules were uncommon, and no case of premalignant hyperplasia was seen. Only further work will show whether this is a genuine epidemiological trend, since population (autopsy) studies common 40 years ago have in general been replaced by more detailed study and follow-up of biopsy material. There is some evidence of changing incidence patterns in non-Western populations as social and dietary conditions change, as discussed in Chapter 19.

PROBLEMS WITH THE CONVENTIONAL VIEW OF BENIGN BREAST DISEASE

When problems are defined, solutions are more easily found. Even just recognizing the problems goes a long way towards resolving them. We see four main problems in the classical approach to benign breast disease:

- Nomenclature
- The borderline between normal and abnormal
- Correlation of clinical symptoms and signs with histological changes
- The assessment of premalignant potential.

Nomenclature

As discussed in Chapter 1, the situation has been beset by multiple loose terminology. Each worker in the past has tended to introduce his or her own terminology, reflecting personal ideas of disease and its underlying pathology, without linking it to earlier studies. At first the terms were mainly clinical, e.g. 'chronic mastitis', but later reflected biopsy appearance, e.g. 'fibrocystic disease', of symptomatic lesions without appreciating the range of histological appearance in patients without symptoms. This leads on to the second problem.

The borderline between normal and abnormal – what determines normality or abnormality?

Many organs under endocrine control show a wide range of appearances associated with cyclical or pulsed hormonal secretion. This is especially true in females, where cyclical changes are set against a background of the broader changes of development and involution at the extremes of reproductive life, and particularly so in the breast. Most of these cyclical changes show a spectrum which on occasions may extend outside the normal range. Clearly it is important to try to define the point, even if blurred, at which normality crosses the line to abnormality.

A number of factors must be assessed in deciding where the boundary of normality lies, including incidence, clinical impact and histology. Macrocysts are an example of the importance of incidence; they are common and commonly multiple, while microcysts are found in almost all breasts if looked for carefully enough. Clearly microcysts must be regarded as normal, and macrocysts – with an incidence of perhaps 10% of all women – are at most an aberration of normality and cannot be considered as disease.

The importance of clinical impact can be illustrated by mastalgia. A large proportion of women experience premenstrual discomfort for a few days, this causes little interference with quality of life, and can be considered as normal. However, when pain persists for 3 out of 4 weeks of the cycle and is of great severity, it must be looked at in a different light. This is quite uncommon, and the clinical impact can be quite severe, hence it can be regarded as an aberra-tion of normality, and perhaps in the most extreme cases, as disease.

Histological appearances have given particular difficulty in this area; even minimal degrees of hyperplasia have been regarded as carrying cancer risk in the past, but recently the high incidence of simple hyperplasias in normal women has caused a reassessment of significance. A number of pathologists, and Page and his co-workers in particular[7], have defined and categorized histological patterns and their significance with considerable precision. This has allowed hyperplasias to be placed in three broad groups: normal (no increased cancer risk), slightly increased risk (equivalent to aberration) and high cancer risk.

Benign breast conditions cannot always be categorized as definitively normal or abnormal using these three criteria because there is usually a spectrum of severity. However it is possible, using considerations such as these, to assess where an individual patient lies along this spectrum, so that an appropriate management policy can be determined.

Correlation of clinical symptoms and signs with histological changes

In the past, a patient with a local clinical abnormality such as an area of painful nodularity has been subjected to biopsy and the histological changes correlated with that clinical nodule. This ignores the fact that the classic changes of 'fibrocystic disease', including fibrosis, adenosis, cyst formation and lymphocytic infiltration, may be seen in the asymptomatic breast, and ignores the dynamic changes within the breast from month to month. Thus, a second biopsy from a clinically identical area a few centimetres away might show different histological changes, as might a biopsy a few months later. (A recent study provides interesting confirmation of this heterogeneity of response within different areas of the breast. Normal volunteers given defined oral contraceptives showed diverse histological changes on biopsy, often with secretory and involutional changes coexisting in different parts of the same breast.[8])

The histology of a clinical lesion must be assessed against the broad spectrum of histological change which might be seen within a 'normal' breast, symptomatic or not. Failure to do so leads to confusion of significance – painful nodularity, a clinical condition which has no distinct radiological or pathological counterpart, has been called fibroadenosis, and correlated with cancer risk.

Only lesions which are both definite clinical and pathological entities, e.g. a macrocyst, can be assessed from both points of view. Terms such as fibroadenosis or fibrocystic disease are misleading, because they imply that these histological patterns are abnormal and that they correlate with clinical conditions. Histological changes are best described by a general term such as ANDI, which correctly indicates pathogenesis without using misleading specific terms, or by the specific individual histological elements present in the biopsy material.

The assessment of premalignant potential

This aspect has understandably dominated the efforts of breast surgeon and pathologist alike. Both have been frustrated by the three factors discussed above and it is not surprising that attempts to assess premalignant potential of fibrocystic disease have given almost infinitely variable results from one study to another. Confusion of nomenclature is particularly great when discussing the epithelial hyperplasias. Because of their pre-cancerous association, the use of different terms in different countries has led to serious misunderstanding, compounded by failure to define the borderline between normal and abnormal. Only recently has this problem been addressed in a uniform and structured manner, as with the work of Page discussed above.[9]

Where do the answers to these problems lie? First, in defining the range of normality, both in terms of clinical symptoms and signs, and of histological appearance. Secondly, recognizing that breast problems may be clinical, physiological or histological, and each problem may sometimes reflect only one of these three: sometimes more than one. Thirdly, by providing a comprehensive framework within which individual clinical or histological situations can be placed so that they are seen within an overall context. This must allow precise placement of a problem within the overall clinicopathological framework of benign breast disease and also encompasses the decision whether an individual clinical situation lies towards the normal or abnormal end of the spectrum of a particular process.

THE PHYSIOLOGICAL PROCESSES UNDERLYING THE ANDI CONCEPT

The physiology of the breast has been described in detail in Chapter 2, but the broad outline is important in understanding ANDI. The main processes are related to hormonal effects on the breast during reproductive life, in the three phases of development, cyclical change and involution. As these three stages are of increasing complexity, it is not surprising that the processes go wrong more often during the long period of cyclical activity than during development, and even more commonly in the long and complex process of involution. Consideration of the impact of these hormonal events on lobules, ducts and stroma sets the scene for an understanding of the clinical conditions which arise from them.

Pathogenesis, clinical presentation and management of benign breast disorders are set out in this chapter only in conceptual terms. The details of clinical features, pathology and management are given in the rest of the book. We hope readers will persevere with the concepts of this chapter – we believe it makes detailed assessment and management of individual clinical problems so much easier.

Hormone-controlled processes of the breast
Breast development

The premenarchal breast consists of a few ducts only. The striking feature of the perimenarchal development of the breast is the addition of lobular structures to the already developing duct system. The lobules develop particularly during early reproductive life at 15–25 years of age. At first 'primitive' type 1 lobules of Russo and Russo (Chapter 2), they are gradually replaced by more mature and less active lobules during the cyclical period, and especially with pregnancy. This explains the frequency of fibroadenoma during early and midreproductive life, for it is a condition analogous to gross hypertrophy of a lobule. Until the age of about 35 years, the luteal phase is also associated with enhanced acinar sprouting from the ductules.

A distinctive element of the lobule is its highly specialized connective tissue, and the close interaction between epithelium and connective tissue separated only by a basement membrane. This lobular connective tissue is pale and loose (Figure 3.1) with mononuclear infiltrate and differs notably from the much less interesting and urbane interlobular fibrous stroma (see Chapter 2).

Cyclical change

Both epithelial and stromal elements of the lobule are under hormonal control and there is evidence that the two work in tandem. In fact, normality seems to be very much dependent on a normal, balanced relationship between both elements. The details of the interaction of hormones and growth factors on epithelium, myoepithelium, basement membrane and stroma are now being elucidated (as discussed in Chapter 2) and give an inkling of the mechanisms underlying this relationship. It is likely that interference with these close relationships is responsible for many of the conditions that are often included under the term 'benign breast disease'. The changes occurring with each menstrual cycle have been

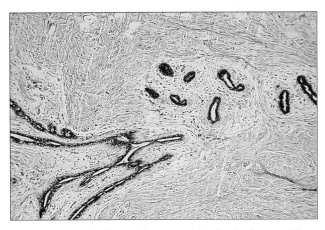

3.1 The perimenarchal breast showing early lobular development. The pale, loose lobular connective tissue contrasts with the denser interlobular fibrous stroma.

summarized by Vorherr,[10] and expanded with more recent studies which demonstrate a peak of mitosis in the late cycle followed by apoptosis (see Chapter 2). They provide a potent opportunity for minor upsets to occur with repetitive cyclical changes.

These cyclical changes are associated with clinical symptoms of heaviness and fullness that are not associated with consistent histological change, but for which a hormonal basis is being elucidated through recent studies. A correlation with prolactin secretion in response to pituitary stimulation, and particularly with bioactive forms of prolactin,[11] brings new supportive evidence not available until recently. This illustrates the need to consider physiological aspects as equally or more important than structural changes in assessing benign disorders. Superimposed on the cyclical changes are the much more radical effects of pregnancy and lactation. With the repeated development and involutional changes of menstruation and pregnancy occurring throughout 40 years of reproductive life, there is abundant opportunity for minor aberrations to occur.

When one studies a section of normal breast from a patient who has no breast complaint or overt clinical disease on examination, the striking feature is the wide spectrum of histological appearance. Figure 3.2 is from an asymptomatic patient in her thirties, and within a small area may be seen well-developed lobules, poorly developed lobules, dilated ducts and normal ducts, lobule-deficient fibrous tissue and fatty tissue.

These normal appearances provide the elements 'fibrosis' and 'adenosis' that have been documented as the histological appearance of biopsies taken from patients with nodular breasts. It has not always been appreciated that the same changes may be evident elsewhere in the same breast, where there is no clinical complaint.

The variability of appearance within the normal breast is illustrated following pregnancy. Under the intense hormonal stimulation associated with pregnancy, a uniform pattern of lobular development and maturation is seen (Figure 3.3), but postlactational involution is patchy (Figure 3.4).

With such variable involution following the total stimulation of pregnancy, it is not surprising that the more minor cyclical changes with menstruation can, compounded over a long period, produce marked differences in the structure and appearance of various areas of the breast tissue on a purely random basis.

Breast involution

Involution starts quite early and changes are obvious by 35 years of age and often earlier. Thus cyclical change and involution run in tandem for 20 years or more, increasing the chance of aberration of normality – as reflected in the high frequency of presentation to a breast clinic during this period. The involution affects the lobules particularly and is much dependent on the relationship between the epithelium and specialized stroma of the lobule. In Figure 3.5, which shows an involuting breast, an orderly regression of lobules and surrounding fibrous tissue can be clearly seen.

During this process of lobular involution, the loose

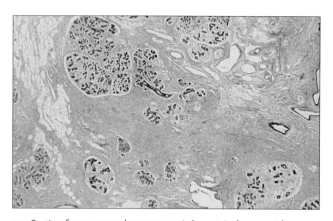

3.2 Section from a normal asymptomatic breast. It shows a wide variety of histological appearances – the changes commonly ascribed to 'fibrocystic disease'.

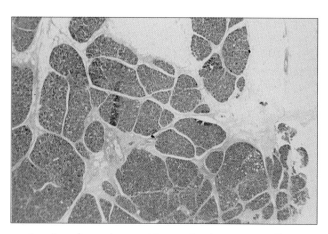

3.3 A section of normal pregnant breast, showing extreme, uniform lobular development.

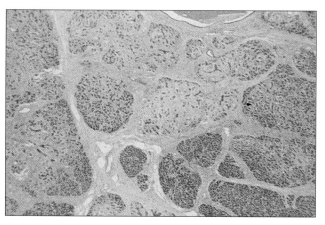

3.4 Histological section from a postlactational breast. Involution is patchy, varying from marked to negligible.

hormone-responsive intralobular connective tissue is replaced by the more standard interlobular type of fibrous tissue. If this replacement is well coordinated with the regression of epithelial tissue, the uniform picture of involution shown in Figure 3.5 is seen. Eventually, by the time the menopause has been reached and passed, involution is extensive (Figure 3.6) with only a few ducts remaining, and few if any lobular structures.

But it does not always happen in that way, and minor aberrations of this process are very common during a period of fluctuating involution extending over 20 years. It appears that normal epithelial involution of the lobule is dependent on the continuing presence of the specialized stroma around it. Should the stroma disappear too early, the epithelial acini remain and may form microcysts. The exact mechanism is not known, but one finding is that the structural protein fodrin (expressed in normal breast epithelium) is not expressed in micro- or macrocysts,[12] although it is not certain whether this is a primary or secondary phenomenon. Microcysts are obviously a prime target for macroscopic cyst formation if pressure disparity occurs between secretion and drainage, as might occur with obstruction of the draining ductule. Microcyst formation is very common in normal breasts (Figure 3.7), as demonstrated by Parks,[4] and, in this process of cystic lobular involution, microcysts may appear even though there is still specialized stroma present.

Presumably this arises from minor obstruction to the duct by kinking or compression from fibrous tissue, or perhaps by vigorous secretion from still active epithelial tissue. (It is interesting that the lobular vein exits from the lobule alongside the ductule so venous compression readily occurs.)

Recent work has shown that there is continual turnover of fluid within cysts, but, paradoxically, that particular molecules (e.g. hormones) may persist in a cyst for months or even years (Chapter 9). As long as some of the specialized stroma remains, the lobule can still involute normally in spite of these microcysts, but should the specialized stroma disappear early then further cystic change is likely (Figure 3.8).

Mechanical duct obstruction leading to macrocysts (Figure 3.9) is almost bound to occur in a proportion of lobules, because there are many possible mechanisms: from internal blockage by epithelial cells or debris, through simple kinking and angulation, to strangulation by the surrounding maturing fibrous tissue.

Recent work on the neonatal breast is of great interest, since it shows that the involution which occurs in the first year of life following withdrawal of maternal hormones follows an identical pattern to that seen over 20 years of adult involution, even to microcyst formation as the stroma reverts to the banal interlobular form. It is now known that the number of ovarian follicles decreases progressively from the age of 35 years, so there is a progressive withdrawal of hormonal stimulation over the full period in which these involutional changes and aberrations occur.

Thus three periods occur and overlap: lobule development

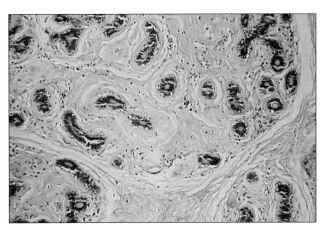

3.5 Section from a normal involuting breast. The orderly regression of both epithelial and stromal elements of the lobule is obvious. The lobular stroma has been replaced by fibrous tissue, and there is little residual epithelial tissue.

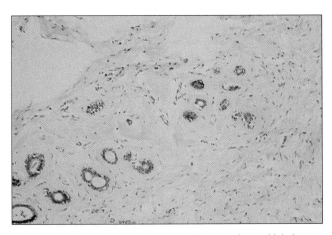

3.6 A section of postmenopausal breast, showing advanced lobular involution.

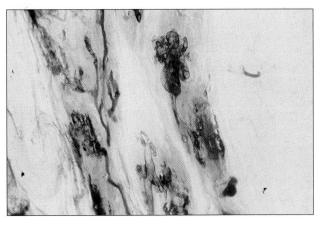

3.7 Involuting breast showing microcystic lobular change (thick section technique).

at 15–25 years, cyclical change at 15–50 years and involution at 35–55 years. Each period has its own clinical presentations, but overlapping and interacting processes also lead to complex clinical situations. The introduction of hormone replacement therapy has complicated the situation by extending these changes beyond the menopause. Thus benign disorders expected to resolve at the menopause may persist, or even arise *de novo*.

A FRAMEWORK BASED ON PATHOGENESIS

Table 3.2 sets out a classification of the more important clinical benign breast disorders that make up the main constituents of ANDI. An important point of the classification is the replacement of the term disease by disorders in the interpretation of 'BBD'. This does not mean that there is no benign breast disease, but recognizes that most breast complaints are due to disorders based on the normal processes of development, cyclical change and involution, and lie towards the normal or aberration end of the spectrum, with only a few severe enough to be placed at the disease end. The concept that conditions such as fibroadenoma and duct ectasia lie within the normal or minor aberration range is foreign to conventional teaching in pathology and surgery. Hence we give the reason in some detail.

REASONS FOR INCLUDING VARIOUS BENIGN BREAST DISORDERS AS PART OF ANDI

Disorders of development

Fibroadenoma

Since it can be shown that fibroadenomas arise from lobules, it is not surprising that these are seen predominantly in women in the 15–25 age group, even though they may not be diagnosed until later, when postpregnancy or involutional changes facilitate clinical recognition in the softer drooping involutional breast, or ultrasound demonstrates impalpable lesions.

What is the evidence to support the contention that fibroadenoma should be placed in the benign breast disorder side of ANDI rather than regarded as a neoplasm? Parks[4] showed that hyperplastic lobules, histologically identical to clinical fibroadenomas, are present so commonly as to be regarded as normal; they can probably be found in all breasts if they are sought sufficiently carefully. A full spectrum can be found between these hyperplastic lobules and clinical fibroadenomas, which do not show the inexorable growth typical of true neoplasms. They usually grow to 1 or 2 cm in diameter and then stay constant in size. They show hormonal dependence similar to normal lobules by lactating during pregnancy (Figure 3.10) and will involute to be replaced by hyaline connective tissue in concert with the rest of the breast in the perimenopausal period.

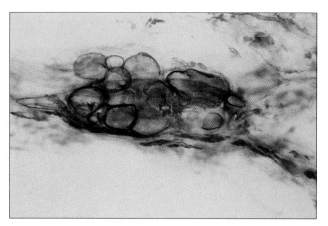

3.8 A further stage in the evolution from microcystic involution to macrocyst formation.

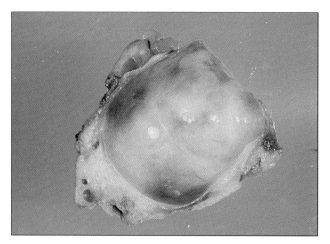

3.9 In a fully developed macrocyst, the bands in the wall reflect the origin from gross distension of number of acini (ductules) within a single lobule.

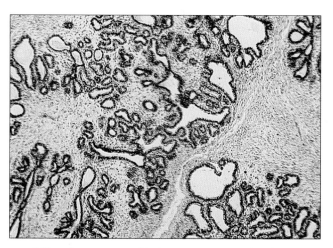

3.10 A fibroadenoma removed in the postpartum period. It shows lactation similar to the normal breast, indicating that fibroadenomas respond readily to normal physiological stimuli.

These hormonal responses are much more complete than those usually seen in benign tumours. Rarely, a fibroadenoma will continue to grow to a size of 3 cm, although this is sufficiently common to be regarded as within the normal spectrum. Growth beyond 5 cm is sufficiently uncommon in Western populations as to justify being regarded as a disease, known as giant fibroadenoma. Similarly, a multiple fibroadenoma (more than five lesions in one breast) is so uncommon in Western populations, and its implications so uncertain, as also to justify being considered a disease. Thus fibroadenoma fits well into the ANDI classification: small fibroadenomas are normal, clinical fibroadenomas are a mild aberration of the normal processes, and giant and multiple fibroadenomas are placed to the disease end of the spectrum.

Good evidence can be put forward to support this view that fibroadenoma should not be regarded as a neoplasm, as discussed in Chapter 7. All the cellular elements of fibroadenoma are normal on conventional and electron microscopy, and epithelium and myoepithelium maintain a normal relationship,[13] while molecular biology studies have shown that fibroadenomas are polyclonal in keeping with hyperplasia, in contrast to phyllodes tumours which are monoclonal in keeping with a neoplastic condition.

Adolescent hypertrophy

This condition is associated with gross stromal hyperplasia at the time of breast development. The aetiology is unknown, and this is not surprising because so little is known about the control of breast stroma – important though this is. Nevertheless, it is likely that there is a hormonal basis to the condition, a view supported by recent reports that danazol (an antigonadotrophin) may have a beneficial effect. The continuous spectrum from a small breast through to massive hyperplasia fits the horizontal element of the ANDI concept, with excessively large breasts an aberration, and the extreme hyperplasia of gigantomastia placed at the disease end.

Disorders of cyclical change
Mastalgia and nodularity

Premenstrual enlargement and postmenstrual involution of the breast occurring with each cycle is so commonly associated with discomfort and nodularity as to lie firmly within the spectrum of normality. We have used the term 'cyclical pronounced mastalgia' or 'severe painful nodularity' to differentiate the clinical disorder from the more common physiological discomfort and lumpiness. A duration of painful nodularity of more than one week of the cycle is a useful definition for differentiation from normal discomfort, and the severity of the pain can be quantified with a pain chart. This is a more pragmatic approach than the innaccurate histological concepts of fibrocystic disease, or the concept of 'non-disease'[14] which is unhelpful to those unfortunate women who suffer from its more severe manifestations. While no histological basis has been defined for these changes, the objection of such women to the concept of non-disease is supported by hormone studies,[11] which show an underlying physiological abnormality demonstrated by excess prolactin release from the pituitary following stimulation of the hypothalamic pituitary axis.

These findings stress the importance of taking a broad view of benign breast disorders, avoiding undue emphasis on non-specific histological changes and giving due attention to significant physiological changes. It is likely that subtle stromal and epithelial changes accompany physiological variations in more severe cases of cyclical nodularity and mastalgia, but more sensitive techniques may be necessary to demonstrate them. Oedema, stromal or lobular, can be demonstrated in the late cycle, but at present good evidence correlating this with clinical symptoms is lacking.

Painful nodularity of the predominantly cyclical phase of reproductive life (20–35 years) merges into and overlaps those symptoms which are more typically part of the involutional phase, especially cyst formation and sclerosing adenosis. While all have been lumped together as fibrocystic disease (or fibroadenosis) in the past, the clinical problems and management differ.

Disorders of involution

Since the process of involution extends over 20 years of monthly cycles of mitosis and apoptosis, it is not surprising that a number of aberrations should arise involving different elements of the normal breast. As discussed below, the evidence favours an aberration of normal processes for most of these. It is interesting that the incidence of these changes is similar in a number of races with widely differing cancer incidences,[15] supporting the 'normal' view against the 'precancerous' view.

Cyst formation

The desirable integrated involution of stroma and epithelium outlined earlier in this chapter is not always seen, and minor aberrations of the process are understandably common during a period of fluctuating involution extending over 20 years. The exact mechanism of this involution is not well understood,[16] but it appears that the normal epithelial involution of the lobule is dependent on the continuing presence of the specialized stroma around it. If the stroma disappears too early, the epithelial acini remain and may form microcysts, setting the pattern for macrocyst development by obstruction of the efferent ductule as discussed above. This concept of the macrocyst as being an involutional aberration (and hence part of ANDI), rather than a disease, fits in with its common occurrence and the fact that it is so frequently multiple and subclinical.

The fact that macrocysts appear to develop in two directions – apocrine and non-apocrine cysts[17] – is something which is as yet poorly understood, but the evidence is strong that both develop from a common origin of microcystic involution.[18]

Sclerosing adenosis

This condition may be considered as an aberration of either the cyclical or the involutional phase of breast activity because it can show histological changes which are both proliferative and involutional. This illustrates the complexity on the one hand, but the simplicity of concept on the other, of regarding these as aberrations of so many interacting normal processes. Considering the complex interrelationship of stromal fibrosis and epithelial regression occurring during involution, superimposed on cyclical changes of ductal sprouting, it is not surprising that this complex picture, in which epithelial acini are strangled and distorted by fibrous tissue, should arise. It is surprising that it does not occur more commonly.

Duct ectasia and periductal mastitis

The second major group of benign breast disorders consists of those associated with duct ectasia and periductal mastitis. The pathogenesis of duct ectasia is obscure. The classic theory, proposed by Haagensen,[19] regards duct ectasia (dilated ducts) as being the primary event leading to stagnation of secretion, epithelial ulceration and leakage of duct secretions containing chemically irritant fatty acids into periductal tissue to give a chemical inflammatory process. This secondary inflammation is then seen as leading to periductal fibrosis, with subsequent fibrous contraction and nipple retraction.

An alternative theory sees the primary process as periductal mastitis, perhaps on an autoimmune basis, leading to weakening of the muscle layer of the ducts and secondary dilatation. It is likely that both processes may occur separately or in conjunction, thus explaining the wide spectrum of clinical behaviour in this condition. Both duct dilatation and duct sclerosis may represent an aberration of involution. Periductal fibrosis can occur in the absence of duct ectasia or of inflammation[20] and probably represents part of the normal involutional process. Duct ectasia is so common in the postmenopausal breast that it must be regarded as part of the normal ageing process.

The wide variety of clinical symptoms associated with this condition – nipple discharge, nipple retraction, inflammatory masses and abscesses (sterile or bacterial) – can best be explained and understood by accepting more than one process in the pathogenesis. Duct ectasia appears to be a simple involutional process in the elderly, and congenital inversion of the nipple is an aberration of nipple eversion during breast development. Both are aberrations of ANDI, which may progress to disease as discussed fully in Chapter 11. Non-bacterial periductal inflammation is multifactorial, due to smoking in some cases, idiopathic and possibly involutional in others. The fact that some aspects of this complex condition are clearly parts of ANDI, some parts probably are not, and others are of unknown cause at present, illustrates the view that the ANDI concept should be utilized where it is appropriate, but that those aspects where an association is not obvious can be left outside until the pathogenesis has been clearly established.

Epithelial hyperplasias

The third element of the benign breast disorder complex, epithelial hyperplasias, has given rise to most confusion and problems in management. Many people would see this lying firmly on the side of disease rather than disorder, but a number of studies have shown that this is not so with simple hyperplasias. Parks[4] showed that lobular and intraductal papillary hyperplasia is common in the premenopausal period and tends to regress spontaneously after the menopause, and hence should be regarded as an aberration of normal involution. Kramer and Rush[21] found in their autopsy study that 59% of women over the age of 70 exhibited some degree of epithelial hyperplasia. Sloss et al.[22] concluded from their autopsy study that 'the mere presence of blunt duct adenosis, apocrine epithelium and intraductal epithelial hyperplasia in the breast of women is insufficient to warrant such tissue being called disease'.

Hence the simple epithelial hyperplasias may be placed firmly within the concept of benign breast disorder. However, careful studies by Page et al.[7] and Wellings et al.[23] have shown that the other ends of the spectrum – atypical lobular hyperplasia and atypical ductal hyperplasia – particularly as seen in the terminal ductal lobular unit (TDLU), are sufficiently commonly associated with malignancy as to be regarded as associated or premalignant conditions. Hence, epithelial hyperplasias with marked atypia belong firmly under the column of BBD.

There is at present insufficient evidence to allow a firm opinion as to whether conditions placed under the benign breast disorder column here present a continuous spectrum, with the implication that the 'disorders' move to 'disease'. They may be entirely separate processes and certainly, at the present time, no such progression of hyperplasias to cancer *in situ* should be assumed; it should be left as an open question. This controversial area is discussed more fully in Chapter 18.

AN EXTENSION OF THE CONCEPT OF ANDI TO INCLUDE MOST BENIGN BREAST DISORDERS?

Since the conceptual thinking prior to ANDI was encompassed in the chronic mastitis/fibroadenosis/fibrocystic disease attitude to BBD, it is not surprising that ANDI is equated sometimes with these conditions and used as a synonym for painful nodularity. This is restrictive, as it has been shown that a majority of benign breast disorders lie within the concept, some clearly do not and some remain inconclusive.[24] Our current view of the classification of all benign disorders is shown in Table 3.2. Most conditions are regarded as part of ANDI, and the old term 'fibroadenosis' is designated 'painful nodularity of ANDI'.

Some of the less common benign breast disorders also fit well into the concept of aberrations of normality and it is useful to consider the arguments for including them within this framework. Briefly, these arguments are as follows:
• *Nipple inversion:* This is an aberration of development

of the terminal ducts, preventing the normal protrusion of ducts and areola.

- *Mammary duct fistula:* Nipple inversion predisposes to terminal duct obstruction, leading to recurrent subareolar abscess and mammary duct fistula – the usual form of periductal mastitis seen in younger women. Extraneous factors such as smoking and oro-nipple contact interact with the processes of ANDI.
- *Epithelial hyperplasia of pregnancy:* Marked hyperplasia of the duct epithelium occurs in pregnancy, and the papillary projections sometimes give rise to bilateral bloody nipple discharge, a condition which is always benign when occurring in pregnancy.
- *Benign duct papilloma:* This is a common condition during the period of cyclical activity and shows minimal if any malignant potential. It is reasonable to regard it as an aberration of cyclical epithelial activity.
- *Adenosis:* For similar reasons it might be considered logical to extend the concept of aberration of normality to encompass adenosis as a manifestation of involution.

IMPLICATIONS FOR THE MANAGEMENT OF BENIGN BREAST DISORDERS

It follows from the foregoing that most of the conditions listed under benign breast disorders can be regarded as minor aberrations of normality and hence do not demand active specific treatment. This being the case, any active management of these conditions should be based on considerations such as accurate diagnosis, patient concern and interference with quality of life. No treatment is required based solely on inherent pathological significance until the disease end of the spectrum is reached. This concept of management is outlined here and details of management are given in the appropriate chapters.

Adolescent hypertrophy
In its more severe forms, treatment is indicated because of psychological and physical morbidity from the size and weight of the breast. It is the degree of this morbidity that determines treatment with hormonal or surgical therapy.

Fibroadenoma
The concept of fibroadenoma being a part of ANDI and not a neoplasm has been one of the conceptual changes behind us moving gradually from active to conservative management over the past 20 years. The results from many centres now justify this approach as discussed in Chapter 7.

Inverted nipple
This is the failure of development of major ducts, and treatment short of severing the ducts is unlikely to give a long-term satisfactory result. Hence treatment is related to the patient's view of the cosmetic deformity, and recommended only after recognizing the uncertain long-term results of

minor surgical procedures for this condition, and the consequences of total duct division for cosmesis and lactation if the defect is to undergo total correction.

Likewise, recurrent subareolar abscess associated with nipple inversion will require eradication of the sump-like dilated duct underlying the recurrent infection.

Cyclical mastalgia and nodularity
It is generally accepted that these manifestations are physiological, and that most cases can be treated by adequate reassurance. But the view that the most severe cases, those lasting perhaps 2 weeks or more of the menstrual cycle, interfere so much with the quality of life as to merit consideration as disease is confirmed by the high incidence of hormonal abnormalities in these patients. It is unhelpful to tell the patient that she has a non-disease if her symptoms interfere with her quality of life. Rather, the severity of her mastalgia should be assessed objectively with pain charts so that her condition can be placed on the normal–aberration–disease scale and appropriate management instituted. There is equally strong evidence that most cases are not psychologically based, and hence endocrine-related treatment is appropriate in those cases severe enough to warrant therapy.[25]

Cysts
Macrocysts and microcysts are so common as to need no active treatment other than that required to allow diagnosis and allay patient concern. It is now well established by practice that simple cysts are satisfactorily treated by aspiration, a policy that might have been predicted from the ANDI concept. The recent differentiation of cysts into apocrine and non-apocrine[17] does not at present alter this conservative therapeutic approach, because any breast cancer risk is a general one, and not related to the individual cyst. Likewise, since the condition is a minor aberration of a normal process, excision is not required for multiple or recurrent cysts, except in the presence of a bloody aspirate or a residual lump, both requiring exclusion of coexisting cancer.

Sclerosing adenosis
This condition causes diagnostic problems to surgeons, radiologists and histopathologists and sometimes problems to the patient in the form of a lump or pain. It requires no treatment other than careful exclusion of cancer, although it sometimes requires symptomatic treatment for pain.

Postmenopausal nipple retraction
The only importance of this is to recognize that it may be caused by the simple involutional process of periductal fibrosis. It requires no active management other than exclusion of cancer. In our experience, nipple retraction is more commonly due to ductal fibrosis than to cancer, and fortunately the diagnosis is easily made in older patients because the postmenopausal breast lends itself to accurate mammography.

Duct ectasia/periductal mastitis complex

The symptoms of this condition that can be categorized under the aberration column cause little clinical upset and require no therapy other than reassurance for opaque, non-bloody discharge.

Rarely, the discharge may be sufficiently profuse to cause social embarrassment. In this case, after a pituitary adenoma has been excluded, the patient may be treated in mechanical fashion by a total duct excision. This approach is rarely necessary, but it again demonstrates the value of assessing the impact of symptoms on quality of life to place them appropriately along the spectrum of severity.

Management of blood-related discharge is directed towards excluding more serious pathology.

Epithelial hyperplasias

Epithelial hyperplasias without atypia usually found as a chance histological finding fall somewhere between normality and an aberration in significance. With atypical hyperplasias, the emphasis moves towards the disease state, and special consideration should be given to assessment of cancer risk, as defined particularly by Page and Dupont.[9]

ABERRATION TO DISEASE?

The ANDI concept is based on the progression from normal to aberration to disease. Sound evidence for the progression from normal to aberration exists, as discussed in the section on fibroadenoma. However, no evidence exists for or against the supposition that giant fibroadenomas arise from the continued progression of small fibroadenomas, i.e. that aberration progresses to disease. It is possible that giant fibroadenoma is a separate condition *de novo*, or an added factor may lead to progression from a 'standard' fibroadenoma. There is certainly evidence from molecular biology that a change from polyclonality occurs with phyllodes tumours, although it is not clear whether this is a secondary change in a fibroadenoma, or is present in a phyllodes tumour *de novo* (see Chapter 7).

Likewise, it is likely that normal epithelium and apocrine changes form a continuum with simple hyperplasias, but there is less evidence to support the direct progression from the latter to atypical hyperplasias or carcinoma-in-situ. Thus, on the basis of present evidence we do not know whether disease in this case is a progression from aberration or whether disease and aberration are two separate conditions.

This is one of the most interesting areas of benign breast disorders, and new evidence is starting to provide answers to some of these questions. For instance, simple fibroadenoma is classified as an aberration, but multiple fibroadenomas are sufficiently rare and troublesome to be classified as disease. It has recently been found that transplant patients on cyclosporin have an increased incidence of multiple fibroadenomas, giving a new insight into progression from aberration to disease. Cigarette smoking has a similar significance for duct ectasia/periductal mastitis, and it is likely that the various factors that lead to atypical hyperplasias will become elucidated in the near future.

The time is approaching when we are likely to have much greater insight into these questions. Meanwhile, this does not compromise the utility of the ANDI classification in helping understand benign breast disorders, and the concepts are sufficiently flexible to allow us to incorporate new information as it becomes available. The past 10 years have seen the concept strenthened and refined by new knowledge.

RECENT DEVELOPMENTS HAVING A BEARING ON THE ANDI CONCEPT

Apocrine metaplasia

Apocrine metaplasia has a particular interest in that it is a frequent finding in ANDI, suggesting normality, yet carrying a slight but definite increase in cancer risk. For that reason, there is much interest in possible mechanisms for indicating cancer risk, and which might throw light on the evolution from normal to aberration to disease.

Haagensen[26] suggested three possible mechanisms by which apocrine metaplasia might relate to cancer.

Apocrine metaplasia is a precursor to malignant transformation.

Apocrine metaplasia may result from a response to the same stimulus as can cause cancer.

Apocrine metaplasia might itself have a higher propensity for malignant change.

Kumar and colleagues[27] demonstrated by an immunohistochemical technique that cells of apocrine metaplasia have very high levels of prolactin not seen in normal ductal cells, blunt duct adenosis, lobules or fibroadenoma. Tschugguel *et al.*[28] found that apocrine metaplastic cells demonstrate endothelial calcium-dependent nitric oxide synthase, unlike other cells of benign breast disorders, suggesting that the vascular effects of nitric oxide might play a part in progression to malignant change. A study of fetal breast tissue has made the situation even more complex.[29] Epithelial cells bearing a biochemical marker for apocrine cells (anti-GCDFP-15 monoclonal antibody) were found in some duct cells of fetal breasts, and in lobules of adult breasts, although no cells with histological or ultrastructural apocrine features were found. This suggests that apocrine cells appear when some unknown stimulus causes apocrine precursor cells to take on the typical morphology.

Cyst formation and duct ectasia

These processes have largely eluded research efforts into pathogenesis, although the absence of fodrin in the wall of cysts may be important.[12] Animal experiments are notoriously irrelevant to human breast disease, although the action of keratinocyte growth factor (FGF-7) commands some interest in such an otherwise sterile field. Yi *et al.*[30] have shown that this stromal cell-derived paracrine mediator for epithelial proliferation causes hyperplastic changes in ducts in rats similar to ANDI. In mice it causes dilatation of ducts along much of their length (duct ectasia?), and when given together with exogenous oestrogen and progesterone, it produces numerous end-buds with a picture resembling the histological changes of ANDI.

Fibroadenoma and hyperplasias

It seems likely that an imbalance between cell proliferation and apoptosis may be involved in the development of ANDI conditions, as breast tissues under hormonal control undergo continuing remodelling, involving a balance between quiescence, proliferation and apoptosis. Evidence supporting this is becoming available: Ferrieres et al[31]. found that bcl-2 levels in normal ducts and lobules varied with the menstrual cycle, being higher in the follicular than luteal phases, with high progesterone levels apparently suppressing bcl-2 activity. Levels of bcl-2 were higher and the progesterone effect absent in fibroadenomas, giving a possible mechanism for excessive lobular growth in this condition. There is also evidence for a role for matrix metalloproteinases in this hormone control of reproductive organs.[32]

Allan et al. studied apoptosis in normal epithelial cells adjacent to pathology (fibroadenoma, fibrocystic disease and cancer), and found reduced apoptosis in the case of the latter two.[33] They suggest that this reduced apoptosis may be the cause of cellular build-up in ANDI, although an alternative is that the pathological tissue could affect apoptosis by a (secondary) paracrine mechanism.

Loss of heterozygosity (LOH) is an indicator of a clonal, neoplastic condition rather than a simple hyperplasia. Lakhani et al. have shown that LOH is a feature of atypical ductal hyperplasia (ADH) as well as ductal and lobular carcinoma-in-situ (DCIS and LCIS), suggesting that the essential step towards malignancy (aberration to disease) has already taken place at the stage of ADH. They have recently shown[34] evidence of LOH in some cases of ductal hyperplasia without atypia, but not in apocrine cysts or benign papillomas. The cases showing LOH could not be distinguished morphologically from those without. This would suggest that progression from aberration to disease may occur early in some cases of hyperplasia without atypia, presumably those that will progress to more severe pathology, or that these cases may be different *ab initio*. However, other workers[35] have found differing results, emphasizing the preliminary nature of these approaches.

These findings as yet raise as many questions as they answer, but they do hold out hope that similar techniques may soon give a much deeper understanding of the mechanisms of ANDI, and of the relationship between aberration and disease.

REFERENCES

1. Hughes LE, Mansel RE & Webster DJTW. Aberrations of normal development and involution (ANDI): A new perspective on pathogenesis and nomenclature of benign breast disorders. *Lancet* 1987; 2: 1316–1319.

2. Hughes LE, Smallwood J & Dixon JM. Nomenclature of benign breast disorders: report of a working party on the rationalisation of concepts and terminology of benign breast conditions. *The Breast* 1992; 1: 15–17.

3. McFarland J. Residual lactation acini in the female breast. Their relationship to chronic cystic mastitis and malignant breasts. *Archives of Surgery* 1922; 5: 1–64.

4. Parks AG. The microanatomy of the breast. *Annals of the Royal College of Surgeons of England* 1959; 25: 295–311.

5. Sarnelli R & Squartini F. Fibrocystic condition and 'at risk' lesions in asymptomatic breasts: a morphological study of postmenopausal women. *Clinical and Experimental Obstetrics and Gynecology* 1991; 18: 271–279.

6. Hutson SW, Cowen PN & Bird CC. Morphometric studies of age related changes in normal human breast and their significance for evolution of mammary cancer. *Journal of Clinical Pathology* 1985; 38: 281–287.

7. Page DL, Vander-Zwag R, Roger LW et al. Relationship between component parts of fibrocystic disease complex and breast cancer. *Journal of the National Cancer Institute* 1978; 61: 1055–1063.

8. DiLieto A, De Rosa G, Albano G et al. Desogestrone versus gestodene in oral contraceptives: influence on the clinical and histomorphological features of BBD. *European Journal of Obstetrics, Gynecology, and Reproductive Biology* 1994; 55: 71–83.

9. Page DL & Dupont WD. Anatomic indicators (histologic and cytologic) of increased breast cancer risk. *Breast Cancer Research and Treatment* 1993; 28: 157–162.

10. Vorherr H. *The Breast. Morphology, Physiology and Lactation.* New York: Academic Press, 1974.

11. Kumar S, Mansel RE, Hughes LE et al. Prediction of response to endocrine therapy in pronounced cyclical mastalgia, using dynamic tests of prolactin release. *Clinical Endocrinology* 1985; 23: 699–704.

12. Simpson JF & Page DL. Loss of expression of fodrin (a structural protein) in cystic changes in the human breast. *Laboratory Investigation* 1993; 68: 537–540.

13. Archer F & Omar N. The fine structure of fibroadenoma of the human breast. *Journal of Pathology* 1969; 99: 113–117.

14. Love SM, Gelman RS & Silen W. Fibrocystic 'disease' of the breast – A non disease. *New England Journal of Medicine* 1982; 307: 1010–1014.

15. Bartow SA, Pathak DR, Black WC et al. Prevalence of benign, atypical and malignant breast lesions in populations at different risk of breast cancer. *Cancer* 1987; 60: 2751–2760.

16. Azzopardi JG. *Problems in Breast Pathology*. London: WB Saunders, 1979.

17. Miller WR, Dixon JM, Scott WN & Forrest APM. Classification of human breast cysts according to electrolyte and androgen conjugate composition. *Clinical Oncology* 1983; 9: 227–232.

18. Dixon JM, Scott WN & Miller WR. An analysis of the content and morphology of human breast microcysts. *European Journal of Surgical Oncology* 1985; **11**: 151–154.

19. Haagensen CD. Mammary duct ectasia – a disease that may simulate carcinoma. *Cancer* 1951; **4**: 749–761.

20. Davies JD. Inflammatory damage to ducts in mammary dysplasia: a cause of duct obliteration. *Journal of Pathology* 1975; **117**: 47–54.

21. Kramer WM & Rush BF. Mammary duct proliferation in the elderly – a histological study. *Cancer* 1973; **31**: 130–137.

22. Sloss PT, Bennett WA & Clagett OT. Incidence in normal breasts of features associated with chronic cystic mastitis. *American Journal of Pathology* 1957; **33**: 1181–1191.

23. Wellings SR, Jensen HM & Marcum RG. An atlas of subgross pathology of the human breast with reference to possible pre-cancerous lesions. *Journal of the National Cancer Institute* 1975; **55**: 231–273.

24. Hughes LE. Classification of benign breast disorders. *British Medical Bulletin* 1991; **47**: 251–257.

25. Pye JK, Mansel RE & Hughes LE. Clinical experience of drug treatments for mastalgia. *Lancet* 1985; **ii**: 373–377.

26. Haagensen DE Jr. Is cystic disease related to cancer? *American Journal of Surgical Pathology* 1991; **15**: 687–694.

27. Kumar S, Mansel RE & Jasani B. Presence and possible significance of immunohistochemically demonstrable prolactin in breast apocrine metaplasia. *British Journal of Cancer* 1987; **55**: 307–309.

28. Tschugguel W, Knogler W, Czerwenka K *et al*. Presence of endothelial calcium-dependent nitric oxide synthase in breast apocrine metaplasia. *British Journal of Cancer* 1996; **74**: 1423–1426.

29. Viacava P, Naccarato AG & Bevilacqua G. Apocrine metaplasia of the breast: Does it result from metaplasia? *Virchows Archiv. A, Pathological Anatomy and Histopathology* 1997; **431**: 205–209.

30. Yi ES, Bedoya AA, Lee H *et al*. Keratinocyte growth factor causes cystic dilatation of the mammary glands in mice. *American Journal of Pathology* 1994; **145**: 1015–1022.

31. Ferrieres G, Cuny M, Simony-Lafontaine J *et al*. Variation of bcl-2 expression in breast ducts and lobules in relation to plasma progesterone levels: Overexpression and absence of variation in fibroadenomas. *Journal of Pathology* 1997; **183**: 204–211.

32. Hulboy DL, Rudolph LA & Matrisian LM. Matrix metalloproteinases as mediators of reproductive function. *Molecular Human Reproduction* 1997; **3**: 27–45.

33. Allan DJ, Howell A, Roberts SA *et al*. Reduction in apoptosis relative to mitosis in histologically normal epithelium accompanies fibrocystic change and carcinoma in the premenopausal breast. *Journal of Pathology* 1992; **167**: 25–32.

34. Lakhani SR, Slack DN, Hamoudi RA *et al*. Detection of loss of heterozygosity (LOH) indicates that mammary hyperplasia of usual type is a clonal, neoplastic proliferation. *Journal of Pathology* 1996; **178**(Suppl): 5A.

35. Kasami M, Vnencak-Jones CL, Manning S *et al*. Loss of heterozygosity and microsatellite instability in breast hyperplasia. *American Journal of Pathology* 1997; **150**: 1925–1932.

The approach to diagnosis and assessment of breast lumps

CONTENTS

KEY POINTS AND NEW DEVELOPMENTS

1. Triple assessment – clinical examination, imaging and pathology – is now the standard approach to all breast lumps.
2. Examination, ultrasound and cytology should normally be available at the first visit, with provision of an immediate diagnosis if the lump is benign.
3. A standard sequence should be followed to exclude normal structures and differentiate normal nodularity from a dominant lump.
4. A further sequence should be followed for lumps recurrent after biopsy.
5. A clear follow-up policy is desirable to prevent clinics being overwhelmed by patients without serious disease.

6. Ultrasound is important in differentiating a discrete lump from general nodularity, in locating deep-seated cysts and in ensuring accurate targeting for cytology specimens.
7. Wide-bore needle biopsy is being used more frequently, due to improved biopsy specimens from spring-loaded needles.
8. Guidelines regarding staffing and organization of breast clinics have been drawn up in the UK to ensure efficient handling of patients by appropriately experienced staff.

PART 1:
THE DIFFERENTIAL DIAGNOSIS AND CLINICAL ASSESSMENT OF BREAST LUMPS

Although imaging and cytology, the second and third aspects of triple assessment, are of increasing importance in reaching a rapid, accurate diagnosis of a breast lump, clinical assessment is still of great value in ensuring that these are used to best advantage. It is also important to be aware of the many minor and less common abnormalities which may simulate a pathological breast lump; this awareness may save the patient much unnecessary investigation.

It is fortunate that, although there are many causes of lumps in the breast (Table 4.1), a few diagnoses cover the large majority.

There are two major problems of diagnosis: first to decide whether the lump is within or outside the spectrum

Table 4.1 Causes of lumps in the breast		
Type	**Cause**	**Frequency of presentation**
Normal structures	Normal nodularity	Common
	Prominent fat lobule	Less common
	Prominent rib	Less common
	Intramammary lymph node	Rare
	Edge of biopsy wound	Less common
	Accessory breast	Rare
ANDI	Fibroadenoma	Common
	Cyclical nodularity	Common
	Cyst	Common
	Galactocele	Rare
	Sclerosing adenosis	Less common
	Stromal fibrosis	Rare
Inflammatory	Chronic infective abscess	Rare
	Fat necrosis	Rare
	Foreign body granuloma	Rare
	Mondor's disease	Rare
Benign tumours	Duct papilloma	Less common
	Giant fibroadenoma	Rare
	Lipoma	Rare
	Granular cell myoblastoma	Rare
Intermediate tumours	Phyllodes tumour	Rare
	Carcinoma-in-situ	Less common
Malignant	Primary tumour	Common
	Secondary tumour	Rare
Lesions of the nipple and areola	Squamous papilloma	Less common
	Leiomyoma	Rare
	Retention cyst	Rare
	Papillary adenoma	Rare
Lesions of the skin	Sebaceous cyst	Less common
	Hydradenitis	Rare
	Benign and malignant skin tumours	Rare

of normality and, secondly, if abnormal, whether it is benign or malignant.

In the past, there has been a tendency to biopsy all breast lumps irrespective of their characteristics. This results in a large number of biopsies. In one series,[1] 75% of benign biopsies showed tissues which can be regarded as normal. Because benign lumps need just as careful assessment as malignant ones in an effort to avoid unnecessary biopsies and, in particular, repeated unnecessary biopsies, the practice of triple assessment has been widely accepted, as set out in this chapter. The introduction of cytology into the breast clinic in one study reduced the overall open biopsy rate by half, and the rate for benign masses by two-thirds.[2]

CLINICAL ASSESSMENT OF A BREAST LUMP

History

The history is particularly important in the assessment of breast lumps, especially in relation to duration of the mass, fluctuation in size with the menstrual cycle and any associated pain. Each must be considered in association with the overall clinical picture and no one feature should be allowed to dominate clinical thinking. In the past, it has been widely thought that a small, painful lump is not malignant; however, pain can be the primary presentation of cancer in around 6% of cases,[3] although it should be noted that the pain indicative of cancer differs in characteristics from that of cyclical mastalgia (Chapter 8).

Inspection

Detailed and systematic examination is of great importance, particularly in elucidating the early signs of malignancy. These are well known, but two of them, skin attachment and nipple retraction, can sometimes be caused by benign conditions.

Cancer is the likely diagnosis when nipple retraction is associated with a lump, but two benign lumps may also cause nipple retraction. A chronic abscess associated with periductal mastitis may cause retraction by a combination of shortening of ducts and areola oedema. A large cyst or fibroadenoma arising centrally among the major ducts can cause relative shortening by displacement and so give rise to apparent nipple retraction (Figure 4.1).

The same mechanism can operate with skin attachment. Haagensen[4] calls this false retraction. Large cysts or fibroadenomas can displace Cooper's ligaments and give rise to apparent skin fixity and distortion, while a chronic abscess associated with periductal mastitis will lead to actual skin attachment, oedema and sometimes *peau d'orange*. Mondor's disease may also give rise to the appearance of skin retraction (see Figure 17.5). Hence the necessity to obtain cytological or histological confirmation in all cases of suspected malignancy.

Palpation

History before palpation has become even more important in recent years because of the increasing use of devices which can confound breast examination, ranging from augmentation prostheses to pacemakers. The patient may forget to mention it, or may assume that the physician will recognize it.

Consistency, surface characteristics and mobility in relation to surrounding tissues are each important in diagnosing benign lesions. A fibroadenoma has a characteristic rubbery consistency, a smooth or smoothly lobulated surface and a degree of mobility within the breast which can only be described as extraordinary; this combination of characteristics provides an unequivocal clinical diagnosis. This classic pattern is usual in young girls, but is often obscured in older women by incarceration of the fibroadenoma in a background of involutional changes such that the fibroadenoma is robbed of its classic discrete, smooth surface and mobility. The diagnosis can be aided by the use of ultrasound.

While palpation of a moderately tense cyst is equally characteristic, the clinical findings vary greatly depending on the degree of intracystic tension, which may vary from normal tissue tension to a hardness which exceeds

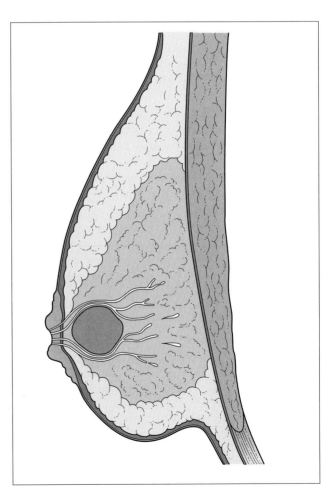

4.1 A large benign cyst may stretch and distort main ducts or Cooper's ligaments, leading to 'pseudoretraction' of skin or nipple.

that of cancer. Thus cysts are commonly misdiagnosed. They may be missed completely because they are soft; in other cases cancer is confidently diagnosed because the cyst is so hard. This alone justifies the passage of a fine needle in every breast lump because the finding of unexpected fluid will save the patient much distress and unnecessary surgery. The surface of a cyst is usually smooth, but a large cyst may be lobulated and occasionally a group of small cysts will feel nodular so as to simulate a fibroadenoma.

Assessment of the mobility of a breast lump within the surrounding tissue provides diagnostic information; as illustrated in Figure 4.2, there are three degrees of mobility of a lump in relation to the surrounding breast tissue.

Because a fibroadenoma has no attachment to surrounding capsule except for a single stalk, its mobility is extreme. The wall of a cyst is confluent with the fibrous breast stroma, hence the surrounding parenchyma can be felt to move with the cyst giving it an intermediate degree of mobility. At the other extreme, an infiltrating cancer fixes the surrounding breast tissue so that the affected quadrant of the breast moves with the mass. But, occasionally, a very large cyst or benign tumour will have a similar effect by stretch-fixation of Cooper's ligaments so that the quadrant of the breast moves with the lump.

Palpation is even more important for ill-defined lumps. By far the commonest problem in breast assessment is to decide whether an area which feels abnormal to the patient is truly abnormal, or whether it is part of general nodularity of the breast. This arises particularly when a woman's attention is drawn to the upper outer quadrant of the breast by premenstrual pain or tenderness. Careful assessment to determine the pattern of nodularity in both

breasts is essential. In doubtful cases it is useful to stand behind the patient and palpate both breasts simultaneously (Figure 4.3).

In this way it is surprising how often an apparent single mass is found to be bilateral and symmetrical when the mirror image sections of the breast are examined together. In this situation, ultrasound is invaluable in deciding if a true discrete abnormality is present or whether the palpable abnormality is simply glandular breast tissue. If an abnormal area is noted on ultrasound it can be sampled cytologically using the probe as a guide for the needle.

A complete physical examination, including axillary and supraclavicular palpation, is important in all breast disease, but rarely provides discriminatory diagnostic information with benign conditions.

Assessment of nodularity
Normal nodularity or dominant lump?
The commonest presenting lump in women during the reproductive period is the normal breast nodularity, or the cyclical nodularity of ANDI, felt in the upper outer quadrant and axillary tail of the breast.

To decide whether a mass is dominant or merely part of normal or cyclical nodularity is critical for an early carcinoma must not be missed; it is equally important that the surgeon does not embark on a series of biopsies of normal nodular breasts in young women, with increasing scarring and repeated worry every time an area of tenderness develops. Yet to avoid missing cancer in the 'at risk' age group (more than 25 years of age), undiagnosed discrete persisting lumps must be excised. Assessment is essentially clinical in young women, supplemented by

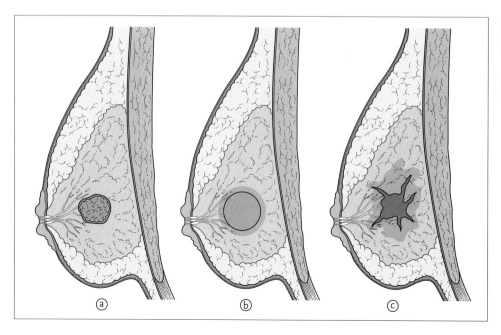

4.2 Mobility of breast lumps in relation to surrounding breast tissue. (a) Fibroadenoma; (b) cyst; (c) cancer. The shaded area indicates the amount of breast tissue 'moving' with the lump.

ultrasound, cytology or core needle histology. In an older woman where there is doubt as to whether or not a dominant mass is present, mammography and ultrasound are indicated.

To avoid unnecessary biopsy, a well-defined approach must be taken to determine whether a mass is dominant and persistent. If a single examination is inconclusive, the following sequence is useful:

- Examine both breasts simultaneously as described (Figure 4.3).
- Examine the patient during the first half of the menstrual cycle.
- Confirm or refute a localized abnormality by ultrasound examination.
- Use cytology and/or core histology repeatedly if necessary.
- Review the patient over a period of 2 months. If doubt still persists or any of the triple assessment tests are discordant, then open biopsy, often under local anaesthetic, should be performed.

Nodularity may be assessed for clinical signs of malignancy and recorded on a 1–5 scale (P1–5) in the same way as cytology, as is discussed below. Where full assessment shows nothing more than general nodularity that is deemed to be within normal limits (P2), reassurance and explanation of the physiological basis of the nodularity is adequate treatment. Specific treatment is only required when pain is the major symptom; this is dealt with in the section on breast pain (Chapter 8).

Particular notice should be taken of a patient who is certain that she can feel an abnormality in her breast, especially if she is over the age of 40. A woman may feel an abnormality some time before her medical attendant is able to do so, and the older the patient, the more likely she is to be right. Such a patient should be subjected to a full triple assessment and if no abnormality is found on examination or investigation, she may be reviewed in 2–4 months.

Assessment of a discrete or dominant mass

Having decided that a lump is not just part of normal nodularity, the physical characteristics should be carefully assessed to make a specific diagnosis. This is useful as a discipline in sharpening a physician's diagnostic acumen, but it is also important because some discrete lumps are due to normal structures. If the clinical features are definitely those of a normal structure and this is confirmed by triple assessment, surgical biopsy can be avoided. Nevertheless, the emphasis must always be on excisional biopsy where doubt persists regarding the diagnosis of any persisting dominant mass in a woman of cancer age group or where one of the elements of the triple assessment is discordant.

FEATURES OF INDIVIDUAL LESIONS

Normal structures (Figure 4.4)
Prominent fat lobule
Fat lobules are often easily palpable and one may become more prominent than another. This is seen most frequently along the inferior margin of the breast or over the axillary tail, due perhaps in both cases to pressure from a brassière. The superficial nature of the lesion, its site, soft smooth consistency and softness to a needle point, will usually allow

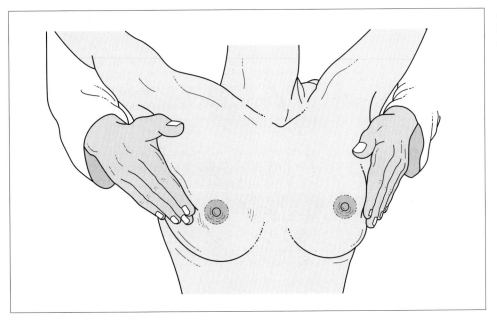

4.3 Mirror image palpation of both breasts simultaneously helps assessment of doubtful lumps.

confident diagnosis. Ultrasound also clearly shows the fat lobules as characteristic fat pockets.

Prominent rib

It is not uncommon for a patient, usually young, to present with a 'breast lump' which appears to be normal breast tissue over a normal prominent rib. Sometimes the rib is asymmetrical, but more often it is identical to the opposite side and it is difficult to know why the patient has suddenly become aware of it. Occasionally, radiology of the rib cage is necessary before reassuring the patient. Ultrasound of the area of patient concern can be reassuring.

Intramammary lymph node

Intramammary lymph nodes are usually confined to the axillary tail of the breast and are impalpable because they are small and embedded in the breast stroma. Sometimes lymph nodes in the outer quadrant of the breast proper may enlarge sufficiently to be palpable. Although they feel cystic, they are slightly elongated and peripheral to the breast area where cysts are commonly found. They have a soft feel to a needle point and have a characteristic appearance on mammography, being smooth ovoid lesions, sometimes with a notch along one margin. Lymphocytes are found on cytology which can be guided by ultrasound for small mobile nodes. It is usually possible to make a diagnosis and to avoid surgery.

Accessory breasts

Accessory breasts occur under the anterior axillary fold, are usually bilateral and come to notice during pregnancy or if the patient gains weight. They may be affected by the full range of breast pathology, including nodularity, or cysts of ANDI, fibroadenoma, carcinoma, etc. The condition is described more fully in Chapter 15.

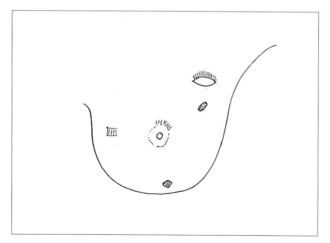

4·4 Normal structures that may be misdiagnosed as a significant dominant mass: prominent fat lobule, prominent rib, intramammary lymph node, accessory breasts, edge of a previous biopsy wound (see text).

Edge of a previous biopsy wound

Patients may present complaining of a 'lump' at the site of a previous scar which is due to the persisting edge of a defect in the breast which sometimes occurs if a biopsy wound is not closed by deep sutures after a large amount of tissue has been removed. These are seen less often now that better localization allows smaller biopsies (the British Association of Surgical Oncology Surgical Guidelines suggest a maximum weight of 20 g for benign biopsies). They are most common deep to the nipple/areola, and the most important aspect is awareness (for further discussion see page 8).

Masses due to ANDI
Fibroadenoma

In its classic form, this tumour is the most easily diagnosed breast lump. When it occurs in the age group of 15–25 years it is rubbery, firm, smooth or lobulated and extremely mobile. Clinical diagnosis is usually accurate and confirmation by ancillary tests is not always necessary. However, ultrasound and histology (FNAC or core needle biopsy) is essential whenever clinical features are atypical, and some clinicians recommend it in all patients, even in this age group. While cytology should be used for women older than 25 years, fibroadenoma is one of the lesions that is well known to cause difficulties in cytopathological diagnosis.

Fibroadenomas are also commonly seen in later life when the diagnosis is much more difficult. The patient has now reached the cancer age group, so definite exclusion of malignancy is mandatory. The fibroadenoma is caught up in the involutional fibrosis of the breast, so that it loses its characteristic smoothness and mobility; it requires full assessment as for any other dominant lump, by clinical assessment, mammography, cytology and biopsy if indicated. Calcified fibroadenomas are often seen on screening mammograms.

The clinical and radiological similarities between fibroadenoma, cyst and some circumscribed cancers (especially medullary cancer) should be remembered. Where an otherwise typical fibroadenoma is softer than expected, a phyllodes tumour should be suspected (see Chapter 7).

Cyclical nodularity ('fibroadenosis')

The problem of cyclical nodularity is that already discussed – the discrimination between general nodularity and a prominent mass in an individual patient. The problem becomes worse as normal nodularity moves across the spectrum to the more severe cyclical nodularity of ANDI.

Perhaps the most interesting aspect of this problem is why some patients with cyclical nodularity develop a dominant lump. In many cases, cyst formation or localized extravagant adenosis with or without fibrosis may underlie the mass, but in other cases, histological findings are no different to adjacent clinically unremarkable breast.

Exaggerated local end-organ response to hormonal stimulation seems the most likely cause.

The recognition of the basic normality of cyclical nodularity as a part of ANDI should be extended to histological assessment. Pathologists should be encouraged to drop the terms 'fibroadenosis' and 'chronic cystic mastitis' following the philosophy of Foote and Stewart[5] who wrote in 1945: 'Chronic cystic mastitis is so ingrained in the minds of some pathologists that this diagnosis of a locally excised portion of breast almost amounts to a surgicopathologic reflex.'

Cysts

A cyst is the commonest discrete mass found in patients presenting to a breast clinic, a fact causing little surprise since it has been estimated that about 1 in 10 of all women will develop a symptomatic breast cyst during their reproductive life, and recurrent or multiple cysts are common.

Clinical diagnosis is surprisingly uncertain; variation in size, variation in shape due to lobularity or multiplicity, variation in consistency due to intracystic pressure mean that cysts can as easily be missed completely as confidently diagnosed as cancer. Fortunately, definite diagnosis is made certain by simple needle puncture; this alone provides the justification for inserting a needle into every suspected dominant breast lump. Aspiration is also the first step in management (Chapter 9) and this process may be aided by ultrasound in deeply set cysts.

Galactocele

Galactocele presents in the same way as a cyst, some time after parturition. It is managed in the same way as other cysts, and is discussed more fully in Chapter 9.

Sclerosing adenosis

Sclerosing adenosis presents most commonly as a radiological abnormality, a chance histological finding or as a cause of mastalgia. When it presents as a lump, it is dealt with as any dominant mass, and requires no specific treatment (see Chapter 10).

The remaining lesions listed in Table 4.1 present in more specific fashion than the manifestations of ANDI and are dealt with in the appropriate sections of the book.

Isolated axillary masses

The possibility of benign axillary pathology mimicking cancer should be remembered. Reactive lymphadenopathy and ANDI in axillary accessory breast tissue are two conditions which may mimic secondary cancer, and both illustrate the importance of separate assessment of axillary masses.

The commonest cause of a clinically significant axillary mass is occult malignancy, either from the breast (often contralateral) or other sites of carcinoma or lymphoid malignancy. Benign causes include reactive lymphadenopathy (temporary or associated with conditions such as rheumatoid arthritis), lipoma or accessory breast tissue containing any pathology (including manifestations of ANDI) that may be seen in the breast itself.[6] Isolated axillary masses are subjected to the same triple assessment as breast lumps.

FOLLOW-UP AFTER ASSESSMENT AND/OR BENIGN BREAST BIOPSY

A clearly defined follow-up policy is particularly important in busy breast clinics because routine follow-up of patients presenting with breast lumps can quickly swamp clinic facilities and interfere with the efficient care of new referrals. The following principles guide our own practice:

- Young girls under the age of 25 should be discharged after assessment.
- Biopsy by FNAC or core should be done in older women at the first attendance and the patient discharged if the results are unequivocally benign, unless there are strong indications of increased cancer risk.
- Patients aged 25–50 with significant cancer risk indicators as set out in Chapter 18, currently have annual checks and at least biennial mammography in some clinics, although there is at present no clear evidence that this is beneficial.
- Patients over the age of 50 should be encouraged to attend the regular population breast screening programme.
- Most patients should be discharged at the first clinic visit, but the possibility of a sampling error with a vague mass is best managed by reassessment after 2 months.

The vexed question of whether it is safe to leave *in situ* a lump after negative triple biopsy was discussed in open forum at the 1993 Nottingham International Breast Meeting.[7] The consensus view was that such a lump could be left *in situ* after negative triple assessment and that this policy could apply to all ages, although preferably after two negative cytology examinations. This approach was considered to be sound from a medico-legal point of view provided the patient was happy with such a course, and had been instructed to return if the mass changed.

Since the time of that conference, the trend has been towards guided core needle biopsy if the diagnosis is equivocal, rather than repeated FNAC.

MANAGEMENT OF RECURRENT LUMPS FOLLOWING BIOPSY

Many breast lumps, such as fibroadenoma, cysts and nodularity, are prone to be multiple over a period of time. However, a new lump may be cancer so any new lump must be reassessed in the same way as the original lump.

A different situation arises when a lump appears in the region of a previous biopsy. It must also be reassessed completely but a number of additional factors need consideration.

Recurrent fibroadenoma may represent inadequate removal of the stalk or involvement of adjacent lobules. Excision biopsy of the recurrent lump rather than enucleation is indicated. Phyllodes tumours are also known to recur locally and the original sections should be checked to be certain that fibroadenoma remains the correct diagnosis.

Recurrent cyst is common and requires no treatment other than reaspiration provided the rules governing aspiration are adhered to (Chapter 9).

The breast parenchyma may fail to heal following a biopsy, leaving a palpable dip with prominent edge in the breast tissue. The prominent edge is frequently mistaken for a new mass.

A recurrent lump following biopsy of nodularity of ANDI may be due to:
- the edge of the biopsy wound,
- scarring,
- pathology that was missed at the original biopsy,
- suture granuloma,
- progression of the original lesion, or
- a new lesion.

Such a lump must be carefully reassessed with a view to avoiding biopsy if (1) or (2) can be confirmed; (3) should always be considered if the interval is short and the operator relatively inexperienced; (4) is particularly important where the initial biopsy showed high-grade epithelial dysplasia or carcinoma-in-situ, because progression is common in these conditions. Cytological diagnosis is often difficult in the case of suture granuloma, particularly if recurrent cancer is a possibility.[8]

BREAST MASSES RELATED TO DIFFERENT LIFE PERIODS

Breast masses in adolescence

A number of papers have reported studies of breast tumours in adolescence (Table 4.2).

Stone *et al.*[9] reported 143 masses between the ages of 10 and 20. The incidence increased steadily throughout the decade with a marked predominance from 16 to 20 years: 70% were fibroadenomas, 6% cysts and 12% 'hyperplasias', presumably nodularity of ANDI. Other diagnoses were seen in only one or two cases.

A second study[10] of 74 cases in a paediatric population (to 18 years) gives a similar distribution and includes prepubertal asymmetrical development of the nipple bud. This is much the commonest swelling of the early part of adolescence. Recognition is vital, because ill-advised biopsy will lead to amastia. A further paper on clinico-pathological correlation in the adolescent group is that by Sandison and Walker,[11] in which 12% of referrals and 3% of histological specimens came from this age group. Among 151 histological specimens were 114 fibroadenomas, three duct papillomas, four cysts and four cases of duct ectasia. This is a particularly helpful paper.

Table 4.2 Summary of breast masses found during adolescence (10–20 years)		
	Breast mass	**Frequency of presentation**
Male	Gynaecomastia	Common
Female	Premenarchal development of breast bud Fibroadenoma Cyst Giant fibroadenoma Phyllodes tumour Adenocarcinoma Metastatic tumour	Common Common Rare Rare Rare Very rare Very rare
Nipple and areola	Retention cysts Inversion Molluscum contagiosum Leiomyoma	Uncommon Uncommon Rare Rare
Other conditions	Duct papilloma Subareolar abscess (periductal mastitis) Virginal hypertrophy Nipple discharge from Montgomery's tubercle	Rare Uncommon Uncommon Rare

Concern is often expressed that fibroadenoma in this age group must be removed because of the possibility of cancer. Although the few cases of cancer in adolescence (it is exceedingly rare and none were seen in Sandison and Walker's series) have usually been misdiagnosed as fibroadenoma, review of case reports and the authors' experience shows that fibroadenoma has been diagnosed because of the age group, not because of typical physical signs of fibroadenoma. Thus, masses with rapid growth, recent nipple retraction, surrounding tissue and lymph node involvement have been diagnosed as fibroadenoma. The risk of cancer can, for practical purposes, be ignored in an adolescent with a lump showing the typical features of the common fibroadenoma. The commonest metastaic tumour in this age group is rhabdomyosarcoma.

Lumps in the male breast in adolescence are less common. One series[9] reported cases over a 15-year period. All were due to gynaecomastia. Unlike girls, there is a marked peak incidence at the age of 13 or 14. Gynaecomastia is much more common than this series would suggest but, like this series, we have seen no other cause for breast mass in an adolescent male (see Chapter 16). Inflammatory masses in human immunodeficiency virus (HIV)-positive males are being reported with increasing frequency, and will undoubtedly appear sooner or later in adolescents.

Breast problems associated with pregnancy and lactation

The enlarging breast of pregnancy typically obscures any underlying pathology, while the softness and dependency of the postlactational breast may reveal pre-existing pathology; hamartoma is a typical example. The conditions that appear in association with pregnancy are listed in Table 4.3.

Fibroadenoma may increase in size quite markedly in early pregnancy, but this is not normally associated with increased malignancy. Pregnancy may precipitate some cases of the very rare condition of gigantomastia due to multiple fibroadenoma (Chapter 7).

Operations on the breast during this period may cause problems; damage to the ducts in late pregnancy or the puerperium may give milk fistula, while pregnancy occurring within a year of total duct excision may cause marked breast engorgement.

Breast lumps in older women

The incidence and nature of benign breast lumps in older women (more than 55 years) differ from those of the reproductive period. In a comprehensive study, Devitt[12] reviewed 581 women in this age group presenting with benign breast disorders. The commonest presentation was with non-specific nodularity, 25% associated with pain. Eight per cent had simple cysts, most under the age of 60, and there was a significant relationship to postmenopausal hormone therapy. Eight patients had fibroadenomas, four of which were calcified. Thus a similar range of benign breast lumps is seen in the older women, but characterized by a much lower incidence and a much lower frequency compared to cancer than that seen during reproductive life.

Prolonged use of hormone replacement therapy results in an increased incidence of benign masses more usually associated with the second half of reproductive life, especially cysts and fibroadenoma, so that the pattern of postmenopausal benign breast disorders is changing.

PART 2:
TRIPLE ASSESSMENT AND ORGANIZATION OF THE BREAST CLINIC

In the past, clinical assessment was not only the mainstay of diagnosis of breast lumps, but usually the only assessment prior to surgical excision or mastectomy. Many investigations have been introduced over recent years, and the three modalities of imaging, clinical assessment and pathological examination, known as triple assessment, have now become standard practice.

Since clinical examination alone is relatively inaccurate for diagnosing cancerous masses and has limited reproducibility (only 73% accuracy in one series of malignant lumps examined by four surgeons[13]) it becomes mandatory to image and sample pathologically any suspicious palpable area in the breast. In women below 35 years the imaging should be by ultrasound, with a combination of mammography and ultrasound in older women.

Ultrasound is now a major technique when used as part of triple assessment for the examination of solid lumps and as a guide for accurate cytological sampling of small solid lesions. Modern specialist breast units should base their diagnostic practices on standard triple assessment and the most accurate results are obtained when the information provided by each individual test is put together to ensure

Table 4.3 Breast problems during pregnancy and lactation	
	Frequency of presentation
Mass	
Enlargement of axillary breast	Uncommon
Enlarging fibroadenoma	Rare
Gigantomastia	Rare
Mastitis/abscess	Common
Galactocele	Uncommon
Other conditions	
Blood-stained nipple discharge	Uncommon

consistency between tests. A recent review has shown a 99% predictive value for the diagnosis of benign breast changes if all three components of the triple assessment are found to be benign.[14]

FINE NEEDLE ASPIRATION CYTOLOGY (FNAC)

In the past, the classic teaching for clinical diagnosis of a lump was to follow the sequence: inspect, palpate, percuss, auscultate. Today the sequence should be: inspect and palpate, image, insert a needle. This sequence forms the classical technique of triple assessment which is now mandatory for the diagnosis of all palpable breast abnormalities.[15]

It is sound policy to insert a needle into every breast lump or suspicious area for three purposes: to assess the consistency of the mass, to aspirate fluid if it proves to be a cyst, and to provide a cytological specimen if the lesion proves to be solid and blood-stained fluid is obtained. The rubbery feel to the needle point of a fibroadenoma or involutional nodularity is as characteristic as the softness and absence of resistance with fat, and the grittiness of cancer. Equally characteristic is the sudden sensation experienced when the needle tip traverses the fibrous wall to enter a cyst.

Technique is important in taking a specimen for cytological study (Chapter 20) and equipment to provide an optimal specimen should always be available. Indeed, the measure of the quality of a surgeon's skill in FNAC is the number of inadequate diagnostic smears produced from aspirating solid masses. The proportion of inadequate smears can be automatically printed off for each surgeon from the modern breast clinic databases such as the British Association of Surgical Oncology Breast database. A specimen is sent for cytological examination from any breast mass with one exception. A cytological examination of cyst fluid is unnecessary unless the fluid is blood stained or a residual mass is palpated.

FNAC results are increasingly reported on a consistent grading scale from 1 to 5 as shown in Table 4.4.

Similar grading systems can be applied to imaging and clinical examination results which then allow a shorthand description of triple assessment (see Chapter 6). For example, a young woman with a fibroadenoma which is classically palpable as a breast mouse, and with a typical ultrasound image and typical benign cytology, would be graded P2 U2 C2. A frank carcinoma could be P5 M5 C5.

The use of this shorthand coding allows immediate identification at a multidisciplinary group meeting and can indicate discordant results between the different modalities, thus giving a higher rate of overall diagnostic accuracy after further or repeated investigations for suspicious results. It is a not infrequent experience that the multidisciplinary discussion allows a small and difficult cancer to be diagnosed by highlighting one of the modalities in a way which might be missed in a routine paper report sent to the clinician from the laboratory.

FNAC has an accuracy of around 99% when carried out by experienced aspirators and read by an expert cytopathologist.[16] In one series of 1104 cases with a false-positive rate of 0.4%, the benign conditions which led to a false-positive diagnosis were postradiation changes, granulomatous mastitis and fibroadenoma.[17] Skilled cytology can contribute to a positive diagnosis of benign conditions, and not just exclude cancer. In an excellent article reviewing the cytological features of 265 benign masses, Maygarden and colleagues discuss those features which are helpful in cytological diagnosis of benign conditions, and those benign conditions which can be diagnosed by cytology.[18]

The technique has a lower accuracy in benign lesions but this is mainly due to the higher rate of acellular smears produced on aspiration of benign lesions. Specimens from masses arising during pregnancy and lactation require

Table 4.4 Results of fine needle aspiration cytology (FNAC)		
C1	Inadequate	A cellular or sparsely cellular or poorly preserved smear
C2	Benign	Adequately cellular with unequivocal benign epithelial cells
C3	Probably benign	Adequately cellular with mainly benign cells present but some mild atypia present
C4	Suspicious/probably malignant	Some features of malignancy in a low cellularity sample or highly cellular with some atypical cells present
C5	Malignant	Frankly malignant cells present Cells showing lack of cohesion with large nuclear to cytoplasmic ratios and nuclear variability Severe nuclear pleomorphism

assessment that takes into account the specific cellular changes in the breast at this time.[19]

Limitations and complications of FNAC

Fine needle aspiration is generally considered to be an innocuous procedure, in spite of occasional local complications such as pneumothorax (see Chapter 20). However, it may also cause local tissue trauma which may interfere with definitive histology of a small lesion. Lee and colleagues[20] studied 184 definitive specimens with a history of preceding fine needle aspiration and were able to find definitely attributable changes in 17 (9.3%). Changes included near-total destruction of the lesion from haemorrhage or infarction, and one of benign papilloma cells implanted in surrounding fibrogranulation tissue causing diagnostic problems.

Mammography should be avoided within the week following fine needle aspiration. In a study of 52 women, repeat mammography was performed within 5 days of FNAC; in three cases significant differences were seen (probably due to haematoma) although the diagnosis was not changed in any case.[21] However, when a mass has been assessed by sonography and FNAC, mammography is normally being used to assess the rest of the breast, rather than the mass in question. If this is the case, it can proceed provided the radiologist is informed.

The presence of an augmentation prosthesis should be excluded in every case, so that ultrasound-guided fine needle aspiration can be performed.[22]

ULTRASOUND IN TRIPLE ASSESSMENT

Ultrasound has several uses in the triple assessment setting. The main uses are to clarify the presence or not of a discrete abnormality within a vague palpable area or an asymmetric density on mammograms. It is of little value as a routine screen of the whole of a breast without any palpable abnormality. It is also useful for differentiating deep cysts from nodularity and allows accurate aspiration of those cysts.

It is excellent as an accurate guide to cytological sampling of a small mobile lesion or a vaguely palpable lesion, as the needle can be moved around the lesion to sample it under direct vision. Similarly, ultrasound can be used to direct a core needle biopsy to ensure that small lesions are properly and accurately sampled.

Ideally, ultrasound is performed in the clinic by a radiological member of the team with a special interest in breast disease. This is not always practicable, and it is possible for an interested surgeon to do much of the diagnostic work achievable with ultrasound. This subject has been dealt with recently by Staren and Fine.[23,24]

New techniques, such as colour Doppler ultrasonography, have been used to differentiate benign from malignant masses.[25] At present these techniques are not particularly discriminating, but the effectiveness of the equipment is improving rapidly.

Two-dimensional ultrasound may be manipulated to give three-dimensional images, with increased information about the nature of a mass, and the characteristics of particular pathological conditions.[26] With this technique, still in an investigative phase, a mass can be considered benign if its rim is continuous in all planes.

WIDE BORE NEEDLE BIOPSY

More recently the use of wide bore needle biopsy (WBN) has increased dramatically (see Chapter 20). This technique has two major advantages over FNAC. First, it supplies a histological section and so the reading only requires histology skills. These are more readily available than skilled cytopathological reading. Secondly, since histology is evaluated the technique can often differentiate between *in situ* and invasive breast cancer, unlike FNAC.

The original wide bore needles, such as the 'Tru Cut®', were actuated manually and rather cumbersome as both hands were required to work the needle. The early needles often produced poor cores from benign breast lesions and were painful for patients. However, the introduction of spring-loaded 'guns' with rapid firing of needles produced much better cores and as the needles cut quickly they are less painful. Several manufacturers now produce this type of needle. Using a gun, a 14-gauge needle will cut through even the toughest breast tissue and has the added bonus that it is easily visible on ultrasound. McMahon and colleagues found such a gun to give a higher success rate with less pain than the older types of needles.[27]

ORGANIZATION OF CLINICS

In order to deliver high-quality triple diagnosis all the three elements of clinical examination, imaging and cytology have to be present. Traditionally these have been performed by the surgeon or gynaecologist although it is unusual to find all three skills in one individual. Thus it is common for the symptomatic patient to be referred first to the surgeon who then arranges (or performs) the other investigations. In the past the three elements were often separated in time but this practice has increasingly come under criticism by patients and the lay media.

As a result of several high-profile media features in the early 1990s which demonstrated wide variations in the efficacy and speed of breast diagnosis, several groups of breast specialists set up working parties to define good practice in breast clinics. In 1994 a working party of the British Breast Group published a document calling for the establishment of multidisciplinary breast specialist units with a core staff of a surgeon, radiologist, pathologist, oncologist and breast care nurse and with a specified caseload of breast referrals, giving a minimum of 50 new breast cancers annually.[28]

This report was followed by a major report published in 1995 by the Breast Surgeons Group of the British Association of Surgical Oncologists (BASO), which laid down guidelines for the management of symptomatic referrals to breast specialists.[29] This report defined both the core multidisciplinary team and the facilities that should be available for rapid and accurate diagnosis of breast lumps (Tables 4.5 and 4.6).

Both reports endorsed the widespread use of triple assessment with mandatory case conferences on a regular basis to discuss the final diagnosis prior to therapeutic surgery. The proposed advantages of this close cooperation would be a high rate of preoperative diagnosis of breast cancer and a concomitant fall in the number of open surgical biopsies.

The cost effectiveness and accuracy of triple assessment have been confirmed in two recent US studies.[30,31] Equivalent UK calculations suggest cost savings of £240 (day case) or £470 (inpatient) per diagnosis. These reports were well received by breast specialists in the UK who were already moving towards similar clinic arrangements.

These arrangements have recently been endorsed by the National Health Service Executive in the UK in a report of good practice published in 1996[32] with central funding support. Similar media and patient pressures have occurred in the USA where additional funding is also being provided.

The aims, problems and outcome of a specialized breast clinic have been reported in a study by Barclay et al.[33]

Table 4.5 Composition of a breast unit recommended by the BASO Guidelines.[29] Each member should have a special interest in breast disease

Surgeon
Radiologist
Pathologist
Clinical oncologist
Medical oncologist
Nurse specialist

Table 4.6 Breast clinic diagnostic services recommended by the BASO Guidelines[29]

1. The breast clinic should diagnose >50 cancers per year
2. Diagnosis should be based on triple assessment
3. Mandatory multidisciplinary review sessions should be carried out
4. The majority of patients without cancer should receive all diagnostic tests at first visit
5. Patients without cancer should be given a diagnosis at first visit
6. Patients with newly diagnosed cancer will usually be given the diagnosis at a second visit
7. A breast care nurse should be present with the surgeon when this occurs, and the patient should be encouraged to bring a partner or friend when the results are being discussed
8. Patients should not receive abnormal results by telephone or letter

---

REFERENCES

1. Cox PJ, Li MKW & Ellis H. Spectrum of breast disease in outpatient surgical practise. *Journal of the Royal Society of Medicine* 1982; **75**: 857–859.
2. Dixon JM, Clarke PJ, Crucioli V *et al*. Reduction of the surgical excision rate in benign breast disease using fine needle aspiration cytology with immediate reporting. *British Journal of Surgery* 1987; **74**: 1014–1016.
3. Preece PE, Baum M, Mansel RE *et al*. Importance of mastalgia in operable breast cancer. *British Medical Journal* 1982; **284**: 1299–1300.
4. Haagensen CD. *Diseases of the Breast*. Philadelphia: WB Saunders, 1986, p 252.
5. Foote FW & Stewart FW. Comparative studies of cancerous versus non-cancerous breasts. *Annals of Surgery* 1945; **121**: 6–53.
6. Moreira De AJ, Cosiski MHR, Filho JM *et al*. Differential diagnosis of axillary masses. *Tumori* 1996; **82**: 596–599.
7. Sainsbury JRC. Item presented at the Nottingham International Breast Meeting. *The Breast* 1994; **3**: 190.
8. Maygarden SJ, Novotny DB, Johnson DE *et al*. Fine needle aspiration cytology of suture granulomas of the breast. *Diagnostic Cytopathology* 1994; **10**: 175–179.
9. Stone AM, Shenker RI & McCarthy K. Adolescent breast masses. *American Journal of Surgery* 1977; **134**: 275–277.
10. West KW, Rescorla FJ, Scherer LR & Grosfield JC. Diagnosis and treatment of symptomatic breast masses in the paediatric population. *Journal of Paediatric Surgery* 1995; **30**: 182–187.
11. Sandison AT & Walker JC. Diseases of the adolescent female breast. A clinico-pathological study. *British Journal of Surgery* 1968; **55**: 443–448.
12. Devitt JE. Benign disorders of the breast in older women. *Surgery, Gynecology and Obstetrics* 1986; **162**: 340–342.
13. Boyd NF, Sutherland HJ, Fish EB *et al*. Prospective evaluation of physical examination of the breast. *American Journal of Surgery* 1981; **142**: 331.
14. Layfield LJ, Glasgow BJ & Cramer H. Fine needle aspiration in the management of breast masses. *Pathology Annual* 1989; **24**: 23.
15. Dixon JM, Anderson TJ, Lamb J *et al*. Fine needle aspiration in cytology in relationship to clinical examination and mammography in the diagnosis of a solid breast mass. *British Journal of Surgery* 1984; **71**: 593–596.
16. Barrows GM, Anderson TJ, Lamb J & Dixon JM. Fine needle aspiration of breast cancer: relationship of clinical factors to cytology results in 689 primary malignancies. *Cancer* 1986; **58**: 1493–1498.
17. Jatoi I & Trott PA False positive reporting in breast fine-needle aspiration cytology: Incidence and causes. *Breast* 1996; **5**: 270–273.
18. Maygarden SJ, Novotny DB, Johnson DE & Frabie WJ.

Subclassification of benign breast disease by fine needle aspiration cytology. *Acta Cytologica* 1994; **38**: 115–129.

19. Finley JL, Silverman JF & Lannin DR. Fine needle aspiration cytology of breast masses in pregnant and lactating women. *Diagnostic Cytopathology* 1989; **5**: 255–259.

20. Lee KC, Chan JKC & Ho LC. Histologic changes in the breast after fine needle aspiration. *American Journal of Surgical Pathology* 1994; **18**: 1039–1047.

21. Horobin JM, Matthews BM, Preece PE & Thompson AJ. Effect of fine needle aspiration on subsequent mammograms. *British Journal of Surgery* 1992; **79**: 52–54.

22. Fornage BD, Sneige N & Singletary SE. Masses in breasts with implants: Diagnosis with U-S guided fine needle aspiration biopsy. *Radiology* 1994; **191**: 339–342.

23. Staren ED. Physics and principles of breast ultrasound. *American Surgeon* 1996; **62**: 103–107.

24. Staren ED & Fine R. Breast ultrasound for surgeons. *American Surgeon* 1996; **62**: 108–112.

25. Holcombe C, Pugh N, Lyons K et al. Blood flow in breast cancer and fibroadenoma estimated by colour flow ultrasonography. *British Journal of Surgery* 1995; **82**: 787–788.

26. Rotten D, Levaillant JM, Constancis E et al. 3-Dimensional imaging of solid breast tumors with ultrasound-preliminary data. *Ultrasound in Obstetrics and Gynecology* 1991; **1**: 384–390.

27. McMahon AJ, Lutfy AM, Matthew A et al. Needle core biopsy of the breast with a spring-loaded device. *British Journal of Surgery* 1992; **79**: 1042.

28. British Breast Group. Working Report. *Breast* 1994 Supplement.

29. BASO Guidelines for surgeons in the management of symptomatic breast disease in the United Kingdom. *European Journal of Surgical Oncology* 1995; **21**: S1–S13.

30. Schmidt WA, Wachtel MS, Jones MK et al. The triple test: a cost effective diagnostic tool. *Laboratory Medicine* 1994; **25**: 715–719.

31. Vetto J, Pommier R, Schmidt W et al. Use of the triple test for palpable breast lesions yields high diagnostic accuracy and cost savings. *American Journal of Surgery* 1995; **169**: 519–522.

32. NHS Management Executive. *Improving Outcomes in Breast Cancer*. EL (96)15, July. London: Department of Health, 1996.

33. Barclay M, Carter D, Horobin JM et al. Patterns of presentation of breast disease over 10 years in a specialised clinic. *Health Bulletin* 1991; **49**: 229–236.

Chapter 5

The relationship between clinician and pathologist in benign breast disorders

KEY POINTS AND NEW DEVELOPMENTS

1. Great progress has been made in providing accurate definitions of individual pathological entities in the breast – allowing more precise assessment of clinical significance.
2. The older problems of communication between clinician, radiologist and pathologist have been resolved by the development of multidisciplinary teams.
3. This chapter attempts to bridge the terminology gap for clinicians unable to confer directly with their pathology colleagues, written from a clinician's point of view.
4. Individual lesions are discussed on the basis of the anatomical element of the breast from which they arise, to enhance the links between clinical presentations and histological descriptions, and to place them within the overall spectrum of breast disorders.
5. More detailed pathology is given in the chapters dealing with each condition.

The first aim of this chapter is to provide an overview of the many benign conditions discussed in this book, to help find the place each occupies in the overall spectrum of pathology of the breast. In an ideal situation, breast clinicians will have weekly interactive multidisciplinary case discussions with a pathologist and a radiologist. This facility is not available to all, and those isolated from direct contact with pathologists may find difficulty in assessing the clinical implications of a histopathology report. Often this arises from the changes in concepts and terminology that have made such major advances in breast disease in the last 30 years.

The second aim of this chapter is to provide a brief general insight, from the perspective of the clinician, into those major changes which affect understanding of benign breast conditions. No attempt is made to provide a comprehensive account of breast pathology, which is better obtained from detailed pathology textbooks; the subject is much too large to be covered in a clinically orientated book such as this.

A number of excellent textbooks are available to the reader who wishes to pursue the subject in greater depth than that provided in standard textbooks of pathology. Haagensen's *Diseases of the Breast*[1] is a classic, and provides clear descriptions of the pathology of most breast disorders based on the author's long experience as a surgeon-pathologist. *Problems in Breast Pathology* by Azzopardi[2] gives clear expositions of many of the diagnostic problems experienced by the pathologist, in language accessible to clinicians. Another useful book is Page and Anderson's *Diagnostic Histopathology of the Breast*,[3] while the recently published volume, *The Breast*, in the third edition of *Symmer's Systematic Pathology* gives welcome prominence to benign disorders.[4] Extensive histological illustrations would not be appropriate in this clinically orientated chapter, but one excellent source for such material is the monograph by Trojani.[5]

DEVELOPMENTS OF THE PAST 30 YEARS

The problems arising from the blanket use of the term 'fibrocystic disease' and its synonyms to describe pathology often found in breast biopsies has been described in detail in Chapters 1 and 3. This usage was an easy way to provide mild justification to a surgeon who performed a biopsy for nodularity, but it had two major defects. First, it did not recognize the fact that all these processes are a spectrum, with no clear differentiation between normal and abnormal. Oberman and French wrote in 1961 'adenofibroma, fibrocystic disease and intraductal papilloma do not appear to represent distinct entities, but rather form a spectrum of conditions having their basis in an abnormality between hormonal stimulus to the breast, principally estrogen, and stromal and epithelial response'.[6] In view of this it is unfortunate that this term is still used as a diagnosis, suggesting both a specific condition and an abnormality.

Secondly, since the main concern of clinician and patient alike was cancer risk, it was inevitable that an attempt would be made to relate such a risk to fibrocystic disease. Hence it is desirable that this term be dispensed with completely, and replaced with one that is accurate and consonant with pathogenesis.

This can be achieved if the general multifaceted manifestations of benign breast disorders are called 'changes of ANDI', and the individual elements, those with more clearly defined significance, are given their individual histological descriptive names when sufficiently overt to warrant mention. Thus a typical report could be: 'Sections show mild (or moderate or severe) changes of ANDI, with microglandular adenosis and small foci of sclerosing adenosis (or microcyst formation; or ductal epithelial hyperplasia without atypia; or any other changes worthy of specific mention).'

The major advances of the past 30 years lie in these two areas. The blanket histological diagnosis has been replaced by detailed descriptions of the individual histological patterns found, so the pathology report should cover only what is actually seen. Then attempts have been made to lay down specific criteria for making a diagnosis, with further criteria for assessing progression from normal to abnormal to disease. These moves towards objective criteria have facilitated quantitative estimates of cancer risks for each pattern. Thus pathology reports now describe as many changes as warrant comment, and the clinical significance is the summation of the significance of each element.

GENERAL CLASSIFICATION OF BENIGN BREAST CONDITIONS

Benign breast disorders can be classified in a number of ways, the most basic being shown in Table 5.1.

The lesions in groups 2, 3 and 4 are outside the scope of this chapter, but call for clear communication between clinician and pathologist, whose histological interpretation may depend on accurate information about diseases outside the breast.

Most breast disorders arise from the glandular tissue, which includes ducts, lobules and associated periductal and perilobular stromal tissue. Few conditions arise solely from the general fibrous tissue of the breast.

BENIGN DISORDERS OF DUCTOGLANDULAR TISSUE

The important benign conditions arising from ductoglandular tissue are presented in Table 5.2.

Individual conditions tend to be related to different areas of the glandular tree and, in general, benign pathological processes in the breast fall into two main groups. Those on a macroscopic scale tend to occur in the larger ducts (especially the terminal 2–3 cm close to the nipple) and also tend to have a segmental distribution based on the glandular distribution of a single collecting duct. These include duct ectasia and macroscopic papillomas. The second group arise on a microscopic scale from the region of the terminal ductal lobular unit (TDLU), the area of most active epithelial proliferation, and also the area where the epithelium and specialized stroma of the lobule are in constant interaction with the hormonally controlled activity of the breast.

It is not surprising that there should be a tendency to different pathology affecting the two regions, for they are both anatomically and functionally distinct. The major ducts extending to the last branching act as collector and expulsor of milk; they contain elastic in their walls, and their lining epithelium is non-secretory. The smallest ducts, consisting of extralobular and intralobular portions, behave more as the acini. They have no elastic in their walls, and their lining cells take on a secretory function during lactation,[3] justifying the composite term TDLU.

Factors such as these are helpful in differentiating the two groups of lesions. For instance the presence of elastic tissue helps to differentiate duct ectasia from cysts (of lobular origin).[2] The lactiferous sinus tends to be involved by the same conditions as are found in the major ducts.

Anatomical factors are also used to assess histological patterns. The fact that the breast ductal system has a two-layer epithelial lining, consisting of continuous luminal epithelial cells and a discontinuous myoepithelial cell layer within an intact basement membrane, is helpful in differentiating benign conditions from malignant. No matter how distorted the pattern, this basic two-layer structure can usually be demonstrated, sometimes with the help of chemical or immunochemical stains.

Certain conditions show a segmental distribution. The best example of this is seen in duct ectasia.[2] While this affects the terminal (subareolar) 2–3 cm first, in more severe cases it extends peripherally to involve subsegmental and even terminal ducts. One or more segments show duct dilatation, but it is rare for more than three or four segmental ducts to be involved. Why only three or four of the 10–15 duct systems in the breast are involved (often bilaterally) is one of the enigmas of breast pathology. Benign duct papilloma is another condition with a segmental distribution. This involves the larger, juxta-nipple portion of the duct. It is quite common to have two or three 'solitary' papillomas in the main duct, and in older patients the process may extend centripetally to involve much of the ductal system of a single segment (see Figure 12.6).

Severe ductal hyperplasias also tend to show a segmental distribution, at least in the early stages, while lobular hyperplasias tend to be more diffuse.

Table 5.1 Benign disorders of the breast

1. Disorders arising from the tissues of the breast
    i)   ductoglandular
    ii) supporting stroma
    These can be further divided into
    a) disorders arising from abnormalities of the normal physiological processes of the breast, such as hormonal influences, cell turnover, etc. (ANDI)
    b) disorders due to well-defined extraneous influences, such as lactational abscess, fat necrosis
2. Disorders of adjacent structures
    e.g. skin, underlying muscle
3. Systemic disorders involving breast tissues
    e.g. diabetes, vasculitis
4. Distant disorders metastasizing to the breast
    e.g. metastatic tumours, typhoid abscess

Table 5.2 Benign disorders of ductoglandular tissue related to different areas of the glandular tree

Nipple ducts	Large ducts	Smaller ducts	TDLU
Nipple adenoma Nipple papilloma Duct fistula	Duct papilloma Duct ectasia Duct adenoma	Tend to be involved by processes arising in and extending from adjacent large ducts or TDLU, e.g. duct ectasia/sclerosis, duct papillomas, duct hyperplasias	Adenosis Ductal epithelial hyperplasia Lobular epithelial hyperplasia Peripheral papillomas Fibroadenoma Phyllodes tumour Cysts Sclerosing lesions Fibrosis ?Granulomatous mastitis

Lesions involving the nipple ducts
Nipple adenoma

This lesion, with typical clinical presentation and appearance described in Chapter 14, is less clear-cut histologically. It may show a variety of histological appearances, including papillomatous, benign hyperplasia and adenotic patterns. Its origin is not clear, but appears to arise in the milk sinus region. A clear histological diagnosis implies a benign lesion. It infiltrates the nipple in a non-malignant fashion.

A duct papilloma, sometimes prolapsing through the nipple duct orifice, can also occur in this region.

The rather heterogeneous group of lesions carrying the word 'adenoma', discussed in various parts of this chapter, are listed in Table 5.3.

Mammary duct fistula

One variant of this condition, discussed in Chapter 11, is associated with abnormally extensive squamous epithelial lining of the terminal portion of the duct in a young woman, often associated with congenital inversion of the nipple, and unrelated to general duct ectasia.

Lesions involving major ducts

Solitary (discrete) duct papilloma

This condition is described under papillary lesions later in this chapter, and in Chapter 12.

Duct ectasia

The pathology of this is described more fully in Chapter 11. The dilated ducts are usually most prominent in the subareolar region, but may extend in severe cases to involve the smaller and even the terminal ducts. Periductal sclerosis may be seen as much as dilatation, and surrounding inflammation is a prominent feature. It carries no malignant potential.

Ductal adenoma

This lesion was described by Azzopardi and Salm[7] and is important because it is a benign lesion, but with a complex histology which may simulate cancer to those unfamiliar with it. It presents as a 1–3-cm mass (without nipple discharge) in women of all ages. It appears to arise from

medium- and small-sized ducts (but short of the TDLU), which may become markedly dilated (although one group found it more commonly close to the nipple[4]).

The histological pattern varies; usually tubular structures lined by a benign double epithelial cell layer can be seen, often with much fibrosis and even calcification. Some authorities consider that some, and perhaps all, of them arise from sclerosis of an intraductal papilloma, associated with infarction. They do not carry an increased cancer risk.

Lesions involving the smaller subsegmental and interlobar ducts

These ducts tend not to have specific pathological processes, but may be affected by extension of adjacent pathology. For example, ductal hyperplasia may extend into them from the TDLU region, and duct ectasia and discrete duct papillomas may extend from their usual situation in the larger ducts.

Lesions involving the TDLU
Cysts

The pathology of cysts is covered in Chapter 9. For the purposes of histological definition of cancer risk, they are classified as microcysts if less than 3 mm in diameter, and macrocysts if greater.

Fibroadenoma and phyllodes tumour

The pathology of these conditions is covered in more detail in Chapter 7. Of interest is the fact that fibroadenoma involves the whole TDLU, both epithelial and stromal elements, maintaining a normal relationship between the two. This, together with the gradation seen from normal lobule to clinical fibroadenoma, supports the view that it is best regarded as an aberration of normal development than a benign tumour (Chapter 3). The application of molecular biology to breast disease is still at an early stage, but it appears that fibroadenomas are polyclonal, consistent with a simple hyperplasia. In contrast, the stromal element of phyllodes tumour is monoclonal, consistent with a neoplasm.

Tubular adenoma and lactating adenoma

These are two variants on fibroadenoma. The first is seen in young women as a well-defined, mobile mass similar to fibroadenoma. Macroscopically it resembles a yellowish fibroadenoma, and histologically it consists of small tubules of benign structure and little stroma. It is sometimes seen in association with a fibroadenoma, suggesting that the two conditions may be related. Its significance is the same.

A lactating adenoma is a similar mass occurring during pregnancy or lactation. Some people consider it to represent no more than a fibroadenoma presenting with lactational features, others that it represents a different lesion, perhaps with similar origins. Lactating adenomas carry no serious significance.

Table 5.3 Conditions carrying the term 'adenoma'
Nipple adenoma
Ductal adenoma
Tubular adenoma
Lactating adenoma
Myxoid adenoma

Carney's syndrome

This peculiar myxoid adenoma is part of an inherited disorder discussed in Chapter 17.

Hamartoma

This lesion has similarities to and differences from fibroadenoma. It is similar in presentation as a firm mass, but it differs in the multiplicity of tissues seen and the lack of a capsule, as well as its probable origin from an embryological rest. Variations in the dominant tissues have been given different names, such as adenolipoma or muscular hamartoma, but without differing significance. The lesion is discussed in Chapter 17.

Hyperplasias

Hyperplasias have given rise to more confusion than any other aspect of benign breast disorders. This has resulted largely from confusion of definition and terminology, compounded by a natural tendency for clinicians to relate terms such as 'hyperplasia' or 'dysplasia' to cancer. Recent histopathological studies, particularly those of Wellings and Page and their co-workers, discussed in Chapters 3 and 18, have led to a much clearer understanding of significance and a better definition of patterns, although this clarity does not always extend to terminology!

The term 'hyperplasia' implies a benign condition, it does not signify cancer or cancer risk. Hyperplasias with atypia tend to be associated with a small or moderate increase in cancer risk. The term 'cancer *in situ*' is used for those patterns which imply a high risk of malignancy.

AN OUTLINE OF TERMINOLOGY AND GROUPINGS OF HYPERPLASTIC LESIONS OF THE BREAST

The terms organoid and non-organoid are often used by pathologists in describing patterns. Organoid hyperplasias are those in which different elements combine to form an organized structure, such as a lobule in adenosis. Thus, in organoid hyperplasias, existing lobules hypertrophy or new ducts and/or lobules are formed. The structure will show the normal lumen of the lobular acinus lined by its two-layer epithelium and surrounded by a loose lobular stromal tissue.

In the non-organoid form, previously called epitheliosis or papillomatosis but now called epithelial hyperplasia, the hyperplasia is of a single tissue, forming masses or sheets of cells without forming a new fully developed structure. Both organoid and non-organoid may be present in combination, for example when hyperplasia invades (or develops within) the lobular structure of adenosis.

Adenosis (organoid hyperplasia)

The concept of adenosis as an organoid hyperplasia, signifying increase in the number or size of glandular elements, should be one readily accessible to all. In fact, adenosis is a nightmare to the clinician trying to understand breast pathology, for many reasons. A very wide variety of patterns are described as adenosis, including a non-organoid form. This apparent contradiction of terms usually raises no queries! Some authorities settle for a minimum of types and terms, others use a very detailed classification; some dismiss commonly used terms as unhelpful. The varying conditions discussed in this chapter to which the term 'adenosis' is applied are listed in Table 5.4 and considered in appropriate parts of the chapter.

The following is a simplification which attempts to provide some meaningful concepts for the various terms used, and the conditions to which those terms are attached. Written as a clinical contribution, it makes no claim to pathological precision or veracity.

The unqualified term 'adenosis' could be taken to mean simply an increase in the number or size of TDLU structures. This is not easy to define as the size and number of lobules in the normal breast vary widely (a normal lobule may have from 10 to 100 acini according to Bonser *et al.*[8]), and the number varies greatly with age. Nevertheless, changes are seen where the pattern is clearly outside that commonly found.

Blunt duct adenosis (simple adenosis)

This has been the commonest term used for adenosis in general since Foote and Stewart introduced the term in 1945.[9] Azzopardi uses it as a convenient term to describe 'all the pathological hyperplasias and hypertrophic processes affecting the parenchyma of the breast which give rise to two-layered epithelial structures…with blunt endings…and associated with…stroma akin to the specialised stroma of lobular and periductal tissue'. In general, this means a lobular structure in which the elements, two-layered epithelium and stroma are hypertrophied and the lumen dilated, without an increase in number of cells or units. There is a spectrum from normal to 'abnormal' in the one breast, and even within different parts of a single lobule. It is not clear whether blunt duct adenosis represents development of new 'abnormal' lobules, or alteration of pre-existing lobules. It is recognized as common in normal breasts with no great significance. For this reason, and because of the lack of clinical correlate or prognostic significance, Page and Anderson[3] dismiss the term, and there is a tendency for it to disappear from recent publications.

Table 5.4 Conditions carrying the term 'adenosis'
Blunt duct adenosis
Sclerosing adenosis
Microglandular adenosis
Apocrine adenosis
'Other types' of adenosis

Sclerosing adenosis

In this form of adenosis, the two-layer epithelial structure persists, but there is marked hypertrophy of the myoepithelial and stromal elements with sclerosis sufficient to distort the lobular architecture and enough to mimic cancer. It varies in extent from a trivial histological finding to a palpable mass. It shows both proliferative and involutional changes, so views about its pathogenesis have been conflicting. Once again it forms part of a spectrum extending from normality[4] and so can be regarded as a process of ANDI. In fact there is some epidemiological evidence that the incidence is increased in women taking the contraceptive pill, and in African women with early and frequent pregnancies, supporting the possibility of a relationship to cyclical hormonal changes, and hence part of ANDI.

Azzopardi maintains, from his own work, that the epithelial outgrowth may occur from small and medium-sized ducts, as well as predominantly from lobules. This outgrowth may be sufficiently vigorous to 'invade' adjacent structures such as nerves. The important feature is that the lesion maintains a 'lobulo-centric' or organoid pattern, in spite of the gross distortion. This basic nodular whorled unit can be seen by the naked eye with a hand lens. The maintenance of this pattern, seen under low-power microscopy, is an important feature for the pathologist in differentiating sclerosing adenosis from cancer.

The lesion itself carries no increased cancer risk, but it may be associated with other changes, such as atypical hyperplasia, which will determine cancer risk. There is some evidence that the lesions may regress spontaneously after the menopause.

Sclerosing adenosis is discussed further in Chapter 10.

Microglandular adenosis

Microglandular adenosis exemplifies the problems of pathological terminology. Although described as adenosis, this lesion is non-organoid, in that the full lobular pattern is not maintained, yet it remains a benign 'adenosis'! It is an uncommon condition where a proliferation of small, acinar structures infiltrate the breast stroma or even adipose tissue. Unlike most benign conditions, in microglandular adenosis the two-layer structure of epithelium is lost and there is a single layer of cells without a myoepithelial layer, and even the presence of a basement layer is controversial.

The lesions are relatively discrete, and occur from chance findings to 2–3 cm in diameter. The diagnostic problem arises from the fact that these isolated incomplete epithelial structures appear in stroma and adipose tissue, without the normal lobule 'periphery', so simulating invasion. Pathologists use benign cytological features and the general pattern to differentiate them from cancer. While generally considered benign, the neoplastic significance remains uncertain at present, some authors finding associated cancer in about a quarter of cases.[10]

Other types of adenosis

Many other variants of adenosis have been described, the names given reflecting minor histological changes that are particularly prominent in each case. They do not have major implications for clinicians, although accurate description is important to pathologists in differentiating benign conditions from malignant. Examples include tubular adenosis, secretory adenosis, adenosis of pregnancy, adenomyoepithelial adenosis, nodular adenosis, mixed and transitional forms of adenosis.

Apocrine adenosis is an area of potential confusion; the term has been used for differing conditions,[4] and recent work has suggested that one type may be associated with aggressive breast cancer.[11]

Ductal and lobular hyperplasias (non-organoid hyperplasias)

In this group of conditions a hyperplasia of the lining epthelium occurs, giving rise to solid or semisolid sheets of a predominantly single cell type which fill small ducts and lobules. Hyperplasia may occur anywhere in the ductal system from within the lobule to the nipple ducts, but it is generally agreed that most significant hyperplasias arise in the smallest ducts of the TDLU from whence they may spread into the small ducts or into the lobule. Significant hyperplasias tend to take one or two forms: ductal or lobular. In British literature, the term 'epitheliosis' has been applied to hyperplasias severe enough to be considered significant, particularly when of the ductal type. In American literature, the term 'papillomatosis' has been used for the same condition. This is confusing because the term is also used to describe a different condition, multiple intraduct papillomas. Recently, the tendency has been to discard both terms; neither is used in the ACP consensus document, which simply uses the term 'hyperplasia'.

Both ductal and lobular hyperplasias arise within the TDLU, the differentiation between the two, and the justification for calling them ductal and lobular respectively, depending on differing histological characteristics and clinical behaviour rather than any demonstrated difference in site of origin or pathogenesis.

Ductal hyperplasia

Ductal hyperplasias are typically divided into three degrees: mild ductal hyperplasia, moderate or florid ductal hyperplasia and atypical ductal hyperplasia (ADH). Although the borderlines between the three are to some extent subjective, good agreement is obtained between different pathologists if specific guidelines are used, and considerable epidemiological data are now available linking the differing degrees to cancer risk.

Mild hyperplasia is typically defined as more than two but less than four cell layers between basement membrane and lumen (without cellular atypia or encroachment on the lumen). Moderate or florid hyperplasia is when the cell layer is of greater thickness, usually enough to distend the ductule, when cells start to bridge the lumen and when some cellular atypia is seen. It is quite commonly found in 'normal' postmenopausal breasts.

ADH relates to the third degree when there is further divergence from normal, but short of the changes justifying the diagnosis of ductal carcinoma-in-situ (DCIS). Pathologists, working particularly from the studies of Page (Chapter 18), have laid down detailed criteria for categorizing the stages, so allowing provision of assessments for clinicians with reasonable reproduceability from one centre to another.

It is generally accepted that mild hyperplasia carries no cancer risk, moderate or florid only a small risk (relative risk (RR) about 1.5). For ADH, the risk increases to fourfold, with an increase to tenfold if there is a marked family history. This is much the same as that for DCIS and is discussed further in Chapter 18.

An interesting difference between ADH and DCIS is that the invasive cancer risk implied for the former applies generally to both breasts, whereas that of DCIS is specific to that breast and usually to the same segment. This carries the implication that DCIS is a much more fundamental step towards invasive malignancy than ADH.

Figures 5.1–5.4 show the low-power general appearance of the range of hyperplasias from simple apocrine metaplasia through hyperplasia without atypia, hyperplasia with atypia and intraduct cancer.

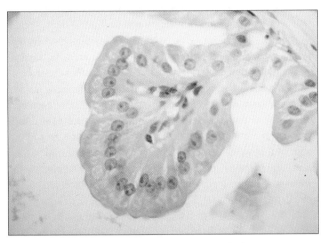

5.1 Apocrine metaplasia within a cyst. This shows the large eosinophilic, cytologically regular apocrine cells projecting as a papillary tuft with a stromal core.

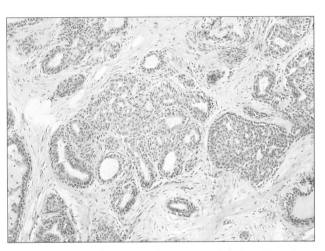

5.2 Hyperplasia (moderate). This demonstrates the filling of ductules with cells which on high power were seen to be cytologically normal. The general architecture of the TDLU can still be seen despite the filling and distension of ducts by cells.

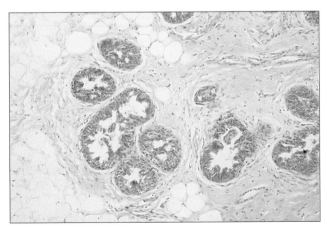

5.3 Atypical ductal hyperplasia. The duct is not plugged with cells but the hyperplasia shows much more darkly staining epithelium, due to increased nuclear size and pleomorphism of the nuclei. The diagnosis of atypical changes was made on the basis of the cytology of the cells studied at high power.

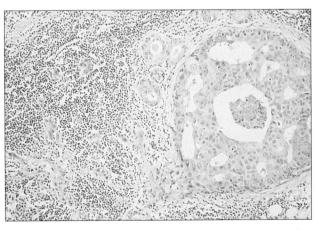

5.4 Intraduct cancer in a duct with an area of invasive cancer around the duct. Note the large paler cells of the intraduct cancer with spaces in the epithelium giving a rather cribriform appearance. There is a small area of central necrosis.

Lobular hyperplasia

Hyperplastic lesions of the lobule show a spectrum from atypical lobular hyperplasia (ALH) through lobular carcinoma-in-situ (LCIS) to invasive lobular cancer. They all differ from adenosis in that there is an increase in proliferation of cells within the acinus, losing the two-cell layer, without necessarily an increase in lobular size.

The proliferating cells within the lobule are distinctive, relatively small and rounded, with remarkable uniformity (monotonous is an apt description), although they include myoepithelial and lymphoid cells as well as luminal epithelial cells.

As with ductal hyperplasia, there are degrees of change. ALH is diagnosed when less than half the acini are expanded, when there are still luminal spaces free of cells, and when different types of cells are intermixed. Changes seen as the condition moves towards LCIS include expanded lobules with the lumen completely obliterated, and replacement of the myoepithelial and lymphoid cells by the single cell type. A category equivalent to mild ductal hyperplasia is not usually included in descriptions, perhaps because such a change in lobules would be similar to adenosis.

The changes frequently extend into the interlobular ducts, sometimes by pagetoid spread between basement membrane and luminal cells. This is in contrast to ductal hyperplasia, which tends to spread intraluminally to interlobar ducts or lobules. It is difficult to assess the true incidence because these conditions are largely silent both clinically and radiologically, and hence discovered mainly as an unexpected change on biopsy.

Multiple foci and bilateral involvement are common. The fact that lobular hyperplasia is seen predominantly in premenopausal women raises the possibility that regression may occur after the menopause. This would fit in with the finding of Page and colleagues that the risk of subsequent cancer, similar to that of ADH and DCIS, is mainly in the 10 years after diagnosis, falling after this period. They found an overall relative risk increase of 4 times, increasing to 10 times for those with a close family history, and greater in those where the process extended into the interlobular ducts.[12] This tenfold risk is the same as for LCIS, but in this case does not increase further with a family history.[4]

Apocrine cell hyperplasia

Metaplasia to apocrine-like cells is very common in the breast, especially lining cysts. Apocrine cells have a typical appearance, with abundant fine granules close to the lumen, eosinophilic cytoplasm, small round nuclei and apical snouts. They frequently form small papillary ingrowths into the cyst lumen (Figure 5.1) and also in small ducts, as well as in association with much other pathology, such as fibroadenoma and sclerosing adenosis. They are generally considered to have a benign outcome, and even to be a sign of benignity. There is some controversy regarding their long-term significance, and whether they might carry a small

increase in cancer risk. This is discussed further in Chapters 9 and 18. Apocrine adenosis is mentioned above.

Papillary lesions

A papilloma is an epithelial lesion whose branches have a fibrovascular core. It may be macroscopic or microscopic, single or multiple, benign or malignant. Papillomas are best considered in terms of clinicopathological groupings, rather than on pathology alone. The various conditions carrying the term papilloma are listed in Table 5.5.

Solitary (discrete) intraductal papilloma

This is the typical well-known lesion of the large subareolar ducts, usually only 3–4 mm in diameter (so difficult to locate in a specimen) and presenting with bloody nipple discharge. When larger, it elongates along the length of the duct, or expands into a diverticulum of dilated duct. It may be multiple in the sense of two to three similar papillomas lying adjacent in the one duct, and occasionally small papillomas will extend into the smaller ducts. Solitary intraductal papillomas usually occur in elderly women, suggesting presence over a long period, and behave as benign lesions. While these 'solitary' papillomas may be multiple, and may even spread to be peripheral, they are very different clinically and biologically from the 'multiple peripheral' group discussed below. Papillomas may show apocrine change, and undergo torsion leading to fibrosis or infarction.

Histology shows typical benign features, with a two-cell-layer configuration, but diagnosis may be difficult in the presence of fibrosis and distortion. Bilateral occurrence and recurrence are rare, and it is generally considered that solitary intraductal papilloma is a benign condition (Chapter 18).

Multiple (peripheral) duct papillomas

This term is best reserved for the rare condition described by Haagensen[1] where multiple papillomas, large enough to be palpable, occur in peripheral ducts and sometimes bilaterally. They arise in the TDLU region, and are often associated with severe hyperplasia or DCIS, or with changes suggestive of papillary carcinoma. It is not surprising that cancer subsequently develops in a considerable proportion.

Table 5.5 Conditions carrying the term 'papilloma'

Solitary (discrete) duct papilloma
Multiple (peripheral) duct papilloma
Juvenile papillomatosis (Swiss cheese disease)
Papilloma of the nipple
Papillary adenoma of the nipple
Papillomatosis

Juvenile papillomatosis (Swiss cheese disease)

This equally rare condition, described by Rosen and Kimel,[13] has many features in common with Haagensen's multiple papillomas. The specific features that overlap with Haagensen's series are young age, bilaterality and family history of breast cancer.

It is clear that both groups of multiple, peripheral papillomas are distinct from the discrete, central lesion, but whether the cases classed in the juvenile group are different to Haagensen's cases, or basically examples of the same condition, will only be determined as larger series are accumulated. Both forms of multiple, peripheral papillomas are discussed in Chapters 17 and 18.

Microscopic papillomas (papillomatosis)

These occur in two forms: apocrine and non-apocrine. Apocrine papillary change has been mentioned above under apocrine cell hyperplasia. Non-apocrine micropapillomas are also common, both in the premenopausal and postmenopausal breast. Most of these are areas of hyperplasia rather than true papillomas (they are without a fibrovascular core) and so are now called hyperplasia of ductal type (mild or moderate). The term papillomatosis was commonly used in the American literature for the condition called epitheliosis in British writings, so this is a terminological rather than a pathological distinction, and should gradually disappear from use.

Radial scar and complex sclerosing lesions

These are two sclerosing lesions often seen in association with sclerosing adenosis, and the three are often linked together under the term 'sclerosing lesions'. They have a distinctive structure, and while their origin is uncertain, they are probably distinct from sclerosing adenosis. They have both lost the lobulocentric configuration of sclerosing adenosis and are characterized by a central fibroelastic core with a stellate arrangement of radiating tubular structures. The cellular, connective tissue around the ductules causes much distortion, but careful examination will demonstrate the two-cell structure of benign lesions. The epithelium sometimes shows varying degrees of hyperplasia, and it is this which determines prognostic significance.

The two types of lesion are differentiated on size, 'radial scar' being used for lesions less than 1 cm in diameter, and 'complex sclerosing' for those greater. They are frequent in normal breasts, and frequently multiple. Their significance lies in the way that they mimic small cancers radiologically, so that they have achieved prominence since the widespread introduction of breast screening.

Thus these lesions can be considered as an aspect of ANDI, but require differentiation from small tubular cancers, and careful evaluation of any associated hyperplasia. They are discussed further in Chapter 10.

Fibrous change (fibrous disease)

Young women in the second half of reproductive life may present with a hard, ill-defined mass continuous with surrounding breast tissue but not fixed to skin or deeply. Biopsy may show unremarkable fibrous tissue. The clinical aspects of this condition are discussed in Chapter 17.

During normal lobular involution, the loose intralobular stroma is gradually replaced by dense fibrous tissue, and the glandular elements become less obvious and eventually disappear. There is no reason to believe that fibrous change is anything other than a local exaggeration of this process[2] and thus one end of the spectrum of involutional changes of ANDI. Although the condition is seen over a wide age range during the reproductive period, involutional changes may also start remarkably early.

Other conditions can give rise to excessive fibrosis, but can usually be identified without great difficulty. Fibrosis can follow gross periductal mastitis or inadequately treated lactational abscess. There is an autoimmune-related type, associated with marked lymphocytic infiltration of the fibrous tissue seen classically in diabetes (Chapter 17). The more cellular process of fibromatosis is rarely seen in the breast, sometimes as part of Gardner's syndrome. With any form of fibrosis a particularly fibrous carcinoma must be excluded by looking carefully for scattered cancer cells.

INFLAMMATORY CONDITIONS OF THE BREAST

The breast is subject to a wide range of inflammatory conditions in addition to lactational abscess. They are listed in outline in Table 5.6.

Obviously the list cannot be comprehensive, and there will be overlap between different groups, but it is useful to see that there is a much wider spectrum than lactational abscess.

Table 5.6 Inflammatory conditions of the breast

Acute inflammatory conditions
Lactational abscess
Subareolar abscess
'Metastatic' abscess
Chronic inflammatory conditions
Unresolved lactational abscess
Foreign body response
?Autoimmune response
Granulomatous responses
Fat necrosis
Periductal mastitis
Cholesterol granuloma
Idiopathic granulomatous disease
Infective conditions
Systemic granulomatous diseases

Lactational abscess

This condition is dealt with in Chapter 13, and is too well known to justify detailed description, but chronic lactational abscess is of some interest. This used to be quite common, and was attributed by surgeons to the inappropriate use of antibiotics. The condition has now largely disappeared, and it seems likely that those cases, which could closely simulate cancer, were due to unresolved abscesses associated with periductal mastitis. The fact that the mixed bacteria in these abscesses require antibiotics effective against anaerobic bacteria was not appreciated in the 1950s. Since these antibiotics have been used, the problem is rarely if ever seen, in spite of the substitution of aspiration for open drainage in early cases. However, this is not the case in developing countries, where chronic lactational abscess still appears high on the list of benign breast conditions. This is probably due to the lack of antibiotics and facilities for surgical drainage in these countries. It may also represent underdiagnosis of periductal mastitis.

Other acute abscesses

Recurrent subareolar abscess may be quite an acute condition in those cases associated with juxta-nipple duct obstruction. Unless treated adequately, it will convert to a more chronic, perhaps granulomatous condition, as is usual with cases arising from duct ectasia in older women. The pathology of the wide range of abscesses (acute, subacute, chronic and recurrent) seen with the duct ectasia/periductal mastitis complex is discussed fully in Chapter 11.

The breast may be involved in 'metastatic' infections, such as in typhoid.

Foreign bodies

These may be complicated by chronic bacterial infections if organisms gain access, or varying types of sterile reactions as seen with silicone prostheses.

Granulomatous reactions

The most important aspect of these processes is to recognize the wide variety of agents which can underly them, from trauma with fat necrosis to 'idiopathic' agents. The various forms of periductal mastitis are an important group, and it is probable that many cases of so-called idiopathic granulomatous mastitis are the result of unrecognized duct ectasia underlying the more obvious lobular involvement. Cholesterol granuloma is another variant of periductal mastitis.

Infective conditions such as tuberculosis are important causes of granulomatous reactions in women in developing countries and in immunocompromised patients in Western countries. Systemic granulomatous conditions, such as sarcoid and Wegener's, disease may first present in the breast. All these conditions are discussed in appropriate chapters elsewhere in the book.

CYTOLOGICAL DIAGNOSIS

This large subject is beyond the scope of this book, but the developments over the past 30 years have been so great that they deserve some comment.

The emergence of cytology as a discipline in its own right has resulted in much greater diagnostic accuracy. Classical errors, such as regarding the active epithelial cells from fibroadenomas in young girls as malignant, and a similar mistake with the epithelial cells in nipple discharge from pregnant women, should not now be made, although these diagnostic pitfalls cannot be ignored completely.

The most important realization is that a diagnosis of malignancy, particularly invasive malignancy, must be made on consideration of all the evidence, cytological, architectural, radiological and clinical. For this reason it is now commonplace and desirable to discuss cytology as one diagnostic element at a multidisciplinary clinic.

This is also one reason for a significant move in the past few years away from FNAC towards core needle biopsy, both in conjunction with or to replace FNAC. Other reasons for this trend towards core needle biopsy include the greater availability of image-guidance techniques in the clinic, and better cores obtained with less pain using newer spring-loaded needles.

Another development has been the recognition that FNAC can make a positive contribution to diagnosis of benign conditions, in contrast to its use solely to exclude malignancy. Maygarden et al.[14] have reviewed their experience of making a positive diagnosis from FNAC in 265 benign mass lesions (excluding ductal and lobular hyperplasias). A specific benign diagnosis was made in 49% of cases and this was correct in 80%. Analysis of findings gave specific patterns for diagnosing fibroadenoma, papilloma, fat necrosis, duct ectasia and fibrocystic change in general. The useful features were overall cellularity, nature of background, bipolar naked nuclei, architectural arrangements of epithelial cells, foam cells and stroma. However, cytology was less reliable in distinguishing between proliferative and non-proliferative changes of ANDI. This paper includes a valuable algorithm for diagnosing benign conditions.

REFERENCES

1. Haagensen CD. *Diseases of the Breast*, 3rd edn. Philadelphia: Saunders, 1986.

2. Azzopardi JG. *Problems in Breast Pathology*. London: WB Saunders, 1979.

3. Page DL & Anderson TJ. *Diagnostic Histopathology of the Breast*. Edinburgh: Churchill Livingstone, 1987.

4. Elston CW & Ellis IO (eds) *The Breast*, Vol 13, *Symmer's Systematic Pathology*, 3rd edn. Edinburgh: Churchill Livingstone, 1998.

5. Trojani AA. *Colour Atlas of Breast Histopathology*. London: Chapman and Hall Medical, 1991.

6. Oberman HA & French AJ. Chronic fibrocystic disease of the breast. *Surgery, Gynecology and Obstetrics* 1961; **112**: 647–652.

7. Azzopardi JG & Salm R. Ductal adenoma of the breast: a lesion which can mimic carcinoma. *Journal of Pathology* 1984; **144**: 15–23.

8. Bonser GM, Dossett JA & Jull JW. *Human and Experimental Breast Cancer*. London: Pitman Medical, 1961.

9. Foote FW & Stewart FW. Comparative studies of cancerous versus non-cancerous breast. 1. Basic morphologic characteristics. *Annals of Surgery* 1945; **121**: 6–53.

10. James BA, Cranor ML & Rosen PP. Carcinoma of the breast arising in microglandular adenosis. *American Journal of Clinical Pathology* 1993; **100**: 507–532.

11. Wells CA, McGregor IL, Makunura CN *et al.* Apocrine adenosis: A precursor of aggressive breast cancer? *Journal of Clinical Pathology* 1995; **48**: 737–742.

12. Page DL, Dupont WD & Rogers LW. Ductal involvement by cells of atypical lobular hyperplasia: a long term follow-up study of cancer risk. *Human Pathology* 1988; **19**: 201.

13. Rosen PP & Kimel M. Juvenile papillomatosis of the breast – a follow-up of 41 patients diagnosed before 1979. *American Journal of Clinical Pathology* 1990; **93**: 599–603.

14. Maygarden SJ, Novotny DB, Johnson DE & Frable WJ. Sub-classification of benign breast disease by fine needle-aspiration cytology – comparison of cytologic and histologic findings in 265 palpable breast masses. *Acta Cytologica* 1994; **38**: 115–129.

Chapter 6

Breast imaging methods

CONTENTS

KEY POINTS AND NEW DEVELOPMENTS

1. The indications for mammography in benign breast disorders have not changed but it should not be done in women under 35 years of age unless there is a strong clinical suspicion or known diagnosis of cancer.
2. The role of ultrasound in benign breast disorders has expanded with the improved image quality of high-resolution, high-frequency scanners. It is the primary investigative tool in women under 35 years of age and is an invaluable adjunct to mammography in the evaluation of lumps or mammographic abnormalities in women over 35 years.

3. Ultrasound-guided fine needle aspiration cytology (FNAC) and, increasingly, wide bore needle biopsy (WBN) are the ideal techniques for diagnosis of abnormalities identified. To diagnose mammographic abnormalities invisible on ultrasound, stereotactic FNAC, WBN or vacuum-assisted biopsy should be performed.
4. Coding imaging findings on reports ensures that an appropriate management plan can be instituted. This should be clearly understood by all members of the multidisciplinary team involved and should be part of a coding system that also involves clinical and cytological/histological findings.

The evaluation of the symptomatic breast requires clinical assessment with imaging and cytology/histology if indicated. There are several techniques available for imaging the breast, some of which are no longer in routine clinical use and others are under evaluation.

IMAGING TECHNIQUES OF PROVEN VALUE

Mammography

Since the publication in 1930 of the first report of the clinical use of mammography, the X-ray examination of the breast, there have been considerable improvements in radiographic technique, image acquisition and display. These have resulted in improved image detail with progressive decrease in radiation exposure. The mean glandular dose for the standard breast, when using a grid, should not exceed 3 mGy per exposure. Using current mammography systems it is possible to achieve doses of approximately half that per view.[1] Today's state-of-the-art mammogram machine has a rotating 'C' arm, a target suitable for soft tissue imaging, appropriate beam filtration, microfocal spot magnification, built-in moving grid, automatic exposure chamber, independent compression device and a high-output generator. The basic technique involves medio-lateral oblique and cranio-caudal views of each breast. Additional views, for example of the axillary tail, can be obtained as indicated.

The main impact of this method, of course, has been on the diagnosis and management of breast cancer but it also has its place in the investigation, evaluation and management of benign breast disorders and benign disease of the breast. Mammography is the imaging technique of first choice in symptomatic patients 35 years of age or older. There is a low incidence of breast cancer in women under 35 years of age[2] and in general the breast is denser and more glandular, limiting the usefulness of mammography. Therefore mammography is not indicated in women under the age of 35 unless there is a clinical, ultrasound or cytological/histological suspicion of breast cancer where it then becomes important in further management.

There is no evidence to indicate that very low doses of radiation such as those from current mammographic techniques induce breast cancer. An increased incidence of breast cancer has been observed in several groups of women exposed to high doses of radiation, e.g. Japanese survivors of atomic bombings at Hiroshima and Nagasaki. This evidence also indicates that women are at most risk of radiation-induced cancer when less than 20 years, the risk being halved at 30 years and less than one-tenth by the age of 40.[3] It is therefore important that mammography is not performed on women under 35 years unless there is a strong clinical suspicion of malignancy, and every effort should be made to ensure that any woman undergoing mammography receives as low a dose as is achievable and consistent with diagnostic-quality mammograms.

Film-screen mammography

Current film-screen combinations provide high-contrast, high-resolution images with dramatic reduction in radiation dose when compared to non-screen film. To achieve and maintain high-contrast images dedicated processing is necessary. A rigorous quality-control programme needs to be in place to maintain the standards of the mammography equipment, the film-screen combination and the processing.

Xeromammography

This technique used electrostatic imaging with dry, powder processing. At the time of its introduction it produced high-contrast, high-resolution images at doses considerably less than the available non-screen film mammography. Its inherent advantages were its ability to penetrate dense breast tissue and its 'edge-enhancement effect', highlighting the margins of microcalcification and mass lesions. However, continuing improvements in film-screen mammography led to declining sales of xeromammography units and production was discontinued in 1989.

Digital mammography

Many of the limitations of conventional mammography could be overcome with a digital mammography system. The image would be acquired, displayed and stored independently, allowing optimization of each stage. The contrast limitations of film-screen mammography could be overcome and computer-aided diagnosis may be feasible. The first such machines are currently undergoing evaluation but the cost, if nothing else, means it will be some time before they are widely available.

Contrast studies

Alteration in clinical practice and the widespread availability of breast ultrasound have resulted in a significant reduction in the use of ductography and pneumocystography.

Ductography

A single duct discharge when it is blood stained, profuse, serous or watery may be secondary to a carcinoma or an intracystic papilloma. Ductography involves cannulating the duct and injecting dilute, water-soluble radiographic contrast slowly until a feeling of fullness in the breast is experienced by the patient. The cannula is withdrawn and the nipple sealed with Micropore. Two mammographic views are taken at right-angles to one another.

Connections with small cysts, enlarged ducts and intraductal filling defects due to papilloma, carcinoma, granuloma or inspissated secretion may be demonstrated. Although it may not be possible to differentiate these conditions using ductography, the technique can demonstrate the location and extent of the abnormality.

Contraindications to ductography are the presence of mammary infection or nipple infection. A rare complication is the development of a localized or generalized mastitis as a result of sensitivity to the contrast medium.

There are considerable variations in the extent to which ductography is used in different units. This is discussed further in Chapter 12.

Pneumocystography

Blood-stained fluid aspirated from a cyst raises the possibility of an intracystic papilloma or carcinoma. Pneumocystography is a technique of cyst aspiration in which the fluid aspirated is replaced with the same amount of air. Mammography is then performed, allowing the lining of the cyst and any filling defects to be viewed. The technique has now been replaced by ultrasound which allows evaluation of the nature of the cyst and its lining.

Ultrasound

The use of ultrasound in breast examination was first described in 1951 and developments in high-frequency, high-resolution, real-time ultrasound since the 1980s have rapidly accelerated the use this technique in the evaluation of breast disease due to a significant improvement in image quality.

State-of-the-art ultrasound equipment should incorporate a real-time, high-frequency (7.5–13 MHz), hand-held linear probe with adjustable focal zones. The patient is scanned in the supine oblique position with the symptomatic side raised and the arm above the head, allowing good compression and a vertical beam (Figure 6.1).

The sensitivity of ultrasound is operator dependent and good technique is essential. The position of the patient and the way the probe is held are very important as there is significant deflection of the beam from fatty tissue, resulting in degradation of the image. This is most marked when the probe is not vertical to the breast tissue being imaged. The use of ultrasound jelly ensures that there is no air between the probe and the skin which would deflect the beam. However, difficulty with contact and achieving a vertical beam can mean that the subareolar area is difficult to image in some women.

The examination is targeted to the area of concern. To endeavour to examine the entire breast or both breasts would be very time consuming and has a substantial false-positive rate, resulting in unnecessary further investigation and morbidity. In a recent review of 12 760 breast ultrasound examinations, 1575 clinically and mammographically occult lesions were detected. Only 44 (2.8%) of these lesions detected on ultrasound alone were malignant.[4]

It is also important to remember that ultrasound does not show some non-palpable cancers that are mammographically visible.[5] For example, detection of microcalcification to significant levels has only been achieved when the operator has been made aware of the location of the microcalcification shown on mammography.[6] It is important to be aware of these false negatives and false positives and to use ultrasound appropriately.

Ultrasound is the primary method of imaging palpable abnormalities in women under 35 years of age.[7] It is an appropriate adjunct to mammography in older women in three specific areas: (1) in the evaluation of palpable masses, (2) in the evaluation of abnormalities detected at mammography, and (3) in the assessment of the augmented breast. It is not a suitable screening tool[8] but used appropriately, by an experienced operator using state-of-the-art equipment, it is an indispensable tool in breast imaging.

IMAGE-GUIDED DIAGNOSIS

Ultrasound-guided diagnosis

Ultrasound is an ideal technique for the accurate guidance of FNAC and WBN. Its utilization in the biopsy of mass lesions identified in an area of nodularity ensures that the cytology or histology obtained is from the lesion rather than the surrounding breast tissue.

Fine needle aspiration cytology (FNAC)

For ultrasound-guided FNAC, the patient is positioned as for diagnostic ultrasound. The operator holds the probe with the left hand and, using the right hand, introduces a cannulated 35-mm 21G needle with a sharp bevel into the skin adjacent to the middle of the right-hand edge of the probe (Figure 6.2).

This is advanced to the lesion in the plane parallel to the middle of the probe and therefore the ultrasound beam, thus ensuring that the entire length of the needle is clearly visualized (Figure 6.3).

The cannula is withdrawn and a low-pressure connection tube with a 5-mL syringe attached is connected to the needle. While an assistant applies 1 mL of suction the lesion is sampled up to 30 times with slight rotating movements. Ultrasound visualization allows the needle to be 'stepped' through the lesion, ensuring that it is adequately sampled. If a lesion is near the chest wall the needle can be advanced in a path that lies parallel to the

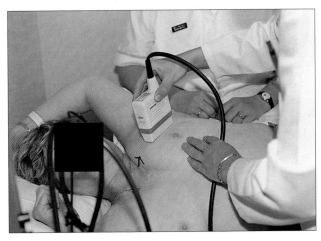

6.1 Patient positioned for ultrasound scan in the supine oblique position with the symptomatic side raised and the arm above the head.

chest wall by introducing it into the skin 1 cm away from the edge of the probe.

Wide bore needle biopsy (WBN)

For ultrasound-guided WBN the patient is positioned as for diagnostic ultrasound. The operator holds the probe with the left hand and, using the right hand, anaesthetizes the skin 2 cm beyond the right-hand edge of the probe. A small incision is made through this area. This allows the introduction of a wide bore needle, bevel edge leading, such that as it is advanced to the lesion it lies parallel to the chest wall. When the tip of the needle reaches the lesion it is rotated 180 degrees to ensure that the bevel edge lies superficial. Thus, as the needle advances, its path is more towards the skin than the lung.

The most effective biopsies are obtained using a spring-loaded biopsy gun with a >2-cm throw and 16- or 14-gauge needles.[9] Two cores are obtained. The cores are put in 10% formalin. If they float it suggests the presence of a high fat content and the biopsy should be repeated. Multiple passes have been shown to increase diagnostic yield, but with an experienced operator two cores should be sufficient for diagnosis in the majority of biopsies performed under ultrasound guidance.[10] Firm pressure over the needle track for 5 minutes avoids any significant haematoma.

Facilitating open biopsy

The use of ultrasound to image and diagnose symptomatic and mammographic breast abnormalities has resulted in a significant decrease in diagnostic open biopsies. There are, however, instances where cytology or histology may not provide a definitive diagnosis and excision biopsy is indicated.

If the lesion is impalpable but visible using ultrasound, a localization wire can be introduced under ultrasound guidance. There are a variety of localization needle–wire assemblies available and the precise one used will depend

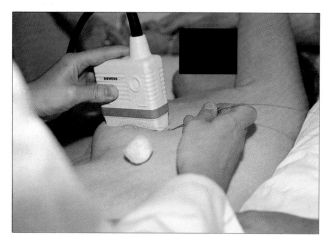

6.2 Ultrasound-guided needle placement.

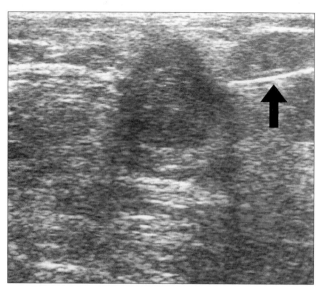

6.3 Ultrasound image showing that the needle (arrow) is clearly visible throughout its length, with its tip at the edge of the lesion to be biopsied.

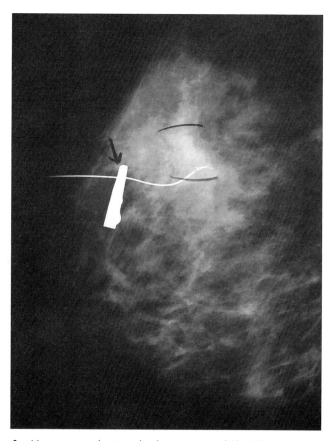

6.4 Mammogram showing a localization wire with the 'X' lying just below the area of asymmetric density/distortion. The clip (arrow) marks the skin entry point of the wire.

on local preference and availability. Using the technique described above, the needle–wire assembly is introduced to lie just behind the lesion. When the needle is correctly positioned the wire is advanced through the needle to release its anchoring device. The needle is then removed, leaving the wire in position. Mammography is then performed in two planes to show the surgeon the relationship of the wire to the lesion, its position and depth from the skin surface (Figure 6.4).

The surgeon cuts down along the wire to its tip and excises the lesion and the wire. The specimen is then radiographed to ensure that the suspicious lesion has been excised (Figure 6.5) and the specimen sent for histological evaluation.

On occasion an ultrasound-guided skin mark over the lesion may be sufficient to indicate the lesion to be removed.

Stereotactic-guided diagnosis

The radiological features of some benign conditions, especially sclerosing adenosis and radial scar, and subclinical malignancy can be identical. Thus, biopsy is indicated to exclude malignancy in these impalpable lesions. Even with state-of-the-art ultrasound equipment, microcalcification without associated soft tissue mass is difficult to visualize, as is distortion. These lesions and mammographically detected, ultrasound-invisible abnormalities require X-ray guidance for biopsy.

The stereotactic technique uses two-plane radiographic views acquired at different X-ray source positions, 15 degrees to the right and left of the midline, to determine the location of radiographically visible objects in three spatial planes: the x horizontal, y vertical and z depth coordinates (Figure 6.6).

The area to be sampled is identified on these images and the computer is used to guide the tip of the biopsy device being used to this point. The stereotactic images are

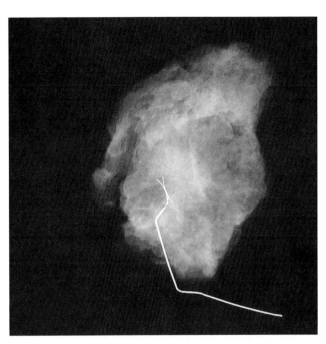

6.5 The specimen X-ray confirms that the suspicious area has been removed.

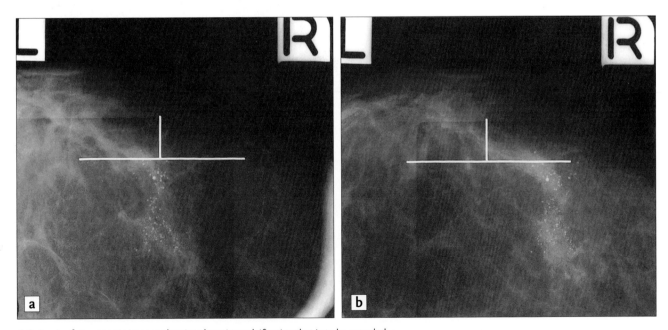

6.6 A pair of stereotactic images showing the microcalcification that is to be sampled.

repeated to confirm that the needle is in the correct position and the lesion is sampled (Figure 6.7).

When doing WBN biopsy of microcalcification or areas of distortion it is advisable to obtain at least five samples to increase the diagnostic yield.[10] Stereotaxis can be performed with a special attachment to upright mammography units or with a dedicated prone biopsy table. The advantages of the add-on units is that they are much less expensive than the dedicated prone units and they can perform standard mammography when not being used for needle guidance. The prone position avoids vasovagal attacks and is better tolerated by the patient. It also allows access to the breast from all angles, which can be difficult with add-on units.

Stereotaxis is used to guide FNAC, WBN or vacuum-assisted biopsy and large-gauge needle biopsy. The vacuum-assisted biopsy device uses vacuum to pull tissue into the probe and to remove the specimen without removing the probe each time. Tissue samples are obtained at consecutive clock positions to achieve contiguous sampling.[11] Large-gauge needle biopsy allows up to a 2-cm core of tissue to be removed percutaneously, allowing the entire lesion to be removed under local anaesthetic and obviating the need for wire-guided localization biopsy. Vacuum-assisted biopsy and large-gauge needle biopsy devices were originally designed for use with prone biopsy tables and the expense and limited use of this equipment means that they are not yet widely available.

Stereotaxis can also be used to place localization wires.

TECHNIQUES OF UNCERTAIN VALUE

Magnetic resonance imaging (MRI)

MRI of the breast has tremendous potential for improving the future treatment and management of breast disorders but its current clinical use is limited and is still the subject of ongoing research. Contrast-enhanced MRI is known to have a high sensitivity for invasive breast cancer but non-specific parenchymal enhancement appears to be a relative limitation, particularly for menstruating women since the rate of intensity of contrast enhancement varies with the cycle, peaking the week prior to menstruation. Contrast-enhanced MRI appears to have little potential to differentiate ductal carcinoma- in-situ from hyperplasia with or without atypia. It does not replace mammography or ultrasound as the primary imaging modality in the symptomatic breast.

Doppler ultrasound scanning

By using Doppler scanning, quantitative assessment of bloodflow can be obtained transcutaneously. When used in combination with ultrasound sector scanning, the technique is known as 'duplex scanning'. The sector scan is used to identify the solid lesion and the Doppler is then used to identify blood flow in and around the lesion. Advances in technology have improved the detection of bloodflow related to breast lesions but it cannot reliably differentiate benign from malignant lesions because of the overlap in the amount of vascularity between some benign

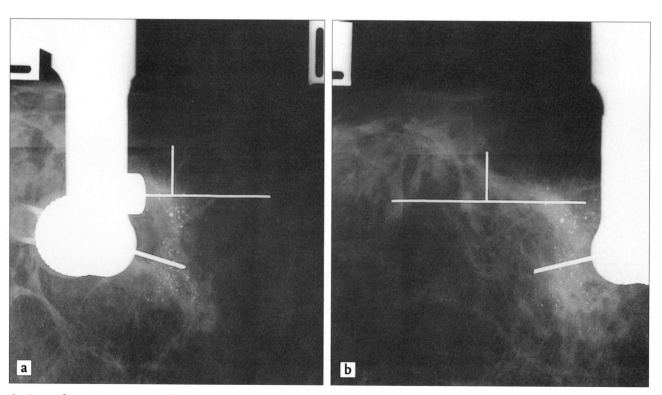

6.7 A pair of stereotactic images confirming that the needle is within the microcalcification.

and malignant lesions and it does not obviate the need for biopsy. It is still largely a research tool.

Thermography

Thermography has been largely discarded as a non-specific technique with high false-positive and high false-negative rates in the diagnosis of breast cancer. It has little demonstrable value in the management of benign disease.

MAMMOGRAPHY IN BENIGN BREAST DISORDERS

In the majority of cases, benign breast lesions present fairly characteristic mammographic appearances. They are usually smooth in outline and rounded, ovoid or lobulated in shape (Figure 6.8).

These lesions may occur singly but more often there are multiple lesions present, usually bilaterally (Figure 6.9).

There may be a surrounding 'halo' of compressed fat, indicating that there is no infiltration. Breast structures such as ducts and trabeculae are displaced rather than disrupted. Most are of equal-to-low density to the surrounding parenchyma but some will be more dense. The most common masses in this category are cysts and fibroadenomas. Calcification, if present, may aid in differentiating a cyst and fibroadenoma. Although infrequent, some cysts demonstrate a thin rim of 'eggshell' calcification in part or all of the wall (Figure 6.10).

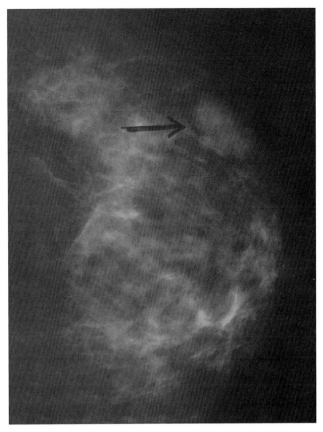

6.8 Mammogram showing a benign lobulated mass lesion (arrow) compatible with a fibroadenoma.

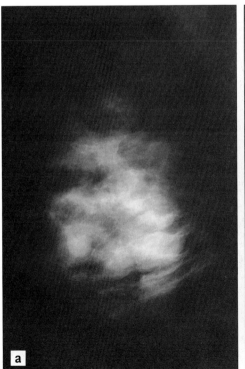

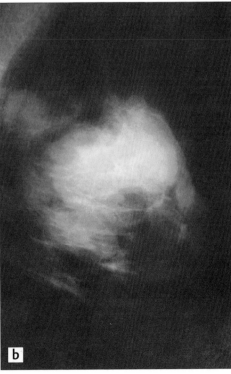

6.9 Mammograms with multiple benign round mass lesions in both breast compatible with multiple cysts.

Fibroadenomas may develop coarse, 'popcorn-like' calcification (Figure 6.11).

Calcifications in benign disease are usually coarse and smooth and occur in characteristic forms in duct ectasia (Figure 6.12). They follow the course of the ducts and are seen as either solid, smoothly marginated cores or hollow cylinders.

Also commonly seen and easy to identify is milk of calcium in microcysts giving a 'teacup' sign on a true lateral film (Figure 6.13). The calcium sediments out in the base of the cyst resulting in a horizontal fluid-calcium level with a curved base. On a craniocaudal view the sedimented calcium has a smudgy appearance.

Fine microcalcifications occur in epithelial hyperplasia, sclerosing adenosis and papillomatosis and then may cause diagnostic difficulties. Benign calcification tends to be round or punctate, occurring in small, widely dispersed groups (Figure 6.14). However, they may vary in size, shape and density with a segmental distribution, thus raising the possibility of malignancy and necessitating biopsy.

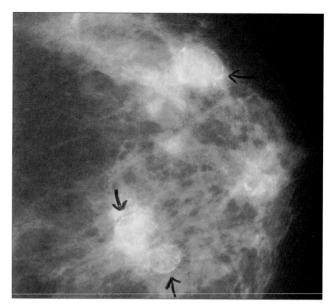

6.10 Mammogram showing curvilinear 'eggshell' calcification in the cyst walls (arrows).

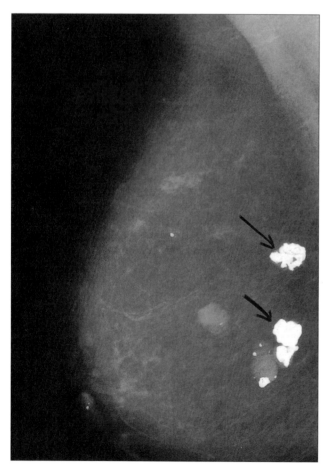

6.11 Mammogram showing multiple fibroadenomas, some with dense 'popcorn' calcification (arrows).

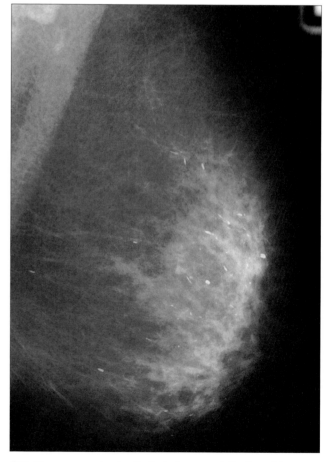

6.12 Mammogram showing the typical coarse calcification of duct ectasia orientated along the line of the ducts. The nipple is retracted.

Duct ectasia may present as enlarged or dense ducts converging on the nipple. Difficulties in interpretation arise with irregular or ill-defined lesions such as abscess, plasma cell mastitis and fat necrosis where they may mimic carcinoma. Lesions giving rise to distortion such as sclerosing adenosis, radial scar or previous biopsy scars can also cause diagnostic difficulties.

Indications for mammography in benign disorders

There are four main indications for the use of mammography in benign disorders of the breast:

- To confirm the clinical diagnosis. The diagnosis of benign disorder on mammography is usually possible. The accuracy of diagnosis was 97% in the authors' unit. Distinguishing between cyst and fibroadenoma is rarely possible unless characteristic calcification is present.
- As an aid in clinically difficult or doubtful cases, e.g. in the common situation of nodular breasts, where multiple palpable lesions are present, and radiological evidence of malignancy might differentiate one lesion from the other.

- To exclude malignancy in patients in the cancer age group in situations such as non-cyclical mastalgia or vague breast symptoms where no lesion is palpable. Fear of cancer is a major cause of morbidity in these cases, and negative mammograms will be very helpful in management.
- In the clinical management of non-operative cases. The added reassurance of benign disease is valuable. Repeat mammographic examination in 6 months' time for microcalcification or asymmetric density of uncertain significance, where biopsy has not been possible, can be useful in a very limited number of cases.

ULTRASOUND IN BENIGN BREAST DISORDERS

Ultrasound in the evaluation of a palpable abnormality identifies if there is a lesion present or not and whether it is cystic or solid. A simple cyst on ultrasound is smooth in outline with a thin wall, it has no internal echoes and it demonstrates posterior enhancement (Figure 6.15).

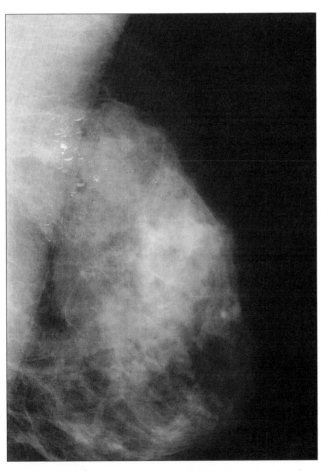

6.13 Lateral mammogram showing milk of calcium layering out in the bases of microcysts, giving the characteristic 'teacup' sign with a convex base and a horizontal line on top.

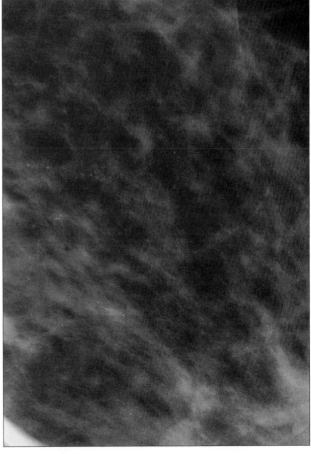

6.14 Magnified mammogram showing widespread benign punctate microcalcification.

Some simple benign cysts do not have this characteristic appearance: internal echoes are found in the presence of proteinaceous material or cellular debris (Figure 6.16); posterior enhancement is not a consistent finding; small cysts 5 mm or less can mimic small carcinomas; and a hypoechoic rim 2–3-mm thick is found around inflamed cysts (Figure 6.17).

It is important to evaluate the cyst wall carefully in two planes to look for projections in the cyst that may indicate the presence of an intracystic papilloma (Figure 6.18) or papillary carcinoma.

Simple cysts with the typical ultrasound findings do not need aspiration unless indicated clinically, but if there is any doubt as to whether the lesion is cystic then aspiration to confirm the nature of the lesion is indicated.

The typical features of a benign solid mass are an ovoid smooth mass, narrower in its anteroposterior than its transverse diameter, with even, low-level internal echoes (Figure 6.19).

Through transmission is variable and hyalinized fibroadenomas are associated with marked attenuation. Some fibroadenomas have an irregular outline and some carcinomas are

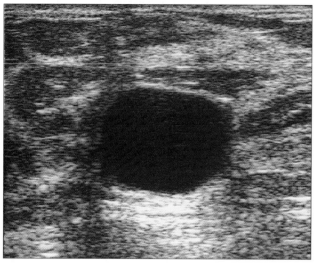

6.15 Ultrasound image showing a simple cyst with no internal echoes and enhancement or 'bright up' deep to the cyst.

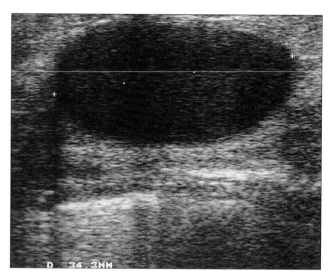

6.16 Ultrasound image of a cyst, confirmed on aspiration, that contains internal echoes secondary to debris in the cyst fluid.

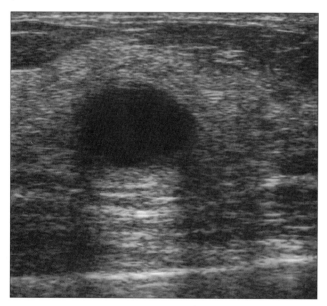

6.17 Ultrasound image of an inflamed cyst. An ill-defined hypoechoic rim can be seen around the edge of the cyst.

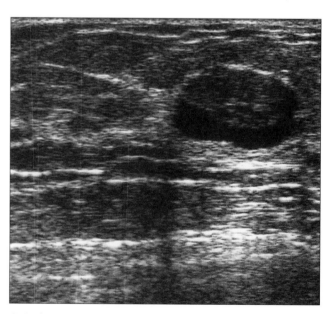

6.18 Ultrasound image showing a lesion projecting into the lumen of a cyst which was proven to be an intracystic papilloma.

circumscribed. This overlap between the ultrasound appearances of benign and malignant lesions means that cytological or histological evaluation of all solid lesions is indicated.

Ultrasound has an important role to play in the management of mastitis. It is also an excellent method for the diagnosis of an abscess cavity and can be used to guide percutaneous drainage.

Indications for ultrasound in benign disorders

There are three main indications for the use of ultrasound in benign disorders of the breast:

- In the evaluation of palpable masses: to identify whether a lesion is present or not, and if there is a lesion to establish whether it is cystic or solid.
- In the evaluation of abnormalities detected at mammography. Ultrasound is invaluable in the evaluation of abnormalities such as mass lesions and areas of asymmetric density. It is important to realize that while ultrasound will detect coarse calcification, a lot of microcalcification is still not detectable and management should be based on the mammographic evaluation.
- In the evaluation of mastitis. Ultrasound is an excellent method for the detection of abscess formation and for guiding percutaneous drainage. Differentiation of inflammatory cancer from mastitis can be difficult clinically as well as radiologically but the presence of a focal abnormality on ultrasound allows targeted biopsy.

REPORTING OF IMAGING FINDINGS

The introduction of the National Breast Screening Programme in the United Kingdom in 1988 focused attention on the multidisciplinary evaluation of breast problems using clinical evaluation, imaging and cytology or histology. It also introduced a national system of categorization for clinical radiological and cytological findings, based on a 5-point scale. This not only allows comparison of results between centres but also ensures effective communication between the members of the individual multidisciplinary teams, thus guiding the appropriate further management of clinically detected or imaging detected abnormalities. The categorization for mammography and ultrasound is shown in Table 6.1.

A corresponding categorization of imaging abnormalities, known as BI-RADS, is used in the United States.[12] The difference between Europe and the United States in the management of categories 2 and 3 is that it is our practice to achieve if at all possible a definitive diagnosis by biopsy in these women. As most of these lesions are benign, and most biopsies are carried out in the clinic the first time the woman is seen, we avoid making patients out of well women. The alternative management is periodic follow-up.[13] The discussion[14,15] is likely to continue, but it is most important that the multidisciplinary members of each and every breast unit have a clear understanding of how and why each category of lesion is managed whichever method is used.

WOLFE PARENCHYMAL PATTERNS

Wolfe[16] described four basic parenchymal patterns on mammography:

- N1 – a parenchyma which is completely or mainly fatty.
- P1 – the presence of prominent ducts occupying 25% or less of the breast.
- P2 – prominent ducts occupying over 25% of the breast.
- DY – the presence of a dense parenchyma, a 'dysplasia'.

Table 6.1 UK National Breast Screening Programme categorization for clinical radiological and cytological findings

		Action[a]
1 or N	Normal	No further action indicated
2 or B	Benign	Solid lesions need cytology
3 or U	Uncertain	Ideally needs histology
4 or S	Suspicion of malignancy	If histology does not indicate malignancy, excision biopsy will be required. If histology indicates cancer, treatment can be offered
5 or M	Malignant	Treatable provided there is cytological or histological confirmation

[a]This column describes the action each category generates in our unit.

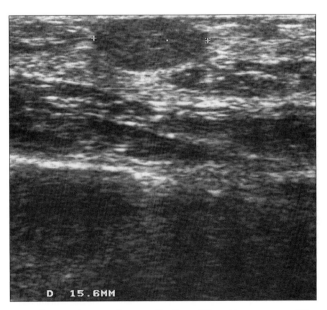

6.19 Ultrasound image showing a benign solid ovoid mass compatible with a fibroadenoma.

He maintained that the risk of developing breast cancer could be predicted using these four basic radiographic patterns in women over the age of 30. The N1 group had the lowest risk and the DY had the highest, at 21–37 times higher risk.

Gravelle et al.[17] have shown an association between these radiographic patterns and epidemiological risk factors. In particular, women with increased risk due to nulliparity or late age of first child showed a significant increase in the P2 and DY patterns. It was also shown that variables such as age and weight were related to the proportion of high-risk mammograms. A further prospective study by Gravelle et al.[18] of parenchymal patterns showed that women with DY and P2 patterns had nearly four times the risk of developing cancer compared with women having N1 or P1 patterns. The combination of the 'high-risk' patterns with age, weight, parity and age at birth of first child may identify groups at particularly high risk. This is discussed further in Chapter 18.

REFERENCES

1. NHS Breast Screening Programme Publication No 24. *Review of Mammography Equipment and its Performance*.

2. Seltzer MH. The significance of breast complaints as correlated with age and breast cancer. *American Surgeon* 1992; **58**: 413–417.

3. Forrest Professor Sir Patrick. *Breast Cancer Screening*. Report to the Health Ministers of England, Wales, Scotland & Northern Ireland, 1986.

4. Gordon PB & Goldenberg SL. Malignant masses detected only by US. A retrospective review. *Cancer* 1995; **76**: 626–630.

5. Potterson AJ, Peakman DJ & Young JR. Ultrasound demonstration of small breast cancers detected by mammographic screening. *Clinical Radiology* 1994; **49**: 808–813.

6. Leucht WJ, Lecht D & Kiesel L. Sonographic demonstration and evaluation of microcalcifications in the breast. *Breast Disease* 1992; **5**: 105–123.

7. Stavros AT, Thickman D, Rapp CL et al. Solid breast nodules: use of sonography to distinguish between benign and malignant lesions. *Radiology* 1995; **196**: 123–134.

8. The W & Wilson ARM. The role of ultrasound in breast cancer screening. A consensus statement by the European Group for Breast Cancer Screening. *European Journal of Cancer* 1998; **34**: 449–450.

9. Hooper KD, Abendroth CS, Sturtz KW et al. Automated biopsy devices: a blinded evaluation. *Radiology* 1993; **187**: 653–660.

10. Brenner RJ, Fajaro L, Fisher PR et al. Percutaneous core biopsy of the breast: effect of operator experience and number of samples on diagnostic accuracy. *American Journal of Roengenology* 1996; **166**: 341–346.

11. Parker SH & Klaus AJ. Performing a breast biopsy with a directional, vacuum-assisted biopsy instrument. *Radiographics* 1997; **17**: 1233–1252.

12. American College of Radiology. *Breast Imaging Reporting and Data System*. Reston, VA: American College of Radiology, 1993.

13. Sickles EA. Nonpalpable, circumscribed, noncalcified solid breast masses: likelihood of malignancy based on lesion size and age of patient. *Radiology* 1994; **192**: 439–442.

14. Wilson R. Management of probably benign breast lesions. *Radiology* 1995; **194**: 912.

15. Sickles EA. Non-palpable, circumscribed, non-calcified solid breast masses: likelihood of malignancy based on lesion size and age of patient. *Radiology* 1994; **192**: 439–442.

16. Wolfe JN. Risk for breast cancer development determined by breast parenchymal pattern. *Cancer* 1976; **37**: 2486–2492.

17. Gravelle IH, Bulstrode JC, Wang DY et al. The relation between radiographic features and determinants of risk of breast cancer. *British Journal of Radiology* 1980; **53**: 107–113.

18. Gravelle IH, Bulstrode JC, Bulbrook RD et al. A prospective study of mammographic parenchymal pattern and risk of breast cancer. *British Journal of Radiology* 1986; **59**: 487–491.

Fibroadenoma and related tumours

KEY POINTS AND NEW DEVELOPMENTS

1. Mixed stromal and epithelial tumours fall into two main types: fibroadenoma (simplex) and phyllodes tumour. These are differentiated by the cellularity and activity of the stromal element.
2. Behaviour is determined by the stroma, with the age of the patient a second important element. The obsolescent term 'cystosarcoma phyllodes' should be abandoned since many are not cystic and most are benign.
3. Fibroadenoma arises from a lobule, probably as the result of increased sensitivity to oestrogen.
4. Molecular biology is providing interesting insights into possible mechanisms. For example, fibroadenomas show the *bcl-2* gene, which delays apoptotic cell death in similar situations.
5. Most fibroadenomas do not show progressive growth, but the growth phase is followed by a static phase in about 80%, regression in about 15% and progression in only 5–10%.
6. Fibroadenomas can be treated conservatively provided diagnosis is confident and the patient compliant; routine excision is no longer appropriate.
7. Triple assessment is by clinical examination, ultrasound and pathology, with fine needle aspiration cytology (FNAC) or core needle biopsy.
8. Fibroadenomas carry a small risk of increased future breast cancer, seen mainly in cases showing a complex histology. The risk is sufficient to be of biological interest, but not to influence management.
9. Up to four fibroadenomas in one breast, and fibroadenomas up to 4 cm in diameter, are not uncommon. Appropriate definition for multiple fibroadenomas is thus five or more in one breast and for giant fibroadenoma is a diameter >5 cm.
10. Giant fibroadenoma and phyllodes tumour in adolescence usually behave in a benign fashion, managed by enucleation without reconstruction.
11. Phyllodes tumours in adults have a high local recurrence rate unless the initial excision is adequate, i.e. 1 cm clearance. Hence, the diagnosis should be made by core needle biopsy before surgery, to ensure an adequate primary excision.

TERMINOLOGY

The World Health Organization has simply defined a fibroadenoma as 'a discrete benign tumour showing evidence of connective tissue and epithelial proliferation'.[1] It has long been recorded and recognized as an entity and as a benign tumour; in the early nineteenth century Sir Astley Cooper used the term 'chronic mammary tumour'. In its classic form, fibroadenoma is one of the commonest, best recognized and most easily managed conditions, yet paradoxically fibroadenomas which are not entirely typical have given rise to more confusion than most breast conditions. This is due to the use of a plethora of terms to describe the more exuberant forms of tumour (in either a histological or clinical sense). Indeed, it is the confusion caused by clinical variants (those of large size or rapid growth) or histological variants (hypercellularity or atypia) which has been the root of the problem.

More recently, there is a better understanding of the wide spectrum of histological appearances and disease behaviour with mixed epithelial and connective tissue proliferation, but the benefits of this better understanding can only be gained by insisting on precise terminology.

The fibrous stromal element of these tumours is the key to classification and behaviour, with any epithelial variant being treated as a secondary problem. Thus, on the basis of the stromal element, the tumours fall into two main groups: fibroadenoma and phyllodes tumour, with a few less common and less important variants. The term 'fibroadenoma' is used for all such tumours in which the fibrous stroma is of low cellularity and regular cytology. It covers tumours of all sizes, because their behaviour is basically similar, i.e. uniformly benign, whatever the size. The group of tumours where the stroma shows markedly increased cellularity and atypia is termed 'phyllodes tumour' (cystosarcoma phyllodes in older terminology).

It is stressed that this diagnosis is made on histological grounds, not size. Thus while most phyllodes tumours are large, the term should also be applied to small tumours if they show the appropriate histological changes in the stroma. Most phyllodes tumours also behave in a benign fashion, although showing a tendency to local recurrence. But there is a spectrum of clinical behaviour as well as of histological atypia, and an occasional case will be frankly malignant and may metastasize.

In summary, fibroadenoma is common, usually small but sometimes large, and for practical purposes always benign. Phyllodes tumour is uncommon, usually large but sometimes small, usually benign but occasionally malignant. The two lesions cannot be distinguished clinically and not always on macroscopic section. Both occur throughout reproductive life; fibroadenoma presents predominantly in the first half, phyllodes tumour more commonly in the second.

Age is an added and important factor in two respects. Tumours of adolescence usually behave in benign fashion irrespective of histology. Tumours of the perimenopausal period which recur may then behave in more serious fashion, even if histologically they look benign at the first presentation.

FIBROADENOMA SIMPLEX

This tumour usually appears in young women as a rubbery-firm, smooth, very mobile mass. These features – and in particular its striking mobility – are so characteristic that a confident diagnosis can be made in most cases in young women. The term 'simplex' differentiates the common, everyday fibroadenoma from the 'complex' fibroadenomas recently delineated, and from multiple and giant fibroadenomas falling outside the range of the simple lesion. The overall incidence is highest in the mid-thirties and early forties, but in this age group diagnosis is more common from imaging or by pathology, and physical signs are less characteristic.

Age and natural history
Clinically, the lesion is predominantly a tumour of young women. This would be expected from its lobular origin, for the time of greatest lobular development is the first years after the menarche. Yet studies have always shown the median age of diagnosis as about 30 years. This seems older than clinical experience suggests but is confirmed in a Cardiff series (Figure 7.1).

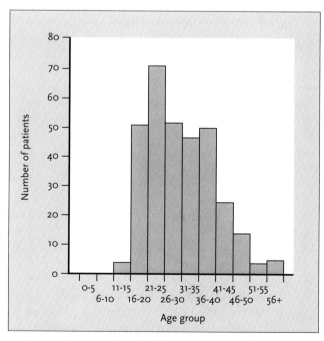

7.1 The age at presentation with fibroadenoma – Cardiff patients. (Reproduced from Foster *et al.*[29] by courtesy of the *Journal of the Royal College of Surgeons of Edinburgh.*)

The older patients are diagnosed in the pathology department, not in the clinic, and this can be explained by the differing physical characteristics of fibroadenomas in different age groups. Lesions with classic physical signs (discrete, smooth, mobile) appear in the 16–25-year age group, being noticed accidently while bathing or dressing. In the older age group the classic clinical symptoms may be obscured by coexisting involutional changes and the histological diagnosis may come as a surprise following excision of a clinical dominant mass, which lacks the notable discreteness and mobility of fibroadenoma in the younger girl.

Widespread use of ultrasound confirms that subclinical fibroadenoma is common throughout reproductive life.

Many fibroadenomas will not be felt in the young firm breast and, if left alone, will remain static or gradually increase in size until 1–3 cm in diameter, taking 1–5 years to do so. During the growth phase, the tumour doubles in size in 6–12 months[2] and is then likely to remain static for the rest of the patient's life or gradually decrease in size. A fibroadenoma may become clinically apparent in the third or fourth decade as the tumour enlarges or the breast becomes softer or more pendulous after childbirth.

A more detailed knowledge of the natural history has come from a number of prospective studies where patients have been followed during conservative management. In the first major study, Dent and Cant[3] followed 63 young women in Capetown with a clinical and cytological diagnosis of fibroadenoma. They found that 31% of 201 lumps disappeared and a further 12% became smaller over 13–24 months' observation, 25% remained static and 32% grew. Regression was slightly more likely with single than multiple lesions. These and similar data must be interpreted with some caution since clinical diagnosis is not absolute and sequential clinical follow-up is subject to observer error. Furthermore, results from a study with a large non-white population and a high incidence of multiple tumours may not be applicable to all Western populations.

Nevertheless, strong general confirmation of these results is provided from a recent study of predominantly white patients from Edinburgh.[4] Two hundred and one patients less than 40 years old were offered conservative management after fibroadenoma diagnosed clinically was confirmed by ultrasound and cytology. The diagnosis was confirmed histologically in all 17 patients opting for surgery, confirming the accuracy of the triple diagnostic assessment. Two-thirds of the tumours were <2 cm in diameter, and one-third were 2–4 cm. Objective assessment of tumour size was obtained by ultrasound measurement. During follow-up, 13% resolved and 85% were unchanged; 2% increased in size and were removed, all four were simple fibroadenomas on histology.

Thus it may be accepted that most fibroadenomas remain static over several years following diagnosis, a few regress and a very small number grow.

To investigate why most fibroadenomas stop growing in this way, Meyer measured cell proliferation in normal breast epithelium, fibroadenomas and epithelial hyperplasias[5] and found that epithelial cells from fibroadenomas differed from the other two. They showed less variation in mitotic rate during the menstrual cycle, and the mitotic rate decreased with age. This may explain why growth stops.

Incidence

In most clinical series the frequency of fibroadenoma is about half that of cancer. In one series of 2005 consecutive outpatient consultations analysed in the authors' unit, 360 patients had discrete lumps requiring excision; of these, 75 were fibroadenomas and 148 were cancers. The ratio in Haagensen's series[2] was 1:4, but this probably reflects the special nature of his cancer referral practice. However, only a minority of fibroadenomas are diagnosed clinically, more are discovered with ultrasound and small histological 'fibroadenomas' can be found in most breasts if looked for carefully enough, so the relative incidence increases considerably when screening with ultrasound is used.

New fibroadenomas are found in about 1:10 000 postmenopausal women undergoing mammographic screening, all in patients having hormone replacement therapy (HRT).

Fibroadenomas are more common in the left breast and predominate in the upper outer quadrants (Figure 7.2).

This distribution reflects the amount of breast parenchyma in the different quadrants.

Fibroadenomas form a much larger proportion of benign lumps in populations where other aspects of ANDI are less common (69% of benign lumps in Nigeria[6]) although the underlying incidence probably remains the same.

In a comparison of the incidence of benign lesions in three ethnic groups with widely differing breast cancer incidence (Anglo-Americans, Hispanics and American Indians), the incidence of fibroadenoma was similar in all three groups, unlike the incidence of severe hyperplasia, which differs in these three groups.[7] Thus the incidence of simple fibroadenomas appears to be fairly constant across many ethnic groups, a pattern which differs from that of hyperplasias, which are more common in Western populations,

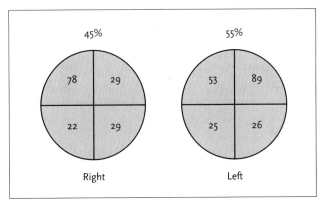

7.2 Distribution of fibroadenomas in breast quadrants – Cardiff series.

and giant fibroadenoma, which is more common in non-Western populations. Whether the apparent increased frequency of fibroadenoma in black populations is real, or merely reflects a large population base, is uncertain.

Pathogenesis

We have already discussed in general terms in Chapters 1 and 3 our reasons for regarding fibroadenoma as part of ANDI, an aberration of normal lobular development rather than a neoplasm. There is good histological evidence that these tumours develop from the breast lobule; for example, elastic tissue is present in ducts but is not present in normal lobules, and elastic tissue is not seen in fibroadenomas.[8] The lobular origin explains many features of fibroadenoma, for instance, why most arise in young women at the time of maximal lobular development and why the stroma forms such a major element in fibroadenomas. This is derived from the hormone-dependent stroma of the lobule and not the simple fibrous stroma of the breast parenchyma. It also explains why many of the (very rare) cases of cancer arising in a fibroadenoma are of the more 'benign' type – lobular carcinoma-in-situ (LCIS).

This concept is supported by the work of Archer and Omar, who found that all the cellular elements of fibroadenoma are normal on conventional histology and electron microscopy.[9] Epithelial and myoepithelial cells maintain a normal relationship. The tumour bulk is due to an increase in fibroblasts, fibrocytes and collagen, and all show normal characteristics. Recent studies give further support from molecular biology.[10,11] Noguchi and co-workers have shown that common fibroadenomas are polyclonal, indicating that they are hyperplasia rather than neoplasia. This is in contrast to fibroadenomas in patients who subsequently developed recurrence in the form of phyllodes tumours, which were found to be monoclonal. The polyclonality of fibroadenomas is seen in both epithelial and stromal elements. The monoclonality of the phyllodes tumour applies only to the stromal element, the epithelial cells remaining polyclonal. These workers suggest that all fibroadenomas begin as polyclonal lesions, but with phyllodes tumours a monoclonal change occurs in the stromal element at an early stage. (If the stroma was monoclonal *de novo*, the phyllodes tumour would be expected to consist of stroma only; this situation is found in the rare pulmonary metastases.) Chromosomal aberrations can be found in 10–20% of fibroadenomas, some of which are also found in breast cancers.[12]

Studies of EGFR (epidermal growth factor receptor) also show a closer relationship between fibroadenoma and normal breast than between fibroadenoma and breast cancer.[13] Study of the expression levels of NM23-H1 messenger RNA in fibroadenoma leads to a similar conclusion.[14] Immunocytochemistry confirms the lobular origin of fibroadenoma, in that the stromal cells show the characteristics of intralobular, as opposed to interlobular, fibroblasts.[15]

Steroid receptors have been studied in fibroadenoma.[16] Oestrogen and progesterone receptors can be demonstrated in relatively low concentrations in both cytoplasm and nucleus. These receptors are more easily demonstrated in fibroadenoma than in other ANDI conditions. Higher levels of oestrogen receptor appear to be associated with epithelial proliferation, and lower levels with stromal cell proliferation.[17] These workers found that progesterone receptors are less related to cellularity, and the overall conclusion was that hormone dependence of fibroadenomas diminishes rapidly as the lesions develop, a further possible explanation for the plateauing in the growth curve. More recently, high levels of oestrogens and their sulphates, as well as sulphatase and aromatase, have been found in fibroadenomas.[18] Prolactin and insulin growth factor 1 receptors are demonstrated in about 50% of cases of fibroadenoma and ANDI.

The aetiology of fibroadenoma is not known, but the fact that lobular proliferation is a response to oestrogen stimulation suggests that it may arise as the result of a lobule becoming unusually responsive to oestrogen. It grows both by proliferation of the lobule and also involvement of adjacent lobules, a fact of relevance to the significant recurrence rate after removal. It is interesting that four fibroadenomas and one phyllodes tumour reported in males from the Armed Forces Institute all occurred in patients with gynaecomastia, who had unusually developed lobule formation.[19] The development of lobules in males apparently requires a greater degree of oestrogenic stimulation than that which commonly induces gynaecomastia.

One interesting hypothesis relates to the finding of increased levels of the *bcl-2* gene in the epithelial cells of fibroadenomas.[20] The gene occurs in a number of tissues and tumours, where it acts to extend cell life by preventing the onset of apoptosis. Thus failure of cell loss by apoptosis could be important in the development of fibroadenoma, although it is surprising that the gene was found only in the epithelial cells, and not in the stromal cells.

The widespread use of the contraceptive pill in young women makes it difficult to obtain accurate data on its role in pathogenesis. There is no evidence that the use of the contraceptive pill increases the risk of developing fibroadenoma and the epidemiological data available suggest that it may be associated with a decreased incidence. A majority of studies show that the risk of developing fibroadenoma is more than halved among those taking the contraceptive pill, particularly long-term users. The epidemiological studies suggest that it is the progestogen element of the combined preparation that is protective.

In this regard, the study by Canny *et al.*[21] is particularly interesting because all ages were investigated in a large case control study, and differing effects were seen. Women less than 45 years showed a decreased incidence of fibroadenoma (OR = 0.57) in association with oral contraceptive use, while those over 45 showed an increased incidence (OR = 1.65 but ns). The difference may be associated with the different age at which oral contraceptive use was started, different formulations or other unknown reasons. Women over 45 taking HRT had a much increased incidence (OR = 2.83

but ns due to small numbers); all patients were on oestrogen alone. No fibroadenoma was seen in seven controls taking a combined pill, again consistent with progesterone being protective.

A negative association between current cigarette smoking (but not former smokers) and fibroadenoma has been reported.[22]

Koerner and O'Connell[23] have taken an opposing view to the ANDI hypothesis and regard fibroadenoma as a neoplasm, largely on the grounds that a human adenovirus 9 may induce a similar lesion in rats.

Pathology

The macroscopic appearance of fibroadenoma is of a sharply demarcated rounded or bosselated tumour with a white, glistening, bulging surface on section (contrasting with the convex cut surface of a cancer). The surface is irregular due to the epithelial-lined clefts which break up the uniformity. It is easily enucleated from its pseudocapsule of compressed breast tissue to which it is attached by a well-defined stalk. If the surface is brownish, phyllodes tumour should be considered.

The histological appearance is very characteristic, consisting of a combination of loose pale stroma and duct-like structures lined by regular epithelial cells. There is a tendency for this to follow one of two broad patterns, to which Cheatle[24] gave the terms 'pericanalicular' and 'intracanalicular'. In the pericanalicular pattern the epithelial structures are abundant, with the appearance of stroma surrounding circular ducts (Figure 7.3a).

In the intracanalicular form (Figure 7.3b), the preponderance of stroma tends to push into elongated epithelial-lined clefts, so that the epithelial clefts now appear to surround islands of stroma. It is now recognized that both patterns are often seen in a single fibroadenoma, and there is no useful purpose in maintaining the differentiation. Varying degrees of epithelial hyperplasia are common and reflected in cytology specimens.

Fibroadenomatoid hyperplasia is a histological pattern of 'microfibroadenomas' occurring as ill-defined areas in the breast, in contrast to the well-defined discrete clinical fibroadenoma. They are best regarded as one part of the spectrum of lobular overgrowth correlating with a spectrum of clinical presentations. While most fibroadenomas in young women are well demarcated and mobile, other areas of lobular overgrowth may be less well demarcated and may even be multicentric; others are no more than a histological finding.

The tissues of a fibroadenoma will respond to external influences in a manner similar to normal breast lobules. Thus they will undergo hyperplastic changes during pregnancy, secrete milk during lactation and involute at the menopause. The hyperplastic changes of pregnancy may outgrow the blood supply, leading to infarction.

It is important to recognize the wide variety of histological changes that may be seen in typical fibroadenomas compared to fewer variations in clinical behaviour. Such histological changes include apocrine and squamous metaplasia, neither of which is significant (except possibly in relation to future cancer risk, as discussed further below). Marked hyperplasia of epithelial elements is also common but does not reflect aggressive behaviour. However, such florid epithelial changes cause trouble to cytologists, and benign fibroadenoma is an important cause of false-positive diagnosis of cancer on cytology in all but the most experienced hands.

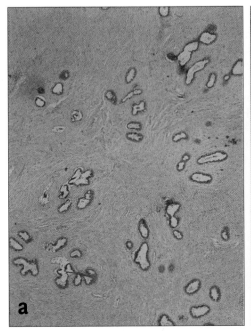 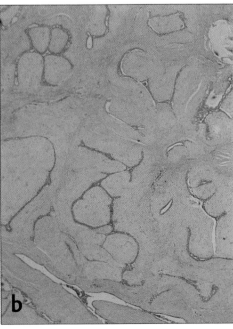

7.3 The histological patterns of pericanalicular (a) and intracanalicular (b) fibroadenomas.

Clinical features

Common clinical presentations

Differing clinical presentations are seen in young girls, during later reproductive life and in postmenopausal women. The clinical features of fibroadenoma are so characteristic in a young woman that the diagnosis can be made with a degree of confidence equalled only by that of a cyst after aspiration. The features are not so characteristic in older women, where the diagnosis should be made with care. One group[25] have reported a diagnostic accuracy of only 50%, reflecting the importance of recognizing the differing clinical signs of fibroadenoma in different age groups.

In the young woman, fibroadenoma is a smooth, round or lobulated, firm discrete swelling with high mobility, giving rise to the term 'breast mouse'. The degree of mobility is truly remarkable, and the diagnosis should be circumspect when a lesser degree of mobility can be demonstrated. One exception to this rule is a fibroadenoma arising behind the nipple, where the surrounding ducts will limit its mobility. (It is not always recognized that there is much lobular tissue behind the areola in many women, explaining the findings that cysts and fibroadenomas, both of lobular derivation, are sometimes found behind the nipple.) The extreme mobility of the tumour in young women is due to encapsulation (Figure 7.4) and to the softness and pliability of breast

stroma in this age group, in spite of the density of the young breast on mammogram.

This also explains why fibroadenomas may appear on palpation to be much more superficial in the breast than their true position, a fact which should lead a surgeon to ensure that adequate facilities are available before embarking on the removal of a fibroadenoma in a young girl under local anaesthetic.

The classic picture is not so obvious in older women, where involutional fibrotic changes surrounding the tumour will decrease its mobility. In this age group, fibroadenoma often masquerades as a dominant mass of ANDI ('fibroadenosis') and is removed as such, the fibroadenoma being revealed only after sectioning (Figure 7.5).

The physical signs of cancer and fibroadenoma may then come much closer together and fibroadenoma should not be diagnosed clinically in this age group until cancer has been excluded unequivocally.

A fibroadenoma is sometimes discovered in an elderly woman as a small, stony, hard, discrete mass, still moderately mobile. At this age the physical characteristics are again so precise that a clinical diagnosis can often be made with confidence. However it can readily be (and must be) confirmed by mammography that the stony-hard consistency is due to calcification (Chapter 6). It is a reasonable assumption that small fibroadenomas discovered in the late reproductive or postmenopausal periods arose many years earlier, remained static, and are then discovered only as a result of involutional changes allowing them to be palpated more readily.

Less common presentations

Very small superficial nodules of fibroadenomatous tissue, 3–4 mm in diameter, are sometimes seen in young women, and often remain unchanged for many years. These are felt only because of their superficial position; similar small static lesions deep in the breast are likely to be present much more frequently than clinically recognized, as borne out by histological study of whole breast sections. Cheatle[24] found small fibroadenomas in 25% of normal breasts.

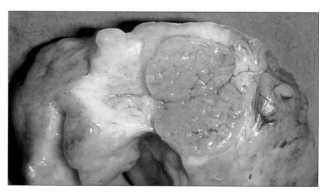

7.4 The typical fibroadenoma of adolescent girls has a well-defined capsule, giving the tumour great mobility.

7.5 A fibroadenoma in a 35-year-old patient. The typical clinical features were obscured by the involutional changes in the surrounding breast tissue.

Increase in size, sometimes marked, is sometimes seen during pregnancy. This may be associated with the general glandular hyperplasia seen in pregnancy, due to infarction or due to stromal hyperplasia.

A few fibroadenomas first become obvious as discrete masses in the late years of reproductive life. These may show a remarkable propensity for growth, rapidly reaching a large size. They have the gross and histological features of a simple fibroadenoma and behave in a benign fashion (but see p. 88). It is interesting that similar rapid growth of a fibroadenoma is also seen in the 13- to 18-year age group, so that 'giant' fibroadenomas tend to have a bimodal distribution at the extremes of reproductive life (Figure 7.6).

Four of the five fibroadenomas in the 11- to 15-year age group in this series were more than 4 cm in diameter, as were about 15% of those between 16 and 25 years. Large tumours are seen less commonly in the next decade but reappear in smaller numbers around the menopause. Even less commonly they may first present during early pregnancy. While giant fibroadenomas in both adolescent and menopausal age groups are uncommon, giant tumours are more common at adolescence than at the menopause.

The infrequency of fibroadenoma after the menopause suggests that they involute with perimenopausal breast involution. During this process they may calcify. Devitt[26] reported a series of 4379 women over 55 years who presented with a breast complaint. Only eight had fibroadenomas, and four of these were calcified. This situation is changing with widespread use of hormone replacement therapy. Occult fibroadenoma in postmenopausal women may be seen to increase in size on imaging when the patients are given unopposed oestrogen as HRT.[27,28]

Thus, simple fibroadenomas fall into four main groups:
- The small, static fibroadenomas of 3–4 mm palpable in the superficial breast.
- The commonest type, which reaches a diameter of 1–3 cm before becoming static. This type comprises 80% of all fibroadenomas and hence must be regarded as the 'norm'.

- The very few giant fibroadenomas of adolescence and the perimenopausal age. These groups are discussed later.
- Fibroadenomas in the 4–5 cm group, which are larger than average but not in the 'giant' range. These comprise about 10% of the total and are distributed fairly evenly over the age range, but form a higher proportion in the perimenarchal and perimenopausal age groups.

Foster et al.[29] investigated whether these larger tumours constitute a different group in terms of histology or behaviour by comparing the cellularity of fibroadenomas of different size groupings. Stromal cells were counted by grey level analysis from a computer-linked TV image. They found no relationship between stromal cellularity and size of fibroadenomas, but cellularity was related to the age of the patient. The mean cell count in patients younger than 20 years was almost double that of older patients, although there was a second lesser increase in stromal cellularity just before the menopause which might be explained by the stimulation of unopposed oestrogen at this time. Thus larger tumours did not appear to be related to cellularity and there is no obvious reason at present why some fibroadenomas should grow to a larger size than average. There is also no reason to treat these larger fibroadenomas differently, nor in our series did they have a particular tendency to recur or to be multiple. Similarly, when Noguchi and co-workers identified fibroadenomas which later recurred as phyllodes tumours, the original fibroadenomas had not shown any peculiarity in relation to size or multiplicity.[11]

Special investigations
Mammography
Mammography is best avoided in younger women, both on grounds of poor diagnostic yield in the dense breast of this age and because of the radiation risk. Certainly it is not indicated in the diagnosis of fibroadenoma under the age of 35.

In the older patient, fibroadenoma can be seen as a solitary smooth lesion, of similar density to the surrounding breast tissue when small, and more dense when large. When small it may be difficult to detect, except as a smooth border

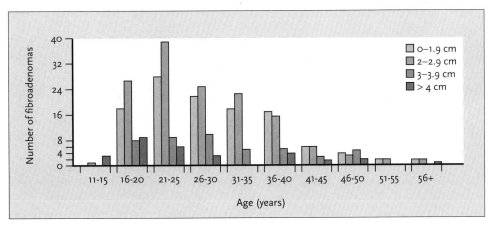

7.6 Size of fibroadenomas related to age at presentation. Large fibroadenomas tend to occur at the extremes of reproductive life. (Reproduced from Foster et al.[29] by courtesy of the Journal of the Royal College of Surgeons of Edinburgh.)

outlined by the mammary fat. It may be surrounded by a halo of compressed fat, when the diagnosis is easier. The radiological appearance may be identical to that of a cyst, but needle aspiration will readily differentiate the two.

In the postmenopausal period, at least half of all fibroadenomas will show typical stippled ('popcorn') calcification, similar to that seen in a uterine fibroid (see Chapter 6).

Ultrasonography (see Chapter 6)

The ultrasonic features of fibroadenoma have been reviewed by Cole-Beuglet et al.[30] They include a round or oval sharp contour, weak internal echoes in a uniform distribution and intermediate attenuation. Ultrasound does not always distinguish these from other masses with certainty. Claims that Duplex spectral Doppler, and more recently colour Doppler, will reliably differentiate from cancer have not been confirmed.[31] At present, a number of new Doppler processing techniques are under investigation.[32]

Cytology

The typical cytological appearance of fibroadenoma can be recognized by experienced cytologists. Aspirates vary greatly in cellularity, from scanty to an abundance of epithelial and stromal cells. The epithelium forms broad sheets that are uniform, equally spaced and cohesive (Figure 7.7).

Cohesive cells typically show branching epithelial structures resembling 'antler horns' and 'bare nuclei' are evident. In less experienced hands, the hyperplastic epithelium typical of fibroadenoma may suggest a malign significance which is not justified by behaviour. Indeed, fibroadenomas are the main cause of false-positive cytology reports. Cytology is not necessary in a young patient (<25 years) with a typical fibroadenoma, but FNAC (and even core needle biopsy) should be used where the features are not entirely typical, because cysts, galactoceles and other lesions are occasionally seen in this age group. Cytology is indicated in older women.

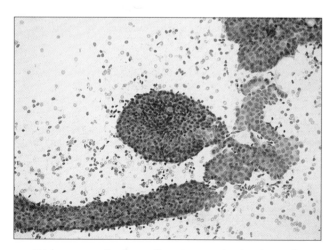

7.7 Cytology preparation from a fibroadenoma, showing sheets of cohesive epithelial cells against a background of 'bare' nuclei.

Management

The management of fibroadenoma is presently in a state of flux, and when this is the case there is a tendency for swings from one extreme to another to occur. With such a common condition, it is important to try to maintain a balance between an excessively reactionary approach (removing every fibroadenoma) and the opposite approach of treating all conservatively, without considering all facets of the problem.

It is useful to look backward as well as forward. Following our postulate that fibroadenoma is a part of ANDI rather than a tumour, we gradually took a more conservative approach during the 1970s and 1980s, as presented in the following extract from the first edition of this book[33]:

> Most textbooks in the past have recommended removal of all fibroadenomas, irrespective of age or other considerations. Yet most fibroadenomas are self-limiting and many go undiagnosed. In practice, solitary fibroadenomas in young women are usually removed on diagnosis, to alleviate patient concern. However, it is not unreasonable to take a flexible attitude related to age group. In women under the age of 25, cancer is so rare that a typical fibroadenoma can be left with impunity. However, our own approach is to remove the tumour if the patient wishes to be rid of it, but to watch it for 6 months if she wishes to avoid operation.

We prefer this flexible approach in patients under the age of 25, and if triple assessment is used and unequivocally benign, the patient may be discharged without follow-up, being advised to return should the lump increase in size. While triple assessment is not mandatory, or even necessary for classical fibroadenomas in this age group, a tendency for inexperienced surgeons to regard all masses in young women as fibroadenomas without assessing the physical signs leads some to consider it safer to investigate all fibroadenomas at any age.

In the past we have preferred a bias towards removal of fibroadenomas in women over 25 years. However, with greater use of core needle biopsy to provide definitive histology, fibroadenomas may be treated conservatively at any age. Wilkinson and Forrest[25] and Dixon and colleagues[34] undertook studies where all fibroadenomas in patients under the age of 35 were observed, provided cytology was negative. This carried some risk of missing cancers, as they found in their preliminary study – they did not utilize image-guided core needle biopsy. Cant et al.[35] considered the same question, and concluded that a conservative policy is safe in women under the age of 25 years, although they found that 'a majority would prefer excision'.

The situation has changed greatly over the past decade as the result of many factors, the influence of the ANDI concept, greater use of sonography and core needle biopsy, and the fruition of the studies following on from the above papers.

If conservative therapy is to be accepted, three requirements need to be satisfied.
- The natural history is consonant with conservation.
- It is safe for the patient.
- The patient finds it acceptable.

The studies outlined above demonstrate that many fibroadenomas are static or regress spontaneously, and so are suitable for conservation.

The safety of conservation has been assessed in a prospective study[34] in which the criteria for conservation were age <40 years and a clinical diagnosis confirmed by cytology and ultrasound (and mammography if >35 years). Ninety per cent of patients opted for conservation and were monitored regularly; excision was advised if the volume increased by 20%, as occurred in 8% of the patients. Patients were discharged after 2 years if the lesion remained static or regressed. No mass under observation proved to be a cancer, and the authors regard the criteria as defining a safe policy. Provision of histology by core needle biopsy can further increase safety. However, some reservations must remain because of the limited follow-up, and 20% of patients defaulted from observation before reaching that point.

Dent and Cant[3] followed a smaller series of patients (<30 years). No cancers were missed or developed, but 53 of the 85 fibroadenomas originally treated conservatively came to excision; none were malignant. Hence, present evidence is that a conservative policy is reasonably safe, with the reservations noted, and recognizing that the results during a special study in a specialized unit may not translate to routine clinical practice.

Different groups interpret patient acceptance in different ways. Dixon and colleagues claim 90% acceptance, in spite of 20% of the patients defaulting. Dent and Cant found that 73% of patients requested operation. Counselling techniques undoubtedly influence patients' preferences and a confident clinician will lead most women to accept conservation. It is also easy to underestimate the ongoing concern experienced by some women who continue to palpate a lump in their breast over years, during repeated campaigns counselling them not to ignore breast lumps.

How can one summarize to give a reasonable, pragmatic policy? Certainly, many fewer fibroadenomas need be removed than was previously the case, but it would be wrong to insist on a rigid conservative policy for all.

For women less than 25 years, risk of malignancy is negligible, especially after triple assessment if clinical features are at all atypical, while the incidence of unsightly hypertrophic scars is higher in this age group. Hence a patient can be reassured and counselled towards a conservative policy. The patient can be instructed to return if the lump increases in size, otherwise there is little point in seeing the patient again.

The situation is similar for women of 25–30, but now the small risk of cancer makes routine triple assessment mandatory.

For patients of 30–40 years the balance is a little different, although management need not differ. Scars are usually excellent, while the risk of cancer is significant, especially if there is a meaningful family history of cancer. The risk of litigation is ever present. Thus the approach to these patients will depend on the demonstrated accuracy of triple assessment in the individual clinic, and the enthusiasm with which the patient accepts conservative management. If there is doubt regarding the nature of the presumed fibroadenoma it is easy to perform ultrasound-guided wide bore core biopsy which will give a definitive histological diagnosis. A minority of patients may prefer a definitive minor procedure under local anaesthesia to the concern of carrying a breast lump. Others will welcome the option of avoiding surgery. Since most patients with a lump attend in order to obtain a definitive exclusion of cancer, they should be allowed to express their own views freely. Two contrasting policies are given by Dixon et al.[34] and Alle et al.,[36] and an individual clinician will be able to assess the data given to form a policy appropriate to the individual institution.

Comparing the policy advocated 10 years ago to that in this second edition, it is clear that the principles have changed very little, and hence are likely to be sound. What has changed practice is the arrival of ultrasound, cytology and core needle biopsy in the clinic, to give a 'one-stop breast assessment' which has led to much better diagnostic accuracy, and with it the opportunity for many more fibroadenomas to be treated conservatively.

Transformation of a fibroadenoma to a phyllodes tumour is an extremely rare occurrence, but it would be desirable to identify such a tumour within a conservative management policy. Noguchi and colleagues have demonstrated that it is not possible to do so on the basis of age, or tumour size, multiplicity or conventional histology.[11] They were able to do so in their small series by clonal analysis, and claim that the technique could be reliably performed on fine needle aspiration specimens. Perhaps this may become a practical procedure in the future, at least in those fibroadenomas that show progression on ultrasound monitoring.

Hormonal therapy

There has been a tendency on the European continent to treat fibroadenomas, along with other breast masses, by hormonal therapy, using tamoxifen, danazol and progestogens among others (e.g. Cupceancu[37]). It is difficult to assess results because of the lack of histological diagnosis or long-term follow-up, and less has been written of this in recent years. We have not followed this practice because of the uncertain long-term effects of hormonal manipulation, especially with tamoxifen, in young women. With technological advances appearing in rapid succession, it is inevitable that new therapies will be tried out; an example is laser treatment.[38]

Recurrence after surgery

New fibroadenomas which appear after removal of a previous tumour are often referred to as recurrent tumours, but this is a loose term and covers at least three groups.

Recurrence at the site of previous removal may represent incomplete removal, or adjacent lobules undergoing the same process. Some surgeons believe that removing the base of the 'stalk' lessens the risk of recurrence and this seems a reasonable step to take.

Newly noted tumours in the same or opposite breast represent the multiplicity of fibroadenomas often seen on careful histological examination of 'normal' breasts. Clinical experience suggests that multiple fibroadenomas may be occurring more frequently in recent years, although there are few firm data to support this.

It is not unknown for the original tumour to be missed and an adjacent area of nodularity excised, particularly if the operation is not carried out by the surgeon who examined the patient before operation. It is important that the surgeon is familiar with the site and characteristics of the lesion before the patient goes to theatre. Ultrasound localization will help in difficult cases.

In the Cardiff series of 322 patients, 23 patients are known to have developed a further tumour during follow-up, with an interval of 1–6 years (mean 2.6 years), 16 in the same breast and 7 in the opposite. Of the 16 'recurrent' tumours in the same breast, 9 were at the same site and 7 elsewhere. Recurrence at the same site was not related to the size of the fibroadenoma, nor to use of the contraceptive pill. Two of these patients have developed a carcinoma during the follow-up period, neither at the site of the fibroadenoma. During the same period, 7 cases of phyllodes tumour were also treated, none of which had recurred at the time of the study, but one has recently recurred after an interval of 8 years.

Local recurrence of fibroadenoma is best excised because of the small risk of a more active tumour.

New tumours elsewhere in the breast are managed on the same principles as for the original tumour. The very rare syndrome of very large numbers of fibroadenomas (i.e. more than five in a single breast) needs to be managed on an individual basis, as discussed below.

Variations in histological appearance of fibroadenoma

Pregnancy

Fibroadenomas frequently show increase in size during pregnancy and secretory changes during lactation, and may show involution after parturition. Moran[39] described 10 cases removed during pregnancy. Azzopardi[8] describes cases showing similar secretory changes to those of lactation in patients receiving large doses of progestogens.

Infarction

Infarction is a complication most commonly seen during pregnancy and lactation. It is usually asymptomatic, but may lead to an increase in size, raising the spectre of lactational cancer. Unrecognized infarction may well be the cause of the calcified fibroadenomas characteristically seen in the elderly patient. Wilkinson and Green[40] report 10 cases of infarction of fibroadenomas but infarction of 'normal' breast tissue can also occur in pregnancy[41] and may be misdiagnosed as cancer. Not surprisingly, infarction has also been reported following fine needle aspiration.

Sclerosing adenosis

This may occur in a fibroadenoma and present some difficulty in histological assessment, but has no other implications for clinical management, except that it is one of the signs of a 'complex' fibroadenoma carrying a slight increased risk of future breast cancer.[42]

Myxoid fibroadenoma

Myxoid change may occur in any fibroadenoma, but a special, hereditary condition in which fibroadenomas may be associated with myxomas of the heart and skin has been described[43] (Carney syndrome). It is important to recognize this condition because of the dangers of atrial myxoma; about 25% of patients present first with the breast lesions.

Juvenile fibroadenoma

Ashikari et al.[44] studied 181 fibroadenomas in adolescent females and picked out 12 which they regarded as being floridly glandular and with a more cellular stroma. They gave these the name of 'juvenile fibroadenoma', but there is no uniformity of opinion among pathologists as to the specificity of this subgroup and it remains to be determined whether the histological picture they describe has a special clinical significance. The term is best avoided in favour of the clinical term of giant fibroadenoma of adolescence, which is considered on page 85.

Adenoma of the breast

There has long been argument as to whether or not a true adenoma of the breast exists, or whether these tumours just represent epithelial dominance in a fibroadenoma. More recently it has been accepted as a distinct entity.[45] Tubular adenoma is a benign, circumscribed, 2–3-cm brownish-yellow tumour occurring mainly in young women. Histologically it shows closely packed tubules of uniform, benign, two-layer epithelium. These lesions may also lactate in association with pregnancy. They are discussed further on pages 52 and 244.

Fibroadenoma with multinucleated stromal giant cells (MSGCs)

MSGCs may be found in otherwise unremarkable breast tissue, but Powell et al.[46] report 11 cases of fibroepithelial tumours containing these cells. They conclude that the presence of MSGCs, whether in simple fibroadenoma or in phyllodes tumour, does not affect behaviour. The tumours should be assessed on the normal criteria applied to the stroma, ignoring the MSGCs.

CANCER AND FIBROADENOMA

Cancer in a fibroadenoma

There are three aspects of the relationship of fibroadenoma and malignancy which require consideration: the association of cancer with a fibroadenoma, the incidence of subsequent breast cancer in patients with a fibroadenoma and the possible progression of fibroadenoma to phyllodes tumour. The last is dealt with elsewhere in this chapter.

The common presence of epithelial hyperplasia in fibroadenomas, which is of no serious import, has led to overdiagnosis of cancer in the past. It is now recognized that exuberant hyperplasia is not of great significance.[8] Cancer is rare; Haagensen found only two true cases in the Columbia records over a 45-year period, both of which were LCIS. He points out that many of the reported cases are cancer adjacent to a fibroadenoma, multifocal cancer also involving a fibroadenoma, or low-grade lobular neoplasia of questionable malignancy. LCIS has classically been regarded as the common type, as would be expected from the lobular origin of fibroadenoma, but a recent series[47] of 105 cases found equal frequencies of lobular and ductal carcinoma-in-situ (95% of cases were in-situ cancer). The mean age of the patients was 44 years, and the clinical characteristics usually did not differ from those without cancer. In the rare cases with invasive cancer, carcinoma-in-situ is usually present also, suggesting this as the origin of the invasive cancer.

Haagensen[2] reports two cases of LCIS treated conservatively, i.e. by local excision, without further trouble. In the series reported by Diaz and colleagues[47] only one of 26 patients treated conservatively for in-situ cancer developed ipsilateral invasive cancer and the prognosis for all patients treated conservatively or by mastectomy was excellent. If LCIS is found in a fibroadenoma after enucleation, it would seem prudent to do a further local excision to determine whether the carcinoma is present in the surrounding breast and then treat it accordingly.

Ductal carcinoma often occurs in association with fibroadenoma rather than confined to it, and takes two forms: (a) direct infiltration from an adjacent cancer and (b) cancerization of the fibroadenoma by tumour growing along the duct into the epithelial clefts, a process analogous to the cancerization of lobules by duct cancer. In either case, the fibroadenoma should be ignored in deciding on a treatment policy for the cancer. In all cases treated conservatively, the patient should be entered into a screening programme for both breasts. The subject of cancer arising in fibroadenoma has been reviewed.[48] A rare oddity is spread of a distant primary tumour to a fibroadenoma, and metastasis of a medulloblastoma to a fibroadenoma has been reported.[49]

Fibroadenoma and subsequent cancer risk

Until recently, there was no strong evidence that the presence of a fibroadenoma is associated with an increased risk of subsequent cancer. In a follow-up of 322 fibroadenomas[29] only two cancers were found, and neither related to the site of the fibroadenoma. Several series have now reported a slight increase in subsequent cancer (with a relative risk <2).

Dupont and colleagues[42] recently reported a large retrospective study of this question and concluded that there is no increased risk for a patient with a simple fibroadenoma and no family history of breast cancer. Patients with a complex fibroadenoma and a family history of breast cancer had a relative risk of 3–4 times. This relative risk persisted for decades after diagnosis. Complex fibroadenoma was defined as those showing cysts, sclerosing adenosis, epithelial calcifications or papillary apocrine change. Patients with a complex fibroadenoma often carried similar changes in the surrounding breast tissue if this was included in the specimen. Since a fibroadenoma carries the same lobular elements as the normal breast, which are under the same influences, it is not surprising that a fibroadenoma should sometimes show the same changes, and carry the same significance.

A second study from Switzerland gave an overall relative risk of 1.6 for all fibroadenomas,[50] and two other studies have given confirmatory results. However, the breakdown of Dupont's study into specific subsets is more meaningful, since this suggests that simple (non-complex) fibroadenomas in patients with no family history of breast cancer carry no excess risk, and this group constitutes a majority of patients.

Ciatto et al.[51] have made the interesting observation that only excised fibroadenomas are associated with an increased risk; those diagnosed and managed conservatively are not.

At present, the bulk of evidence indicates an increased incidence of breast cancer to a degree which is of biological interest, but not sufficient to alter management. The definition of a significant subgroup by confirmation of the work of Dupont and colleagues should be a priority for further research.

MULTIPLE FIBROADENOMAS

Fibroadenomas are often multiple to the extent of three or even four developing concurrently or successively in both breasts. This is sufficiently common to be regarded as part of the 'normal spectrum', so that a pragmatic definition of multiple fibroadenomas as a separate entity would be more than five separate lesions in an individual breast. Haagensen[2] reported an incidence of more than one tumour of 16% among both white and black patients in his series, and points out that this is a minimal figure because the patients are not followed long term.

Our experience in Cardiff is similar. Seven per cent of patients had 2–4 tumours on presentation, and 7% had a further fibroadenoma either before or after the diagnosis for this survey.[29] One-third of the metachronous tumours occurred in the same quadrant as the first fibroadenoma, with an average time of 4 years to the second presentation. The mean age of these patients was 4 years less than those with single tumours. All these figures must be regarded as understatements, because complete follow-up of patients is very difficult in this age group and many tumours undoubtedly go unnoticed. It has been suggested that multiple fibroadenomas are more common in non-white populations. While we have seen this in a very small number of such cases there are few hard data to quantify this.

Multiple fibroadenomas as a distinct entity

If a cut-off point of more than five fibroadenomas in one breast is used to define a specific entity, such an entity is very uncommon in white populations in Western countries, although much higher numbers of fibroadenomas are sometimes reported in black and oriental populations. In spite of this general perception of a high frequency in black and oriental patients, attempts to obtain hard confirmatory data from those working among such populations has proved unrewarding. Otu[6] reported 8% fibroadenomas as multiple in Nigeria, a figure similar to the 7% reported in Cardiff, although the actual numbers in each case are not given. Personal enquiries we have made from West Africa, India, China and the West Indies suggest that the situation does not differ greatly from that seen in Western populations, with most cases of multiplicity falling into the 2–4 range (and some cases being small numbers of giant fibroadenomas rather than more than five). Such cases as have been reported tend to have a familial basis, and are not associated with the contraceptive pill.[2,52] An exception to this is South Africa: Cant and Dent have provided us with unpublished data from their clinic where 11 patients aged 15–29 had more than five fibroadenomas in one breast out of a total of approximately 350 non-white patients with fibroadenoma. This would suggest an increased incidence in their population. None had been on the contraceptive pill before developing a fibroadenoma.

Individual patients may show bizarre features. One 28-year-old Indian woman from Trinidad has had a total of 200 fibroadenomas removed over 6 years from the left breast and 10 (6 years earlier) from the right breast. They continue to form in the left breast, but not in the right. The patient's sister had a smaller (normal range) of fibroadenomas. As this surgeon has seen three cases of multiple fibroadenomas, it would seem possible that this condition is also more common in the West Indies (Dr Naraynsingh, Trinidad, personal communication).

The situation in white populations in Western countries is poorly documented. Williamson et al. from Cardiff[53] reported a single case, and proposed that a register of such cases should be set up. Only two further cases were submitted in response to this request, one in Britain and one in Australia. A recent follow-up is available on all three patients.

The patient originally reported,[53] a single, white, nulliparous female with no family history of breast disease, developed three fibroadenomas at the age of 18. At the time of development she had not been taking oral contraceptives. When removed, each lesion was a simple fibroadenoma.

Over the following 10 years, she developed a further 22 between 5 and 30 mm in diameter, well distributed through both breasts. All have been treated conservatively, and have been followed with ultrasound assessment. Over the past 8 years, only one new lesion has arisen in a quadrant of the breast previously unaffected, while the other 22 have remained static or shown slight regression.

A second similar patient has had each lesion excised as it has become obtrusive. Over 50 lesions have been excised over 20 years and she continues to develop further lesions. The third patient presented with six typical lesions in one breast at the age of 30. A single lesion had been removed from the opposite breast at the age of 21. There has been no recurrence 6 years after excision of the six lesions.

In all three cases the fibroadenomas were typical on clinical, ultrasound and histological examination. All three patients were white, none had a history of breast cancer, and none had been taking oral contraceptives at the time the first lesions presented. Haagensen reported a single case in his book, and the few other reports have been of a single case. It is hoped that future prospective studies will make these anecdotal data redundant.

An interesting recent development is the recognition that multiple fibroadenomas may occur in patients taking cyclosporin as an immunosuppressive agent. This was first noted briefly in 1980[54] but a recent paper[55] gives clearer evidence. The study reported on 29 women (none of African or Asian origin) taking cyclosporin for more than one year. Of these, 43% had fibroadenomas, usually more than one and often bilateral, which were palpable in 11, and found only on ultrasound in two. No breast abnormality was found in 10 patients on azothiaprine/steroids alone; fibroadenomas were multiple in 10 of 13 patients, and bilateral in five. Four patients had more than five fibroadenomas in total. The patients with fibroadenomas tended to be younger and with more recent transplants compared to those without, but there was no clear relationship to dosage or duration of cyclosporin. The masses resolved in one patient in the first study after ceasing cyclosporin, but this was not seen in the second study.

A further patient recently notified to us from Switzerland developed multiple fibroadenomas (17 in the left breast and 6 in the right) after 4 years of treatment with cyclosporin following liver transplantation.

Although the mechanism is not clear, it is considered to be hormonal. Serum follicle-stimulating hormone (FSH) levels were significantly lower, and prolactin and oestradiol levels tended to be higher in patients with fibroadenoma. Such a hormonal effect could be a direct effect of cyclosporin, or a secondary one.

Multiple giant fibroadenomas

This is a rare condition which combines features of both multiple and giant fibroadenomas.[56] It occurs mainly in young adolescent, usually black, girls. Growth of the masses is rapid during adolescence, but slows during adult life. It is usually bilateral, but can be unilateral.[57] Rapid enlargement of multiple giant fibroadenomas may be one of the causes of gigantism of pregnancy.[58]

Any form of conservative management is problematical because of the high incidence of new lesions during the active growth phase. Management should be individualized on the basis of the extent of morbidity, with initial policy concentrating on attempts to conserve breast tissue by enucleating individual lesions.[59] However, in general, it is inevitable that some will need mastectomy to obtain reasonable symptomatic control.

GIANT FIBROADENOMA

Giant fibroadenoma is predominantly a condition of the extremes of reproductive life, the first 5 years after the menarche and a decade before the menopause, and occurs when a fibroadenoma keeps growing beyond the usual l–3 cm diameter. Fibroadenoma is designated 'giant' on the basis of its clinical size alone. This is a matter of definition which has varied widely in the past, some authors suggesting a weight of 500 g, some a diameter of 5 cm and others a 10-cm diameter. In practice, most tumours are closer to 10 cm than 5 cm and sudden growth in size is a dominant feature of adolescent tumours. Since the great majority of common fibroadenomas reach only 2–3 cm in size, greater than 5 cm seems a reasonable definition to pick out this group, particularly when associated with rapid growth. Ashikari et al.[44] combined cellularity of the stroma with size but this is confusing. Size and histology are better kept separate, because clinical behaviour in young girls does not parallel histological appearance. Giant fibroadenomas should be considered in relation to age: adolescent or perimenopausal.

Nomenclature

The nomenclature and definition used for this disorder are often confused due to the loose employment of three terms: giant and/or juvenile fibroadenoma, cystosarcoma phyllodes and sarcoma. Haagensen[2] set out clearly the histological features of the main groups, showing that giant fibroadenoma, phyllodes tumour and sarcoma should be defined on histological features only. His classification has been endorsed by Azzopardi[8] with a significant modification, that the term 'cystosarcoma' be dropped because these tumours are so rarely malignant.

This view is now achieving general acceptance and three terms are thus used for breast tumours with a conspicuous stromal element:

(1)   fibroadenoma;
(2)   phyllodes tumour and sarcoma;
(3)   'pure' sarcoma of the breast.

Phyllodes tumour carries a benign connotation but phyllodes sarcoma is malignant, the differentiation being made on the degree of cytological aberration; both are tumours showing a combination of stromal and epithelial tissues. The term 'phyllodes sarcoma' should be used sparingly and take cognizance of the benign behaviour of most phyllodes tumours, especially in the young. Pure sarcoma is a tumour of connective tissue only. It behaves in a much more malignant fashion than phyllodes sarcoma, and is outside the scope of this book.

The entity of 'juvenile fibroadenoma' is not easily defined. The term has usually been used to designate a fibroadenoma in adolescence which grows rapidly and often reaches a large size, but some authors (e.g. Ashikari et al.[44]) describe histological features which they feel are specific to a subgroup of fibroadenomas in this age group. However, as discussed above, this histological specificity is not generally accepted and there is at present no agreement that juvenile fibroadenoma is a distinct histological group. There is no advantage to the term over a simple classification on the basis of size alone.

Giant fibroadenoma of adolescence[60]

This is a rare but important condition where an unusually large fibroadenoma occurs at or within a few years of puberty. It may be defined more precisely as a fibroadenoma-like tumour greater than 5 cm in diameter and presenting between the ages of 11 and 20 years. The importance of the group lies in the presentation and management. At presentation the diagnostic problems range from failure to detect an abnormality, to confusion with malignancy or virginal hypertrophy. Management has been obscured by unnecessary confusion with other related clinicopathological entities, including phyllodes tumour, and particularly the fibroadenomatous tumours seen later in life.

Giant fibroadenomas in this age group may be associated with multiple fibroadenomas, but usually only one enlarges to a great degree. Nambiar and Kannan-Kutty[61] regarded giant fibroadenoma as a more or less distinct clinicopathological variant, but our own studies show no great difference (apart from the size) in disease behaviour or cellularity when compared with smaller fibroadenomas.[29] It is important that this condition be recognized as benign and that it be separated from phyllodes tumour or phyllodes sarcoma.

Nambiar and Kannan-Kutty[61] reported 25 cases and found a further 61 in the literature. They reported no recurrence or distant metastases, but their own 25 patients were all Chinese, Malays or Indians. Haagensen reports seven cases, of which five were in black patients. Cases reported from Hong Kong do not show great differences between Chinese and white patients; this is discussed further in Chapter 22. We have treated four patients aged 14–16 and one aged 18,[60] all white. Further more recent reports are given below.

An extreme form of single giant fibroadenoma is also occasionally seen in pregnancy as one form of gigantomastia, and is discussed in Chapter 15.

Clinical features

Although the clinical features of giant fibroadenoma of adolescence are varied, there is a remarkable overall similarity in the features described in all publications on this subject. Onset at or soon after puberty, sudden growth, prominent veins and occasional skin ulceration due to pressure are typical. Patients frequently report cyclical changes in the affected breast with premenstrual pain and increased breast size and tension during menstruation. The growths are unilateral, but it is not uncommon for a fibroadenoma of conventional size to present at the same time or later in the opposite breast.

It might be thought that a giant tumour would be diagnosed without difficulty, but this is not always the case. It often occurs at the time of rapid breast development and the mass is obscured by this development. If the consistency of the mass is similar to that of normal breast it may be regarded merely as asymmetry of the breasts (Figure 7.8).

In other cases it may be clear that there is a well-defined mass, firmer than the rest of the breast (Figures 7.9 and 7.10).

In the third group, malignancy is simulated by such rapid growth that there are large dilated veins present over the mass (Figure 7.11).

Pressure necrosis of the overlying skin may occur, so that carcinoma or sarcoma is diagnosed.

Multiple giant tumours are uncommon, as discussed on page 84

Pathology

A wide spectrum of changes in both epithelial and connective tissue elements is found in these tumours. The epithelial element may show varying degrees of hyperplasia, while the stroma varies from fibrous to cellular, with or without mitotic activity, and thus may embrace the spectrum of phyllodes tumour. However, significant cellular atypia is not a feature, and this is important. In our experience, a number of cases have been referred with cytology or histology reports where the pathologist has considered the appearance as sufficiently worrying to recommend wider excision or mastectomy. Where such a report is given in an adolescent patient, further opinions should be sought from pathologists of great experience as these tumours act in a clinically benign fashion, even though clinical and histological features at first sight may suggest malignancy.[8]

The aetiology is obscure, and although a hormonal basis would be expected, there is little direct evidence to support this. There is no clear relationship to the contraceptive pill, with none of the Durban patients taking it.[62]

Race

A review of the literature implies that these tumours are more common in black and oriental races, and discussion with surgeons working in countries with these populations would suggest that this might be true in some parts of Africa and the West Indies, but the situation is not clear-cut (see Chapter 22). The series of 47 cases (25% of all fibroadenomas in this age group) treated in a single unit in Durban over a 6-year period were all black or Indian.[62] It is significant that any reports of malignancy in tumours in this age group have been in black or oriental races, so the tumours should be treated more cautiously in these groups than need be the case in white patients. However, it would still appear that the vast majority of adolescent tumours in all races are benign in their clinical behaviour.

Management

Age is of great importance in assessing giant breast tumours; for practical purposes these lesions in adolescence are always benign. Our small series of six cases[60] showed no recurrence, and the literature supports the view that in

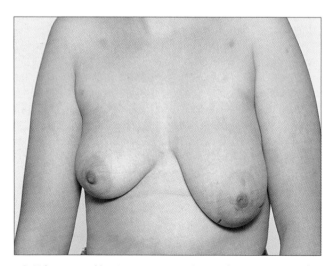

7.8 Eighteen-year-old patient presenting with recent breast asymmetry. She was unaware of the presence of a large discrete mass in the left breast.

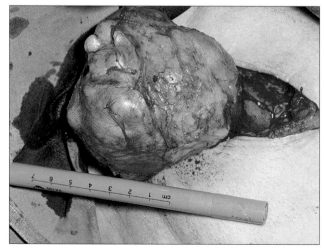

7.9 An 8-cm fibroadenoma at operation.

white adolescent patients, discrete giant tumours, which contain both epithelial and connective tissue elements, have a uniformly benign clinical behaviour even though they may have a wide spectrum of histological appearances.[63] Some of the tumours in our series had a typical fibroadenoma appearance on histology, others had an appearance indistinguishable from benign phyllodes tumour. There do not appear to have been any reports of local recurrence or malignancy in such tumours in white patients of this age group, and age takes precedence over histological assessment in adolescence.

It is reasonable to treat these lesions, on the basis of clinical diagnosis, by enucleation. Mammography and biopsy do not influence the treatment and may even lead to a false diagnosis of malignancy and consideration of unnecessarily radical treatment. Clearly a different attitude will be taken to tumours in patients over the age of 20, and perhaps young patients of non-white races, although the available evidence from black and Indian patients suggests that malignancy is rare in these groups.[61,62]

Giant fibroadenomas tend to be deeper in the breast than is clinically apparent and, for this reason, are best approached from behind through a submammary incision (the Gaillard–Thomas approach; see Chapter 20). This gives an excellent cosmetic result, and with negligible damage to breast ductal tissue. With large tumours, the remaining breast exists only as a compressed rim around the periphery, but this may be expected to expand and lead to a breast of roughly normal size and contour (Figures 7.12 and 7.13).

More radical surgery is not indicated in this age group, irrespective of histological findings, because recurrence is a clinical curiosity in white patients, even when histological features cause concern. Nambiar and Kannan-Kutty recommend excision with a margin of normal tissue, similar to that which many authors, including ourselves, would advocate for phyllodes tumour in older patients. They recommend this in contradistinction to enucleation, which they advise against. However, it is not clear how local excision is achieved. With larger tumours the normal breast exists as a thin compressed rim around the tumour and excision would be tantamount to a simple mastectomy, the operation that is necessary for large phyllodes tumours in older women. No recurrence was reported in the Durban series, although follow-up was incomplete.[62]

Simple mastectomy as recommended and practised in the case reported by Holbrook and Ramsay[64] is certainly to be condemned. Complex reconstructive procedures, such as the insertion of a de-epithelialized flap and silicone prosthesis as recommended by Hoffman,[65] are also inappropriate. Such an approach ignores the fact that the breast remnant rapidly returns to normal after removal of the fibroadenoma (Figure 7.13), a process which might well be inhibited by an implant. Even closure of the cavities by sutures is unnecessary and may lead to breast distortion. Any reconstructive approach should be left until full spontaneous recovery has occurred, since this may be expected with considerable confidence.[60,62]

Giant breast tumours of the perimenopausal period

Giant tumours of the breast show a second peak of incidence in the pre- and perimenopausal period. Such tumours

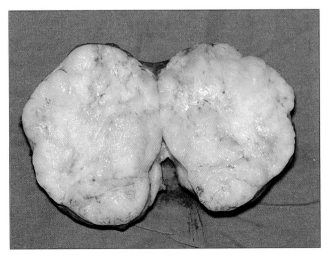

7.10 Macroscopic cut surface of tumour seen in Figure 7.9.

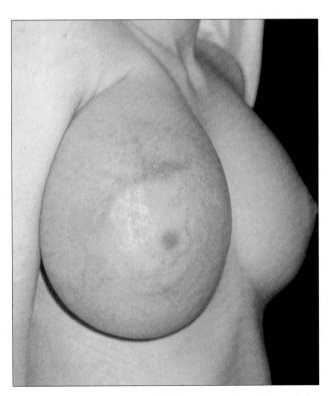

7.11 Benign giant fibroadenoma of adolescence. Rapid growth, vascularity and pressure skin necrosis raised the question of malignancy.

need careful clinical and histological assessment to put them in one of five categories:

- Giant fibroadenoma
- Recurrent and progressive fibroadenoma
- Phyllodes tumour and phyllodes sarcoma
- Pure sarcoma
- Carcinoma.

The last two are outside the scope of this book.

Giant fibroadenoma

A large tumour which clearly has the histological features of a benign fibroadenoma will usually behave in a benign fashion. It may be treated as a fibroadenoma of normal type in younger age groups, although it may not enucleate because of associated involutional fibrosis in the surrounding breast.

Recurrent and progressive fibroadenoma

This is a rare but important variant characterized by multicentricity and recurrence after surgical excision. In reported cases, there has been a tendency to increasing histological activity on succeeding biopsies. One case under our care is typical of cases reported in the literature.

A female patient, born 1935, presented in 1964 with a 3 x 2-cm nodule, which was excised and reported on histology as a benign fibroadenoma. In 1967 she presented

again with gross nodularity of the breast. Most of the tissue of the right breast was involved in a nodular process, which was treated by removal of three-quarters of the breast tissue. Histologically it was found to consist of 'fibroadenosis' mixed with nodules of benign fibroadenoma up to 5 cm in diameter. In 1973 the breast was back to its original size (Figure 7.14) and gross nodularity led to removal of one-quarter of the breast mass.

The macroscopic description was 'tough fibroadenosis' but the histology again showed benign fibroadenomatous tissue.

In 1978 the patient was seen in our unit. Further gross nodularity of the breast and marked discomfort led to a biopsy of the largest (5-cm) mass which showed a fibroadenoma in which 'the spindle cell fibrous stroma differs from previous biopsies and now has undoubted hallmarks of malignancy'. Simple mastectomy was performed and the whole breast was found to be replaced by a huge fibroadenomatous mass. In 1987 the patient was well, with no evidence of local or distant recurrence.

This very rare case probably represents a progression of benign fibroadenoma to malignancy that constitutes the exception rather than the rule. Even so, the degree of malignancy is low, unlike that of primary sarcoma of the breast.

Fibroadenomatoid hyperplasia

This is a condition in which the breast contains multiple foci that are histologically identical to fibroadenoma, but not necessarily well defined from the surrounding breast. The spectrum extends from a minor histological finding, where fibroadenoma and 'fibroadenosis' overlap, to multiple distinct areas of considerable size. Hanson et al. found it in 11% of consecutive breast biopsies[66] and considered it to be a benign condition requiring histological diagnosis, without having any clinical significance. While this is commonly

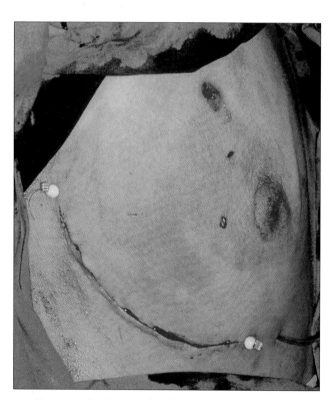

7.12 The tumour has been enucleated via a submammary (Gaillard–Thomas) approach, leaving only a thin rim of compressed breast tissue.

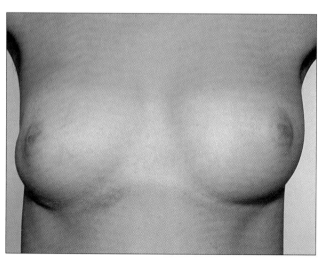

7.13 One year later, the breast has regained almost normal size.

true, especially from a histological point of view, there can be grosser examples of clinical significance in which it overlaps with the condition of recurrent and progressive fibroadenoma discussed above.

A bilateral variant has been described in a male with bilateral gynaecomastia following prolonged treatment with digoxin and spironolactone.[67]

PHYLLODES TUMOUR AND PHYLLODES SARCOMA (CYSTOSARCOMA PHYLLODES)

Although phyllodes tumour and phyllodes sarcoma are dealt with under the heading of giant breast tumours of the perimenopausal period, this is only because they are seen most commonly in this form and at this stage of life. Tumours can occur in any age group, as may tumours as small as a centimetre or so across. The pathology and management of these smaller tumours are similar to the more classic presentation discussed here.

This is a tumour with a dramatic clinical picture and aggressive histological features, so it is not surprising that it has received attention beyond any it deserves in view of its predominantly benign behaviour. It was Johann Muller who first gave it the name 'cystosarcoma phyllodes' in 1838, because it is often cystic and classically has leaf-like projections into it. While these terms were accurately descriptive, the term 'sarcoma' is not justified in a majority of cases, hence the suggestion that the term 'phyllodes tumour' be substituted, with the term 'phyllodes sarcoma' restricted to the small proportion that justify this designation on histological grounds or by clinical behaviour. This is another condition where confusion reigns, and much of the blame must again be directed against imprecise terminology. Since the tumour may be neither cystic nor sarcomatous, 'cystosarcoma' should be abandoned in favour of phyllodes tumour

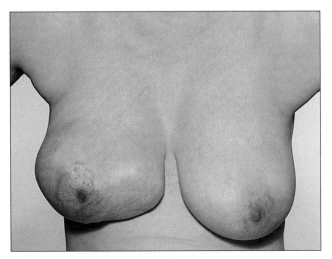

7.14 Recurrent giant fibroadenoma of the perimenopausal period. See text for details.

(benign) or phyllodes sarcoma (malignant). This case is well argued by Azzopardi.[8]

Phyllodes tumour is distinct from giant fibroadenoma both macroscopically and histologically, but it must be reiterated that the diagnosis is a histological one and may apply to any size of tumour. The histological features may be seen in small as well as large tumours. Likewise, it is the pathologist who should decide (on histological grounds) whether the term 'sarcoma' is justified. To diagnose the tumour, both epithelial and fibrous stromal elements must be present, with the stroma showing cellularity, irregularity, hyperchromatism and significant mitosis. Stromal changes are patchy, so many sections need to be studied in the assessment of a large tumour. Contrasting histological pictures of fibroadenoma and phyllodes tumour are shown in Figures 7.15 and 7.16.

The stroma is notably more cellular than in a fibroadenoma, and is dominant in relation to the epithelial component. The stroma is concentrated around the epithelial clefts. An excellent description of the histological details assessed by the pathologist is provided by Azzopardi.[8] The typical macroscopic appearances of giant fibroadenoma and phyllodes tumour are contrasted in Figures 7.10 and 7.18.

Aetiology

Phyllodes tumour is clearly related to fibroadenoma in some cases, because patients may develop both lesions and histological features of both lesions may be seen in the same tumour. However, whether phyllodes tumour develops from a fibroadenoma or both develop simultaneously, or whether phyllodes tumour may arise *de novo*, is not clear. Noguchi and colleagues[11] have studied this question by clonal analysis in three cases where fibroadenoma and phyllodes tumour were obtained sequentially from the same patients. In each case, both tumours were monoclonal and demonstrated the same inactivated allele. They argue cogently that the phyllodes tumour had the same origin as the fibroadenomas, so that certain fibroadenomas can progress to phyllodes tumours.

An intriguing study by Yamashita *et al.*, looking at immunoreactive endothelin 1 (irET-1), exemplifies the manner in which modern science is elucidating mechanisms that will obviously prove to be important in understanding both normal breast function and pathology, while allowing a shift in emphasis from rodent models to human study.[68] Tissue levels of irET-1 were measured in extracts from four phyllodes tumours and 14 fibroadenomas. Immunoreactive endothelin 1 was demonstrable in all cases, but levels were very much higher in phyllodes tumour than in fibroadenoma. Endothelin 1 is primarily a potent vasoconstrictor, but has many other functions. It causes a modest stimulation of breast fibroblast DNA, but can combine with insulin-like growth factor 1 (IGF-1) to produce potent stimulation. ET-1 is not present in normal breast epithelial cells, but specific ET-1 receptors are present on the surface of normal

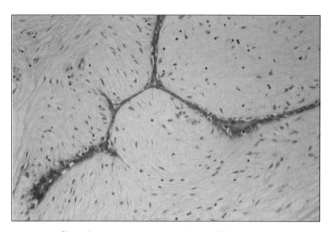

7.15 Giant fibroadenoma – microscopic, hypocellular stroma.

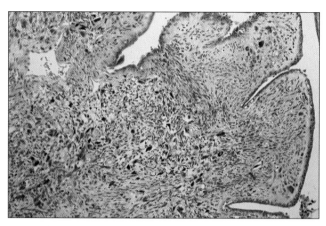

7.16 Phyllodes tumour (sarcoma) microscopic. Cellular stroma with marked pleomorphism.

stromal cells. ET-1 receptors are found on the cell surface of phyllodes tumour stromal cells but immunoreactive cells were found within the epithelial cells but not the stromal cells, suggesting that ET-1 is synthesized by the epithelial cells of phyllodes tumours. Hence this provides a possible paracrine mechanism for the stimulation of rapid stromal growth often seen with phyllodes tumours.

What is important is that phyllodes tumour should not be confused with pure sarcoma (without any epithelial element), for these have a greater degree of malignancy and lumping the two together can obscure the essentially benign nature of many phyllodes tumours. Immunocytochemistry and electron microscopy show that the stromal cells in both benign and malignant phyllodes tumour are a mixture of fibroblasts and myofibroblasts.[69] These techniques allow differentiation from leiomyosarcoma and myoepitheliomas, which can mimic phyllodes tumours but behave differently.

Clinical features

Haagensen[2] reports approximately one phyllodes tumour to every 40 fibroadenomas. Our own hospital experience is similar; seven phyllodes tumours were diagnosed during one period when 332 fibroadenomas were treated. The age distribution is broad, being from 10 to 90 in Haagensen's series of 84 patients, but with a majority between 35 and 55 years. Bilateral tumours are very rare, although an unusual case of three separate tumours in bilateral axillary ectopic breast tissue as well as a normal breast has been reported.[70] Phyllodes tumour is rare in patients before the age of 20, when it appears to behave in a particularly benign fashion, regardless of the histological features.[71] It has also been described in mammary-like glands in the vulva, in the male breast and in the prostate and seminal vesicle.

Most tumours grow rapidly to a large size before the patient presents, but the tumours are not fixed in the sense of a large carcinoma. This is because they are not particularly invasive; the bulk of the tumour may occupy much of the breast, or the whole of it, and produce pressure

ulceration of the skin, but still show some mobility on the chest wall (Figure 7.17).

The tumours are usually softer than fibroadenomas, grossly bosselated and the skin over them shows large, dilated veins. The axillary lymph nodes are not usually involved; a reasonable estimate of the incidence in the malignant subgroup is 10%, so overall the figure is very low.

There is evidence that phyllodes tumours detected in screening programmes are smaller, and histologically 'more' benign, than those presenting clinically.[72]

On section, the tumour is well defined, but histologically may show limited invasion of the pseudocapsule of compressed breast tissue, accounting for the tendency to local recurrence. On cut surface, it has a moist, necrotic, characteristically brownish appearance (Figure 7.18), sometimes with obvious mucoid, haemorrhagic or necrotic areas, and a softer consistency than a fibroadenoma.

The brown colour is notable even with smaller tumours (Figure 7.19) and should alert the surgeon to this diagnosis.

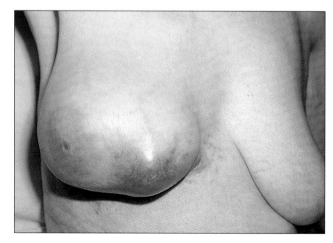

7.17 Typical phyllodes tumour in a middle-aged woman. Pressure has led to thinning of the overlying skin.

Behaviour

While phyllodes tumour shows a distinct tendency to recur locally if excised by a close margin, local or distant metastasis is uncommon. In fact, those tumours assessed as benign after comprehensive histological study can be expected to have an excellent prognosis, especially if treated initially by complete excision. Those which are histologically malignant (phyllodes sarcoma) are unpredictable in behaviour. A single-centre study of 32 cases provides a fair indication of behaviour.[73] Benign tumours showed no recurrence if completely excised, but half (6 of 13) incompletely excised recurred locally. No recurrence was seen after complete excision of four borderline and four malignant tumours, but incomplete excision of a malignant tumour led to uncontrolled chest wall disease.

In Treves and Sunderland's study[74] of 77 cases, 50% of those classified as malignant metastasized. A number of workers[74–76] have tried to assess the malignant potential. It is generally felt that mitotic rate is the best guide, although far from uniformly predictive. A mitotic rate less than 4 per 10 high power fields (HPF) carried an excellent prognosis, 5–9/10 HPF is intermediate and more than 10/10 HPF carries a worse prognosis. Small tumours (less than 4-cm diameter) have an excellent prognosis, and a 'pushing' margin is favourable. Rhodes et al.[77] have recently reviewed the histological assessment of malignancy.

In general, local recurrence of benign tumours remains benign, but transformation to malignancy can occur[73] and explosive malignancy has been reported after 15 episodes of benign local recurrence.[78]

The overall favourable prognosis is shown by Haagensen's series, in which only four out of the 84 patients are known to have metastasized. While we have seen local recurrence in patients, none has as yet metastasized. A recent series of 66 cases from the Mayo Clinic[79] confirms that most behave as low-grade, nonmetastasizing tumours, but neither histological evaluation nor DNA analysis by flow cytometry gives a reliable assessment of behaviour in an individual tumour.

Treatment

Age is important in the management of these lesions. Under the age of 20, all should be treated by enucleation, because they almost invariably behave in a benign manner.[71]

Aspiration cytology can suggest the diagnosis of phyllodes tumour[80] but the more definitive histology of core needle biopsy is needed before planning treatment.

The situation is less clear-cut in older patients. Few surgeons have sufficient experience to be dogmatic about management. Haagensen reports one of the largest series, and recommends wide local excision as the primary approach to treatment of benign phyllodes tumours. He had a local recurrence rate of 28% among 43 patients treated by local excision, with a minimum 10-year follow-up. But only three of the recurrences required secondary mastectomy, and none has died from the tumour. Only 1 in 21 patients treated by mastectomy (simple or radical) developed local recurrence; this was a phyllodes sarcoma which rapidly produced both local and systematic metastases. Higher recurrence rates for benign than malignant phyllodes tumour have been reported in a number of series, reflecting a more casual surgical approach for the tumours considered less serious.

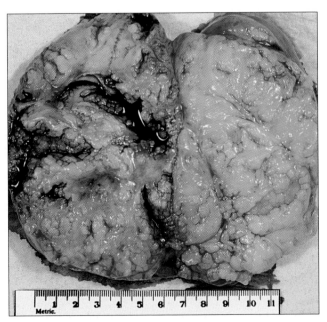

7.18 Giant phyllodes tumour – macroscopic brown, irregular, cellular, leaf-like masses, necrosis and haemorrhage.

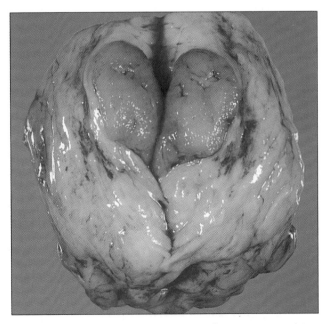

7.19 Small benign phyllodes tumour. Note similarity to Figure 7.5, but distinct brownish colour.

It is clear that incomplete excision is the main determinant of recurrence in benign and intermediate lesions. Why are high recurrences reported from most series when this is so well demonstrated? There are two main reasons: the failure to anticipate the possibility of a phyllodes tumour and the failure to define a technique which will ensure complete excision. The first can be met only by a high level of suspicion, and triple assessment of all masses before surgery. It is particularly important to avoid excision biopsy as a diagnostic procedure because it is almost impossible to effect a defined excision margin of a biopsy cavity, whereas this is easily done as a primary procedure while the tumour is still *in situ*. For this reason, histological diagnosis should be made by core needle biopsy, or at least no larger procedure than incision biopsy.

Complete macroscopic excision, with a suggested margin of 1 cm, can be ensured by appropriate technique. With the usual technique of excision while applying traction to the mass, it is easy to dissect too close to the tumour at some point of the dissection. A reliable way to avoid this is for the surgeon to place the left fingers on the mass, and dissect outside the fingers, with traction only on the surrounding breast tissue. The inherent reluctance to cut one's own finger will ensure a full centimetre clearance around the whole circumference of the tumour!

For small lesions where the diagnosis is suggested by triple assessment or macroscopic appearance (soft, brown, fleshy appearance), the tumour should be excised with a 1-cm margin of normal breast tissue. If histology is benign, this would be sufficient treatment, with a quadrantic excision for intermediate lesions. Where the diagnosis is first recognized on histological examination of an excision biopsy specimen, quadrantic excision of the scar is recommended as a means of ensuring adequate local clearance. For large lesions and recurrent lesions, a good clearance inevitably involves near total mastectomy and we prefer simple mastectomy, with immediate reconstruction should the patient wish it. Mastectomy is a small price to pay for freedom from local recurrence, and reconstruction can readily lessen the price. We are reinforced in this policy by the fact that the stroma sometimes shows increased malignancy with recurrence.

Zurrida and colleagues take a more conservative approach,[81] recommending a 'wait and see' policy after a phyllodes tumour is first diagnosed after excision, provided it is assessed as benign on histology. This is on the basis that only 10% of such cases recurred in their series. However, this figure is lower than other series, and the avoidance of unnecessary surgery has to be set against the psychological stress to the patient of frequent follow-up, knowing that they have had a suboptimal procedure, and the small but definite risk of developing a more malignant recurrence. Clearly the optimal management is to make a preoperative diagnosis and ensure total excision at the primary operation.

The histological association of carcinoma with phyllodes tumour is similar to that discussed under fibroadenoma (see page 83): a predominance of LCIS, and occasionally involvement of the lesion from adjacent cancer. There is some evidence for an increased incidence of related breast carcinoma, simultaneous or subsequent, in patients with phyllodes tumour and this is an added reason for careful long-term follow-up of such patients.

REFERENCES

1. World Health Organization. *Histological Typing of Breast Tumours*, 2nd edn. Geneva: WHO, 1981.
2. Haagensen CD. *Diseases of the Breast*, 3rd edn. Philadelphia: WB Saunders, 1986.
3. Dent DM & Cant PJ. Fibroadenoma. *World Journal of Surgery* 1989; 13: 706–710.
4. Dobie V, Walsh J, Lamb J & Dixon JM. Natural history of fibroadenoma of the breast. In: Mansel RE (ed.) *Recent Developments in the Study of Benign Breast Disease*, pp 75–81. London: Parthenon Publishing, 1994.
5. Meyer JS. Proliferation in normal breast ducts, fibroadenomas and other ductal hyperplasias measured by nuclear labelling with tritiated thymidine. *Human Pathology* 1977; 8: 67–81.
6. Otu AA. Benign breast tumours in an African population. *Journal of the Royal College of Surgeons*, Edinburgh 1990; 35: 373–375.
7. Barton SA, Pathak DR, Black WC *et al*. Prevalence of benign, atypical and malignant breast lesions in populations at different risk of breast cancer. *Cancer* 1987; 60: 2751–2760.
8. Azzopardi JG. *Problems in Breast Pathology*. London: WB Saunders, 1979.
9. Archer F & Omar M. The fine structure of fibroadenoma of the human breast. *Journal of Pathology* 1969; 99: 113–117.
10. Noguchi S, Motomura K, Inaji H *et al*. Clonal analysis of fibroadenoma and phyllodes tumour by means of polymerase chain reaction. *Cancer Research* 1993; 53: 4071–4074.
11. Noguchi S, Yokouchi H, Aihara T *et al*. Progression of fibroadenoma to phyllodes tumour demonstrated by clonal analysis. *Cancer* 1995: 76: 1779–1785.
12. Petersson C, Pandis N, Risov H *et al*. Karyotypic abnormalities in fibroadenoma of the breast. *International Journal of Cancer* 1997; 70: 282–286.
13. Zeladahedman N, Werer G, Collins P *et al*. High expression of the EGFR in fibroadenomas compared to breast carcinomas. *Anticancer Research* 1944; 14: 1679–1688.
14. Goodall RJ, Dawkins HJS, Robbins PD *et al*. Evaluation of the expression levels of NM23-H1 messenger RNA in primary breast cancer, benign breast disease, axillary lymph nodes and normal breast. *Pathology* 1994; 26: 423–428.
15. Atherton AJ, Monaghan P, Warburton MJ *et al*. Dipeptidyl peptidase IV expression identifies a functional subpopulation of breast fibroblasts. *International Journal of Cancer* 1952; 50: 15–19
16. Nardelli GB, Lamaina V & Siliotti F. Steroid receptors in benign breast disease, gross cystic disease and fibroadenoma. *Clinical and Experimental Obstetrics and Gynecology* 1987; 14: 10–15.

17. Martin PM, Kutten F & Serment H. Progesterone receptors in breast fibroadenomas. *Journal of Steroid Biochemistry* 1979; **11**: 1295–1298.

18. Pasqualini JR, Cortes-Prieto J, Chetrite J *et al.* Concentration of estrone, estradiol and their sulphates, and evaluation of sulfatase and aromatase activity in patients with breast fibroadenoma. *International Journal of Cancer* 1997; **70**: 639–643.

19. Ansahboatene Y & Tavassoli FA. Fibroadenoma and cystosarcoma phyllodes of the male breast. *Modern Pathology* 1992; **5**: 114–116.

20. Ferrieres C, Cuny M & Simony-Fontaine J. Variation of bcl-2 expression in breast ducts and lobules in relation to plasma progesterone levels: overexpression and absence of variation in fibroadenomas. *Journal of Pathology* 1997; **183**: 204–211.

21. Canny PF, Berkowitz GS, Kelsey JL & Livolsi VA. Fibroadenoma and the use of exogenous hormones. *American Journal of Epidemiology* 1988; **127**: 454–461.

22. Berkowitz GS, Canny PF, Vivolsi VA *et al.* Cigarette smoking and benign breast disease. *Journal of Epidemiology and Community Health* 1985; **39**: 308–313.

23. Koerner FC & O'Connell JX. Fibroadenoma: morphological observations and theory of pathogenesis. *Pathology Annual* 1994; **29**(Part 1): 1–19.

24. Cheatle GL. Hyperplasia of epithelial and connective tissues in the breast: its relation to fibroadenoma. *British Journal of Surgery* 1923; **10**: 436–455.

25. Wilkinson S & Forrest APM. Fibroadenoma of the breast. *British Journal of Surgery* 1985; **72**: 838–840.

26. Devitt JE. Benign disorders of the breast in older women. *Surgery, Gynecology and Obstetrics* 1986; **162**: 340–342.

27. Cyrlak D & Wong CH. Mammographic changes in post-menopausal women undergoing hormone replacement therapy. *American Journal of Roentgenology* 1993; **161**: 1177–1183.

28. Myer JE, Frenna TH, Polger M et al. Enlarging occult fibroadenomas. *Radiology* 1992; **183**: 639–641.

29. Foster ME, Garrahan N & Williams S. Fibroadenoma of the breast – a clinical and pathological study. *Journal of the Royal College of Surgeons (Edinburgh)* 1988; **36**: 16–19.

30. Cole-Beuglet C, Soriano RZ, Kurtz AB & Goldberg BB. Fibroadenoma of the breast. Sonomammography correlated with pathology in 122 patients. *American Journal of Radiology* 1983; **140**: 369–375.

31. Holcombe C, Pugh N, Lyons K *et al.* Blood flow in breast cancer and fibroadenoma estimated by colour doppler ultrasonography. *British Journal of Surgery* 1995; **82**: 782–788.

32. Cosgrove DO. Doppler ultrasound of the breast. *Imaging* 1994; **6**: 185–196.

33. Hughes LE. In: Hughes LE, Mansel RE & Webster DJT. *Benign Disorders and Diseases of the Breast*, p 64. London: Baillière Tindall, 1989.

34. Dixon JM, Dobie V, Lamb L *et al.* Assessment of the acceptability of conservative management of fibroadenoma of the breast. *British Journal of Surgery* 1996; **83**: 264–265.

35. Cant PJ, Madden MV, Close PM *et al.* Case for conservative management of selected fibroadenomas of the breast. *British Journal of Surgery* 1987; **74**: 857–859.

36. Alle KM, Moss J, Venegas RJ *et al.* Conservative management of fibroadenoma of the breast. *British Journal of Surgery* 1996; **83**: 992–993.

37. Cupceancu B. Short term tamoxifen treatment in benign breast diseases. *Endocrinologie* 1985; **23**: 169–177.

38. Lai LM, Mumtaz H, Ripley PM *et al.* Laser treatment of breast fibroadenomas. *Lasers in Medical Science* 1997; **12**: 296.

39. Moran CS. Fibroadenoma of the breast during pregnancy and lactation. *Archives of Surgery* 1935; **31**: 688.

40. Wilkinson L & Green WO Jr. Infarction of breast lesions during pregnancy and lactation. *Cancer* 1964; **17**: 1567–1572.

41. Hasson J & Pope CH. Mammary infarcts associated with pregnancy presenting as breast tumours. *Surgery* 1961; **49**: 313–316.

42. Dupont WD, Page DL, Parl FF *et al.* Long term risk of breast cancer in women with fibroadenoma. *New England Journal of Medicine* 1994; **331**: 10–15.

43. Carney JA & Toorkey BC. Myxoid fibroadenoma and allied conditions (myxomatosis) of the breast. A heritable disorder with special associations including cardiac and cutaneous myxoma. *American Journal of Surgical Pathology* 1991; **15**: 713–721.

44. Ashikari R, Farrow JH & O'Hara J. Fibroadenomas in the breast of juveniles. *Surgery, Gynecology and Obstetrics* 1971; **132**: 259–262.

45. Hertel BF, Zaloudek C & Kempson RL. Breast adenomas. *Cancer* 1976; **37**: 2891–2905.

46. Powell CM, Cranor ML & Rosen PP. Multinucleated stromal giant cells in mammary fibroepithelial neoplasms – a study of 11 patients. *Archives of Pathology and Laboratory Medicine* 1994; **118**: 912–916.

47. Diaz NM, Palmer JO & McDivitt RW. Carcinoma arising within fibroadenomas of the breast – a clinicopathological study of 105 patients. *American Journal of Clinical Pathology* 1991; **95**: 614–622.

48. Yoshida Y, Takaoka M & Fukumoto M. Carcinoma arising in fibroadenoma. Case report and review of world literature. *Journal of Surgical Oncology* 1985; **29**: 132–140.

49. Brydon HL & Carey MP. Medulloblastoma metastasising to a breast fibroadenoma. A case report. *British Journal of Neurosurgery* 1991; **5**: 73–75.

50. Levi F, Randimbison L, Te VC & Lavecchia C. Incidence of breast cancer in women with fibroadenoma. *International Journal of Cancer* 1994; **57**: 681–683.

51. Ciatto S, Bonardi R, Zappa M & Giordi D. Risk of breast cancer subsequent to histological or clinical diagnosis of fibroadenoma. *Annals of Oncology* 1997; **8**: 297–300.

52. Naraynsingh V & Raju GC. Familial bilateral multiple fibroadenomas of the breast. *Postgraduate Medical Journal* 1985; **61**: 439–440.

53. Williamson MER, Lyons K & Hughes LE. Multiple fibroadenomas of the breast – a problem of uncertain incidence and management. *Annals of the Royal College of Surgeons of England* 1993; **75**: 161–163.

54. Rolles K & Calne RY. Two cases of benign lumps after treatment with cyclosporin A. *Lancet* 1980; **2**: 795.

55. Baildam AD, Higgins RM, Hurley E *et al.* Cyclosporin A and multiple fibroadenomas of the breast. *British Journal of Surgery* 1996; **83**: 1755–1757.

56. Musio F, Mozingo D & Otchy DP. Multiple giant fibroadenoma. *The American Surgeon* 1991; **57**: 438–441.

57. Kuusk U. Multiple giant fibroadenomas in an adolescent breast. *Canadian Journal of Surgery* 1988; **31**: 133–134.

58. Stavrides S, Hacking A, Tiltman A & Dent DM. Gigantomastia in pregnancy. *British Journal of Surgery* 1987; **74**: 585–586.

59. Schneider B, Laubenberger J, Kommoss F *et al.* Multiple giant fibroadenomas. Clinical presentation and radiological findings. *Gynecolologic and Obstetrics Investigation* 1997; **43**: 278–280.

60. Raganoonan C, Fairbairn JK, Williams S & Hughes LE. Giant breast tumours of adolescence. *Australian and New Zealand Journal of Surgery* 1987; **57**: 243–247.

61. Nambiar R & Kannan-Kutty M. Giant fibroadenoma (cystosarcoma phyllodes) in adolescent females. A clinico-

pathological study. *British Journal of Surgery* 1974; **61**: 113–117.

62. Naidu AG, Thomson SR & Nirmul D. Giant fibroadenomas in black and Indian adolescents. *South African Journal of Surgery* 1989; **27**: 171–172.

63. Mies C & Rosen PP. Juvenile fibroadenoma with atypical epithelial hyperplasia. *American Journal of Surgical Pathology* 1987; **11**: 184–190.

64. Holbrook WA & Ramsay JH. Giant fibroadenoma of the breast. *Bulletin of the School of Medicine of the University of Maryland* 1956; **41**: 58–63.

65. Hoffman SH. Giant fibroadenoma of the breast: immediate reconstruction following excision. *British Journal of Plastic Surgery* 1978; **31**: 170–172.

66. Hanson CA, Snover DC & Dehner LP. Fibroadenomatosis (fibroadenomatoid hyperplasia): a benign breast lesion with composite pathologic features. *Pathology* 1987; **9**: 393–396.

67. Neilsen BB. Fibroadenomatoid hyperplasia of the male breast. *American Journal of Surgical Pathology* 1990; **14**: 774–777.

68. Yamashita J, Ogawa M & Egami H. Abundant expression of immunoreactive endothelin-1 in mammary phyllodes tumour – possible paracrine role of endothelin-1 in the growth of stromal cells in phyllodes tumour. *Cancer Research* 1992; **52**: 4046–4049.

69. Auger M, Hanna W & Kahn HJ. Cystosarcoma phylloides of the breast and its mimics. An immunohistochemical and ultrastructural study. *Archives of Pathology and Laboratory Medicine* 1989; **113**: 1231–1235.

70. Saleh HA & Klein LH. Cystosarcoma phyllodes arising synchronously in right breast and bilateral axillary ectopic breast tissue. *Archives of Pathology and Laboratory Medicine* 1990; **114**: 624–626.

71. Anderson JR. Cystosarcoma in adolescent females. *Annals of Surgery* 1970; **171**: 849–858.

72. Ockrim JB & Watkins RM. Screen detected phyllodes tumours: are they important? In: Mansel RE (ed.) *Recent Developments in the Study of Benign Breast Disease*. Carnforth: Parthenon Press, 1999. In press.

73. Moffat CJC, Pinder SE, Dixon AR *et al.* Phyllodes tumour of the breast. A clinico-pathological review of 32 cases. *Histopathology* 1995; **27**: 205–218.

74. Treves N & Sunderland D. Cystosarcoma of the breast – a malignant and a benign tumour. A clinico-pathological study of 77 cases. *Cancer* 1951; **4**: 1286–1332.

75. Lester J & Stout AP. Cystosarcoma phyllodes. *Cancer* 1954; **7**: 335–353.

76. Norris HJ & Taylor HB. Relationship of histological features to behaviour of cystosarcoma phyllodes. Analysis of 94 cases. *Cancer* 1967; **20**: 2090–2099.

77. Rhodes RH, Frankel KA, Davis L & Tatter D. Metastatic cystosarcoma phyllodes. *Cancer* 1978; **41**: 1179–1187.

78. Kuipers T, Stark GP & Spilker G. Explosive malignant transformation of a primarily benign phyllodes tumour. *European Journal of Plastic Surgery* 1992; **15**: 233–236.

79. Keelan PA, Myers JL, Wold LE *et al.* Phyllodes tumour: Clinicopathologic review of 60 patients and flow cytometric analysis of 30 patients. *Human Pathology* 1992; **23**: 1048–1054.

80. Shabb NS. Phyllodes tumor: Fine needle aspiration cytology diagnosis of 8 cases. *Acta Cytologica* 1997; **41**: 321–326.

81. Zurrida S, Bartoli C & Galimberti V. Which therapy for unexpected phyllodes tumour of the breast? *European Journal of Cancer* 1992; **28**: 654–657.

Breast pain and nodularity

CONTENTS

KEY POINTS AND NEW DEVELOPMENTS

1. Mastalgia is now accepted as a common cause of morbidity, occasionally severe enough to interfere with quality of life, and then sufficient to justify careful investigation and treatment.
2. The basic cause of cyclical mastalgia is clearly endocrine in nature, but the precise mechanism(s) continues to elude investigators.
3. Cancer, sclerosing adenosis and postsurgery scars are rare but important causes, while referred pain often presents as mastalgia.
4. Most mild to moderate cases are seeking reassurance, and this is usually all that is required.
5. Management of more severe cases follows classification into cyclical and non-cyclical cases, with the latter further divided into true non-cyclical and musculoskeletal pain. Pain charts are an important aid to assessment.
6. Evening primrose oil for the mild to moderate case and danazol for the moderate to severe case are the mainstays of treatment. Bromocriptine and tamoxifen are used for resistant and recurrent cases.
7. Lower than usual dosage has improved the therapeutic ratio with danazol and tamoxifen. Short courses, repeated if necessary, are preferred to longer, continuous therapy.
8. Cases refractory to standard treatment need careful individual assessment; some patients may benefit from psychological assessment and therapy.
9. Results of surgery, including mastectomy, are unpredictable, and surgery should be used only exceptionally.
10. Mastalgia in the postmenopausal period is being seen more frequently in women on hormone replacement therapy (HRT); it is usually self-limiting and not of great severity.
11. There is considerable overlap between cyclical mastalgia and premenstrual syndrome (PMS) but there are also significant differences, requiring differing approaches.

Mastalgia is one of the commonest symptoms in patients attending a breast clinic and is also the most frequent reason for breast-related consultation in general practice.[1,2] Many terms have been used to describe mastalgia in the past, including the term 'mastodynia' introduced by Heineke in 1821 and 'mazodynia' used by Birkett in 1850. The mixing of pathological with clinical terms noted in Chapter 3 has caused confusion in the past and it is better to use 'mastalgia' to denote the symptom of pain in the breast without any specific pathological connotation being implied.

HISTORICAL NOTE

The literature amply demonstrates that breast pain is the commonest presenting symptom of breast conditions and it would be natural to assume that it was a well-documented subject with clear definitions and guidelines for management. Until recently this was not the case; the literature devoted to mastalgia has been poor both in quality and in clarity. Most of the problem has been due to attempts to relate poorly defined clinical presentations with pathological terms as previously discussed in Chapter 3.

Birkett in 1850 in his textbook of breast diseases[3] described breast pain as 'mazodynia' and noted two subtypes: with induration (nodularity) or without induration. He noted premenstrual exacerbation of tenderness in the nodular group and suggested aperients and tonics as treatment. Cheatle and Cutler[4] in 1931 used the term 'mazoplasia' to describe bilateral painful nodular breasts, and suggested it was present to some degree in all women's breasts. Later authors used the all-embracing term 'chronic mastitis' to denote painful nodular breasts,[5,6] with some attempting to define degrees of severity.[7] Carl Semb described various degrees of painful nodularity in his exhaustive study of 1928,[8] but also mixed symptomatic terms with pathological descriptions. Geschickter devoted a whole chapter in his 1945 book to the subject of mastodynia (painful breasts) and described many of the clinical features of mastalgia,[7] but concluded, as had others before him, that mastodynia progressed into the various forms of chronic cystic mastitis.

Thus, despite a small number of exhaustive studies by these eminent clinicians and pathologists, there was no clear account of mastalgia as a symptom. In 1971, a special research clinic was set up within the Cardiff Breast Clinic in order to answer some of the questions regarding mastalgia and benign breast disease. The findings of this mastalgia clinic, which has continued to study this problem to the present, form the substance of this chapter.

FREQUENCY OF BREAST PAIN

The frequency of breast pain as a presenting symptom of breast disorders in various clinics is shown in Table 8.1.

The exact frequency is difficult to ascertain as many studies do not state the population from which the study group is drawn. An example is Geschickter's detailed account which described 375 cases of mastodynia seen in Baltimore over a period of 50 years, but the incidence of other breast conditions is not stated.[7]

A recent study from the USA[11] shows a significant impact among a population of 1171 women attending a general obstetrics and gynaecology clinic. Sixty-nine per cent suffered regular discomfort and 36% had consulted about their breast pain. Current moderate-to-severe pain was found in 11% of women. Mastalgia interfered with usual sexual activity in 48% and with physical (37%), social (12%) and work (8%) activity.

In general, it can be concluded that breast pain is present in about 50% of patients presenting to surgical clinics with breast problems but higher levels of around 65–70% were volunteered by women interviewed at a screening clinic and at screening carried out on site in a group of working women at a large retail chain store (the Cardiff Marks and Spencer Study).

MASTALGIA IN BREAST CANCER

Although this book does not deal with cancer, the role of breast pain in the diagnosis of early breast cancer is of considerable importance. Classic teaching was that early cancers were not painful, so that patients presenting with pain were unlikely to have cancer. While this is generally true for bilateral cyclical mastalgia, more detailed work has shown that pain does not exclude cancer, and may occasionally be the only presenting symptom of a subclinical cancer. Several papers make the point that although breast pain is an uncommon symptom in breast cancer, it does not exclude the diagnosis.

Table 8.1 Frequency of breast pain as a presenting symptom in benign and malignant breast disease	
Study	Percentage of patients attending complaining of mastalgia
Semb[8]	85
Southampton Breast Clinic[9]	50
Cardiff Breast Clinic	45
General practice[12]	47–52
Working population (Cardiff Marks & Spencer Study)	66
Screening clinic[10]	70
Obstetric and gynaecology clinic[11]	69

Preece *et al.*[12] noted that mastalgia indicating an underlying cancer differed from cyclical premenstrual mastalgia in that it was unilateral, persistent and constant in position. Of 17 patients who presented with mastalgia alone out of a population of 240 operable breast cancers, they found five were T0 tumours and five T1 tumours, suggesting that mastalgia as a *sole* presenting symptom is associated with smaller tumours. Preece's work has been confirmed by an Italian study[13] of 200 patients presenting with local breast pain and negative physical examination. Mammography detected subclinical cancer at the site of the pain in five patients.

The literature on this topic is generally consistent, as is shown by Table 8.2.

The converse side of this question is whether cyclical mastalgia reflects a hormonal environment which predisposes to breast cancer. Studies attempting to answer this question raise many difficulties, but the bulk of evidence suggests that any such predisposition is minimal. However, one matched case control study of 420 women showed a relative risk of cancer of 2.12 (95% CI = 1.31–3.43) in those who gave a history of cyclical mastalgia, after allowing for confounding risks such as oral contraceptive use and pregnancies.[18] This apparent increase in risk needs confirmation by larger and prospective studies.

CLASSIFICATION

Previous attempts at classification based on pathological terms did not give any practical help in the understanding or management of mastalgia. A pressing need was to classify accurately the symptom of mastalgia and this was initially done by drawing up a protocol in the Cardiff Mastalgia Clinic describing significant features of the symptom (Table 8.3).

In addition, a comprehensive gynaecological history was taken and careful physical examination performed. All the patients studied in the Mastalgia Clinic had already been examined clinically by an experienced breast surgeon and by mammography (when indicated) to exclude carcinoma of the breast and extramammary causes ranging from cervical spondylosis to biliary pain. These patients thus presented with painful breasts with or without nodularity. Cases with a discrete lump were managed as detailed in Chapter 4.

Analysis of the initial 232 patients studied with this protocol defined certain patterns of mastalgia.[19] The frequency of each type is shown in Table 8.4.

The general validity and utility of this classification has been confirmed, with some modifications, in 25 years' experience in the Cardiff Mastalgia Clinic.

Table 8.2 Frequency of breast pain as a presenting symptom of operable breast cancer

Study	Percentage of cancers presenting with pain
Preece *et al.*[12]	7
River *et al.*[14]	24
Haagensen[15]	5
Smallwood *et al.*[9]	18
Yorkshire Group[16]	5
Chiedozie and Guirguis[17]	8

Table 8.3 Contents of the Cardiff Mastalgia Protocol

Feature	Examples
Descriptive terms	Tenderness/heaviness/burning
Periodicity	Continuous, intermittent
Duration	
Distribution in breast	
Radiation	
Aggravating factors	Physical contact
Relieving factors	Analgesics/drugs/well-fitted brassière
Diurnal pattern	
Disturbance of lifestyle	Sleep loss/marital problem/can't hug children
Dominant hand	

Table 8.4 Frequency of patterns in 232 prospectively documented mastalgia parients

Pattern/diagnosis	Number (%)
Cyclical pronounced	93 (40)
Non-cyclical	62 (27)
Tietze's syndrome	25 (11)
Trauma (post-biopsy)	19 (8)
Sclerosing adenosis	11 (4.5)
Cancer	1 (0.5)
Miscellaneous/non-breast	21 (9)
From Preece *et al.*[19]	

Cyclical pronounced pattern

The commonest type of pain is related to the menstrual cycle, and particularly to ovulation (Figure 8.1). Clearly, many women experience 2 or 3 days of premenstrual breast tenderness or heaviness every month and this should be regarded as normal (Figure 8.2).

Fine nodularity which begins a short time before menstruation and regresses postmenstrually is equally normal; the difficult problem is deciding where normality ends and disease begins. When the normal discomfort is exceeded, we have used the term 'cyclical pronounced mastalgia'.

The cyclical group has been given the adjective 'pronounced' to denote the increased intensity of the symptom defined either by duration (>1 week per cycle), or by severity documented using a pain chart (Figure 8.3).

Severity is necessarily a subjective assessment, as is all assessment of pain in clinical practice, but obtrusive features in the lifestyle, such as sleep loss, work disturbance or interrupted sexual activity, can give some guide. This group probably represents the 'mastodynia' group of previous reports, although some authors state that associated nodularity excludes mastodynia. The cyclical pronounced patient

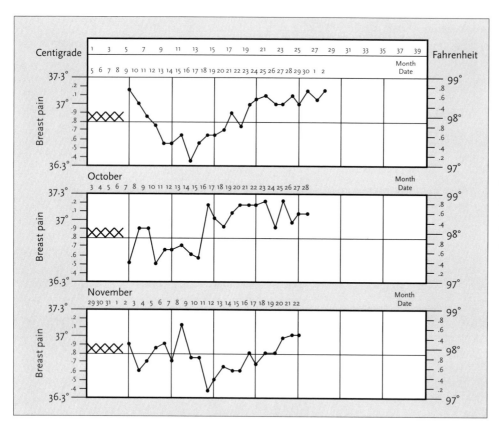

8.1 Basal body temperature chart recorded by a patient with mastalgia. The first two cycles show a biphasic ovulatory pattern and breast pain occurred for about 2 weeks premenstrually in the first cycle (top level) and for about 4 days in the second cycle. No pain occurred in the third cycle (lower panel) which appears to have a non-ovulatory temperature pattern. This chart demonstrates the association of mastalgia with ovulation and the variation in one woman from cycle to cycle. XXX = menstrual period.

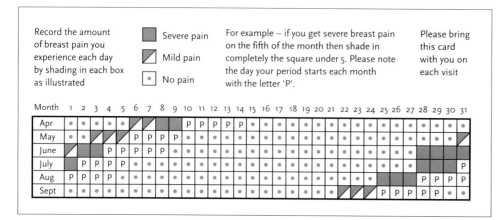

8.2 Breast pain chart showing daily recording of breast pain. The chart shows 3–4 days of mild premenstrual pain per cycle which would be regarded as normal. P = period.

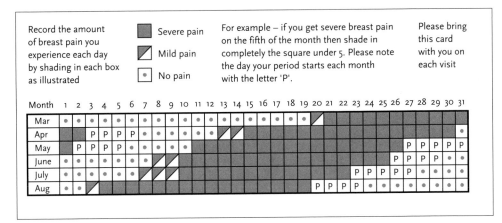

Record the amount of breast pain you experience each day by shading in each box as illustrated

■ Severe pain

◪ Mild pain

⊡ No pain

For example – if you get severe breast pain on the fifth of the month then shade in completely the square under 5. Please note the day your period starts each month with the letter 'P'.

Please bring this card with you on each visit

8.3 Pain chart of a patient with cyclical pronounced mastaglia showing 2–3 weeks of severe premenstrual mastalgia per cycle over 6 months.

almost invariably has nodularity of a varying degree which is maximal in the upper outer quadrant, and shows similar cyclicity to the pain.

Other characteristics of the cyclical pronounced group are shown in Figure 8.4 and it is worth noting that the terms 'heaviness' and 'tenderness to touch' are used frequently to describe symptoms of the pattern.

Bilateral pain and nodularity are also common. The pain often radiates to the axilla and down the medial aspect of the upper arm, presumably as a referred pain via the intercostobrachial nerve. A well-taken history will often reveal the temporal association with the menstrual cycle, but we have found a simple pain chart to be extremely useful in displaying this pattern (see Figure 8.3). This is essential in patients who have had a hysterectomy. A pain chart is readily completed by most patients and has the added advantage of giving a simple quantitation to the symptom (days of pain) which is useful for assessing effectiveness of therapy.

Mammography has proved unhelpful in the cyclical pronounced pattern, as the nonspecific changes of radiological density ascribed to 'fibroadenosis' have been the main feature, and no specific radiological appearance correlates with the site or side of pain.

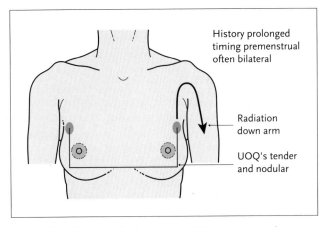

History prolonged timing premenstrual often bilateral

Radiation down arm

UOQ's tender and nodular

8.4 The clinical features of cyclical mastalgia. It is premenopausal; mean age = 34 years. Descriptive terms are 'heaviness' and 'tenderness to touch', relieved by menstruation and menopause. UOQ, upper outer quadrant.

Non-cyclical pattern

The second largest group (27%), the non-cyclical pattern, is distinguished principally by its lack of relationship with events in the menstrual cycle and again is well shown by the pain chart (Figure 8.5).

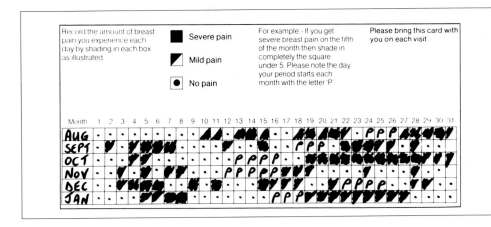

Record the amount of breast pain you experience each day by shading in each box as illustrated

■ Severe pain

◪ Mild pain

⊡ No pain

For example:- If you get severe breast pain on the fifth of the month then shade in completely the square under 5. Please note the day your period starts each month with the letter 'P'

Please bring this card with you on each visit

8.5 Pain chart showing a non-cyclical pattern of mastalgia. There is no demonstrable relationship to any phase of the menstrual cycle.

Detailed analysis of 72 non-cyclic patients has shown that they fall into two main groups: true non-cyclical mastalgia and musculoskeletal pain (Figure 8.6).[20]

The two groups are roughly equal in frequency of presentation, although this varies with the efficiency of screening before reaching the mastalgia clinic. The mean age of the musculoskeletal group is greater (39 years versus 34 years) and the duration of pain shorter (15 months versus 35 months).

True non-cyclical breast pain

This pattern occurs in both pre- and postmenopausal women in contradistinction to the cyclical pattern but the mean age of these patients is similar at 34 years. The non-cyclical pattern differs in several respects from the cyclical. The pain tends to be well localized in the breast and is more frequently subareolar or upper outer quadrant. Simultaneous bilateral pain is not uncommon and the descriptive terms of 'burning, drawing or abscess-like' are different. Other terms indicative of a transient sharp quality, such as pricking or stabbing, have also been commonly used which may last for minutes or days at a time. When the pattern was assessed quantitively using a linear analogue scale (see later), it was scored by the patients at a lower intensity than the cyclical pattern. Nodularity is less prominent than in the cyclical group, but is still seen in 54% of patients. When differentiated from musculoskeletal pain, non-cyclical breast pain has a better response to hormonal therapy than previously thought. About half will have a useful response to danazol, with a similar response rate reported for tamoxifen.[21] Half will have a spontaneous remission, but after a mean period of 27 months.

Mammography has been of some interest in the non-cyclical group, as the radiological changes of coarse calcification and ductal dilatation attributed to duct ectasia or periductal mastitis have been commonly seen in this group. Of the 62 patients documented, no less than 42 showed radiological evidence of duct ectasia somewhere in the painful breast and of these 20 showed the typical coarse calcification at the site of complaint. These findings led us initially to describe the non-cyclical pattern as the 'periductal mastitis' pattern, but we prefer to use the 'non-cyclical' term, first because it conforms to our principle of not mixing symptomatic with pathological terms, and secondly because we have no histological evidence that non-cyclical pain is due to the pathological changes of duct ectasia.

A further term, 'the trigger spot', has been introduced for this pattern, or at least a subgroup of it,[22] based on the special feature that pressure by palpation at the indicated site of pain will reproduce the patient's pain. However, in our experience, while this picture is seen in some patients, it does not describe the overall group and there is no correlation with any histological finding at the site of complaint.[23] We feel it is best reserved as a small subtype of non-cyclical mastalgia.

Chest wall (musculoskeletal) pain

Musculoskeletal pain is almost always unilateral (92%) and falls into two groups: Tietze's syndrome and lateral chest wall pain.[20] A good response is often obtained with an injection of steroid and local anaesthetic.

Tietze's syndrome[24] or painful costochondral junction syndrome is not a true breast pain but the pain is often felt in the region of the breast overlying the costal cartilages, which are the source of the pain (Figure 8.7).

It has a characteristically chronic time course and, on examination, one or several costal cartilages are tender and feel enlarged. Typically the pain is felt within the medial quadrants of the breast and increased pain occurs on pressure over the affected cartilage. Radiological examination of these patients reveals no abnormality in the costal cartilages or specific features in the breast.

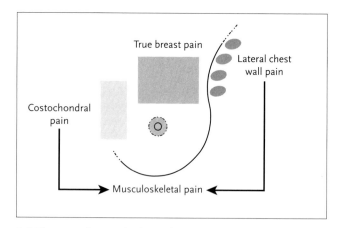

8.6 The types of non-cyclical mastalgia. (From Maddox et al.[20])

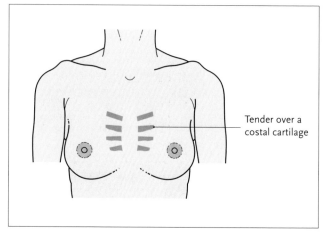

8.7 The clinical features of Tietze's syndrome. It is often unilateral; any age; no time pattern; no palpable abnormality; chronic course.

Trauma

The trauma group, 8% of the total, complained of a persistent non-cyclical type pain localized to a previous benign biopsy scar. There were no specific findings apart from the presence of the scar, but on enquiry it was revealed that several of the biopsies had been complicated by infection or haematoma, and some of the painful scars had been made across Langer's lines of tension. However, prolonged breast discomfort of annoying degree can follow even simple, uncomplicated biopsy. Indeed, the considerable incidence of long-term pain after all forms of breast surgery is not always appreciated. In a study of 282 patients undergoing major breast surgery, one-third to one-half still had pain after a year.[25] It was particularly troublesome after mastectomy with reconstruction, and after subpectoral implant insertion.

Sclerosing adenosis

Eleven patients had pain at the site of sclerosing adenosis (seven proved histologically and four shown on mammography), but there were no clear diagnostic features to the descriptive terms used by the patients.

Sclerosing adenosis was unusually common in a study of benign breast disorders in Nigeria, both in absolute terms and in the frequency with which it was associated with mastalgia.[26] It was seen in 52 of 657 women with benign disorders, and associated with mastalgia in no fewer than 68%, whereas mastalgia was a complaint in only 10% of those with 'mammary dysplasia'.

Other causes

Cancer was an uncommon cause of pain in the Cardiff series as these cases were filtered out in the general breast clinic. Thus only one case of a cancer developing during observation in the Mastalgia Clinic was seen in Preece's original study.. This patient had a well-localized pain with no lump at presentation and negative mammography, but the pain persisted for 1 year and a repeat mammogram showed an impalpable cancer. Cancer usually shows a non-cyclical pain chart, as illustrated in Figure 8.8.

The miscellaneous group (Table 8.4) consisted of patients who were unclassifiable into the preceding groups or were shown to have pain due to a non-breast cause, such as gallstones or angina. About 10–13% of patients presenting with breast pain will be found to have a cause outside the breast, particularly of musculoskeletal origin, such as cervical spondylosis.[27]

Other general findings for the whole group of patients were that mastalgia is commoner in the left breast and half of the patients had experienced pain for over 1 year prior to consultation. Thus mastalgia is often prolonged and seems to have a predilection for the left breast as does cancer and most breast pathology.

In summary, there are three major pain patterns: the cyclical pronounced, non-cyclical and chest wall pain, and only these three will be considered further in the discussion of therapy.

AETIOLOGY OF MASTALGIA AND NODULARITY

History

Many of the surgeons who wrote about the clinical description of mastalgia also speculated on the cause of the condition, but modern hormone estimations were unavailable and most of the conclusions remained pure speculation. Several workers suggested that some ovarian influence was responsible for the cyclical pattern of mastalgia as they had noted the association with the menstrual cycle and also the absence of the problem after the menopause.[4,7] Perhaps we should not be too critical of these scientists because aetiological terms coined by them have a very familiar ring today and endocrinology was far less advanced. Cutler proposed a luteal abnormality and Geschickter described a relative hyperoestrogenism.

Other theories were those of excessive water retention and, more importantly, neuroticism. As early as 1829, Astley

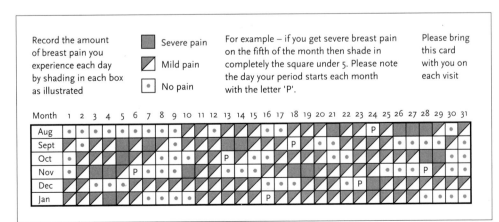

8.8 Pain chart of a patient who subsequently developed a small palpable cancer at the site of pain. The chart shows a typical non-cyclical but persistent pattern.

Cooper began the trend of describing mastalgia patients as 'being of a nervous disposition' but also added that this was a personal impression.[28] Unfortunately, this trend continued, without any rational scientific basis, and was brought up to date almost a century and a half later by a leading gynaecologist with the comment in an influential gynaecology textbook that mastalgia patients were 'frustrated, unhappy nulliparae'.[29] Even such an authority as Haagensen wrote that women with severe breast pain were 'in general, unstable and hypochondriacal although they are not frankly psychotic'.

These impressions and hypotheses have now been examined scientifically.

Studies of aetiology

Water retention

Oedema due to water retention has been suggested as a cause of both mastalgia and the premenstrual syndrome because women had reported weight gain and breast and ankle swelling in late cycle. As a result, treatment with diuretics was proposed.[30] There was, however, no study in the literature showing that general oedema was associated with mastalgia. At the Cardiff Mastalgia Clinic, we therefore carried out estimations of total body water using tritiated water in mastalgia patients and asymptomatic normal women.[31] The results clearly showed that there were no significant differences in water gain between the fifth and twenty-fifth days of the cycle when mastalgia patients were compared with normal controls, and this was true even for the cyclical group who displayed the typical premenstrual increase in breast pain. This suggests that simple retention of body water does not seem to be correlated with mastalgia, although it might be argued that intramammary oedema is more important. Breast swelling is common in the luteal phase when assessed volumetrically.[32,33] This work has been confirmed since it has been possible to study the water component of breast volume changes using MRI.[34]

Psychoneurosis

We next turned our attention to the hypothesis that mastalgia patients were more neurotic than other patients as suggested

by Astley Cooper. Using the well-validated Middlesex Hospital Questionnaire (MHQ), specifically designed as a rapid screening test for differentiating between 'normals' and psychiatric cases,[35] the psychoneurotic profiles of 300 patients presenting to hospital with mastalgia (cyclical and non-cyclical) and 156 patients presenting with varicose veins were tested.[36] The scores of the varicose vein and mastalgia patients were significantly lower than those of psychiatric outpatients, which had been published by the MHQ designers (Table 8.5).

Moreover, the only differences between mastalgia cases and varicose vein patients were in favour of the former (although a different pattern has been shown in treatment-resistant cases – discussed later in this chapter). This study showed conclusively that there is no scientific foundation for the impressions of those who believed mastalgia patients to be psychoneurotic. Psychological aspects of mastalgia are discussed more fully in Chapter 22.

Endocrine abnormalities

The advent of accurate radio-immunoassays for estimation of blood hormones and the discovery of human prolactin as a separate entity from growth hormone caused a rapid upsurge in interest in the 'hormonal imbalance' hypotheses previously discussed. From previous work, three main theories emerged regarding the aetiology of painful nodular breasts:

- Increased oestrogen secretion from the ovary
- Deficient progesterone production ('relative hyperoestrogenism'[37])
- Hyperprolactinaemia.

Early studies failed to support the first two theories, as steroid levels were found to be no different in patients and controls,[38–40] but a French group in 1979 showed a significantly depressed level of luteal progesterone,[37] thus supporting the second theory. Furthermore, the same group obtained symptomatic relief by correcting the depressed progesterone level with an exogenous progestogen. Unfortunately, no other group has been able to find a definite defect in luteal phase progesterone and in all British and American studies there was no significant difference between mastalgia patients and controls.[39,41]

Table 8.5 Neuroticism scores of mastalgia patients compared with patients with varicose veins, and psychiatric outpatients – mean (SD)

	Mastalgia (n = 300)	Varicose veins (n = 156)	Psychiatric outpatients (n = 173)
Anxiety	7.6 (0.23)	7.8 (0.30)	11.0 (0.26[a])
Depression	4.2 (0.16)	5.1 (0.21)	7.6 (0.29[a])
Phobia	5.0 (0.16)	5.7 (0.22)	6.8 (0.29[a])

[a] Significantly greater than mastalgia or varicose vein groups. High scores imply abnormality (MHQ questionnaire) .

Our experience is similar, and in a study of 50 mastalgia patients and 18 controls we failed to show any difference in luteal phase progesterone between the two groups.[42] Further studies of the free fraction of progesterone measured daily in the saliva failed to reveal any differences between controls and mastalgia patients in Wales or Scotland.[43,44] In contrast, a study of 671 patients on parenteral medroxyprogesterone acetate for contraception and 1433 controls showed a halving of clinically significant mastalgia in the contraception group.[45] The case for a luteal defect therefore remains unproven and the therapeutic value of progestogens is also debatable (see later). One review concludes that there are no significant differences in basal levels of ovarian steroids and gonadotrophins in women with benign breast conditions compared with controls.[46]

Prolactin was only accepted as a separate hormone from 1970 onwards, and a specific radioimmunoassay became available a year later, but has since received a great deal of attention. As the major lactogenic hormone, there are *prima facie* reasons for believing that it may play a role in a condition which is thought to be due to overstimulation of a normal physiological process. However, although several studies of random basal prolactin levels showed no significant differences between normals and patients with benign breast disorder (review by Wang and Fentiman[46]), analysis of prolactin secretion in normal women has shown that the hormone is secreted in a pulsatile manner and has a diurnal variation.[47] These factors suggest that random sampling of basal prolactin is inappropriate. In order to avoid these problems, Malarkey *et al.* measured 24-hour profiles, but again failed to find any differences between controls or biopsied benign disease cases at any time of the day or night.[40] One further study of daily sampling at a fixed time throughout the menstrual cycle revealed a small but statistically significant difference between women with cystic disease and controls.[48]

The above studies were performed on random or 24-hour basal prolactin levels, but a more recent approach is the examination of the dynamics of the pituitary release of prolactin.

Prolactin is almost unique in that its secretion is tonically inhibited by dopamine (Figure 8.9), but neural control of prolactin is extremely complex.[49]

However, prolactin secretion by the pituitary can be stimulated by the use of thyrotrophin-releasing hormone (TRH) and domperidone. Both agents produce an immediate rise in serum prolactin in normals and test different sections of the control system, as TRH is directly stimulatory to the lactotrophs while domperidone antagonizes the inhibitory action of dopamine on prolactin secretion. Peters and colleagues examined the stimulated prolactin response to TRH in a mixed group of benign disease patients and found that the patients with mastalgia had a significantly greater rise in prolactin compared with controls.[50]

We also examined the pituitary control of prolactin secretion in 17 patients with cyclical mastalgia compared with 11 controls and confirmed Peters' findings that the TRH-induced rise of prolactin is significantly greater at 20 minutes (Figure 8.10) and is maintained for up to 60 minutes postinjection.[51]

The basal prolactin levels were not significantly different between the groups. The enhanced prolactin response is also seen after domperidone administration (Figure 8.11), whereas the thyroid-stimulating hormone (TSH) response to TRH is not different between mastalgia patients and controls.

These studies strongly suggest that there is a disturbance of hypothalamic control in women with cyclical mastalgia and this 'fine tuning' defect may be the primary problem in painful nodular breast disease. It is of interest that a similar defect has been demonstrated in the cyclical oedema syndrome, which has many similarities to cyclical mastalgia although they are distinct conditions.[52]

Caffeine and methylxanthines

Other theories that have been put forward include the overstimulation of breast cells due to interference with ATP degradation by methylxanthines consequent on high caffeine intake.[53] There is some biochemical evidence to support this contention, but caffeine intake appears to be much lower in British women than is common in the USA and may not be relevant in the UK. Even in American women the serum caffeine and theobromine levels were found to be identical, although the catecholamines were significantly

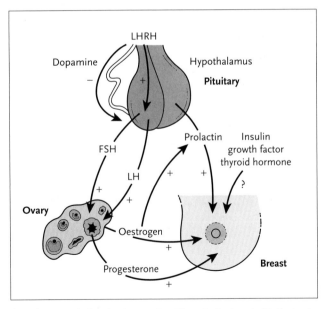

8.9 The control of prolactin secretion. The principal control is the tonic inhibitory effect of dopamine, but note that oestrogen acts to elevate prolactin levels. In practice, the relationships are more complicated than depicted in this simple diagram.

raised in women with mastalgia.[54] The epidemiological evidence for the potential role of caffeine has been conflicting as case control studies have both supported[55,56] and opposed[57-59] any association.

The methylxanthine intake varies between different cultures and a proper trial of withdrawal of a dietary substance is difficult to control, so these results need further study.

However, if a patient with mastalgia was found to have an intake in excess of 10 cups of coffee a day, it would seem worth suggesting a change to decaffeinated coffee.

The caffeine methylxanthine hypothesis has been challenged by several investigators. Two case control studies, one of histologically diagnosed benign breast disease and one of 'fibrocystic' disease, both failed to show an association with coffee consumption.[59,60] A randomized trial of caffeine reduction with non-blind assessment showed some reduction in breast nodularity in the coffee abstaining group, but the changes were minor and there was no correlation of palpable nodularity at entry to the study with coffee consumption at that time.[61]

Several studies of caffeine restriction in the treatment of mastalgia have been performed, although some of these have

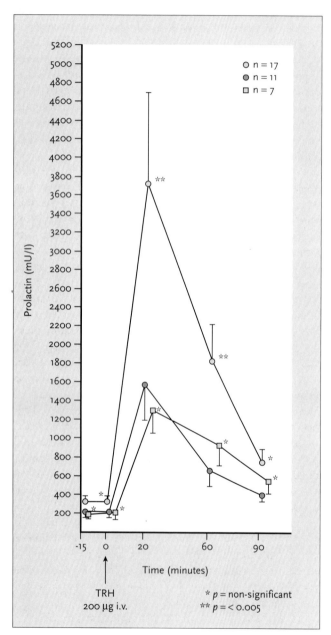

8.10 TRH test in women with cyclical and non-cyclical pain and controls. The cyclical mastalgia patients (n = 17) show a significantly increased peak release of prolactin at 20 minutes. The non-cyclical patients (n = 7) have a similar response to controls (n = 11). Values given are the mean (1 SEM. Mann–Whitney U test: (From Kumar et al.,[51] with permission of *Cancer*.)

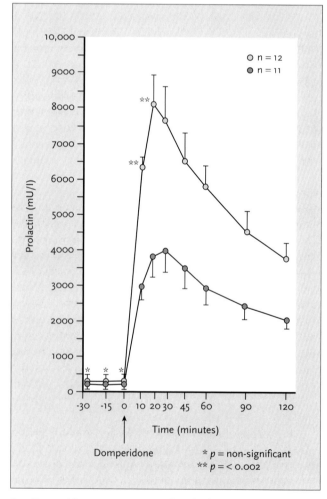

8.11 Domperidone test in women with cyclical mastalgia (n = 12) compared with controls (n = 11). Domperidone 10 mg i.v. (bolus) gives a typical high peak of prolactin secretion but the cyclical mastalgia patients show a significantly higher peak prolactin release at 20 minutes. Values given are the mean (1 SEM. Mann–Whitney U test:. (From Kumar et al.,[51] with permission of *Cancer*.)

been directed at reduction of benign proliferative disease. Minton and co-workers originally reported that caffeine restriction produced improvement in symptoms, but these studies were uncontrolled.[62] Subsequent randomized trials have failed to demonstrate a clear advantage for caffeine restriction.[61,63] Despite this, recommendations on caffeine restriction still appear in official publications on fibrocystic disease (American Cancer Society leaflet, 1992).

Prostaglandins and essential fatty acids

A recent hypothesis proposes an abnormality of prostaglandin synthesis secondary to deficient essential fatty acid (EFA) intake in the diet.[64] This is supported by circumstantial evidence that other stigmata of EFA deficiency, such as increased sebum secretion, are commoner in benign breast disorder patients.[65] Measurements of plasma fatty acids[66] have confirmed abnormal profiles in patients with mastalgia, with proportions of saturated fatty acids increased, and EFA reduced. Treatment with evening primrose oil improved the profiles towards normal, but this was not necessarily associated with a clinical response. The end result of EFA deficiency is postulated to be amplification of prolactin effects on breast cells because of deficient production of prostaglandin E1.

Other workers have reported lipid abnormalities unrelated to EFAs, with elevation of HDL-C in cyclical mastalgia patients, but not in non-cyclical.[67] They also report an improvement in symptoms consequent on a low fat dietary regimen.

Miscellaneous factors

Mastalgia is reported in a wide and diverse range of conditions, mainly associated with events during reproductive life. Examples range from a 17% incidence of new or more severe mastalgia following tubal ligation[68] to the expected association with macromastia (Chapter 15). An excess in patients who have not breastfed and in women not undertaking active exercise has been reported.[69] Mastalgia is sometimes precipitated by prescription of drugs, especially psychotropic drugs, such as phenothiazines, or herbal remedies, such as ginseng. These examples illustrate the importance of taking a comprehensive history, even though the majority of patients will have no specific underlying cause.

Pain in the nipple and areola, including that due to vasospasm, is discussed in Chapter 14.

In summary, it is clear that the cherished and widely accepted hypotheses of neuroticism and general water retention have found little support in experimental results and modern work suggests that control mechanisms of pulsatile secretion of gonadotrophins and/or prolactin are abnormal in patients with painful nodular breasts. This, of course, just moves the basic questions back one stage, leaving the aetiology of such hormonal abnormalities as the next question to be answered. The possibility of an end-organ abnormality remains to be investigated in detail.

MANAGEMENT OF PATIENTS WITH MASTALGIA

The first consideration in management is the taking of a careful history and examination of the breast. If a dominant or discrete lump is present, management is as detailed in Chapter 4. The group of patients remaining comprises those with mastalgia and nodularity and those with diffusely nodular breasts that are painless. The latter group requires nothing other than exclusion of significant pathology and can be discharged if there are no other indications for follow-up. The next section on therapy deals with patients with mastalgia irrespective of the presence of nodularity and the term 'mastalgia' is used to denote pain with or without nodularity.

Each patient must have her symptomatology assessed carefully so that the pain can be designated as cyclical or non-cyclical, and if the latter, true non-cyclical breast pain or musculoskeletal pain.

Reassurance and other supportive measures

For patients with mastalgia of whatever pattern, the first and most successful treatment is reassurance that their symptoms are not due to cancer. Geschickter stated that 'cancer should be excluded; rule out infection, reassure and give support' and Billroth emphasized that 'friendly advice, reassurance and the banishment of suspicion and fear of dread disease is of great importance'. These quotations have been emphasized because the manner of delivery and conviction of the reassurance are very important, as it is certainly true that many women consult surgeons about their mastalgia because they fear there is cancer in their breasts. Reassurance of these patients does not cure their breast pain but it does alter their attitude to the pain, so that it is no longer a serious problem.

One of the difficulties with active reassurance is that many surgeons dislike using the term 'cancer' in the patient's presence (even when discussing the absence of the condition), and so resort to various euphemisms, which are open to misinterpretation. For example, the following statement of reassurance was actually made to a patient with painful nodularity: 'You have something in your breast; don't worry about it and as there is nothing I can do about it, there's no point in me seeing you again.' Most clinicians would translate this sentence as: 'You have fibroadenosis (ANDI); it is harmless and the cause is unknown, but as I don't know of any useful treatment for the pain, I don't think you need to come to Outpatient's for a repeat visit.' However, the patient's translation was: 'I have cancer; it is incurable and the surgeon is abandoning me!'

These points are made to underline that sympathetic, detailed reassurance is required and in our Mastalgia Clinic we have successfully treated 85% of 1000 mastalgia patients by simple reassurance. In a recent review of the Edinburgh Breast Clinic McFayden *et al.* found that of 797 patients referred to the breast clinic only 213 were deemed to have sufficiently severe pain to be referred to the Mastalgia Clinic.[70]

Some clinicians agree with Geschickter's recommendation of support for the painful breast. We generally find that our patients with persistent mastalgia have already fitted themselves with the most comfortable brassière they could find. However, there is a report of the therapeutic value of a well-fitting brassière,[71] although the placebo effect of fitting a specially designed brassière in the hospital must have played a considerable part in the good results obtained.

It is inevitable that patients attending a breast clinic with breast pain will be anxious, and the effectiveness of relaxation therapy has been investigated in Aberdeen.[72] Patients were randomized to receive relaxation therapy (via an audio tape) during the middle month of a 3-month observation period, against no therapy for the controls. Sixty-one per cent of the intervention group had a response at a Cardiff Breast Score grade I or II, compared with 25% in the control group.

The next step in management is concerned with those patients who have been reassured, but still find that mastalgia causes considerable interference to their lives. This group, in our experience, is about 5% of the new patient referrals to a breast clinic and the mastalgia in this group may be so severe as to cause relationship problems within the family because a husband is unable to touch his wife's breasts for 3 weeks every month or children are unable to hug their mother.

Since there is no clear-cut diagnostic pathophysiology in mastalgia, hormonal investigations have little place in management apart from a routine prolactin level in cases with galactorrhoea or amenorrhoea, to exclude a prolactinoma. It should also be remembered that a common presentation of both mastalgia and amenorrhoea is pregnancy, but this should have been excluded by an accurate history, and if necessary by a pregnancy test.

In cases where the onset of pain corresponds to institution of drug therapy, consideration should be given to stopping or substituting the drug, depending on the indications for the drug, and taking into account the fact that mild mastalgia of this type will frequently decrease spontaneously with time.

The contraceptive pill

The role of the oral contraceptives in the epidemiology of breast cancer is hotly debated and, due to the long lag between hormonal events and breast cancer occurrence, the matter remains unresolved. However, in terms of benign breast disorders, most reports have indicated a protective effect.[73,74] We have recorded the type of oral contraceptive taken by our mastalgia patients but on analysis there are no correlations between pain patterns and brands. Some women may experience mastalgia for the first time on starting a new oral contraceptive but most mastalgia then tends to disappear or is minimal.

In a study of 44 patients suffering from mastalgia/nodularity at the time of starting oral contraception, 53% found an improvement in their mastalgia, but nodularity improved in only 8%.[75]

If a patient has severe mastalgia that starts for the first time on commencing oral contraception, it is worth advising either a change to a lower dose or, if already on a 30 μg pill, a change to a different brand. Little is known of the exact effects of exogenous 'balanced' mixtures of oestrogens and progestogens as the controversy regarding the 'potency factors' of different progestogens has shown.[76,77] If mastalgia remains a major problem, then occasionally a change to mechanical methods of contraception may be helpful, but there is no guarantee of response and the risks of an unwanted pregnancy are increased. In our experience, the severity of the mastalgia dictates whether the patient will readily agree to stop taking the oral contraceptive.

Drugs available for treating mastalgia

The many different hypotheses of aetiology of benign breast disorders discussed in the previous section have given rise to a number of specific therapies which are perhaps more logical than the previous empirical treatments (Table 8.6). However, it is important to distinguish clearly between controlled and uncontrolled studies because there is a powerful placebo effect in subjective symptoms such as pain. Our

Table 8.6 Mastalgia: aetiological hypotheses and treatments	
Hypothesis	**Treatment**
Hyperoestrogenism	Androgens/anti-oestrogens (tamoxifen)/LHRH agonists
Luteal insufficiency	Progesterone/progestogens
Hyperprolactinaemia	Bromocriptine (dopamine agonist)
Increased gonadotrophin	Danazol (antigonadotrophin)
Dietary methylxanthines	Caffeine restriction
Dietary essential fatty acids (EFA) deficiency	Evening primrose oil (EFA supplement)
Local inflammation or fibrosis	Local steroid injection
Miscellaneous	Pyridoxine/thyroid hormones/vitamin A/HRT

benchmark for studies is the double-blind, placebo-controlled trial and we have used this technique in nearly all of our therapeutic studies.

We have devised a number of objective methods of assessment which can be analysed and submitted to statistical analysis, including pain charts indicating number of days of symptoms per month, visual linear analogue (VLA) scales for patient assessment of severity, and clinician assessment of tenderness and nodularity. The results can be expressed in absolute and comparative terms, pre- and post-treatment, for each individual (Figure 8.12).

We have also found it helpful to have an overall response grade – the Cardiff Breast Score (CBS) – to assess the benefit of treatment (Table 8.7).[78]

Doppler measurement of breast vascularity has been used to monitor response to drug therapy in mastalgia, with a good correlation reported.[79] This may prove a useful approach, but requires wider confirmation in view of the operator dependency of these techniques.

Diuretics

One of the popular treatments, certainly among primary healthcare physicians, is the administration of diuretics. These have no rational basis, as was demonstrated by the lack of correlation between retention of body water and symptoms.[31] As no placebo-controlled trial has shown any beneficial effect, it is likely that their apparent 'efficacy' in general practice is due to the placebo effect. Pain is the subjective symptom *par excellence*, and for this reason all studies in mastalgia should be at least placebo controlled and preferably randomized between the active and placebo therapies.

Progestogens

The luteal deficiency hypothesis, recently championed by Mauvais-Jarvis and his colleagues,[37] had also been considered by earlier workers and attempts were made to correct the progesterone deficiency by administration of luteal extracts with varying success. The apparent demonstration by the Paris group of a definite progesterone deficiency in benign breast disorders gave rise to hopes that simple correction by progestogens would be useful. Other groups had also failed to find a progesterone deficiency.

Progestogens have been compared with placebo in the PMS and failed to show any benefit greater than the placebo effect.[80] A randomized controlled trial of medroxyprogesterone acetate in patients with cyclical mastalgia showed no significant improvement in pain, tenderness or nodularity.[81] A recent double-blind randomized study of 80 mastalgia patients using vaginal micronized progesterone showed a greater than 50% reduction in pain in 65% of the active group compared with 22% in the placebo group.[82] Breast nodularity was not affected. In a double-blind placebo-controlled study of the application of progesterone gel to the breast, von Fournier *et al.* were unable to find an active effect despite the known absorption of progesterone through the skin[83] and a similar study in Edinburgh gave similar results. Thus the precise role of progesterone and progestogens remains unclear.

Bromocriptine

The discovery of a small elevation of basal prolactin in patients with benign breast disorders[48] and the availability of a specific prolactin-lowering agent, bromocriptine, suggested that the first truly specific treatment for mastalgia was attainable. In fact, a report of the effectiveness of bromocriptine had already appeared, describing a good response in 10 or 15 patients in an open study.[84] Soon afterwards a controlled study showed that the drug was effective in relieving breast swelling in patients with the premenstrual syndrome.

Table 8.7 The Cardiff Breast Score	
CBS I	An excellent response leaving no residual pain
CBS II	A substantial response leaving some residual pain but considered by the patient to be easily bearable
CBS III	A poor response leaving substantial residual pain
CBS IV	No response
Thus CBS I and II are considered useful responses, III and IV as non-responders.	

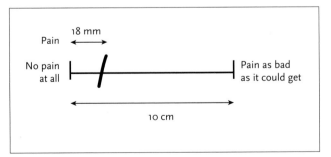

8.12 A typical VLA scale. The patient has made a mark 18 mm from the 'no pain' end and so a reading of 18 is obtained. This scale is sometimes known as an LAS scale (linear analogue scale).

These encouraging results were tested in the Cardiff Mastalgia Clinic in a double-blind, placebo-controlled trial carried out on 53 patients using a bromocriptine dosage of 2.5 mg twice daily.[85] Assessment of response, which had been sketchy with the previous two bromocriptine trials, was improved by using a simple scale for the clinician's assessment, and a subjective, self-rating VLA scale for the patient's response (Figure 8.12).

The VLA scales were completed independently of the clinician's assessment. Unlike the previous studies, the patients were randomized into their respective pain patterns to see if any pattern responded preferentially. The results of this trial showed that the cyclical pattern of pain was significantly reduced by bromocriptine compared with placebo, but that the non-cyclical pattern failed to respond (Figure 8.13).

This trial demonstrated for the first time that patients classified according to a simple symptomatic classification responded differentially to a precise manipulation of the pituitary output of prolactin. Blood sampling during the trial confirmed the depression of prolactin levels on bromocriptine to subnormal levels as these patients were initially normoprolactinaemic as expected.

It is currently not understood how lowering of prolactin levels produces amelioration of mastalgia, but the mechanism is presumed to be due to a reduction in the overall stimulation of breast cells by prolactin, because it is known that bromocriptine does not lower sex steroid levels. When the data on serum prolactin levels were analysed to see if there was a correlation between amount of depression and symptom improvement, no correlation could be found. This suggests that the effects may be more complicated than was first thought. As bromocriptine is a dopamine agonist, it is possible that there is a direct effect on breast tissue, independent of prolactin effects, if breast cells have dopamine receptors similar to those found on pituitary cells. However, recent studies in our laboratories have failed to detect dopamine receptors on human breast cells grown in monolayer culture.

Confirmation of the Cardiff results has come from other controlled trials,[86–88] and it is clear from review of the literature that this drug is consistently effective in reducing the symptoms of mastalgia.[89] The problem with bromocriptine is that some women experience severe side-effects, the commonest being nausea, vomiting and dizziness, which have caused a 20% drop-out rate in many trials. The severity of side-effects can be reduced by introducing the drug slowly in an incremental scheme and avoiding doses higher than 2.5 mg twice daily (Table 8.8).

The incidence of side-effects is variable and some women have no problems even at high dosage. In our experience, of 216 patients treated with bromocriptine, 75 (35%) had significant adverse effects and 46 had to stop treatment (although 13 of these had already had a clinically useful response).

Danazol

Danazol was introduced in 1971 by Greenblatt and co-workers, who suggested it may have a role in mastalgia.[90] This agent, like bromocriptine, is unique in its action on the pituitary–ovarian axis. It was originally described as an impeded androgen and in monkeys it was shown to act as an antigonadotrophin, as it depressed serum follicle-stimulating hormone (FSH) and luteinizing hormone (LH) and prevented ovulation. Its action in humans is not so clearly defined because it only interferes with FSH and LH levels at high dosage. It may have a local tissue effect as it has been shown to bind to both progesterone and androgen receptors but not to oestrogen receptors.

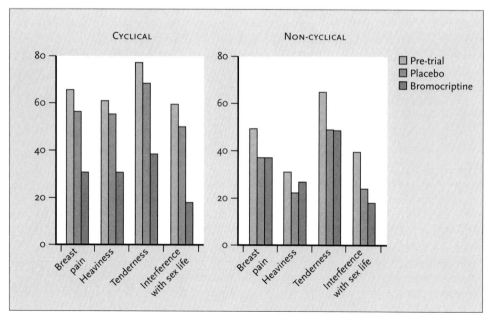

8.13 VLA results of the Cardiff controlled trial of bromocriptine in mastalgia. Note the placebo response in both cyclical and non-cyclical patients, but the significantly lower scores, i.e. improvement, on bromocriptine in the cyclical patients. (From Mansel et al.,[85] with permission of the British Journal of Surgery.)

Table 8.8 Recommended incremental dosage scheme for bromocriptine therapy

Days	Dose
1–3	1.25 mg at night with food
4–7	2.5 mg at night with food
8–11	1.25 mg in the morning and 2.5 mg at night (with food)
12 onwards	2.5 mg in the morning and 2.5 mg at night (with food)

Greenblatt's group initially used the drug for treating endometriosis but a number of papers soon followed from the same group showing the usefulness of danazol in painful nodular breast disease.[91,92] All these reports were of uncontrolled studies and appeared to be cumulative, and were thus open to the criticisms of lack of placebo control. We therefore carried out a double-blind placebo study in the Cardiff Mastalgia Clinic on 28 patients with cyclical mastalgia, using a detailed protocol similar to that described earlier.[93] This study showed that danazol was clearly beneficial in cyclical mastalgia, producing both relief of symptoms and reduction in nodularity and these effects could be obtained with doses as low as 200 mg. The lower dose gave much lower side-effects and only a 10% drop-out rate was recorded in the trial.

The hormonal effects of danazol treatment were a low luteal progesterone (suggesting anovulation) and an unchanged prolactin, so it appears the drug is working on the ovary or pituitary although only 30% of these patients were amenorrhoeic on the drug. The side-effects are mainly amenorrhoea, the incidence of which increases with dose up to 100% at 600–800 mg, and various mild androgenic effects such as weight gain, acne and hirsutism. All of these effects are dose related and can be minimized by low-dose therapy.[94] Our current practice is to start at 200 mg daily and then use a maintenance dose of 100 mg daily on alternate days.

In our experience, of 295 patients treated with danazol, 88 (30%) complained of significant adverse events and 43 had to stop treatment. However, many of these were before we had developed the low-dose regimen. A recently reported side-effect has been a lowering of the voice pitch which has been permanent in a small number of cases, but our experience is that only 5% of patients notice this symptom and it is generally reversible on stopping the drug. Danazol currently appears to be the best agent for severe breast pain and nodularity with an overall improvement rate of 70% in our total group of 295 treated patients.

Another double-blind, controlled study from Nottingham reported that danazol was superior to bromocriptine for cyclical breast pain.[95] A paper reporting the experience of a Brisbane mastalgia clinic also confirmed the efficacy of danazol in practice with an overall success rate of 67% compared with the rates of 30–40% for other agents.[69]

Both Peters[96] and Stein et al.[97] showed a significant benefit from the somewhat similar agent gestrinone, which has androgenic, anti-oestrogenic and antiprogestogenic properties, and some androgenic side-effects. Both double-blind, randomized placebo-controlled studies used 2.5 mg twice weekly for 3 months, with benefits and side-effects similar to danazol. The lower dosage necessary has potential advantages regarding side-effects, but the drug does not yet have the benefit of the extensive and prolonged experience with danazol.

Evening primrose oil

The fatty acid deficiency hypothesis has led to the testing of treatment by supplementing the diet with an EFA. One preparation which has proved valuable is the oil of evening primrose (EPO) which is unique in containing 7% (-linolenic acid and 72% linoleic acid and represents the richest natural source of EFAs known (Figure 8.14).

Several trials have shown EPO to be useful for treating mild cases of cyclical mastalgia.[98] This agent is potentially useful in mild to moderate cases as it has virtually no side-effects. Patient acceptance is high as it is viewed as a 'natural substance' rather than a hormone or drug. Interestingly, the EPO trial also showed that non-cyclical pain was unresponsive to this therapy, as had been found in the bromocriptine trial, although this conclusion has been modified with further analysis of the non-cyclical group, as discussed later. The positive balance of moderate effectiveness and minimal side-effects leads us to use it as the first-line treatment in patients with mastalgia of moderate severity. In our own experience, of 85 patients treated with EPO as first-line therapy, 58% had a clinically useful response (CBS I or II). In our overall experience of 241 patients treated only 9 (4%) complained of a significant adverse effect.

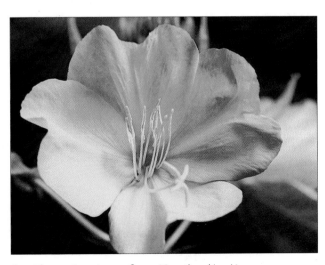

8.14 The evening primrose flower (*Oenothera biennis*).

Tamoxifen

The anti-oestrogen drug tamoxifen was reported to be helpful in mastalgia in an Italian study,[99] but this drug is currently only licensed for the treatment of breast cancer in the UK. A recent double-blind study of tamoxifen in Guy's Hospital, London, showed that tamoxifen 10 mg daily significantly improved mastalgia, with response rates of 98% for cyclical and 56% for non-cyclical pain. Side-effects were reported to be 'minimal', but in this study about 15% of the patients dropped out on therapy.[100]

A further study from the Guy's group showed that 20 mg of tamoxifen was equally effective, but gave the same relapse rate and caused much higher side-effects.[21] This study also compared 3- versus 6-month treatments; the longer period did not increase response rate, nor did it reduce the relapse rate (seen in up to half the patients by 2–3 months). The same group have investigated various metabolic side-effects of tamoxifen in their patients, and found no significant alteration with short-term treatment.[101,102]

In the largest trial to date,[103] the dose has been reduced further to 11 days per cycle. Three hundred and one women were randomized to receive 10 mg or 20 mg daily from day 15 to day 25 in the cycle over a period of 3 months. There were no placebo controls. The response rate was no different in the two groups: three-quarters obtained a useful response. One-quarter had recurrence by one year, again with no difference between the groups. However, side-effects were significantly greater in the 20 mg group, 66% versus 50%, although only 8% and 2% stopped treatment because of side-effects.

A potential problem of tamoxifen therapy in premenopausal women is an elevation of serum oestradiol on tamoxifen, although this was not found by Ricciardi and Ianniruberto.[99] A further problem has been raised by a toxicology study which showed that a small number of rats developed liver tumours on high-dose tamoxifen. Although the drug is currently mainly indicated for malignant disease, it is being used increasingly as a third-line drug for mastalgia, while recognizing that relapse is a significant problem at the end of the course. The appropriate dose on present experience is 10 mg daily for 3 months, repeated for relapse if necessary, with further courses given only after full consideration of the possible long-term effects. The latest trial suggests that treatment in the luteal phase only may be successful, further reducing the likelihood of adverse long-term effects.

LHRH analogues

These are dealt with below in the section on refractory mastalgia.

Other therapeutic approaches

A number of groups report varying degrees of success with different dietary measures, particularly a low fat diet.[67,104] Boyd and colleagues[104] have reported marked improvement in breast symptoms after a diet which limits fats to 15% of caloric intake. However, the practical difficulties in maintaining and monitoring such a diet probably explain the less enthusiastic interest among all but the most dedicated patients and centres.

The evidence for many other varied therapeutic approaches is generally poor and it is likely that the results reported are due to the placebo effect.

Leis has reported excellent results in a series of 721 mastalgia patients outside a formal study.[105] The low-fat, high-fibre diet, supplemented with vitamins A, C and selenium, gave an 81% response for pain and tenderness and 39% response for nodularity.

The caffeine/methylxanthine theory suggests that withdrawal of dietary coffee, cola and chocolate would help the symptoms of benign breast disorder, and this has been found in an open study by Minton et al.[62] While this may be relevant to cultures with a very high coffee intake, other experience is less convincing. This question is discussed earlier in this chapter with consideration of aetiology.

A small number of studies have suggested that pyridoxine (vitamin B_6) may be useful in treating mastalgia on the basis that pyridoxine will enhance the decarboxylation of dopa to dopamine and so inhibit prolactin levels. Most studies have been uncontrolled and further it has been shown that pyridoxine treatment does not lower serum prolactin in patients with the amenorrhoea–galactorrhoea syndrome.[106] In contradistinction, a recent study has shown that pyridoxine lowers exercise-induced prolactin secretion.[107] A double-blind study using pyridoxine at a dose of 200 mg daily in cyclical mastalgia found that the vitamin did not significantly improve breast pain compared with placebo.[108]

Other studies of vitamin A administration and treatment with thyroid hormone[109] have been reported to show improvement of mastalgia, but the studies were open and involved a small number of heterogeneous patients and are thus difficult to interpret.

Vitamin E has been studied in a controlled trial using mammographic change as the outcome measure in 105 women, but no changes were found compared to the placebo group.[110]

Treatments for non-cyclical mastalgia

All the above treatments have been directed at the cyclical group of patients whether the authors have realized this or not, but our studies suggest that the cyclical group appears to have an endocrine basis and, in turn, appears to respond to endocrine-directed therapy. It also seemed at first that the non-cyclical group appeared to be unresponsive to manipulation of the endocrine system but results have been more encouraging when true non-cyclical mastalgia has been differentiated from musculoskeletal pain of chest wall origin.

Our results show that it is worthwhile treating true non-cyclical mastalgia in the same way as for cyclical mastalgia. This then leaves musculoskeletal pain, localized 'trigger-spot' pain, and refractory mastalgia. A report of five cases of breast pain relieved by surgical decompression of the thoracic outlet [111] emphasizes the need to exclude referred pain in general, and musculoskeletal pain in particular in all cases. These patients all had typical arm pain as well as breast pain, so differentiation from mastalgia should not be difficult.

Attempts have been made to treat the generalized non-cyclical group with non-steroidal anti-inflammatory agents but there is no published evidence of their efficacy. Our experience of non-steroidal anti-inflammatory drugs (NSAIDs) is similarly disappointing. As an extension of this approach, Crile suggested that a local injection of lignocaine and prednisolone may be effective in relieving the localized non-cyclical pain.[112] His description corresponds to the trigger-spot subgroup mentioned previously and he found the steroid/local anaesthetic injection gave initial relief in two-thirds of the patients with continued relief in about one-half of the patients followed. Our experience has been similar; we have obtained a 70% response rate.

Surgical excision

More extensive surgical excision for mastalgia as a symptom is uncommon but prophylactic excision for premalignant disease has been performed more commonly and is considered in Chapter 4. For most types of mastalgia, except the trigger spot mentioned above, the symptom extends so widely in the breast that segmental resection is insufficient. Thus most surgeons have used subcutaneous mastectomy, or total mastectomy in earlier times. Most of these operations are carried out for 'prophylaxis' of breast cancer by plastic surgeons and documentation of the numbers and results of operations performed solely for mastalgia is very poor, although nearly all authors list mastalgia as an indication for the operation. The Nottingham Breast Clinic reported that only four patients underwent subcutaneous mastectomies for mastalgia in 12 years, with only two patients obtaining relief and one patient developing a fibrous capsule.

Our experience is of only 12 cases over 25 years, all with severe mastalgia resistant to medication, and drawn from a pool including many tertiary referrals as well as our own cases.[113] They represent less than 1% of cases of mastalgia severe enough to require detailed investigation and treatment. The median age at time of surgery was 35 years (29–53) and duration of pain prior to surgery 6.5 (2–16) years. The procedures were two quadrantectomies, one bilateral subcutaneous mastectomy without reconstruction, and subcutaneous mastectomy with implant in eight patients, three bilateral. The results were not encouraging, only five patients (50%) were free of pain after mastectomy, and pain recurred in both patients with quadrantectomy. Five patients having mastectomy developed complications, wound dehiscence in two (eventually requiring musculocutaneous flap reconstruction), and capsular contraction in five. However, on review those patients who were pain-free were happy long term with the outcome, and considered the cosmetic deficiencies well justified by the relief of pain.

Surgery should only be undertaken after all drug therapies have been exhausted and have failed. The patient should be reviewed by a psychologist prior to surgery, and the complications of the procedure, which are common both early and in the long term, outlined by the surgeon. Particularly troublesome is fibrous contracture around implants, especially if they are placed subcutaneously (Figure 8.15).

Additionally, nipple or areolar necrosis and infection of the prosthesis are not uncommon. Our view is that this operation is rarely indicated for breast pain because it has a modest chance of therapeutic success and a high incidence of complications. A review of the detailed results of this operation performed for mastalgia is urgently needed but perhaps the paucity of published figures reflects other surgeons' disquiet about surgery for this indication.

NATURAL HISTORY OF MASTALGIA

One of the problems of therapeutic trials in mastalgia is that the natural history of the condition is poorly documented. Because spontaneous remissions can occur, these may give a false impression of treatment benefit. Geschickter[7] briefly described some features of the natural

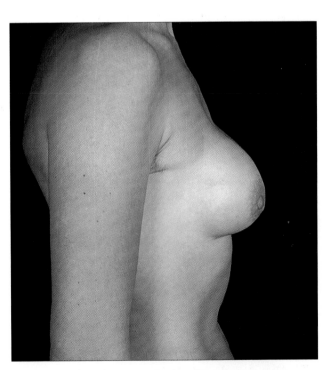

8.15 Patient with a subcutaneous implant after subcutaneous mastectomy for benign breast disease. The breast is hard to palpation and projects rigidly from the chest wall. Although this complication is now seen less frequently with more modern techniques and prostheses, it has not been eliminated.

history of his mastodynia cases and noted that the majority found relief of pain at the menopause.

In an effort to correct this lack of knowledge, we undertook a review of all our mastalgia cases documented between 1973 and 1976 in the Cardiff Mastalgia Clinic.[114] There were a total of 258 patients and a follow-up of 66% was obtained by direct interview or postal questionnaire. Details regarding the duration of pain and spontaneous remission were obtained. The results showed that cyclical pain was most commonly relieved by hormonal events such as pregnancy and the menopause but this was not the case with non-cyclical pain. It also appeared that patients with cyclical pain who started having symptoms at an early age (<20 years) tended to have persistent pain often throughout reproductive life, whereas a late age of onset was associated with a shorter overall duration of pain. This implies that younger patients may require treatment for prolonged periods as we had previously found that post-treatment recurrence of pain is common. In view of these findings, we aim to treat young patients with severe mastalgia in short intermittent bursts rather than continuous periods. However, patients near the menopause may be treated for longer periods in the expectation that their pain will be naturally resolved in the near future by their menopause.

It should be noted that patients investigated in the Mastalgia Clinic were by definition severe cases of long duration, so these findings do not apply to the many women who develop mild to moderate mastalgia in the fourth and fifth decades. In many of these patients, natural remission occurs within a few months.

PLAN OF MANAGEMENT FOR PATIENTS WITH MASTALGIA

Our detailed management protocol and experience of treatment in nearly 300 mastalgia patients has been published[115] and recently updated for 500 patients.[78] The improved response rate (92% with cyclical and 64% with non-cyclical) in the second report compared with the earlier one reflects improved understanding of the diagnosis and classification of mastalgia, along with more accurate assessment of each of the drug therapies for particular patients (Figures 8.16 and 8.17).

The corresponding response rates to placebo have been CBS I 4%, CBS II 15%, CBS III 6% and CBS IV 75%.

The important points in management are shown in Table 8.9.

The first priority is exclusion of cancer by appropriate tests and firm reassurance of the patient. This will be adequate treatment for around 85% of patients with mastalgia presenting to hospital and probably higher in family practice.

The 15% of mastalgia patients with severe mastalgia who are not helped by reassurance should then be assessed initially by a pain chart to define the pain pattern to give a baseline measurement of the number of days of pain per cycle. Patients who are still troubled by their mastalgia after 2–3 months of charting (to allow for spontaneous remission) should be treated by one of the three main agents.

Cyclical mastalgia
Our current first choice for treatment of cyclical mastalgia is EPO as it has a reasonable response and is almost free of side-effects. In addition it does not interfere with the menstrual cycle, but cost can be a problem in some countries. Our next option is danazol which has the best response rate overall (around 80%) but has significant side-effects (Table 8.10), especially on the menstrual cycle.

However, low-dose maintenance regimens of danazol using 25 or 50 mg per day have much lower side-effects. The third agent we use is bromocriptine which has an efficacy midway between danazol and EPO (Figure 8.16), but also gives side-effects in some 20% of patients (Table 8.10), principally nausea and dizziness. The drug does not disturb the menstrual cycle

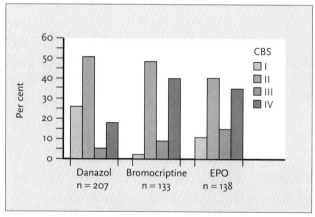

8.16 Overall response of patients with cyclical mastalgia to drug treatment (EPO, evening primrose oil; CBS, Cardiff Breast Score). (From Gateley et al.[78])

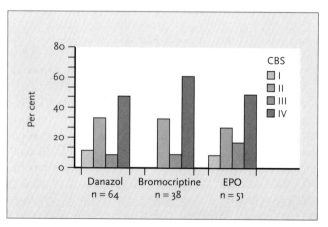

8.17 Overall response of patients with non-cyclical mastalgia to drug treatment (EPO, evening primrose oil; CBS, Cardiff Breast Score). (From Gateley et al.[78])

and this is a positive advantage to some patients. Our review of treatment has shown that failure of response to one drug does not predict subsequent failure on another drug, so it is worth trying all three drugs in turn in an individual before concluding that the mastalgia is unresponsive.

Patients are assessed after 2 months of treatment (4 months for EPO) and given a CBS grade. If a clinically useful grade (CBS I and II) has been achieved, treatment is continued for a full 6-month course (if danazol, on a reduced maintenance dose). With a CBS III score, treatment is continued for a further 2 months then reassessed. CBS IV patients are considered for an alternative therapy at 2 months.

Non-cyclical mastalgia

The overall response with true non-cyclical mastalgia to the three principal drug therapies is lower at around 50%

overall, but rises to 64% if patients are carefully divided into true non-cyclical and musculoskeletal. The order of efficacy of the agents is still danazol, bromocriptine and EPO (Figure 8.17); because the response rates are lower, we recommend using danazol first as this offers the best chance of response.

Again it is worth trying the other agents in turn, but the evidence from the controlled studies shows that bromocriptine and EPO effects are only slightly better than placebo in non-cyclical patients.

The use of local anaesthetic and steroid injection in non-cyclical mastalgia is well worth while if a persistent localized painful area can be demonstrated on repeat visits to the clinic, and the same is true for musculoskeletal chest wall pain. We use Depo-Medrone with lidocaine injection (Upjohn) which contains methylprednisolone 40 mg and lignocaine (lidocaine) hydrochloride 10 mg/mL. Medially located injections are conveniently performed with the patient supine, laterally located injections are best made in the lateral position, affected side uppermost, in each case so that the breast falls into a dependent position, minimizing the thickness of traversed breast tissue. The localized tender area is marked and 1 mL of the injection is carefully infiltrated at the level of the pectoral fascia. (The injection should not be subcutaneous as this will cause skin atrophy.) The only side-effect is mild local discomfort but this is quickly relieved by the local anaesthetic. Care should be exercised to make sure the injection is not too deep as we have seen one small pneumothorax following an injection into the axillary tail.

Choice of drug with regard to side-effects

The choice of drug should be generally as recommended in Table 8.9 but the attitude of the patient may indicate the final choice. Patients who are fertile must take mechanical precautions against pregnancy if taking bromocriptine or danazol as both of these agents are potentially teratogenic and may interfere with concomitant oral contraception

---

Table 8.9 Principles of mastalgia treatment

1. Exclude cancer
2. Reassurance
3. Define pattern (pain chart or history)
4. Cyclical mastalgia (overall response 92%)
   (a) EPO: six capsules daily
   (b) Danazol: 100–300 mg daily then reduce
   (c) Bromocriptine: 1.25 mg, increasing to 3.75–5 mg daily
5. True non-cyclical mastalgia (overall response 64%)
   (a) Danazol
   (b) EPO
   (c) Bromocriptine
6. Musculoskeletal chest wall pain
   Lignocaine/steroid injection to trigger spots and Tietze's syndrome
7. Consider surgery only as a last resort.

Table 8.10 Side-effects of the principal therapies

Therapy	Common side-effects	Incidence(%)
Danazol (100–400 mg)	Weight gain Acne Amenorrhoea Hirsutism Reduction in breast size Voice change	25
Bromocriptine (2.5 mg twice daily)	Nausea Dizziness Headache	20
Evening primrose oil (6 capsules daily)	Mild nausea	<2

pills. Thus, a patient who is unable or refuses to use barrier contraception should be treated with EPO, which can be taken with the oral contraceptive. If patients dislike the idea of drug-induced amenorrhoea, the choice of agents will be between EPO and bromocriptine, neither of which alters the menstrual cycle. These choices are illustrated in the flow diagram in Figure 8.18.

Length of drug treatment
It appears from our studies that the good response obtained with most of the endocrine treatments was short lived, as might be expected if the postulated endocrine defect is long term. In the danazol trial, recurrence of symptoms was appearing 3 months after finishing active treatment (Figure 8.19).

We have found that about one-half of the patients have recurrent mastalgia at 6 months but some of these had milder pain than before. Other authors have similar experience.[116]

Our current policy is to treat for 2 months (danazol and bromocriptine) or 4 months (EPO) initially. If a clinically useful response (CBS I or II) is obtained, treatment is continued for a full 6 months (with reduced dose for danazol). If there is a CBS III response, treatment is continued for a further 2 months (provided side-effects are not troublesome) with review after a further 2 months.

Of the 50% that recur, some will not require further therapy as the pain is milder but the patients with severe recurrences can be put back onto the original therapy if there had been a previous good response, or on to an alternative if the

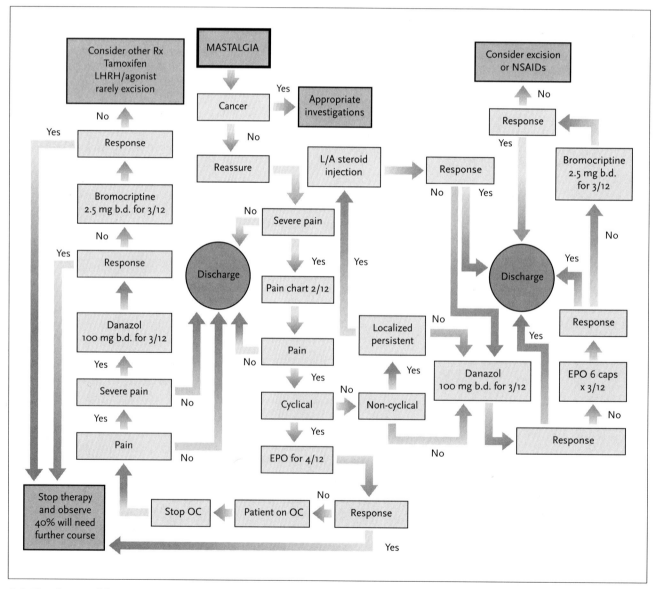

8.18 Flow diagram of the management of mastalgia. (L/A, local anaesthetic; OC, oral contraceptive.)

initial response had been poor.[78,117] (This change of therapy often had occurred already if the response had been poor.) These short treatment bursts limit drug costs and may be less suppressive to the pituitary–ovarian axis than continuous treatment, although studies of long-term usage and high dosage in both bromocriptine and danazol have not indicated any permanent suppression.

What happens to patients who defect during treatment? Of 71 such patients contacted from the Longmore Breast Clinic in Edinburgh, 36 said they were better, 19 felt no more could be done, 18 had learnt to live with their pain, 14 did not want more treatment even if the pain recurred, 5 were still taking the medication prescribed, 2 were pregnant and 5 postmenopausal.

MASTALGIA IN THE POSTMENOPAUSAL PATIENT

Although mastalgia is seen much less frequently after the menopause, in recent years the widespread use of HRT is leading to an increased incidence. The basic principles of assessment and management are similar to those in premenopausal patients, with some provisos.

Non-breast causes such as biliary pain, cervical spondylosis and shoulder lesions are more common and need careful exclusion. Likewise, the higher incidence of breast cancer requires careful assessment of persisting focal pain. Fortunately, diagnostic imaging techniques are more accurate in this age group, although HRT may cause obscuring parenchymal densities more typical of premenopausal women. Because true breast pain is uncommon in postmenopausal women (except on HRT), most are due to musculoskeletal pain (Figure 8.20).

Management is the same as for premenopausal women.

Patients on HRT

In postmenopausal women, continuous oestrogen administration may stimulate ductal cell proliferation resulting in mild discomfort with fullness and nipple paraesthesia, but these symptoms do not persist.[118] In contrast, combined oestrogen and progesterone stimulates both ductal and alveolar cells to give fullness and tenderness. While this is usually modest and temporary, it may be severe and persist. Paradoxically, women who have breast tenderness at the start of HRT tend to have relief, whereas those without it before tend to develop tenderness after HRT, although this usually resolves by 6 months.[119] Where this requires active management, the following options can be tried:

* Stop the HRT, if this is appropriate.
* Try progesterone alone. As the level of oestrogen/progesterone receptors decreases, breast symptoms rapidly resolve as the cells undergo apoptosis. This option may not be acceptable to some women because progesterone may cause bloating, weight gain and depression.
* Try a medium dose of unopposed progestogens. This needs to continue for 3 months, as the initial effect is to cause a surge of mitosis, making symptoms worse, but then going on to secretory effects. Bromocriptine has proved ineffective in mastalgia due to HRT, and there are inadequate data on the efficacy of danazol in this situation.

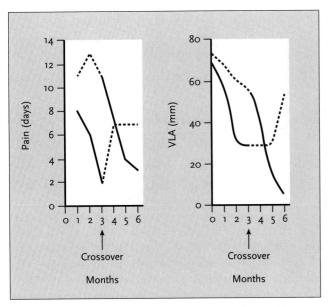

8.19 The results of the Cardiff danazol trial for days of pain and VLA scores for tenderness. Note that symptoms return after 1–3 months when the patients took placebo (----) after a course of danazol (——).

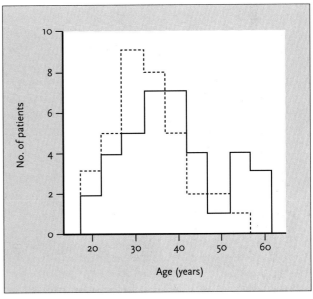

8.20 The age incidence of true non-cyclical mastalgia compared with musculoskeletal pain. ---- , Non-cyclical mastalgia; —— , musculoskeletal pain. (From Maddox *et al.*[20])

PATIENTS WITH REFRACTORY MASTALGIA

Every breast clinic has a small group of patients who appear refractory to normal therapeutic approaches and recognition as a centre with an interest in mastalgia leads to increasing numbers of such referrals from an increasingly wide geographical area. There is no single or simple answer to the management of these patients, but each needs to be assessed in greater than usual depth, and in an individual manner.

First, the classification and severity of the pain should be reassessed with the benefit of a new period of pain chart recording. Many such patients have had inadequate standard treatment, as a result of inadequate assessment, inappropriate prescription or failure to comply. Such patients merit a further episode of conventional treatment with full explanation. Our study of 126 patients who failed to respond to first-line therapy with bromocriptine, danazol or EPO, showed a 57% response to a second drug and a 25% response to a third drug.[120] The corresponding figures for non-cyclical pain were 24% and 21% (little better than placebo). However, most of these secondary responses were to danazol; in patients who had previously had one of the other drugs, response rates were very low in patients who had failed to respond to danazol. Analysis of responders and non-responders to first-line therapy failed to identify any factors which might help predict a secondary response.

When a patient fails to respond to danazol, it is probably best to move to tamoxifen or possibly an LHRH analogue if the patient wishes to try further therapy, recognizing the possible side-effects, especially with prolonged therapy. Tamoxifen can be given as 10 mg daily for 3 months, and possibly only on days 15–25 of the cycle. As it induces ovulation, contraception is particularly important if appropriate. Zoladex, a depot LHRH analogue, is given as a rod containing 3.6 mg zoladex delivered into the subcutaneous space of the abdominal wall each 28 days for six doses. Although it has proved to give some beneficial effect,[121] the unpleasant menopause-like side-effects and the risks to bone metabolism limit its general use.

Can psychological testing help? Preece et al.,[36] using the MHQ to assess psychoneurotic tendency, identified an abnormal subgroup of patients (4%) who had failed to respond to reassurance and three treatment options. Their scores were close to those of psychiatric patients, in contrast to the normal scores of the average mastalgia patient. This test might be useful as a predictor of failure of response, but has not been tested in this way prospectively.

Jenkins et al.[122] carried out a similar study of patients with severe, refractory mastalgia using a structured, diagnostic psychiatric interview. In this group, they found a significant incidence of psychiatric abnormality, including anxiety, panic disorder, somatization disorder and depression, patterns common in other groups suffering from various types of chronic pain. They suggest that this subgroup might benefit from psychiatric assessment and trial of tricyclic antidepressants, particularly before any surgical approach for refractory mastalgia.

Can endocrine evaluation help? Kumar et al.[123] showed that the results of dynamic pituitary function testing correlated with the response to hormonal therapy in cyclical mastalgia patients, but this invasive test would not be suitable for routine use. Its efficacy raises the possibillty that a simpler, non-invasive endocrine assessment may become available.

The example given here illustrates the diverse factors that can underlie refractory mastalgia. Such 'one-off' factors become more likely with increasing refractoriness, and require patient 'listening' to elucidate.

A 35-year-old woman attending the breast clinic of a major institution was asked to undergo an open breast biopsy as part of an ongoing research project at that time. She reluctantly agreed, and the biopsy was complicated by a major haematoma requiring drainage under general anaesthesia and delayed healing. She did not see the original surgeon again, and staff were unwilling to discuss her complication, the details of the research project or her constant pain at the site of the scar. She consulted three breast surgeons of repute in different institutions, by whom she was treated unsuccessfully with a variety of hormonal and non-hormonal measures. Each lost interest when she failed to respond to their prescriptions, and her pain escalated.

It was clear that the patient suffered from modest pain in the scar (a common occurrence) but the severity and persistence of her pain were related to her anger at the unwillingness of the original team to accept responsibility for the complications of an unnecessary and unwanted procedure. After discussion of the background, the patient was able to tolerate the annoying discomfort.

A summary view of the extent of the clinical problem of mastalgia as seen in the Cardiff Breast Clinic 1973–1998 is given in Figure 8.21.[124]

THE RELATIONSHIP OF CYCLICAL MASTALGIA TO PMS

PMS has been defined as physical or psychological symptoms appearing during the luteal phase of the menstrual cycle, which improve during menstruation, but interfere with the person's well-being. On this definition, cyclical mastalgia is part of PMS, but in practice it is often seen in isolation from other aspects of PMS. Horrobin and Manku regard both as disorders of EFA metabolism.[64]

In general, PMS is a multisymptomatic complex which is dealt with by gynaecologists, and cyclical mastalgia by surgeons, although this varies from country to country. What is surprising is how little interaction there has been between the two specialties dealing with apparently closely related conditions, and how little interest has been shown in the relationship between PMS and cyclical mastalgia.

Some degree of PMS is extremely common,[125] and it probably affects all women. For example, 96% of 400 nurses surveyed in a Nairobi teaching hospital were affected, with 80% complaining of breast tenderness and 75% of abdominal bloating.[126] However, most did not consider it an illness, but rather part of their femininity. Only 6% changed their activities, and only 3% took medication.

It is clear from general clinical experience that PMS and cyclical mastalgia overlap, but equally that the two may occur independently, especially in the impact of the various elements on the patient's life.

Yet while progestogens have generally been the mainstay of treatment for PMS, most trials of progestogens for mastalgia have shown no benefit over placebo. Danazol, on balance the most efficacious treatment for cyclical mastalgia, has also been advocated for PMS.[127] It has been found to work best in those with a marked cyclical mastalgia element but not effective in those with some of the other elements

of PMS, particularly the psychological symptoms. This would suggest fundamental differences between the two.

Only recently have workers looked specifically at this problem. Goodwin et al. looked at the similarities, and not surprisingly found that PMS symptoms, and concern about breast problems, were more common in women with cyclical mastalgia.[128] Ader et al.[129] studied this relationship in 30 women with a recent history of cyclical mastalgia. As would be expected, PMS was significantly more likely when cyclical mastalgia is present than when it is not. But other PMS symptoms were not present in most cycles with mastalgia. They concluded that cyclical mastalgia is a chronic pain disorder where presentation, aetiology and effective therapy differ from those of PMS, and the two need to be investigated independently.

This is in keeping with our own experience; in most

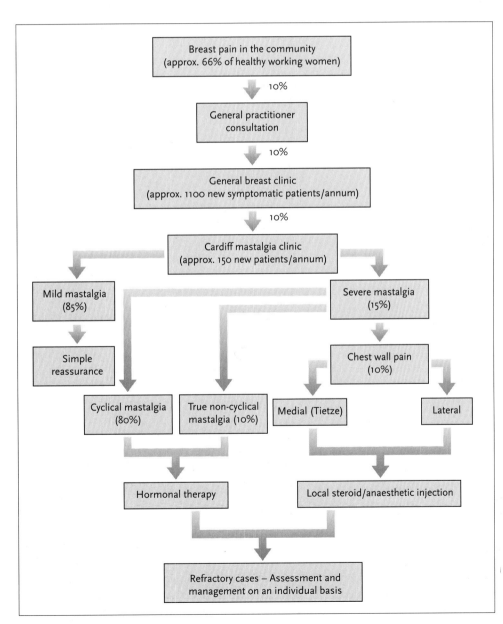

8.21 An overall view of the clinical problem of mastalgia as seen in the Cardiff Breast Clinic.

women presenting with cyclical mastalgia this is the dominant concern, rather than other aspects of PMS. It is important that those with cyclical mastalgia (and also non-cyclical mastalgia) are assessed by a physician with experience of the full range of breast disease, and in particular by one who can confidently exclude the patient's fear of malignancy. It seems likely that a considerable degree of selection has already been undertaken by the referring physician, and this may be why the two conditions have been considered in isolation for so long. It is likely that the uncertainties relating to these two important conditions will soon be elucidated by further investigation.

REFERENCES

1. Nichols S, Waters WE & Wheeler MJ. Management of female breast disease by Southampton General Practitioners. *British Medical Journal* 1980; **281**: 1450–1453.

2. Roberts MM, Elton RA, Robinson SE & Erench K. Consultations for breast disease in general practice and hospital referral patterns. *British Journal of Surgery* 1987; **74**: 1020–1022.

3. Birkett J. *The Diseases of the Breast and their Treatment*, p 164. London: Longman, Brown, Green and Longmans, 1850.

4. Cheatle GL & Cutler M. *Tumours of the Breast*. London: Edward Arnold, 1931.

5. Atkins HJB. Chronic mastitis. *Lancet* 1938; **i**: 707–712.

6. Patey DH. Two common non-malignant conditions of the breast. *British Medical Journal* 1949; **i**: 96–99.

7. Geschickter CF. Mastodynia (painful breasts). In: *Diseases of the Breast*, 2nd edn, p 183. Philadelphia: JB Lippincott Co., 1945.

8. Semb C. Pathologico-anatomical and clinical investigations of fibro-adenomatosis cystica mammae and its relation to other pathological conditions in mamma, especially cancer. *Acta Chirurgica Scandinavica* 1928; **64** (suppl. 10): 1–484.

9. Smallwood JA, Kye DA & Taylor I. Mastalgia: is this commonly associated with operable breast cancer? *Annals of the Royal College of Surgeons* 1986; **68**: 262.

10. Leinster SJ, Whitehouse GH & Walsh PV. Cyclical mastalgia: clinical and mammographic observations in a screened population. *British Journal of Surgery* 1987; **74**: 220–222.

11. Ader DN & Browne MW. Prevalence and impact of cyclical mastalgia in a United States clinic-based sample. *American Journal of Obstetrics and Gynecology* 1997; **177**: 126–132.

12. Preece PE, Baum M, Mansel RE *et al.* The importance of mastalgia in operable breast cancer. *British Medical Journal* 1982; **284**: 1299–1300.

13. Fariselli S, Lepera G, Viganotti P *et al.* Localised mastalgia as presenting symptom in breast cancer. *European Journal of Surgical Oncology* 1988; **14**: 213–215.

14. River L, Silverstein J, Grout J *et al.* Carcinoma of the breast: the diagnostic significance of pain. *American Journal of Surgery* 1951; **82**: 733–735.

15. Haagensen CD. *Diseases of the Breast*, 3rd edn, p 502. London: WB Saunders, 1986.

16. The Yorkshire Breast Cancer Group. Symptoms and signs of operable breast cancer. *British Journal of Surgery* 1983; **70**: 350.

17. Chiedozie IC & Guirguis MN. Mastalgia and breast tumour in Nigerian women. *West African Journal of Medicine* 1990; **9**: 54–58.

18. Plu-Bureau G, Thalabad JC, Sitruk-Ware R *et al.* Cyclical mastalgia as a marker of breast cancer susceptibility. *Brit J Cancer* 1992; **65**: 945–949

19. Preece PE, Hughes LE, Mansel RE *et al.* Clinical syndromes of mastalgia. *Lancet* 1976; **ii**: 670–673.

20. Maddox PR, Harrison BJ, Mansel RE & Hughes LE. Non-cyclical mastalgia – an improved classification and treatment. *British Journal of Surgery* 1989; **76**: 901–904.

21. Fentiman IS, Caleffi M, Hamed H *et al.* Dosage and duration of tamoxifen for mastalgia. A controlled trial. *British Journal of Surgery* 1988; **75**: 845–846.

22. Bishop HM & Blamey RW. A suggested classification of breast pain. *Postgraduate Medical Journal* 1979; **55**: 59–60.

23. Dowle CS. Breast pain: classification, aetiology and management. *Australian and New Zealand Journal of Surgery* 1987; **57**: 43–48.

24. Tietze A. A peculiar accumulation of cases with dystrophy of the cartilages of the ribs. *Berliner Klinische Wochenschrift* 1921; **30**: 829–831.

25. Wallace MS, Wallace AM, Lee J & Dobke MK. Pain after breast surgery: a survey of 282 women. *Pain* 1996; **66**: 195–205.

26. Ihekwaba FN. Benign breast disease in Nigerian women; a study of 657 patients. *Journal of the Royal College of Surgeons of Edinburgh* 1994; **39**: 280–283.

27. La Ban MM, Meerschaert R & Taylor S. Breast pain: a symptom of cervical radioculopathy. *Archives of Physical Medical and Rehabilitation* 1979; **60**: 315.

28. Cooper A. *Illustrations of the Diseases of the Breast*, Part I, p 76. London: Longman, Rees, Orme, Brown and Green, 1829.

29. Jeffcoate N. *Principles of Gynaecology*, 4th edn, p 550. London: Butterworths, 1975.

30. Israel SL. *Menstrual Disorders and Sterility*, 5th edn, p 160. New York: Harper & Row, 1967.

31. Preece PE, Richards AR, Owen GM & Hughes LE. Mastalgia and total body water. *British Medical Journal* 1975; **iv**: 498–500.

32. Ingelby H & Gershon-Cohen J (eds) *Comparative Anatomy, Pathology and Roentgenology of the Breast*. Philadelphia: University of Pennsylvania Press, 1960.

33. Milligan D, Drife JO & Short RV. Changes in breast volume during normal menstrual cycle and after oral contraceptives. *British Medical Journal* 1976; **iv**: 494–496.

34. Fowler PA, Casey CE, Cameron GG *et al.* Cyclic changes in composition and volume of the breast during the menstrual cycle, measured by magnetic resonance imaging. *British Journal of Obstetrics and Gynaecology* 1990; **97**: 595–602.

35. Crown S & Crisp AH. A short clinical diagnostic self-rating scale for psychoneurotic patients: the Middlesex Hospital questionnaire (MHQ). *Journal of Psychology* 1966; **112**: 917–923.

36. Preece PE, Mansel RE & Hughes LE. Mastalgia: psychoneurosis or organic disease? *British Medical Journal* 1978; **i**: 9–30.

37. Sitruk-Ware R, Sterkers N & Mauvais-Jarvis P. Benign breast disease. 1: Hormonal investigation. *Obstetrics and Gynecology* 1979; **53**: 457–460.

38. Swain MC, Hayward JL & Bulbrook RD. Plasma oestradiol and progesterone in benign breast disease. *European Journal of Cancer* 1973; **9**: 553–556.

39. England PC, Skinner LG, Cottrell KM & Sellwood RA. Serum oestradiol-17[b] in women with benign and malignant breast disease. *British Journal of Cancer* 1974; **30**: 571–576.

40. Malarkey WB, Schroeder LL, Stevens VC *et al.* Twenty four hour preoperative endocrine profiles in women with benign and malignant breast disease. *Cancer Research* 1977; **37**: 4655–4659.

41. Walsh PV, Bulbrook RD, Stell PM. *et al.* Serum progesterone concentration during the luteal phase in women with benign breast disease. *European Journal of Cancer and Clinical Oncology* 1984; **20**: 1339–1343.

42. Preece PE. A study of the aetiology, clinical patterns and treatment of mastalgia, pp 94–124. MD thesis, University of Wales, 1982.

43. Kumar S, Mansel RE, Wilson DW *et al.* Daily salivary progesterone levels in cyclical mastalgia patients and their controls. *British Journal of Surgery* 1986; **73**: 260–263.

44. Read GF, Bradley JA, Wilson DW *et al.* Evaluation of luteal-phase salivary progesterone levels in women with benign breast disease or primary breast cancer. *European Journal of Clinical Oncology* 1985; **21**: 9–17.

45. Euhus DM & Vyehara C. Influence of parenteral progesterones on the prevalence and severity of mastalgia in premenopausal women. *Journal of the American College of Surgeons* 1997; **184**: 596–604.

46. Wang DY & Fentiman IS. Epidemiology and endocrinology of benign breast disease. *Breast Cancer Research and Treatment* 1985; **6**: 5–36.

47. Nokin J, Vekemans M & L'Hermite M. Circadian periodicity of serum prolactin concentration in man. *British Medical Journal* 1972; **3**: 561–562.

48. Cole EN, Sellwood RA, England PC & Griffiths K. Serum prolactin concentrations in benign breast disease throughout the menstrual cycle. *European Journal of Cancer* 1977; **13**: 597–603.

49. Lancranjan I & Friesen HG. The neural regulation of prolactin secretion. In: Veale WL & Lederis K (eds) *Current Studies of Hypothalamic Function*, Vol I, p 131. Basel: S Karger, 1978.

50. Peters F, Pickardt CR, Zimmerman G & Breckwoldt M. PRL, TSH and thyroid hormones in benign breast disease. *Klinische Wochenschrift* 1981; **59**: 403–407.

51. Kumar S, Mansel RE, Hughes LE *et al.* Prolactin response to thyrotropin-releasing hormone stimulation and dopaminergic inhibition in benign breast disease. *Cancer* 1984; **53**: 1311–1315.

52. Young JB, Krownjohn AM, Chapman C & Lee MR. Evidence for a hypothalamic disturbance in cyclical oedema. *British Medical Journal* 1983; **286**: 1691–1693.

53. Minton JP, Abou-Issa H, Reiches N & Roseman JM. Clinical and biochemical studies in methylxanthine-related fibrocystic breast disease. *Surgery* 1981; **90**: 299–304.

54. Farrar WB, Walker MJ & Minton JP. Common benign conditions of the breast. In: Donegan WL & Spratt JS (eds) *Cancer of the Breast*, 4th edn, p 48. Philadelphia: WB Saunders, 1995.

55. Odenheimer DJ, Zunzunegui MV, King MC *et al.* Risk factors for benign breast disease. A case control study of discordant twins. *American Journal of Epidemiology* 1984; **120**: 565–571.

56. Boyle CA, Berkowitz GS, LiVolsi VA *et al.* Caffeine consumption and fibrocystic breast disease: A case control epidemiologic study. *Journal of the National Cancer Institute* 1984; **72**: 1015–1019.

57. Marshall J, Graham S & Swanson M. Caffeine consumption and benign breast disease. A case control comparison. *American Journal of Public Health* 1982; **72**: 610–612.

58. Lawson DH, Jick H & Rothman KJ. Coffee and tea consumption and breast disease. *Surgery* 1981; **90**: 801–803.

59. Lubin F, Ron E, Wax Y *et al.* A case control study of caffeine and methyl xanthines in benign breast disease. *Journal of the American Medical Association* 1985; **253**: 2388–2392.

60. Heyden S & Fodor JG. Coffee consumption and fibrocystic breasts: an unlikely association. *Canadian Journal of Surgery* 1986; **29**: 208–211.

61. Ernster VL, Mason L, Goodson WH *et al.* Effects of caffeine free diet on benign breast disease: a randomised trial. *Surgery* 1982; **91**: 263–267.

62. Minton JP, Foeking MK, Webster DJT *et al.* Response of fibrocystic disease to caffeine withdrawal and correlation with cyclic nucleotides with breast disease. *American Journal of Obstetrics and Gynecology* 1979; **135**: 157.

63. Russell LC. Caffeine restriction as medical treatment for breast pain. *American Journal of Primary Health Care* 1989; **14**: 36–37.

64. Horrobin DF & Manku MS. Premenstrual syndrome and premenstrual breast pain: disorders of essential fatty acid metabolism. *Prostaglandins, Leukotrienes and Essential Fatty Acids* 1989; **37**: 255–261.

65. Goolmali SK & Shuster S. A sebotrophic stimulus in benign and malignant breast disease. *Lancet* 1975; **i**: 428.

66. Gateley CA, Maddox PR, Pritchard GA *et al.* Plasma fatty acid profiles in benign breast disorders. *British Journal of Surgery* 1992; **79**: 407–409.

67. Sharma AK, Mishra SK, Salila M *et al.* Cyclical mastalgia – is it a manifestation of aberration in lipid metabolism? *Indian Journal of Physiology and Pharmacology* 1994; **38**: 267–271.

68. Saraiva J, Carvalho V, Almeida C *et al.* The quality of life after tubal ligation. *Acta Medica Portuguesa* 1995; **8**: 347–353.

69. Wetzig NR. Mastalgia: A 3 year Australian study. *Australian and New Zealand Journal of Surgery* 1994; **64**: 329–331.

70. McFayden IJ, Forrest APM, Chetty U *et al.* Cyclical breast pain: some observations and the difficulties in treatment. *British Journal of Clinical Practice* 1992; **46**: 161–164.

71. Wilson MC & Sellwood RA. Therapeutic value of a supporting brassière in mastodynia. *British Medical Journal* 1976; **ii**: 90.

72. Fox H, Walker LG, Heys SD *et al.* Are patients with mastalgia anxious, and does relaxation therapy help? *The Breast* 1997; **6**: 138–142.

73. Ory H, Cole P & MacMahon B. Oral contraceptives and reduced risk of benign breast diseases. *New England Journal of Medicine* 1976; **294**: 419–422.

74. Royal College of General Practitioners Study. *British Medical Journal* 1981; **282**: 2089–2093.

75. DiLieto A, De Rosa G, Albano G *et al.* Desogestrel versus gestodine in oral contraceptives. *European Journal of Obstetrics, Gynaecology and Reproductive Biology* 1994; **55**: 71–83.

76. Pike MC, Henderson BE, Krilo MD *et al.* Breast cancer in young women and use of oral contraceptives: Possible modifying effect of formulation and age at use. *Lancet* 1983; **ii**: 926–929.

77. Anderson TJ. Mitotic and apoptotic response of breast tissue to oral contraceptives. *Lancet* 1984; **i**: 99–100.

78. Gateley C, Miers M, Mansel RE & Hughes LE. Drug treatments for mastalgia: 17 year experience in the Cardiff Mastalgia Clinic. *Journal of the Royal Society of Medicine* 1992; **85**: 12–15.

79. Madjar H, Vetter M, Prompeler H *et al.* Doppler measurement of breast vascularity in women under pharmacologic treatment of benign breast disease. *Journal of Reproductive Medicine* 1993; **38**: 935–940.

80. Day JB. Clinical trials in the premenstrual syndrome. *Current*

Medical Research and Opinion 1979; **6** (Suppl 5): 40–45.

81. Maddox PR, Harrison BJ, Horobin JM *et al.* A randomised controlled trial of medroxyprogesterone acetate in mastalgia. *Annals of the Royal College of Surgeons of England* 1990; **72**: 71–76.

82. Nappi C, Affinito P, DiCarlo *et al.* Double blind controlled trial of progesterone vaginal cream treatment for cyclical mastodynia in women with benign breast disease. *Journal of Endocrinological Investigation* 1992; **15**: 801–806.

83. von Fournier D, Junkermann H, Warendorf U *et al.* In: Kubli F *et al.* (eds) *Breast Diseases*, pp 499–506. Berlin: Springer-Verlag, 1989.

84. Schulz KD, Del Pozo E, Lose KH *et al.* Successful treatment of mastodynia with the prolactin inhibitor bromocriptine (CB 154). *Archiv für Gynaekologie* 1975; **220**: 83–87.

85. Mansel RE, Preece PE & Hughes LE. A double blind trial of the prolactin inhibitor bromocriptine in painful benign breast disease. *British Journal of Surgery* 1978; **65**: 724–727.

86. Blichert-Toft M, Anderson AN, Henriksen OB & Mygind T. Treatment of mastalgia with bromocriptine. A double blind crossover study. *British Medical Journal* 1979; **I**: 237.

87. Durning P & Sellwood RA. Bromocriptine in severe cyclical breast pain. *British Journal of Surgery* 1982; **69**: 248–249.

88. Mansel RE & Dogliotti L. European multicentre trial of bromocriptine in cyclical mastalgia. *Lancet* 1990; **335**: 190–193.

89. Mansel RE. A review of the role of bromocriptine in symptomatic benign breast disease. *Research Clinical Forum* 1981; **3**: 61–65.

90. Greenblatt RB, Dmowski WP, Mahesh VB & Scholer HFL. Clinical studies with an antigonadotrophin-Danazol. *Fertility and Sterility* 1971; **22**: 102–112.

91. Asch RH & Greenblatt RB. The use of an impeded androgen-Danazol in the management of benign breast disorders. *American Journal of Obstetrics and Gynecology* 1977; **127**: 130–134.

92. Greenblatt RB, Nezhat C & Ben-Nun I. The treatment of benign breast disease with danazol. *Fertility and Sterility* 1980; **34**: 242–245.

93. Mansel RE, Wisbey JR & Hughes LE. Controlled trial of the antigonadotrophin danazol in painful nodular benign breast disease. *Lancet* 1982; **i**: 928–931.

94. Harrison BJ, Maddox PR & Mansel RE. Maintenance therapy of cyclical mastalgia using low dose Danazol. *Journal of the Royal College of Surgeons of Edinburgh* 1989; **34**: 79–81.

95. Hinton CP, Bishop HM, Holliday HW *et al.* A double blind controlled trial of danazol and bromocriptine in the management of severe cyclical breast pain. *British Journal of Clinical Practice* 1986; **40**: 326–330.

96. Peters F. Multicentre study of gestrinone in cyclical breast pain. *Lancet* 1992; **339**: 205–208.

97. Stein RC, Rawson NSB, Gazet J-C *et al.* Gestrinone in mastalgia. *The Breast* 1994; **3**: 90–94.

98. Pashby NL, Mansel RE, Hughes LE *et al.* A clinical trial of evening primrose oil in mastalgia. *British Journal of Surgery* 1981; **68**: 801.

99. Ricciardi I & Ianniruberto A. Tamoxifen induced regression of benign breast lesions. *Obstetrics and Gynecology* 1979; **54**: 80–84.

100. Fentiman IS, Caleffi M, Brame K *et al.* Double blind controlled trial of tamoxifen therapy for mastalgia. *Lancet* 1986; **i**: 287–288.

101. Fentiman I, Caleffi M, Rodin A *et al.* Bone mineral content of women receiving tamoxifen for mastalgia. *British Journal of Cancer* 1989; **60**: 262–264.

102. Caleffi M, Fentiman IS, Clark GM *et al.* Effect of tamoxifen on oestrogen binding, lipid and lipoprotein concentrations and blood-clotting parameters among premenopausal women with breast pain. *Journal of Endocrinology* 1988; **119**: 335–339.

103. GEMB Group. Tamoxifen therapy for cyclical mastalgia. Dose randomised trial. *The Breast* 1997; **5**: 212–213.

104. Boyd NF, Maguire V, Shannon P *et al.* A clinical trial of low fat high carbohydrate diet in patients with cyclical mastalgia. *Breast Cancer Research and Treatment* 1987; **10**: 117.

105. Leis HP. Recommended current management of mastalgia. *British Journal of Clinical Practice* (Symposium Suppl) 1989; **68**: 50.

106. Lehtovirta P, Ranta T & Seppala M. Pyridoxine treatment of galactorrhoea-amenorrhoea syndromes. *Acta Endocrinology* 1978; **87**: 682–686.

107. Moretti C, Fahri A, Gressi L *et al.* Pyridoxine (B6) suppresses the rise in prolactin and increases the rise in growth hormone induced by exercise. *New England Journal of Medicine* 1982; **307**: 444.

108. Smallwood J, A-Kye D & Taylor I. Vitamin B6 in the treatment of premenstrual mastalgia. *British Journal of Clinical Practice* 1986; **40**: 532–533.

109. Estes NC. Mastodynia due to fibrocystic disease of the breast controlled with thyroid hormone. *American Journal of Surgery* 1981; **142**: 764–766.

110. Meyer EC, Sommers DK, Reitz CJ *et al.* Vitamin E and benign breast disease. *Surgery* 1990; **107**: 549–551.

111. Sutton GCJ, Palmer JD & Royce GT. Breast pain and the thoracic outlet compression syndrome. *The Breast* 1993; **2**: 250–252.

112. Crile G. Injection of steroids in painful breasts. *American Journal of Surgery* 1977; **133**: 705.

113. Lloyd Davies E, Cochrane RA, Sweetland HM & Mansel RE. Is there a role for surgery in mastalgia? *The Breast* 1998; In press.

114. Wisbey JR, Kumar S, Mansel RE *et al.* Natural history of breast pain. *Lancet* 1983; **ii**: 672–674.

115. Pye JK, Mansel RE & Hughes LE. Clinical experience of drug treatments for mastalgia. *Lancet* 1985; **ii**: 373–377.

116. Rasmussen T, Doberl A, Rannevik G & Tobiassen T. The Hjorring project on fibrocystic breast disease. In: Baum M, George WD & Hughes LE (eds) *Benign Breast Disease*, p 135. London: Royal Society of Medicine Symposium Series, 1984.

117. Holland PA & Gately CA. Drug therapy of mastalgia. What are the options? *Drugs* 1994; **48**: 709–716.

118. Blankenstein MA, Szymczak J & Daroszewski J. Estrogens in plasma and fatty tissue from breast cancer patients and women undergoing surgery for non-oncological reasons. *Gynecology and Endocrinology* 1992; **6**: 13–17.

119. Marsh MS, Whitcroft S & Whitehead MI. Paradoxical effects of HRT on breast tenderness in post-menopausal women. *Maturitas* 1994; 97–102.

120. Gately CA, Maddox PR, Mansel RE & Hughes LE. Mastalgia refractory to drug treatment. *British Journal of Surgery* 1990; **77**: 1110–1112.

121. Hamed H, Chaudary MA, Caleffi M & Fentiman IS. LHRH analogue for treatment of recurrent and refractory mastalgia. *Annals of the Royal College of Surgeons of England* 1990; **72**: 221–224.

122. Jenkins PL, Jamil N, Gateley C & Mansel RE. Psychiatric illness in patients with treatment resistant mastalgia. *General Hospital Psychiatry* 1993; **15**: 55–57.

123. Kumar S, Mansel RE, Hughes LE *et al.* Prediction of response to endocrine therapy in pronounced cyclical mastalgia using dynamic tests of prolactin release. *Clinical Endocrinology* 1985; **23**: 699–704.

124. Davies EL, Gately CA, Miers M & Mansel RE. The long term course of mastalgia. *Journal of the Royal Society of Medicine*

1998; **91**: 462–464.

125. Lurie S & Borenstein R. The premenstrual syndrome. *Obstetrical and Gynecological Survey* 1990; **45**: 220–228.

126. Rupani NP & Lema VM. Premenstrual tension among nurses in Nairobi, Kenya. *East African Medical Journal* 1993; **70**: 310–313.

127. The role of danazol in relieving the premenstrual syndrome. *Journal of Reproductive Medicine* 1990; **35**(1 Suppl): 97–102.

128. Goodwin PJ, Miller A, DelGuidice ME & Ritchie K. Breast health and associated premenstrual symptoms in women with severe cyclical mastalgia. *American Journal of Obstetrics and Gynecology* 1997; **176**: 998–1005.

129. Ader DN, Shriver CD & Browne MW. Relation of cyclical mastalgia to premenstrual syndrome. *Psychosomatic Medicine* 1997; **59**: 104.

Cysts of the breast

CONTENTS

KEY POINTS AND NEW DEVELOPMENTS

1. Macrocysts constitute the commonest discrete benign breast mass, estimated to occur in 7–10% of all women.
2. Microcysts develop from apocrine metaplasia of a single lobule throughout most of reproductive life; a few go on to form macrocysts, mainly in the last decade of reproductive life.
3. Macrocysts fall into two broad groups: those with a persisting apocrine cell lining and active secretion/concentration of many substances; and those lined by flattened cells and metabolically much less active.
4. Gross cysts are associated with a small but definite increase in subsequent breast cancer, but opinions about, and evidence for, the details of the associated cancer risk are not uniform.
5. Simple cysts are adequately treated by aspiration; ultrasound is helpful with poorly defined cysts and to ensure complete emptying of recurrent cysts.
6. Cysts yielding blood-stained fluid are investigated by cytology and sonography, and warrant exploration even if triple assessment is negative. Most are due to intracystic papillary tumours of benign histology or low-grade malignancy.
7. Recurrent cysts may be aspirated as often as necessary, without further therapy or investigation.
8. Leakage from a cyst gives surrounding inflammation with altered sonographic appearances (complex cyst) and may give a residual mass after aspiration. Where painful cysts are a problem, a trial of danazol is worthwhile.
9. Since the increased risk of cancer is small, and most patients are in their fifth decade, standard breast screening is appropriate follow-up for most cases.
10. Cysts *per se* are not premalignant, so do not need excision, and screening should be directed at both breasts.
11. Galactoceles cause few clinical problems, being readily managed by aspiration. They may cause greater problems with imaging, because of the variety of appearances seen on sonography and mammography.

Cysts are the commonest abnormality found in patients presenting to a breast clinic, a fact of little surprise since it has been estimated that 7–10% of all women will develop a symptomatic breast cyst during their reproductive life.

Like many other breast lesions, cysts were described by Sir Astley Cooper in 1831.[1] The French surgeon Reclus provided a comprehensive account in 1883[2] in an account so accurate that the disease is still known by his name among French surgeons. Bloodgood[3] has achieved surgical immortality more easily than most with his attention-catching description of the 'blue-domed cysts' which bear his name.

A large majority of breast cysts are a manifestation of ANDI – aberrations of normal lobular involution as described in Chapters 1 and 3. Unless otherwise specified, this chapter refers to these lesions. Some of the less common forms of cysts and pseodocysts shown in Table 9.1 are dealt with in Chapter 17.

The reasons for regarding cyst formation as an aberration of normal involution, and therefore part of the spectrum of ANDI, have been set out in Chapter 3. Haagensen[4] uses the term 'cystic disease' to include other elements of ANDI such as mastalgia and cyclical nodularity, but this can further confuse the issue, and it is preferable to consider each aspect separately. The management of macroscopic cysts is specific to that clinical presentation and unrelated to the other elements of ANDI.

PATHOLOGY

The pathology of breast cysts was only too familiar to surgeons when biopsy excision was the standard management of all cysts. Now the surgical trainee brought up on needle aspiration will see only the small cysts encountered by chance during breast surgery. These vary in size from those just visible to the naked eye to others up to 4–5 mm in diameter. They often occur in a cluster over an area 2–3 cm in diameter. These are the 'blue-domed' cysts (Figure 9.1) which have classically been considered to denote benign disease.

These small cysts have no intrinsic significance except the potential to form larger cysts in due course.

Larger cysts are thin walled and more brown than blue in colour, from the brownish opalescent fluid within them. They usually present as an individual cyst but the single palpable cyst is likely to be the overt presentation of multiple, bilateral cysts, the majority of which are impalpable (Figure 9.2).

The cysts may be uni- or multilocular but, even in unilocular cysts, constricting fibrous bands provide evidence of their origin from a single lobule or group of lobules (see Chapter 3). Cysts are lined by a single layer of epithelium that may be of two types: tall columnar secretory epithelium or attenuated flattened cells. Sometimes they have no epithelial lining at all.

Table 9.1 Breast cysts

True breast cysts
1. ANDI
   - Microcysts
   - Apocrine macrocysts
   - Non-apocrine macrocysts
2. Juvenile cysts
3. Secondary cysts
   - Galactocele
   - Oil cysts of fat necrosis
   - Liquefied haematoma
   - Implant-related loculated fluid collections
4. Papillary cystadenoma

Conditions that require differentiation from breast cysts
1. Dilated ducts/chronic abscess associated with duct ectasia/periductal mastitis
2. Cysts of the dermis and areola
3. Cysts associated with tumour necrosis
   - Phyllodes tumour – benign and malignant
   - Necrotic carcinoma
4. Hyatid cysts

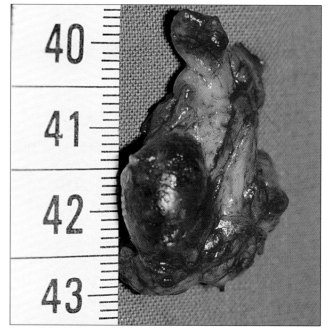

9.1 A typical 'blue-domed cyst of Bloodgood' discovered by chance at biopsy for dominant nodularity. It has already reached the size when its colour is closer to brown than blue. It should have been found by a needle point!

The fluid content of the cysts shows a wide range of appearances from clear to heavily turbid, and from light brown, through grey, to almost black (Figure 9.3).

These fluids consist of a variety of chemical substances, including pigmented products of apocrine secretion, lipofuscin products of peroxidated lipoprotein, breakdown products of haemoglobin and possibly secretory products related to diet.[5] They do not contain blood unless there is an associated neoplasm. Crystal clear watery fluid is not seen in the common cysts of ANDI.

Multiple cysts are frequently impalpable due to the laxity of the cyst, allowing it to merge into surrounding breast tissue of similar consistency. But a very small increase in volume has a disproportionate effect on the intracystic pressure, explaining how a small increase in fluid can cause a large cyst to become tense and clinically apparent in a few days. This also explains the surprising fact that most cysts do not recur after aspiration. In fact, many do not disappear after aspiration but merely revert to their lax, impalpable state, as is readily shown by repeat imaging. Both increase and decrease in size may be seen on serial imaging over a short period, suggesting that the balance between secretion and reabsorption or duct obstruction must be variable, so obstruction of the ductule draining the cyst is not a complete or irreversible process. Little is known of the dynamics of secretion and reabsorption of fluid by the cyst epithelium or through the cyst wall, the other process which might lead to rapid volume change.

There is a rapidly expanding literature on the biochemistry of cyst fluid. It contains many steroid hormones,[6,7] beta human chorionic gonadotrophin (βHCG)[8] and relaxin,[9] tumour markers such as fetoprotein and carcinoembryonic antigen (CEA)[10] and 'gross cystic disease proteins',[11] many of which are found in much higher concentrations than in blood, suggesting an active secretory process.

There is growing evidence that first, breast cyst fluid is not merely the result of filtration from plasma, its composition being strikingly different from that of plasma or extracellular fluid, and secondly, active (though not yet clarified) secretory and/or concentrating mechanisms are involved.[12] Epidermal growth factor (EGF) can also be measured and its level appears to act as a marker for epithelial proliferation elsewhere in the breasts.[12] The biochemistry of breast cyst fluid and its significance has been extensively reviewed.[13]

INCIDENCE

There are surprisingly few satisfactory data on incidence of cysts in the general population. One autopsy study[14] of 225 women without overt clinical breast disease showed a 19% incidence of macroscopic cysts 1–2 mm or more in diameter; in half of these cases the cysts were bilateral. Ultrasound examination will show further impalpable cysts in 1 in 5 patients with a palpable cyst. Foote and Stewart[15] reported 27% incidental cysts in 300 breasts removed for cancer. Haagensen[4] estimates that 7% of white women in Western countries will develop a palpable cyst, because this is the incidence of cancer, and in his practice cyst and cancer are seen with equal frequency. This must be a very rough approximation, although the figure of 7% is quoted almost universally. Others believe 10% to be a better estimate.

PATHOGENESIS AND CYST TYPES

There is such a large body of research data relevant to the aetiology of breast cysts that it is easier if a summary of the conclusions are given first, and the data follow.

The current view is that all macrocysts start with an area of apocrine epithelium in a terminal ductal lobular unit (TDLU). Excessive secretion of the apocrine epithelium,

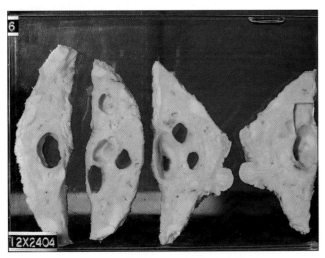

9.2 A breast autopsy. The breast was asymptomatic during life. This illustrates the multiplicity of macroscopic cysts and the diffuse nature of the involutional stromal changes of ANDI.

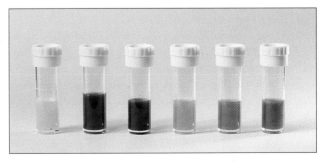

9.3 The range of colours of cyst fluid. The first specimen of opalescent fluid is common; the blood-stained fluid is uncommon and requires further investigation.

probably compounded by osmotic effects of the secretion products, leads to progressive dilatation of the TDLU to give a microcyst. The dilatation is at first confined to the acini containing apocrine epithelium. (These contrast with involutional microcysts, without apocrine epithelium and common in postmenopausal patients.)

If the apocrine microcyst enlarges, it does so in one of two directions: type 1 macrocyst containing actively secreting apocrine epithelium and with contents similar to intracellular fluid, and type 2 macrocysts, with flattened epithelium and contents more akin to extracellular fluid. Type 1 cysts are more prone to occur in patients with multiple or recurrent cysts, and carry a small increase in subsequent cancer risk.

Many early workers and some recent writers have regarded cysts as dilated ducts. However, the clinical course and complications of duct ectasia and involutional cysts are very different, as is the underlying pathology of the two conditions. They should not be linked in any way, although they frequently coexist as different aberrations of involution.

Sir Alan Parks was one of the first workers to shed light on the problem when he described the process of cystic lobular involution.[16] In this process, lobules develop microcysts during their involution, while maintaining some of the specialized lobular stroma around the epithelial acini. As long as this remains, the lobule may go on to complete involution, but if the specialized stroma is replaced by fibrous tissue before the small cysts have regressed, the cystic change is likely to persist. With time, the many small cysts representing the acini of the lobule will coalesce to form a smaller number of larger cysts (see Chapter 3). This is the simplest form of microcystic change, and is common in postmenopausal women. The lobular origin of macroscopic cysts is described by Azzopardi,[17] who shows the value of elastic stains in demonstrating that each cyst derives from a lobule, enormously distended in the case of large macrocysts. Most macrocysts are seen in premenopausal women and disappear at the menopause.

Many workers have noticed a second type of microcyst lined by apocrine metaplastic epithelium, and concluded that obstruction of the outflow from the lobule leads to distension, and conversion of the columnar apocrine cells to a flat cuboidal epithelium, or little epithelium at all. It was assumed that all macrocysts arose by this single mechanism.

Recent work has cast doubt on this simplistic approach from a number of directions, but there is still much uncertainty about detailed mechanisms. Studies from Bradlow's unit[18] have shown that cysts fall into two main groups, dependent on the ratio of Na^+ and K^+ in the cyst fluid. One group of cysts has a low Na^+ and high K^+, resembling intracellular fluid, and is designated type 1; the other (type 2) has a high ratio, resembling extracellular fluid. Different cut-off points for classifying type 1 and 2 cysts have been used, using Na:K ratios varying from 1.5 to 3. In a large study,[19] 52% had type 1, 41% had type 2, and 7% had both.

Type 1 cysts occurred more in younger women who had fewer births. Estimation of the Na^+/K^+ ratio in our own series of 725 patients shows a similar bimodal distribution (Figure 9.4).

Measurement of pH has been reported as distinguishing between the two types of cyst, high K^+ cysts having a higher pH. Dixon and co-workers[20] regard a pH of 7.4 as the cut-off point, whereas Bradlow's group[21] recommend a pH of 7.0. Androgen conjugates are also found to be high in some cyst fluids, and low in others.[22] These findings, now confirmed by other workers, suggest that there may be at least two populations of cysts, possibly corresponding to those lined with apocrine epithelium (Figure 9.5) which is actively secreting in the high K^+ group, while in the others the flat epithelium (or no epithelium lining at all) acts more as a passive membrane (Figure 9.6).

The type 1 apocrine cysts are characterized by tight junctions, so all transport is by cellular pore, while type 2 have loose junctions and secretions can move directly, to some extent, from plasma into cyst fluid.

This would suggest that the progression from micro- to macrocyst is dependent on the balance between secretion and outflow or reabsorption, and this balance might be upset in two ways. In one, obstruction of the ductule draining the original lobule would lead to back pressure and dilatation. A number of possible obstructing mechanisms have been suggested, including benign epithelial hyperplasia and fibrous obliteration of the lumen. But in many cases, the normal involutional fibrosis around the ductule, perhaps augmented by kinking, may alone be sufficient. It seems likely that some obstructive element is important, particularly with large,

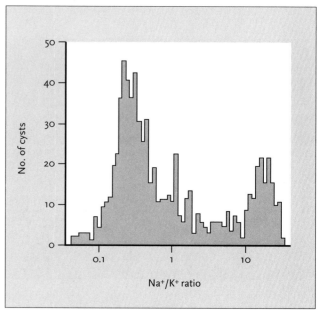

9.4 The bimodal distribution of breast cysts when characterized by Na+/K+ ratio of cyst fluid – Cardiff series.

tension cysts. In the second group, apocrine secretion in excess of the reabsorptive capacity of the cyst may be important. Patients with apocrine-lined cysts are more likely to have multiple cysts and to develop further cysts.[23]

It is these cysts with apocrine lining, particularly where the lining is papillary, which Haagensen[4] has suggested have a small but definite increase in malignancy associated with macroscopic cyst disease. This view has long been disputed, but many studies of this question have now been performed, and there is increasing acceptance that gross cystic disease is associated with a small, but definite, increase in cancer risk[24] (see also Chapter 4).

In this context, it is interesting to note that type 1 cysts have higher concentrations of hormones, androgen and oestrogen congugates, as well as EGF. Conjugated bile acids can also be detected in breast cyst fluid, with significantly higher concentrations in the apocrine-type cyst (with the higher cancer risk) than the flattened walled cyst.[25] Torrisi *et al.* found that EGF levels in breast fluid were a better indicator of proliferative epithelial hyperplasia elsewhere in either breast than Na^+/K^+ ratio.[12] Mannello *et al.* have shown that breast cyst epithelium secretes and accumulates large amounts of prostate-specific antigen.[26] In recent work[27] Dixon *et al.* have shown that intravenously administered tritiated hormone (dihydroepiandrosterone sulphate) appears in the fluid of apocrine cysts within 2 hours, and persists within the cysts for up to 2 years. Furthermore, danazol, spironolactone and evening primrose oil (EPO) can inhibit this process,[28] opening possible therapeutic approaches. A majority, but not all, of type 1 cysts are metabolically active in this way; type 2 cysts are inactive. In contrast, type 2 cysts have been found to concentrate transforming growth factor beta 2,[29] which is reported to have an inhibitory effect on epithelial tumour cell growth. Thus breast cysts, with their active transluminal transport

mechanisms, may well act as a 'window' on what is going on within the rest of the breast.

However, the diversion of cysts along the two paths of high or low Na^+/K^+ ratio occurs during macrocyst development, and not from the beginning. Dixon and co-workers[30] have studied 40 microcysts, and found that all had high concentrations of androgen conjugates and a high K^+/Na^+ ratio. They have shown that microcysts form a single population lined by apocrine secretory epithelium. The two types of macrocysts thus appear to develop from a single, apocrine type of microcyst. Even the type 2 cysts with flattened epithelium may show gradients with protein concentrations higher than serum, showing that they do not act as pure passive membranes.

Wellings and Alpers[31] have contributed further to our understanding of this process with their elegant technique of subgross whole organ sampling. The definitive lesion is the apocrine cyst, in which apocrine metaplasia occurs in hyperplastic/hypertrophic cystically dilated lobules. At first only part of a TDLU may contain tufts of apocrine epithelium, and only this portion of the lobule will show dilatation. They postulate that pressure of apocrine secretion, compounded by the osmotic effects of breakdown products, leads to progressive 'unfolding' of the acini, until the whole lobule may be affected. As patients grow older, the cyst tends to enlarge, and the lining epithelium flattens or atrophies. This confirms the general view of the pathogenesis of cysts, but does not elucidate the mechanism for progression to macrocyst, or the differentiation into types 1 and 2.

Surprisingly, they have shown that the extralobular terminal duct (ETD) is dilated, so that any obstructive element must be beyond the TDLU/ETD junction. Alternatively, the dilatation may be due only to secretory pressure, and Molina *et al.*[32] add evidence that secretion from hyperplastic apocrine epithelium initiates microcysts, and osmotic mechanisms lead to progression to macrocysts.

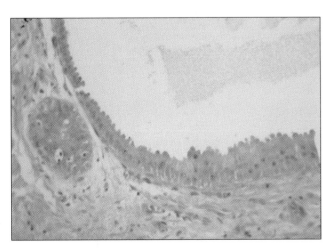

9.5 Wall of apocrine cyst, lined by tall, pink columnar epithelium.

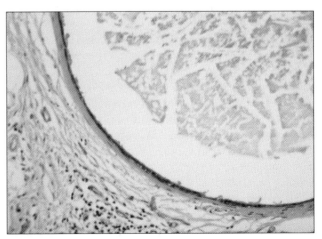

9.6 Cyst lined by flattened epithelium (sometimes the epithelial lining of the cyst wall is lost completely).

Bundred et al.[33] showed that zinc alpha-2 glycoprotein, a marker of apocrine epithelium, is raised in breast fluids, highest in microcysts, intermediate in type 1 cysts, and lowest in type 2 cysts. Nevertheless, levels are still 10 times higher than in serum, confirming the view that all cysts are derived from apocrine epithelium. Levels were also higher in cyst fluid of patients who subsequently developed recurrent cysts.

AETIOLOGY

Cyst formation can be regarded as a minor aberration of normal lobular involution, but the specific aetiological factors responsible for this aberration are unknown. There is some indirect evidence to implicate hyperoestrogenism, either absolute or relative. There is also evidence that acini dilate towards the end of the menstrual cycle, and that this is an oestrogen effect. It has been suggested that excess unopposed oestrogen in premenopausal patients maintains the acini in a dilated state which is accentuated by the pressure of apocrine secretion. A number of cases seem to be related to oestrogen therapy, particularly in postmenopausal patients. Haagensen[4] regards the administration of oestrogen for menopausal symptoms as a potent cause of cysts in women over the age of 50, although Fechner[34] was unable to confirm this. Oestrogen also produces cysts in some rodents but since there are great differences between individual strains of mice, it hardly seems logical to transpose the findings to humans, although the fact that oestrogens also produce cysts in primates[35] is more convincing.

There is also some direct evidence in that England et al.[36] demonstrated raised mean levels of serum oestradiol-17β in 13 women with cysts, although among these patients seven had high levels, four were normal and two were reduced. Both basal and stimulated levels of biologically active prolactin are raised in patients with breast cysts, and this may prove important.[37] At present, a hormonal basis for involutional cysts remains unproven. The cause of this condition is undetermined, and there is no conclusive evidence to support hormonal therapy for cysts, although it is reasonable to withdraw oestrogen supplements in such patients if it otherwise seems appropriate.

Simpson and Page[38] have demonstrated the absence of fodrin in the wall of all cysts. Since fodrin is a cytoskeletal structural protein which binds actin and plays a role in the establishment of cellular orientation and polarity it is attractive to suggest that this loss may be a significant factor in cyst formation, although the loss could be a secondary rather than primary phenomenon.

At present there does not seem to be an animal model for human cysts. Keratinocyte growth factor has been put forward as causing cystic change in mice,[39] but the change demonstrated is cystic dilatation of ducts, and hence different to the lobule-derived cysts of the human breast.

CLINICAL FEATURES

Macroscopic cysts are frequently asymptomatic, the patient often noting the mass accidentally when touching the breast. In other cases, sudden pain draws the attention of the patient to a large cyst, probably due to sudden distension or to leakage of fluid into the surrounding tissue, giving chemical irritation. Pain may also be associated with disappearance of the cyst, which has presumably ruptured or discharged its contents into a duct. Pain is not usually related to the menstrual cycle, nor is variation in the size of the cyst. Nipple discharge is uncommon but does occur and duct injection has sometimes demonstrated communication with a cyst in such a case. The discharge will then be typical of cyst fluid.

Fifty-five per cent of cysts are found in the left breast and 45% in the right, a ratio identical to that for fibroadenoma. Two-thirds occur in the upper outer quadrant, with the upper inner quadrant being next most common. Cysts are uncommon in the lower half of the breast.

On examination, the physical characteristics vary widely according to a number of factors: size, intracystic pressure, depth and situation in the breast, and the characteristics of surrounding breast tissue.

Large cysts are frequently visible when the patient lies down (Figure 9.7).

Generally the cyst is felt as a smooth, tense structure, readily palpable against the chest wall, and to some extent attached to breast tissue (see Chapter 5). Large cysts may be palpably multilocular. Lax cysts are palpated only with

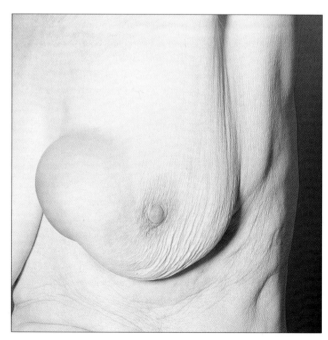

9.7 A large, visible cyst. This is an extreme example, but smaller cysts may also produce an eccentric contour when the patient lies down.

difficulty or not at all. Very tense cysts are so hard that carcinoma may be simulated closely. A large cyst may displace surrounding Cooper's ligaments, producing apparent skin attachment or even retraction (false retraction of Haagensen[4]). The diagnostic problem is fortunately solved readily by routine use of needle aspiration and ultrasonography for all lumps.

A deep cyst may feel much more superficial in a youngish patient with pliable breast tissue and be missed entirely by timorous needling. Likewise, only the foremost loculus of a lobulated cyst may be felt from the surface, so that needling produces surprisingly more fluid than expected. Conversely, needling of one of a cluster of cysts will produce less fluid than expected.

There is a strong clinical impression that multiple cysts are seen most commonly in larger breasts, but no habitus is exempt and simple cysts are common in patients with small, dense breasts. There seems to be no relationship between age and multiplicity or recurrence.

It is difficult to obtain a representative study group to assess the true incidence of subclinical cysts, since all populations are biased to some extent. Of women presenting with painful nodularity to a breast clinic, ultrasound examination will show about 20% to have cysts, of which 20% will be small (<5 mm), and 40% medium (5–15 mm) or large (>15 mm).

AGE

Cysts occur predominantly in the middle and late reproductive period, increasing in frequency from 35 years to a maximal incidence between 40 and 50 years. They are rarely seen before the age of 30, although we have seen a 5-cm cyst behind the areola in a 16-year-old girl, which did not recur after a single aspiration. Perhaps the pathogenesis differs in such juvenile cysts, although the clinical features were typical in this case. Cysts disappear rapidly after the menopause, unless the patient is taking hormone preparations. Of Haagensen's 2511 patients, 78% presented between 35 and 50 years and only 2.3% before the age of 30.[4]

The rare cysts seen in the elderly tend to be large, and associated with a papillary tumour, when the fluid will be blood stained. It seems likely that the even rarer cysts in the elderly not associated with tumour have a different aetiology to the premenopausal cyst, although little has been written about large non-neoplastic cysts in the elderly. Devitt[40] found that only 6% of symptomatic women over the age of 60 had breast cysts, compared with 15% of those less than 55 years presenting to a breast clinic. Furthermore, a majority of the older patients with cysts were taking hormone supplements. It is interesting that this premenopausal concentration of clinical cysts is not seen with histological apocrine microcysts, which are much more uniformly distributed from 25–30 years until the ninth decade.[31]

Brenner studied the development of new cysts in women undergoing mammographic screening, and found that 1% of women developed new cysts between screens, with a clear relationship to hormone replacement therapy (HRT) in those over the age of 50.[41] Only one of 20 women with cysts under the age of 50 was on HRT, compared with 17 of 33 over 50.

NATURAL HISTORY

The natural history can be presented no better than through the results of Haagensen's unique study,[4] in which he has followed 2511 patients, 2235 for 5–30 years. Seventeen were multiple at first presentation on clinical examination (ultrasound or surgery would show much higher figures); 40% developed new cysts, the interval to a further cyst being progressively shorter with age from an average of 10 years in the third decade to 2 years in the sixth. As would be expected, the greater the number of cysts, the shorter the interval to recurrence. With a minimum 5-year follow-up, 30% had only one cyst, 30% had 2–5 cysts, and the remainder had 6 or more. Fifty or more cysts over a prolonged period is not excessively rare. A further excellent paper is that of Jones and Bradbeer, who followed 322 cases for a minimum of 5 years, and obtained similar results.[42]

In our clinic, half the patients develop a further palpable cyst (new or recurrent) in the 12 months following aspiration, and 6% will develop a new cyst for the first time more than 5 years after the initial aspiration. The number of new cysts presenting clinically (i.e. not detected only by imaging) within a period of 5 years after aspiration is shown in Table 9.2.

Only half will not develop a further cyst.

There is considerable controversy about the homogeneity of cyst type for any given patient with multiple recurrent cysts. One group[43] found that concentrations of EGF and insulin growth factor 1 (IGF-1) were concordant when taken from multiple cysts, whether ipsi- or contralateral.

Table 9.2 Number of clinically detected cysts (after aspiration) per patient with a minimum follow-up of 5 years

No. of cysts	No. of patients (%)
1	164 (46.6)
2	66 (18.8)
3	31 (8.8)
4	25 (7.1)
5	22 (6.2)
6 or more	44 (12.5)
Total	352 (100)

Brenner *et al.* showed that only 1:8 new cysts detected between mammographic screenings increased in size, while 60% of the cysts had resolved by one year, and 80% by 4 years without treatment.[41] All those that increased in size did so within 2 years, and this was twice as likely to occur in patients on HRT.

INVESTIGATION (*SEE ALSO* CHAPTER 6)

In practice, cysts are adequately managed by ultrasound, needle aspiration and inspection of the aspirated fluid. Radiological examination is not strictly necessary for cysts, but we utilize mammography for all cyst patients over the age of 35 years as a form of screening, to exclude an incidental cancer. We found five incidental cancers in 357 patients presenting for aspiration of a breast cyst (1.4%).

Ultrasound will usually show cysts to be multiple and bilateral with numbers in excess of those detected clinically or mammographically. Cysts are rounded, ovoid or lobulated with characteristics so similar to fibroadenoma as to make radiological differentiation impossible, emphasizing the superiority of ultrasound in managing cysts. Leakage of cyst fluid into the surrounding tissues gives altered sonographic appearances due to an inflammatory reaction (termed complex cyst by sonographers). Ultrasound of the abnormal rim can confirm inflammation rather than neoplasm.

Pneumocystography has been used when cyst aspiration reveals blood-stained fluid, but has been largely replaced by ultrasound. When used, a minimal amount of fluid should be removed so that the radiologist can easily locate the cyst. Irregularity of the surrounding tissues at one edge suggests infiltration in the rare cystic carcinoma. Such information is not essential because all cysts with blood-stained fluid should be excised, but it gives useful information for preoperative assessment and planning. (The bright red, partial blood staining of a traumatic tap should be easily differentiated from the uniform, old blood of a cystic tumour.)

Ultrasound may provide similar information more easily, and has a place in localizing small, deep impalpable lesions, which may be cystic or solid, for needling under vision.

DIFFERENTIAL DIAGNOSIS

Cysts are readily differentiated from solid lesions by ultrasound and needling. Three other cystic conditions need to be considered: the cystic form of fat necrosis (page 232), galactocele (page 132) and cystic papillary tumours, adenoma and carcinoma (page 133). It cannot be stressed too often that a tense cyst can closely simulate cancer on palpation. The question of cancer should never be raised with a patient before a cyst has been excluded by ultrasound and/or needling.

MANAGEMENT

The last 40 years has seen the management of cysts pass from mandatory excision, through selective aspiration with cytological examination, to routine (and if necessary repeated) aspiration alone. Patey and Nurick[44] had an early influence in the UK in managing cysts conservatively, and this development of a conservative regimen for managing breast cysts has been one of the truly major advances in breast surgery. Like penicillin, it needs no controlled trial to prove its efficacy, and it is unfortunate that some conservative surgeons still insist on excising recurrent cysts. Nevertheless, no aspect of breast disease management is without pitfalls and strict rules must be followed to avoid an occasional disaster.

Aspiration
The first investigation of every easily palpable lump in the breast should be the insertion of a needle, and if this is practised cysts will be diagnosed at first consultation. (Some radiologists prefer to see ill-defined masses prior to aspiration, since needling may produce artefacts which make assessment more difficult.) A 21-gauge needle with a syringe of appropriate size to the estimated cyst volume is plunged directly into the cyst, fixed by two fingers of the opposite hand (Figure 9.8).

No anaesthetic is necessary. The average cyst volume is 5–10 mL, but this varies from less than a millilitre to 75 mL or more. A 10-mL or 20-mL syringe is usually convenient. Tong[45] has argued strongly in favour of the use of evacuated glass tubes (e.g. 'Vacutainer'), but the benefit is probably marginal, particularly with large cysts. (Cysts are often more easily palpated with the patient sitting up. In such cases, the lump is localized and held while the patient lies down for aspiration.) If the mass proves to be solid, a cytological specimen is obtained, and this is facilitated if a

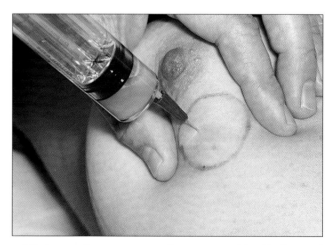

9.8 Technique of aspirating a cyst. The cyst is immobilized by fingers of the left hand.

syringe holder designed for obtaining cytology specimens is used. If the fluid is not blood stained, the cyst is aspirated to dryness, the needle removed and the fluid discarded. Cytological examination of cyst fluid is not useful or cost effective unless the fluid is blood stained. Many early workers advocated cytological examination of all cyst fluid,[44,45] but it is now recognized to be unnecessary and most large units have abandoned it except when blood stained.[46,47]

The breast is carefully palpated to exclude a residual mass. If one exists, it is reneedled under ultrasound guidance for cytology (and to exclude a further cyst) prior to arrangements being made for excision biopsy. An exception to mandatory biopsy is the inflammatory reaction to leakage of cyst fluid seen occasionally, with typical sonographic appearance and inflammatory cells on fine needle aspiration (FNA). These cases are suitable for observation.

If the mass is difficult to palpate, prior visualization by ultrasound is useful and can be used to guide the needle to a deeply placed cyst. Ultrasound is also useful for confirming that the cyst is fully emptied after aspiration.

If the fluid is blood stained, 1–2 mL only of fluid is taken for cytology in Cytospin fluid. The mass is then imaged with ultrasound and any solid area in the cyst is sampled cytologically under vision. The presence of blood is usually obvious, but in cysts with black fluid (usually not due to blood), any doubt should be eliminated by examining the fluid for blood by microscopy or a chemical occult blood test. Blood must be regarded as synonymous with tumour (usually benign, but sometimes malignant). Malignancy is more likely to occur in the elderly but even then the prognosis is favourable.

Mammography is best deferred for a week after aspiration as the trauma may cause diagnostic difficulty, although if the lump has been adequately assessed by sonography, and the main purpose of mammography is to assess the rest of the breast, it need not be delayed.

To summarize, there are two cardinal rules for safe cyst aspiration and these must always be observed:

- The mass must disappear completely after aspiration. If it does not, it must be treated as any other persistent mass, with reneedling, cytology, mammography, needle biopsy and open biopsy as indicated by individual circumstances.
- The fluid must not be blood stained. If it is, ultrasound and cytology as outlined above will be helpful but open biopsy should be stongly considered in all such cases, even if prior triple assessment is negative.

Many workers have recommended that all cysts should be excised if the cyst refills after aspiration. This is not necessary or desirable if the above two rules are met, although it should be regarded as a further indication for mammography if this is not used routinely in cyst patients. We have seen no carcinoma associated solely with refilling of a cyst without blood-stained fluid, except as an incidental finding adjacent to the cyst.

Recurrent cysts

Early recurrence is not rare but is less common than might be expected. Because aspiration might not be expected to influence the natural history, one might anticipate universal recurrence. In fact, only about 10% of cysts refill to become palpable, although almost one half of patients will develop another cyst elsewhere in the breast, and about one-third will develop more than one. We treat a recurrent cyst by repeated aspiration, and are not particularly concerned at the number of aspirations required. Fortunately, cysts rarely refill after two or three aspirations. Recurrence is an indication for mammography but not for excision. Because recurrence usually occurs in patients with multiple cysts, excision is not appropriate treatment. A persistent mass, or blood-stained fluid, remains the only indication for excision.

If recurrence becomes tedious for the patient, we will consider pneumocystography, for this seems to have a clinical benefit in lessening recurrence. Dixon and co-workers[23] have found that apocrine-lined cysts, characterized by a high K^+/Na^+ ratio, are more prone to be multiple and to recur than non-apocrine cysts. Bundred (personal communication) studied 82 women to determine the best predictive factors for cyst recurrence within 2 years of aspiration. A high K^+ level, a K^+/Na^+ ratio greater than 3, and a low Cl^- level in the cyst fluid were all predictive of recurrence. The greater the number of cysts requiring aspiration at the first visit, the greater the chance of recurrence.

Follow-up

This is another area of clinical practice undergoing re-evaluation as the result of increased knowledge over the past decade. Although Haagensen[4] gave evidence many years ago that macroscopic cysts are associated with a definite, but quite small, increase in cancer risk, other workers did not confirm this. Now 12 studies have demonstrated a definite, though relatively small, increase in risk. Bundred et al.[24] showed an increase in subsequent cancer of 4.4 times in women having a cyst aspirated over the expected risk. The risk was even greater in women with multiple or bilateral cysts. This finding has recently been confirmed by a prospective study[19] in which the cyst type was determined by fluid examination at entry. These workers found a similar degree of overall risk, but this was confined to type 1 apocrine cysts, and there was no increase with multiple cysts.

Thus, while the small increase in overall cancer risk seems definite, the further effect of individual factors remains controversial. A further, larger study by Dixon and colleagues[48] showed a similar increase in overall risk, but no relation to cyst type. The main factor affecting cancer risk in this study was age, with the greatest risk in women presenting with a cyst before the age of 45. The differences in these studies – age versus multiplicity versus cyst type – will probably prove to be due to methodological problems. For example, Dixon relied on cancer registry data for his follow-up.

These data provide some basis for devising a follow-up

policy. The overall risk is still not great: only 14 cancers occurred in 352 patients followed an average of 7 years in the Bundred series. It would be reasonable to enter such women in a screening programme at the age of 40, rather than the age of 50 generally recommended in the UK. This would be an appropriate age since cysts are uncommon before 40, but screening should not be long delayed since the median interval between cyst diagnosis and cancer detection was only 3 years in the Italian study. Follow-up of all patients with cysts below the age of 40 is not cost effective, so at present patients are usually discharged after assessment.

Haagensen et al. have recently reported the prognostic influence of the presence of high blood levels of the cyst fluid protein GCDFP-15.[49] Over a 10-year follow-up period, the relative risk of cancer for women who developed 10 or less cysts increased from 1.8 to 4.2 if they showed elevated plasma levels of the protein. The corresponding figures for those developing more than 10 cysts were 2.0 and 7.1. Since this protein is secreted by apocrine epithelium, it is further evidence for the influence of apocrine metaplasia on cancer risk.

There is considerable scope for defining a high-risk population even more closely by adding data on family history, age and cyst type, and with further study of hazards associated with various constituents of cyst fluid. It is important to appreciate that a cyst is an indicator of increased risk, and is not itself a premalignant condition; hence there is no need to excise cysts, and screening must encompass both breasts.

This problem is discussed further in Chapter 18.

Several studies have suggested an increased incidence of benign duct papilloma in women who have had a cyst aspirated. We found five such cases among 352 patients followed for 5 years or more after cyst aspiration.

Hormone therapy

The hormonal background to cysts is not defined sufficiently precisely to justify any form of hormone therapy on a routine basis. One study of patients with recurrent cysts has reported a remarkable reduction (75%) in the number of cysts requiring aspiration after a course of danazol, 100 mg three times per day for 3 months.[50] Benefit was even greater at 6 months, i.e. 3 months after cessation of therapy, and persisted at 3-year follow-up, but had disappeared at 5 years. This indicates that this treatment might prove worthwhile in severe cases with recurrent painful cysts. A controlled trial of EPO in our unit had no effect on the incidence of recurrent cysts.

Mastectomy

Some surgeons recommend subcutaneous mastectomy with silicone implant for extensive or recurrent cystic disease, either on the basis of reduction of cancer risk or for the physical and psychological benefit of the patient. We believe this practice should be condemned except in the most exceptional circumstances. Although cysts are a nuisance, they cause the patient relatively little morbidity when they are managed conservatively by repeated aspiration. This is entirely different to the complications, short and long term, which may trouble patients after bilateral subcutaneous mastectomy with silicone implants or autogenous tissue reconstruction. Until reconstructive techniques improve, mastectomy is difficult to justify on grounds of benefit to the patients. The presence of cysts alone would not justify mastectomy on grounds of cancer risk, and should be considered as one aspect only of cancer risk, in weighing up the very difficult decisions in this area.

GALACTOCELE

A galactocele is an uncommon lesion in which a cyst filled with milky material develops after a period of lactation. There is a surprising paucity of information about this condition, compared with other aspects of breast pathology. Such literature as exists is often obscured by a tendency to confuse galactocele with duct ectasia and recurrent subareolar abscess. The confusion extends down to some of the most recent papers, particularly those which state that galactoceles are prone to lead to chronic sinuses. The first use of the term 'galactocele' has been attributed by Fitzwilliams to de Lambell, who defined it in 1845 as a 'form of tumour which springs from one of the milk ducts, forming a cyst'.[51]

The term is best confined to a specific clinical syndrome in which a woman develops a painless swelling of the breast from a few weeks to some months after ceasing lactation. The swelling is smooth and mobile and in fact has the exact physical characteristics of the usual breast cyst. Aspiration produces what is clearly milk, instead of one of the variety of fluids commonly found in breast cysts. The lesion disappears completely and is usually cured by a single aspiration, but like ordinary cysts, will occasionally require two or three aspirations. It may be found anywhere in the breast, but commonly towards the areola.

In a recent series of 10 cases[52] the age range was from 27 to 36, the duration one week to 6 months; six cases were post partum and five still feeding.

The mammographic appearances have been described[53] and are complex, with three distinctive radiological patterns. Ultrasound is more appropriate as the first examination in this group, and again the appearances are complex, with 50% cystic or multicystic, 37% mixed cystic/solid and 13% solid.[52]

The aetiology and pathology are obscure. Lactation is an essential antecedent in the typical case (although the condition has been described in male infants!). It is usually stated to follow abrupt artificial cessation of lactation.

A simple explanation of the pathogenesis is that a pre-existing cyst which connects with the duct system fills with milk, either by secretion or retrograde filling, but the ductule draining the cyst becomes blocked, trapping the milk. This may become slightly thicker by absorption of water, but retains the obvious characteristics of milk. Since some cysts can be demonstrated to connect with the duct system, it is surprising that galactocele is not more common given the frequency of cysts in the breasts. Presumably the reason is that cysts are an aberration of involution and less common during the usual child-bearing period. It also has been reported that macroscopic cysts resolve during pregnancy along with the well-recognized improvement in mastalgia and nodularity.

Other cases where cysts contain inspissated pus or infected material are better regarded as a separate group, most of which fall into the categories of duct ectasia, periductal mastitis or chronic cystic disease.

PAPILLARY TUMOURS ASSOCIATED WITH MACROCYSTS

Pathology

Papillary tumours within the wall of a cyst are rare, yet by no means excessively so. We see approximately one such tumour a year, yet there is remarkably little written on this subject. Attention was first drawn to the subject by Hart in 1927.[54] He described 124 cases and emphasized that the majority were benign. However, the report does not differentiate between duct papillomas and intracystic tumours, but since 69 of 95 benign cases had nipple discharge and 75 a lump, it must have included both. That confusion, or at least lack of differentiating the two groups, persists to today.

Haagensen[4] regards them all as duct papillomas within grossly dilated ducts, yet this is not consistent with our experience. Cystic dilatation of ducts due to intraductal papilloma (sometimes also called papillary cystadenoma) is commoner than the true isolated cyst containing a tumour, but in our experience the two conditions are clinically distinct, and this is important in management. Cyst puncture and pneumocystography shows no connection with the duct system with the isolated lesion, nor is there any nipple discharge. Azzopardi[17] mentions that papilloma can be seen within cysts, i.e. of lobular derivation, but gives no details apart from mentioning a single case he had encountered. Devitt[55] discusses the problem of carcinoma *in association with* a cyst.

Perhaps the most important point is whether they are single or multiple. Intracystic tumours in the elderly are usually solitary and of low-grade malignancy. Intraductal tumours are usually multiple, and more likely to be associated with multifocal intraduct cancer. Calvert *et al.*[56] described a solitary huge intracystic papillary lesion (18 cm in diameter) which they regarded as intraductal, in spite of the lack of nipple discharge, because fragments of elastic tissue could be identified in its wall. Whether this finding is definitive in such a large lesion is probably less important than the fact that it was solitary, and hence likely to behave as an intracystic tumour and more likely to be suitable for local excision.

A second problem causing confusion is the use of the term intracystic cancer, since this by definition excludes benign lesions. A series of 48 cases of intracystic cancer was reported from the Mayo Clinic[57] where it constituted 0.5% of all breast cancers. However, 31 cases were excluded because they were benign, suggesting that intracystic papilloma has approximately the same incidence as the malignant version. The report gives evidence of the excellent prognosis of the lesions regarded as malignant; only 1:3 showed invasion of the cyst wall, and only 6% had axillary metastases. A series of 16 cases reported in 1969[58] were all reported as malignant, although 12 showed 'orderly papillary epithelium with little mitotic activity', reflecting the tendency to err on the side of diagnosisng cancer at that time.

Carter *et al.*[59] describe 41 cases of intracystic cancer without mention of benign cases. They divide them into three groups: (1) non-invasive intracystic cancer and with no surrounding ductal carcinoma-in-situ (DCIS), (2) intracystic cancer with cyst wall invasion but no DCIS, and (3) intracystic cancer with associated DCIS. They point out the differing prognosis for the first group; none had recurrence, including eight who had biopsy only. It is clear that these form a biologically favourable group.

In summary, intracystic papillary tumours need to be differentiated from multiple ductal papillomas, to be assessed very carefully in terms of malignancy, and assessed in terms of tumour invasion into the surrounding breast.

Clinical features

Papilliferous cysts usually arise in patients a decade or more after the menopause. The patient presents with a soft mass that is usually large and often apparently of recent onset. Aspiration yields old, blood-stained fluid and cytology will usually show epithelial cells of benign or degenerate appearance. Pneumocystography will demonstrate the cyst, and a small papilloma within its wall (Figures 9.9 and 9.10).

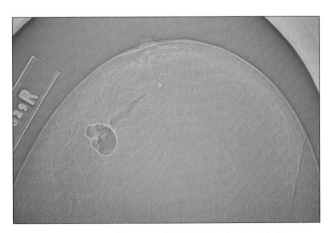

9.9 Pneumocystogram for a cyst containing blood-stained fluid, demonstrating an intracystic papilloma.

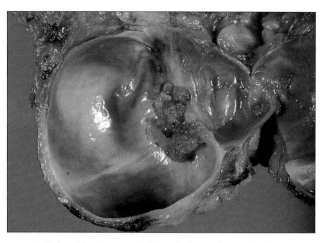

9.10 Typical papillary tumour in the wall of a cyst in an elderly woman.

This technique can also give a fair indication as to whether there is invasion outside the cyst wall to indicate malignancy. Estabrook *et al.* reported mammographic features in 10 such cases.[60]

Ultrasound with guided biopsy can give considerable information regarding differential diagnosis and malignancy of the cyst and its contained tumour, and is replacing pneumocystography as the main diagnostic technique. Invasion of the wall can be assessed, although caution is needed in relying entirely on ultrasound for assessment. It can help target any suspicious area for FNA cytology. The series of 56 tumours with a cystic appearance on ultrasound studied by Omori *et al.* contained a wide variety of pathology. Ten of the 56 were intracystic cancers; other lesions included necrotic cancers and phyllodes tumours, simple cysts and abscesses.[61]

Management

Fortunately the majority of papillary tumours associated with macrocysts are benign, even (or especially) in the elderly. The local nature of the lesion, as a confined cyst, will usually be apparent on clinical examination, and ultrasound. Mammography will give some indication of the presence of invasive cancer or DCIS.

Where the lesion appears to be a confined cyst, in this age group it is best treated by total cyst excision, with a 1-cm resection margin as for phyllodes tumour. This will provide material for adequate histological assessment in all cases, and definitive treatment in the majority proved benign or with minimal invasion on histology.

REFERENCES

1. Cooper A. On diseases of the breast. *Cooper Lectures* 1831; **2**: 125.

2. Reclus P. La maladie kystique des mammelles. *Revue de Chirurgie* 1883; **3**: 761.

3. Bloodgood JC. The bluedomed cyst in chronic cystic mastitis. *Journal of the American Medical Association* 1929; **93**: 1056.

4. Haagensen CD. *Diseases of the Breast*. Philadelphia: WB Saunders, 1986.

5. Dixon JM & Mansel RE. Pigments in breast fluid. *British Medical Journal* 1995; **310**: 403.

6. Bradlow HL, Rosenfeld RS, Kream J *et al.* Steroid hormone accumulation in human breast cyst fluid. *Cancer Research* 1981; **41**: 105–107.

7. Miller WR, Humeniuk V & Kelley RW. DHAS in breast secretions. *Journal of Steroid Biochemistry* 1980; **13**: 145–151.

8. Bradlow HL, Schwartz MK, Fleisher M *et al.* Accumulation of hormones in breast cyst fluid. *Journal of Clinical Endocrinology and Metabolism* 1979; **49**: 778–782.

9. Narde E, Bigazzi M, Agrimonti F *et al.* Relaxin and fibrocystic disease of the mammary gland. *First International Conference on Human Relaxin*, Florence, Italy, 1982.

10. Fleisher M, Oettgen HF, Breed CN *et al.* CEA like material in fluid from benign cysts of the breast. *Clinical Chemistry* 1974; **20**: 41–42.

11. Haagensen Jr DE, Mazoujian G, Dilley VG *et al.* Breast gross cystic disease fluid analyses. I: Isolation and radioimmunoassay for a major component protein. *Journal of the National Cancer Institute* 1979; **62**: 239–244.

12. Torrisi R, Zanardi S, Pensa F *et al.* Epidermal Growth Factor content of breast cyst fluids from women with breast cancer or proliferative disease of the breast. *Breast Cancer Research Treatment* 1995; **33**: 219–224.

13. Angeli A, Bradlow HL, Chasalon FI & Dogliotti L. Biochemistry of breast cyst fluid. *Annals of the New York Academy of Sciences* 1990; **586**: 1–296.

14. Frantz VK, Pickren JW, Melcher GW & Auchinloss H. Incidence of chronic cystic disease in so-called normal breasts. *Cancer* 1951; **4**: 762–783.

15. Foote FW & Stewart FW. Comparative studies of cancerous versus non-cancerous breasts. *Annals of Surgery* 1945; **121**: 6–53.

16. Hayward JL & Parks AG. Alterations in the microanatomy of the breast as a result of changes in the hormonal environment. In: Currie AR (ed.) *Endocrine Aspects of Breast Cancer*, pp 133–134. Edinburgh: Livingstone, 1958.

17. Azzopardi JG. *Problems in Breast Pathology*. London: WB Saunders, 1979.

18. Bradlow HL, Fleisher M, Schwartz D *et al.* Biochemical classification of patients with gross cystic breast disease. *Annals of the New York Academy of Sciences* 1990; **586**: 12–16.

19. Bruzzi P, Dogliotti L, Naldoni C *et al.* Cohort study of risk of breast cancer with cyst type in women with gross cystic disease of the breast. *British Medical Journal* 1997; **314**: 925–928.

20. Dixon JM, Miller WR & Scott WN. pH of human breast cyst fluid. *Clinical Oncology* 1984; **10**: 221–224.

21. Bradlow HL, Breed CN, Nisselbaum J *et al.* pH as a marker of breast cyst fluid biochemical type. *European Journal of Surgical Oncology* 1987; **13**: 331–334.

22. Miller WR & Forrest APM. Androgen conjugates in human breast secretions and cyst fluids. In: Angeli (ed.) *Endocrinology of Cystic Breast Disease*, pp 77–84. New York: Raven Press, 1983.

23. Dixon JM, Miller WR & Scott WN. Natural history of cystic disease: the importance of cyst type. *British Journal of Surgery* 1985; **72**: 190–192.

24. Bundred NJ, West RR, Dowd JO *et al.* Is there an increased risk of breast cancer in women who have had a breast cyst aspirated? *British Journal of Cancer* 1991; **64**: 953–955.

25. Mannello F, Sebastiani M, Amati S & Gazzanelli G. Conjugated bile acids in breast cyst fluid. Relationship to cation-related cyst sub-populations. *Cancer Letters* 1997; **119**: 21–26.

26. Mannello F, Bocchiotti G, Bianchi G *et al.* Quantification of prostate-specific antigen immunoreactivity in human breast cyst fluids. *Breast Cancer Research and Treatment* 1996; **38**: 247–252.

27. Dixon JM, Telford J, Elton RA & Miller WR. Uptake of dihydroepiandrosterone sulphate into human breast cyst fluid. *The Breast* 1997; **6**: 12–16.

28. Dixon JM, Telford J & Miller WR. Effects of spironolactone, danazol and efamast on the uptake of tritiated dihydroepiandrosterone sulphate into human breast cyst fluid. In: Mansel RE (ed.) *Recent Developments in the Study of Benign Breast Disease*, pp 265–270. Carnforth: Parthenon Publishing.

29. Lail C, Siraj AK, Erbas H & Lennard TWJ. Relationship between basic fibroblast growth factor and transforming growth factor beta-2 in breast cyst fluid. *Journal of Clinical Endocrinology and Metabolism* 1995; **80**: 711–715.

30. Dixon JM, Scott WN & Miller WR. An analysis of the content and morphology of human breast microcysts. *European Journal of Surgical Oncology* 1985; **11**: 151–154.

31. Wellings SR & Alpers CE. Apocrine cyst metaplasia: Subgross pathology and prevalence in cancer associated versus random autopsy breasts. *Human Pathology* 1987; **18**: 381–386.

32. Molina R, Fillella X & Herranz M. Biochemistry of cyst fluid in fibrocystic disease of the breast. *Annals of the New York Academy of Sciences* 1990; **586**: 29–42.

33. Bundred NJ, Scott WN, Davies SJ *et al.* Zinc alpha-2 glycoprotein levels in serum and breast fluids: a potential marker of apocrine activity. *European Journal of Cancer* 1991; **27**: 349–342.

34. Fechner RE. Benign breast disease in women on oestrogen therapy. *Cancer* 1972; **29**: 273–279.

35. Engle ET, Krakower C & Haagensen CD. Oestrogen administered to aged female monkeys with no resultant tumours. *Cancer Research* 1943; **3**: 858.

36. England PC, Skinner LG, Cottrell KM & Sellwood RA. Sex hormones in breast disease. *British Journal of Surgery* 1975; **62**: 806–809.

37. Gately CA, Maddox PR, Jones DL *et al.* Biologically active prolactin in patients with macroscopic breast cysts. *British Journal of Surgery* 1992; **79**: 1238.

38. Simpson JF & Page DL. Loss of expression of fodrin (a structural protein) in cystic changes in the human breast. *Laboratory Investigation* 1993; **68**: 537–540.

39. Eunhee S, Bedoya AA, Lee H *et al.* Keratinocyte growth factor causes cystic dilation of the mammary glands of mice. *American Journal of Pathology* 1994; **145**: 1015–1021.

40. Devitt JE. Benign disorders of the breast in older women. *Surgery, Gynecology and Obstetrics* 1986; **162**: 340–342.

41. Brenner RJ, Bein ME, Sarti DA & Vinstein AL. Spontaneous regression of interval benign cysts of the breast. *Radiology* 1994; **193**: 365–368.

42. Jones BM & Bradbeer JW. The presentation and progress of macroscopic breast cysts. *British Journal of Surgery* 1980; **67**: 669–671.

43. Wang DY, Hamed H & Fentiman I. Epidermal growth factor and insulin growth factor 1 in human breast cyst fluid. *Annals of the New York Academy of Sciences* 1990; **586**: 158–160.

44. Patey DH & Nurick AW. Natural history of cystic disease of the breast treated conservatively. *British Medical Journal* 1953; **I**: 15–17.

45. Tong D. The treatment of solitary cysts in the breast: A new technique. *British Journal of Surgery* 1969; **56**: 885–890.

46. Forrest APM, Kirkpatrick JR & Roberts MM. Needle aspiration of breast cysts. *British Medical Journal* 1975; **3**: 30–31.

47. Cowen PN & Benson EA. Cytological study of fluid from benign breast cysts. *British Journal of Surgery* 1979; **66**: 209–211.

48. Dixon JM, McDonald C, Elton RA & Miller WR. Breast cancer risk with cyst type in cystic disease of the breast. Larger study found no association between cyst type and breast cancer [letter]. *British Medical Journal* 1997; **315**: 545–546.

49. Haagensen DE, Kelly D & Bodian CA. GCDFP-15 blood levels for stratification of risk of breast cancer development in women with active gross cystic disease. *Breast* 1997; **6**: 113–119.

50. Locker AP, Hinton CP, Roebuck EJ & Blamey RW. A long term follow up of patients treated with a single course of Danazol for recurrent breast cysts. *British Journal of Clinical Practice* 1989; **43**: 100–101.

51. Fitzwilliams DCL. *On the Breast*, p 173. London: William Heinemann, 1924.

52. Stevens K, Burrell HC, Evans AJ & Sibbering DM. The ultrasound appearance of galactoceles. *British Journal of Radiology* 1997; **70**: 239–241.

53. Gomez A, Mata JM, Donozo C *et al.* Galactocele: 3 distinctive radiological patterns. *Radiology* 1986; **158**: 43–44.

54. Hart D. Intracystic papillomas of the breast – benign and malignant. *Archives of Surgery* 1927; **14**: 793–835.

55. Devitt JE. The clinical recognition of cystic carcinoma of the breast. *Surgery, Gynecology and Obstetrics* 1984; **159**: 130–132.

56. Calvert RJ, Kashi SH & Quinn CM. Giant intra-duct papilloma of the breast. *The Breast* 1994; **3**: 193–194.

57. Gatcher FG, Dockerty MB & Clagett OT. Intracystic carcinoma of the breast. *Surgery, Gynecology and Obstetrics* 1958; **106**: 347–352.

58. McKittrick JE, Doane WA & Failing KM. Intracystic papillary carcinoma of the breast. *American Surgeon* 1969; **35**: 195–202.

59. Carter D, Orr SL & Merino MJ. Intracystic papillary carcinoma of the breast. *Cancer* 1983; **52**: 14–24.

60. Estabrook A, Asch T, Gump F *et al.* Mammographic features of intracystic papillary lesions. *Surgery, Gynecology and Obstetrics* 1990; **170**: 113–116.

61. Omori LM, Hisa N, Ohkuma K *et al.* Breast masses with mixed cystic-solid sonographic appearances. *Journal of Clinical Ultrasound* 1993; **21**: 489–495.

Sclerosing adenosis, radial scar and complex sclerosing lesions

CONTENTS

KEY POINTS AND NEW DEVELOPMENTS

1. All three lesions are important because they may be confused radiologically, macroscopically and histologically with cancer.
2. Sclerosing adenosis may present with mastalgia or as a mass, as well as an incidental radiological or histological finding.
3. Radial scar (RS) and complex sclerosing lesion (CSL) are similar, probably the same process, and are differentiated on size, CSL being 1 cm or more in diameter.
4. With all three, the pathologist finds diagnosis easier on a low-power view than assessing high-power cytology.

5. Because cancer and RS/CSL cannot be differentiated reliably on radiological appearances, all such lesions should be biopsied.
6. The cancer risk associated with an individual lesion is that of associated pathology, such as atypical hyperplasia. The likelihood of such coexisting pathology is related to the size of the lesion and the age of the patient.
7. Whether stereotactic core needle or open surgical biopsy is utilized depends to some extent on the facilities and experience available; many units prefer open biopsy.
8. Oxytocin receptors are prominent in the myoepithelial cells seen in these conditions – possibly playing an aetiological role.

These three lesions have long been recognized by pathologists under a variety of names. They have more recently attracted clinical attention (and some degree of uniformity of terminology) because they are diagnosed more frequently on mammography as screening abnormalities which simulate cancer. Simultaneously, pathologists have subjected them to greater scrutiny because of the intensified interest in differentiating histological patterns into those which may, or may not, be precancerous.

SCLEROSING ADENOSIS

This lesion was first described by Masson in 1923[1] and a number of excellent pathological descriptions have since been published, one such being that by Dawson.[2] It may be regarded as one of the manifestations of ANDI (an aberration of lobular involution; see Chapter 3), in which a well-ordered lobular involution is distorted by excessive myoepithelial proliferation, and accompanied by pronounced fibrous alteration of the specialized lobular stroma.

This is in keeping with the fact that sclerosing adenosis is present (unrecognized) in the breast much more frequently than it presents clinically. Among surgeons it has received little attention, being known mainly through notoriety as a cause of difficulty for pathologists in the diagnosis of cancer on frozen section. Its surgical implications extend over a wider field for it may simulate cancer clinically, macroscopically and radiologically, as well as histologically. In addition, the condition shows an association with breast pain.

Clinical presentation

The condition has four distinct modes of clinical presentation:

- Presentation as a mass
- Presentation with pain
- Presentation on mammography
- Chance histological finding.

Presentation as a mass

This may occur at any age from the mid-20s to the postmenopausal age group. The mass tends to be small, 2 cm or less, firm, poorly delineated and attached to surrounding breast tissue. There are no gross signs of cancer, such as skin retraction or lymphadenopathy, but these would not necessarily be expected with a small mass.

Presentation with pain

This is discussed in more detail in Chapter 8. In brief, sclerosing adenosis produces the same type of localized persisting pain that is seen in cancer, but sometimes having premenstrual exacerbation. Pressure also often causes exacerbation and, in some patients, it is severe enough to interfere with sleep.[3,4] The perineural invasion demonstrated histologically in some cases may be an explanation of the association with pain (Figure 10.1).

In a series of 316 consecutive and unselected cases of benign mammary disorders, Davies found that sclerosing adenosis was the condition most frequently found to show neural invasion by mammary epithelial cells.[5]

Presentation on mammography

With increasing use of mammography as a screening or semi-screening procedure, the radiological features typical of sclerosing adenosis are being detected more frequently, either in association with a mass or in asymptomatic patients. Where the radiological pattern is indistinguishable from cancer, biopsy is mandatory. Where unequivocal radiological signs of sclerosing adenosis are seen on mammography, 90% will have the condition on histology. Thus in our experience, there is a 10% false-negative rate for the mammographic diagnosis.

Chance histological finding

Small patches of sclerosing adenosis are frequently found on histological section of breast tissue. It has been estimated that these occur 20–30 times more commonly than palpable lesions. These small areas found on histology can be ignored.

Frequency of presentation

In our clinic 43 patients were encountered over a 5-year period. The age range extended from 24 to 64 years. Eleven presented primarily with pain, although 25 of the patients experienced some pain at the site of the lesion. Nine presented with a mass and four were chance histological findings. The rest were detected on mammography. Undoubtedly, there would have been other cases detected on histological examination during this period which the pathologist did not bother to report.

Sclerosing adenosis appears to be particularly common in some developing countries, where it is also frequently associated with mastalgia. Ihekwaba found it in 52 of 657 women with benign breast disorders in Nigeria, and associated with mastalgia in 68% of them.[6]

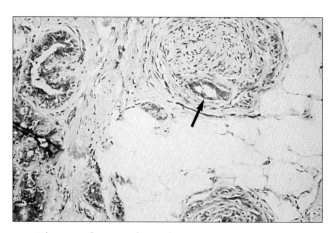

10.1 Sclerosing adenosis with neural invasion (arrow).

Radiological criteria

Three patterns of radiographical change are seen[7] (see also Chapter 6):

- Increased density with irregular margins, very similar to cancer but without fine microcalcification.
- Fine, smooth calcification scattered widely throughout the breast, usually bilateral.
- Smooth microcalcifications, up to 10 in number, arranged in a small group (Figure 10.2). This may or may not be associated with widespread calcification. This pattern cannot be differentiated from that of cancer and biopsy is mandatory.

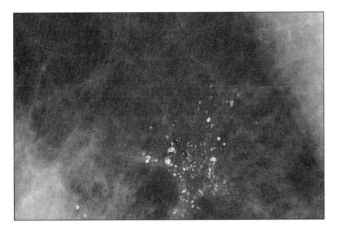

10.2 Mammogram showing microcalcifications typical of a focus of sclerosing adenosis – variable in size, shape and density in a segmental distribution.

Pathology

Careful macroscopic examination will suggest the diagnosis. Sclerosing adenosis occurs as a firm, ill-defined fibrotic mass, but is not as hard, cartilaginous or gritty as cancer and it has a nodular, circumscribed appearance rather than the stellate pattern of cancer. Azzopardi[8] points out that examination with a fine hand lens will often demonstrate clearly the nodular and whorled appearance. The nodules have a brownish tinge and the greyish or creamy streaks of necrotic debris in ductules typical of cancer are not seen.

The microscopic criteria outlined by McDivitt et al.[9] have been summarized by Davies[5] as nodular epithelial lesions in which lobular units are enlarged by an increased number of acini, but the normal two cell population and basement membrane are maintained. The normal lobular structure is distorted by the fibrosis, particularly in the centre of the lesion, where epithelial cells may appear to be isolated and simulate the appearance of invasive malignancy, especially on frozen section. The problem is compounded by mitoses sometimes seen in the early cellular phase, and neural and vascular invasion may occur occasionally. Microcalcification, similar to that seen in malignancy, is common. The problem is now well recognized by experienced pathologists, but was the cause of much overdiagnosis of malignancy in the past.

The histological similarities between sclerosing adenosis and cancer are illustrated in Figure 10.3, in which the two are shown side by side.

The maintenance of a lobular architecture on low-power evaluation is an essential feature used to differentiate the two lesions. Figure 10.4 shows the extensive microcalcification which is the basis of one of the radiological patterns.

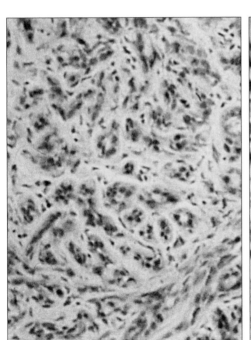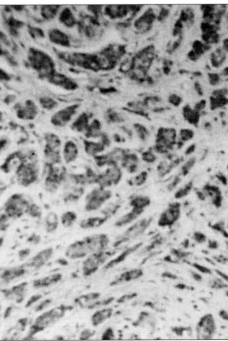

10.3 Sclerosing adenosis (left) and invasive cancer (right) shown side by side, illustrating difficulties encountered in differentiation on frozen section.

The recent development of techniques for localizing oxytocin receptors has shown these to be prominent in the myoepithelial cells, which themselves are prominent in sclerosing adenosis.[10] This raises the possibility that oxytocin and its receptors may play a role in the aetiology and evolution of sclerosing adenosis.

Management

When cancer cannot be excluded in a patient with a mass or mammographic findings, the area must be biopsied. The mass is excised and treated in the usual way for any lump of doubtful pathology. The question of routine needle biopsy does not usually arise because of the small size of the mass, and even localization for fine needle aspiration may be difficult. Some form of stereotactic localization is necessary for needle biopsy in most cases, and whether stereotactic or open biopsy is used depends on the facilities and experience of the individual unit, and the perceived likelihood of cancer from the radiological appearances, as discussed further in the next section. It is generally agreed that subclinical lesions are better submitted to paraffin section, and frozen section avoided because of the difficulty of interpretation. With a macroscopic mass, frozen section may be used, but it is our view that, if there is any discrepancy between the macroscopic and frozen section assessments, it is better to wait for a paraffin section than to proceed to any radical form of surgery on the basis of frozen section. Local excision is adequate management for sclerosing adenosis.

When biopsy is required for a non-palpable, mammographic lesion a standard prearranged procedure involving surgeon, radiologist and pathologist must be followed to ensure that the correct tissue is removed. The steps are described in Chapter 18.

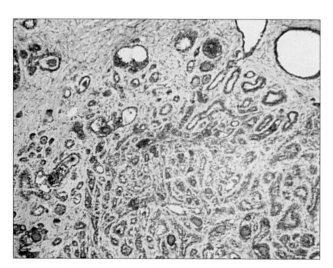

10.4 Sclerosing adenosis showing numerous areas of microcalcification, providing the pathological basis for the typical X-ray appearance.

RADIAL SCAR (RS) AND COMPLEX SCLEROSING LESIONS (CSL)

These conditions are similar to sclerosing adenosis in that they present most commonly as mammographic or incidental histological findings simulating malignancy, and may also present as a mass. However, they differ histologically; sclerosing adenosis lacks the elastosis and epithelial proliferation notable in these two lesions, while the maintained lobular orientation typical of sclerosing adenosis is lost in the greater complexity and distortion of RS and CSL.

These terms were defined much more recently than sclerosing adenosis, the term radial scar being used first by Linell et al. as recently as 1980,11 although the lesions had been described previously under various names by a number of workers.

RS and CSL are considered to be the same process, and are differentiated arbitrarily on the basis of size, lesions smaller than 1 cm being designated as RS, and those larger as CSL. They may be multiple.

The reported incidence in screening programmes is from 0.1 to 0.5 per 1000 women attending. The incidence is much higher in autopsy studies; Nielsen et al. found RS in 28% of unselected autopsies, two-thirds multiple and one-half bilateral.12 It is well recognized that typical pathological lesions may show no mammographic abnormality, even though in practice the majority are found in this way.

Pathology

Macroscopically, small RS may be unremarkable, but larger lesions show the induration, retraction and greyish-white colour typical of cancer. There has been a tendency to regard RS/CSL as impalpable, the presence of a mass being considered to indicate cancer. However, Wallis et al.[13] found a quarter of benign lesions detected on screening to be palpable.

Microscopically, the lesion has a stellate appearance around a central core. The core is of fibrous and elastic tissue with entrapped distorted glandular elements. Radiating from this central core are ducts which may show cystic dilatation. This arrangement suggests that the lesion may develop by sclerosis around a small duct where it branches into terminal ducts. Page and Anderson[14] describe the typical appearance 'the arrangement of parenchyma around a fibrosing spindle, rather in the manner of a central purse string having been pulled'. The distortion of the epithelial cells caught in the central sclerosis is the reason for the confusion with malignancy. The surrounding ducts frequently show benign hyperplasias, adenosis or sclerosing adenosis.

As the lesion becomes larger, the complexity of the surrounding tissues drawn in makes the term complex sclerosing lesion appropriate. The histological appearances of RS are reproduced in the larger lesions, but the greater complexity arises from other changes being drawn in, such as papilloma, sclerosing adenosis and apocrine change.

As with sclerosing adenosis, pathologists report that they make the diagnosis by viewing at low power, rather than by studying high-power cytological detail. In a multicentre study where pathologists reviewed slides of breast screening abnormalities 'blind', RS and CSL were lesions which were diagnosed by different pathologists with a high degree of consistency.[15]

Davies and Kulka[16] have drawn attention to small false arterial aneurysms associated with these lesions. They believe them to be traumatic, resulting from diagnostic needle puncture.

Diagnosis

The lesion is seen in a wide pre- and postmenopausal age group, typically 35–65 with a mean of 55 years.[17] They rarely present as a lump, but after identification on a mammogram, a quarter can be palpated. The typical radiological features are a lucent centre with radiating spicules, with or without microcalcification, and varying appearances on different mammographic views (Figure 10.5). These typical features may also occur with early cancers.

Management

The diagnostic workup is similar to that for sclerosing adenosis, stereoscopic or open biopsy depending on the facilities and experience available, and the perceived risk of malignancy from the radiological appearance. However, it is widely accepted that it is not possible to differentiate with certainty cancer from RS/CSL on mammographic features. Frouge et al.18 reported the pathological findings in 40 RS lesions diagnosed on mammography. Pathology showed 20 pure RS, 12 pure cancers and 8 cancers (7 tubular) associated with an RS. On review of the mammograms, it was not possible to differentiate the three groups on the size and shape of the spicule, the size of the central core or the calcifications.

The experience from our own screening unit is similar: 32 lesions showing radiological features of RS were excised after detailed mammography, ultrasound and FNA; four were well-differentiated cancers and three had small areas of in-situ cancer in the breast tissue adjacent to an RS (Moneypenny, Lyons, Dallimore and Horgan, personal communication). On this evidence, most believe that all RS/CSL lesions should be excised. Those who advocate stereotactic biopsy and watch policy in doubtful cases point out that the associated cancers are excellent prognosis lesions, and the patient is unlikely to suffer if progression is awaited before excision.

Significance

The implications for malignancy of these lesions have been the subject of some controversy, but the balance of opinion at present is that they are not precancerous, and that local excision to ensure accurate diagnosis and eliminate the lesion is appropriate management. It is generally agreed that the cancer risk is that of the individual elements; thus if an area of atypical hyperplasia or cancer-in-situ is included, the prognosis would be that of the individual processes[19]. Sloane and Mayers have drawn attention to the importance of the size of the lesion and the age of the patient in the likelihood of such associated pathology being present[20]. In a study of 126 radial scars in 91 women, atypical hyperplasia and intralesional cancer were rare in lesions less than 6–7-mm diameter and in women younger than 50 years old, but was much higher with larger lesions in older women.

The suggestion that the central epithelial cells represent the earliest stage of a tubular or other breast cancer cannot be excluded – autopsy studies have shown that RS is significantly commoner in cancerous than non-cancerous breasts[19]. On the other hand, follow-up studies have shown no increase in cancers after excision of radial scars[21] and there is insufficient evidence to support a precancerous potential.

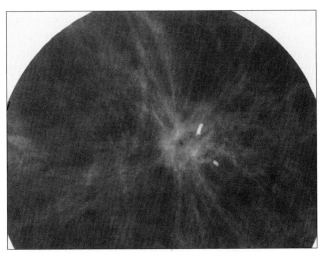

10.5 Mammogram of a radial scar, showing the typical features of central lucent area and long, radiating strands described in the text.

REFERENCES

1. Masson P. *Traite de Pathologie-Medicale*. Paris: A. Malione, 1923.

2. Dawson EK Fibrosing adenosis: a little recognised mammary picture. *Edinburgh Medical Journal* 1954; **61**: 391–401.

3. Preece PE, Fortt RW, Gravelle IH, Baum M & Hughes LE Some clinical aspects of sclerosing adenosis. *Clinical Oncology* 1979; **2**: 192.

4. Preece PE. Sclerosing adenosis. *World Journal of Surgery* 1989; **13**: 721–725.

5. Davies JD Neural invasion in benign mammary dysplasia. *Journal of Pathology* 1973; **109**: 225–231.

6. Ihekwaba FN. Benign breast disease in Nigerian women: a study of 657 patients. *Journal of the Royal College of Surgeons of Edinburgh* 1994; **39**: 280–283.

7. Evans KT & Gravelle IH. *Mammography, Thermography and Ultrasonography in Breast Disease*. London: Butterworths, 1973.

8. Azzopardi JG. *Problems in breast pathology*. London: W B Saunders, 1979. p168.

9. McDivitt RW, Stewart FW & Berg JW. Tumours of the breast. *Atlas of Tumour Pathology*, Vol 2, pp 133–137. Washington DC, 2nd Series Fascicle, 1968.

10. Bussolati G, Cassoni P, Ghisolfi G *et al*. Immunolocalisation and gene expression of oxytocin receptors in carcinomas and non-neoplastic tissues of the breast. *American Journal of Pathology* 1996; **148**: 1895–1903.

11. Linell F, Ljungberg O & Andersson I. Breast carcinoma: aspects of early stages, progression and related problems. *Acta Pathol Microbiol Immuno Scand* 1980; **272**: 199–217.

12. Nielsen M, Jensen J & Andersen JA An autopsy study of radial scars in the female breast. *Histopathology* 1985; 9: 287–295.

13. Wallis MG, Devakumar R, Hosie KB *et al*. Complex sclerosing lesions (radial scars) of the breast can be palpable. *Clinical Radiology* 1993; 48: 319–320.

14. Page DL & Anderson TJ. *Diagnostic Histopathology of the Breast*. p91. Edinburgh: Churchill Livingstone, 1987.

15. Sloane JP, Ellman R, Anderson TJ *et al*. Consistency of histopathological reporting of breast lesions detected by screening. *European Journal of Cancer* 1994; **30A**: 1414–1419.

16. Davies DJ & Kulka J. Traumatic arterial biopsy after fine needle aspirational cytology in mammary complex sclerosing lesions. *Histopathology* 1996; **28**: 65–70.

17. Patel A, Steel Y, McKenzie J *et al*. Radial scars: a review of 30 cases. *European Journal of Surgicical Oncology* 1997; 23: 202–205.

18. Frouge C, Tristant H, Guinebretiere JM *et al*. Mammographic lesions suggestive of radial scars: microscopic findings in 40 cases. *Radiology* 1995; 195: 623–625.

19. Nielsen M, Christensen L & Andersen J. Radial scars in women with breast cancer. *Cancer* 1987; 59: 1019–25

20. Sloane JP & Mayers MM. Carcinoma and atypical hyperplasia in radial scars and complex sclerosing lesions : importance of lesion size and patient age. *Histopathology* 1993; 23: 225–231.

21. Andersen JA & Gram B. Radial scar in the female breast: a long term follow-up of 32 cases. *Cancer* 1984; 53: 2557–60

The duct ectasia/periductal mastitis complex

CONTENTS

KEY POINTS AND NEW DEVELOPMENTS

1. The duct ectasia/periductal mastitis (DE/PDM) complex covers a number of processes which may exist alone or in combination. Some are subclinical and minor variants of normality (ANDI) while the spectrum extends to disease with severe morbidity.
2. Much confusion has arisen through failure to differentiate between histological findings (not clinically overt) and the very overt syndromes of the clinical disease entities.
3. The processes include duct dilatation (ectasia), histological PDM, bacterial mastitis and periductal fibrosis. Associated conditions are nipple inversion and squamous metaplasia of the ducts.
4. Clinical manifestations include nipple discharge (bloody and non-bloody), inflammation, abscess, fistula, mastalgia and nipple retraction. Bilateral involvement is not uncommon.

5. Secondary bacterial invasion shows mixed flora (aerobes and anaerobes) typical of (and probably coming from) those in the mouth and vagina.
6. Cigarette smoking is a powerful facilitator of severe inflammatory complications.
7. Established infections are rarely cured without surgery to the underlying duct abnormality, directed towards a single duct or to multiple ducts, depending on the individual findings.
8. Recurrence is not uncommon, often due to inappropriate or inadequate surgery. Management of recurrence requires a planned sequential approach to find and deal with the persisting pathology.
9. Granulomatous mastitis shows a close resemblance to peripheral perilobular mastitis, and at least some cases are best managed by surgery directed to proximal ectatic ducts.

The terms 'duct ectasia' and 'periductal mastitis' cover the second major group of benign breast disorders – the most important group after those of ANDI. 'Mammary duct ectasia' introduced by Haagensen in 1951[1] is a useful term in that it has a single simple connotation – the presence of dilated mammary ducts, using terminology consistent with that of bronchiectasis and sialectasis. To this has been added periductal mastitis to describe the frequent occurrence of periductal inflammation in association with duct ectasia. This term has advantages over others used such as plasma cell mastitis or comedo mastitis because these specific elements are not present in all cases. Hence the condition is best known as the duct ectasia/periductal mastitis complex even though this by no means covers all the pathological or clinical aspects of the disease.

Until recently, there has also been a lack of awareness of the condition and its less common manifestations among both surgeons and pathologists.[2] This is surprising, for a very comprehensive description of the condition was given by Bloodgood, with typical flamboyant style, in 1923[3] and a further description by Haagensen in 1951.[1] We will show later that understanding of disease has been held back by attempts to confine the clinical manifestations within the straight-jacket of a single all-embracing disease process or, alternatively, attempts to remove the straight-jacket completely and regard the condition as one aspect of 'fibrocystic disease'. Both approaches are incompatible with the breadth of clinical manifestations or the observed pathology.

While the exact aetiology is still uncertain, recent work has demonstrated that a number of pathological processes contribute to the clinical manifestations, including duct dilatation, stagnant secretions, duct obstruction by nipple inversion or epithelial squames, epithelial metaplasia, non-bacterial inflammation, bacterial inflammation and periductal sclerosis. These diverse processes, individual but interrelated, explain the protean clinical presentations. Evolution of thought and practice continues and quite recent demonstration of anaerobic bacteria in many cases is having a major impact on understanding and management, as is the recognition that infective complications are much more common and severe in cigarette smokers. This disease complex presents clinically in many ways, at times giving rise to all three common breast symptoms: lump, nipple discharge and pain. The main manifestations are set out in Table 11.1 and any concept of the disease complex must be able to encompass this wide range of clinical presentations.

There are a number of other chronic inflammatory conditions, such as lymphocytic mastopathy and granulomatous mastitis, which may be unrelated, but which also may overlap with PDM. These are further discussed in Chapter 17. In view of the confusion in nomenclature and understanding, it is useful and salutary to look at it from a historical point of view.

HISTORICAL SURVEY

This condition has been recognized and well described in the surgical literature over many decades, yet remained unrecognized in clinical practice to a surprising degree. It was recorded by many early writers but they were unable, on the whole, to conceive it as a distinct process, confusing it with tuberculosis, galactocele, cystic disease and fat necrosis. Even today, many endocrinological texts confuse the nipple discharge of duct ectasia with galactorrhoea.

John Birkett, surgeon to Guy's Hospital and President of the Royal College of Surgeons of England in 1877, gave a description of the condition in his book on breast disease[4]: 'In the breast of a middle-aged woman it is not uncommon to find the ducts dilated and filled with mucous greenish fluid.' Bloodgood described several cases in 1921[5] in a paper dealing primarily with chronic cystic disease. He returned to the subject in 1923, presenting 31 cases. His description of an advanced case could hardly be bettered[3]: 'The characteristic picture when the dilated ducts are situated in the nipple zone is the palpation of a doughy, worm-like mass beneath the nipple. When explored, one can recognize large and small dilated ducts with distinct wall, containing brown, green, milky or cream-like material, of various degrees of viscosity and consistency.' He went on to describe nipple discharge, palpable tumours, some with skin and nipple fixity resembling malignancy, others resembling subareolar abscesses and peripheral

Table 11.1 The clinical spectrum of duct ectasia/periductal mastitis	
Underlying pathology	**Clinical manifestations**
Duct ectasia	Nipple discharge – thick, creamy, bloody
Periductal mastitis	
Single duct	Recurrent subareolar abscess
	Mammary duct fistula
Multiple ducts	Inflammation and/or abscess formation
	– evanescent
	– recurrent
	– chronic
	Duct fistula
	Mastalgia
Periductal fibrosis	
Inflammatory	Nipple retraction
Involutional	Nipple retraction
Secondary to nipple discharge	Eczema of the nipple/areola
All the above manifestations may rarely occur in the male.	

breast masses. He even described a case of eczema of the areola apparently due to nipple discharge.

Bloodgood made no contribution to aetiology and stated that the condition could be classed as part of chronic cystic mastitis, an area of confusion which persists in some present-day literature. He noted that patients with dilated ducts were often postmenopausal and that the condition seemed to have no relation to parity or breastfeeding. He recognized that the condition could present as nipple discharge or a mass which could be evanescent, but that it could also simulate cancer exactly, that it often settled spontaneously and that it had a tendency to be bilateral.

According to Cutler,[6] it was James Ewing, of the Memorial Hospital in New York, who drew attention to 'plasma cell mastitis' in the 1920s. It is not surprising that a pathologist should so do, for radical mastectomy was not infrequently carried out mistakenly for a chronic inflammatory mass simulating cancer. He used this term because he was impressed with the number of plasma cells infiltrating these lesions. Cheatle and Cutler[7] recorded it in the literature survey in their book on breast tumours. Adair[8] reported 10 cases from the records of the Memorial Hospital, highlighting the clinical problem of inappropriate mastectomy. Further reports added the names comedo mastitis and mastitis obliterans. Each name stressed one particular aspect of the condition, but the different terminology did little to develop a unifying concept of the condition.

The subject was reviewed from the Mayo Clinic in 1948.[9] This paper gave a good review of the literature and reflected the usual attitude at that time: of 172 cases, the great majority had been identified from a retrospective study of pathology specimens usually found as a chance finding in mastectomy specimens for cancer. Only 19 of this series had undergone treatment for clinical manifestations of the condition. The consequences of failure to appreciate the pathology in the past is vividly illustrated in Sandison and Walker's paper from Glasgow.[2] Of 38 juxta-areolar inflammatory lesions studied, eight were incorrectly considered to be neoplastic and seven to be tuberculous, with nine inappropriate mastectomies. In this series, 12 had shown PDM without DE, 12 had shown DE with PDM, and 14 cases had shown ectopic squamous epithelium. These figures may reflect the relative frequency of the different pathologies underlying periareolar infection.

The increasing recognition of the clinical manifestations was not matched by understanding of pathogenesis, or even of pathology. Rodman and Ingleby[10] tried to produce it experimentally, claiming that a similar condition was produced by injection of pancreatized milk into the mammary duct of rabbits.

Three important papers appeared in 1951 which was a vintage year for this condition. Frantz and her colleagues[11] reported an autopsy study of apparently normal breasts, and found an incidence of substantial DE of 25% and almost 50% in women over the age of 60. It was clear that the condition of DE was common, a disease of ageing, and often subclinical.

Zuska et al.[12] described the condition now known as recurrent subareolar abscess or mammary duct fistula, recognizing its pathological basis for the first time, and reporting successful management by simple excision or laying open of the fistula. Earlier, Deaver and McFarland[13] had noted that persistent sinuses were sometimes seen after drainage of non-lactational abscesses, but they could only advise wide drainage, antiseptics and simple mastectomy for resistant cases. Even earlier cases of fistula have been reported in France and England in 1835 and 1892.[14,15] Zuska and his co-workers considered the condition to be a complication of DE ('comedo mastitis') because they saw dilated ducts containing the typical material seen in DE, which in its thicker form resembles a comedo. They also noted that it occurred in younger women, could be bilateral and was associated with squamous cell lining of the affected duct.

Haagensen[1] completed the 1951 trio by publishing his first paper on the subject, and suggested the term 'mammary duct ectasia'. His views are expanded in his textbook.[16] It is surprising that the youngest patient he had seen with the disease was 34 years old, and the mean age of the group was 55. He saw only 67 patients with clinical disease in 30 years' practice, reflecting either the specialized nature of his practice with a bias towards cancer, or suggesting that the disease is becoming more common, because we operated on some 200 cases in 15 years.

Haagensen supported the classic view that duct dilatation was the primary abnormality, leading to stagnation of secretion and nipple discharge, with leakage of material outside the duct leading to a chemical PDM. He regarded it as a rather benign condition and did not discuss severe abscesses, or recurrent inflammation or fistula after surgical excision. He also regarded recurrent subareolar abscess as a separate condition of trivial importance and criticized Zuska et al. for 'confusing it with duct ectasia'.

Atkins[17] drew the attention of British surgeons to recurrent subareolar abscess with a report of 28 cases. He introduced the unfortunate term 'mammillary fistula', suggesting a fistula into the nipple, which soon became corrupted to mammillary duct fistula. The term seems inappropriate because the external opening of the fistula is along the edge of the areola (or more peripheral) and the internal opening is into a duct under the areola rather than within the nipple. It is a term better dropped in favour of the simpler and more accurate term 'mammary duct fistula'. Atkins saw the condition in simple mechanistic terms as an obstruction to the exit of the duct, with build up of secretions leading to infection which burst out through the skin. Again he reported it in younger patients, often with inverted nipples, and sometimes beginning during pregnancy and lactation. He recommended a simple laying open technique, allowing the wound to heal by granulation. He noted no recurrence but gave no details of follow-up.

Three years later, Patey and Thackray[18] reported a detailed histological study of the ducts excised from seven specimens. They found the terminal portion of the involved duct lined by squamous epithelium instead of the normal columnar epithelium and believed this replacement to be congenital rather than acquired, partly because one case also showed multiple sebaceous glands opening into the track.

Hadfield[19] introduced the operation of major duct excision for a number of benign breast conditions, including DE. He paid tribute to having learned the operation from Adair and Urban at the Memorial Hospital of New York, and 3 years later Urban[20] reported his own technique and results, again giving precedence to Adair. The operation slowly became the standard management for all the syndromes of DE/PDM except localized mammary duct fistula.

Two papers from Sandison and Walker in Glasgow in 1962 and 1964[2,21] did much to increase the knowlege of chronic inflammatory conditions of the breast. They helped to fit PDM into an overall picture of breast disease and also suggested that recurrent subareolar abscess might have more than one aetiology. It is well worth while studying their papers in detail for their description of the disease complex. However, they do not appear to have used duct excision, preferring wide *en bloc* excision of diseased tissue. They infer that the results were satisfactory but give no details of follow-up.

Ewing[22] reviewed the syndrome and the relevant literature to move full circle away from Haagensen, suggesting that mammary duct fistula is not a separate entity, but just a manifestation of DE. Habif and his colleagues[23] came down strongly in favour of the other view, reporting 146 cases of mammary duct fistula without seeing a single case with dilated ducts. They were all associated with squamous metaplasia of the terminal duct, and it is clear that these authors fell into the classic error of expecting all manifestations to be based on a single pathological process.

Davies[24] carried out elegant studies of the role of inflammatory cells in the genesis of periductal disease and provided new insights into the frequency of subclinical periductal inflammation, and the possible role this might play in normal duct involution, as well as the clinical manifestations of this condition.

The last 20 years have seen two new developments with an impact on management: the recognition of the importance of cigarette smoking in inflammatory complications, and recognition of the importance of anaerobic bacteria (particularly those normally found in the mouth and vagina). Both of these are leading to the possibility of control by more conservative measures than have been necessary in the past.

Most of the advances in past years have come from detailed correlations of clinicopathological findings with outcome in individual cases, in studies that have emphasized the diversity of the clinical and pathological spectra of these conditions. More recent studies utilize computer analyses of large databases of retrospective case material, with a resulting simplification of concept and management which does not sit comfortably with clinical experience. It remains important to respect the diversity seen in clinical practice, so that individual patients are assessed and managed on an individual basis.

PATHOLOGY AND PATHOGENESIS OF DE/PDM

This condition exhibits a paradox. The pathology of the disease at a point in time – surgical biopsy or autopsy – is well established and well described, yet there is almost total ignorance of the sequence of events leading to or from that point in time. It is useful to summarize the position as understood at present and important to recognize that no single pathological process can explain, or should be asked to explain, the whole clinical spectrum. As with other benign breast disorders, it must be considered in relation to interaction of a number of aberrations of normal processes with added complications sometimes pushing it from the area of disorder to disease (see Chapter 3). There are a number of pathological processes that require consideration, all closely interrelated: DE with stagnation of secretion, and periductal inflammation which may be histological or clinically overt and in the latter case may be sterile or bacterial. Squamous metaplasia of the terminal duct epithelium may be an aetiological factor in some cases, and periductal fibrosis a common outcome.

Stagnation of duct contents, obstructive or passive, is the common factor in all cases, while the tough structure of the nipple/areolar complex obstructs the direct drainage which allows abscesses elsewhere in the body to cure themselves.

Ectatic ducts – pathology

The dilatation seen in ectatic ducts may be considerable, varying from just above normal diameter (about 0.5–1 mm) up to 5 mm or more. Typically three or four of the ducts are ectatic. It is unusual for more than a few of the ducts to be involved and it is not clear why only some are dilated. Similarly, dilatation is often confined to the 2–3 cm closest to the nipple, although it may extend further into the breast; occasionally the dilated ducts extend right to the periphery. Not surprisingly, the older the patient the greater the number of ducts affected, and the further ectatic ducts are likely to extend into the breast. Sometimes the wall of the dilated duct is thin and uninflamed; much more commonly the wall is thickened with fibrosis and disruption of the elastic lamina.

Although ectatic ducts may look like cysts on section, the ducts are more uniformly dilated than cystic. It is now realized that the two conditions are quite separate, though they frequently coexist. Cystic disease is a condition of lobules, DE of the ductal system.[25] The secretion in the ducts may be amorphous, representing cellular debris and fatty acid crystals, or cellular, packed with colostrum cells and inflammatory cells. These colostrum cells are thought by many to be macrophages and by others to be myoepithelial cells. Changes in the epithelial cells lining the ducts tend to be non-specific; sometimes they are hyperplastic in the early stages, later flattened and atrophic or shed completely. Our studies of the duct epithelial cell surface by scanning electron microscopy showed a normal microvillous surface in most cases.

Ectatic ducts – pathogenesis

A number of possible mechanisms for the development of ectatic ducts have been suggested.

Hormonal effect

Endocrine-induced relaxation of contractile, myoepithelial elements of the duct wall, similar to relaxation of the ureter in pregnancy, has been suggested to be implicated in the development of ectatic ducts, and in the past, pregnancy and breastfeeding have frequently been considered as important in the aetiology of DE. However, the evidence of this is poor and Dixon et al.[26] found no relation between parity or breastfeeding and DE.

Obstruction

A second theory incriminates duct obstruction by epithelial squames. Patey and Thackray[18] investigated seven cases of duct fistula and found the terminal portion of the duct to be blocked by squamous epithelium. They concluded that obstruction of the terminal duct due to desquamation of squamous cells was the cause and that the squamous lining was probably a congenital abnormality.

Other authors have not confirmed this finding, and cases are commonly seen where secretion can readily be expressed through the terminal duct with no obstruction to the passage of a probe, although this does not exclude stagnation due to desquamated cells. The common association of subareolar abscess with congenital inversion of the nipple in young girls suggests that the inversion contributes to stagnation. It is not clear whether this is due to mechanical blockage or a greater frequency of squamous metaplasia.

Tedeschi et al.[27] produced experimental evidence which combines obstruction and hormonal effects but suggested that hormonal effects were more important than obstruction in the pathogenesis. They found that ligation of the mammary ducts in rabbits produced no DE, whereas administration of hormones (oestrogen, progesterone or gonadotrophin) produced DE equally alone, or combined with duct ligation. No rabbits developed PDM.

Secondary to inflammation

A third theory is that dilatation results from destruction of the duct wall elastica and myoepithelial cells by inflammation. Two suggested causes of the inflammation are autoimmunity and bacterial infection. Davies induced an autoimmune model in mice[28] and he has also described widespread periductal inflammation with muscle disruption in the normal breast, although often associated with duct obliteration.[29] Whatever the exact pathogenesis at cellular level, this would appear to be part of the normal ageing or involutional process. More overt inflammation is discussed below.

Lymphatic blockage

Yet another theory incriminates failure of absorption of duct secretions due to inadequate lymphatic flow.

The bulk of evidence supports squamous metaplasia/ nipple inversion as the cause of mammary duct fistula in the young, while DE in older life seems to be an aberration of the processes of normal duct involution

Squamous metaplasia and nipple inversion

Squamous metaplasia requires more detailed consideration, especially in relation to mammary duct fistula. Normal squamous epithelium extends into a nipple duct no further than 2 mm from the surface with a sharp linear junction between squamous and columnar epithelium.[30] Patey and Thackray[18] describe this squamous epithelium extending down the duct in surgical specimens for a variable distance into the dilated portion of the duct; they found no significant squamous downgrowth in the fistula itself. Finding fully developed sebaceous glands in the area in two cases led them to come down on the side of congenital aetiology and their arguments are convincing for at least some cases. They found the affected duct lined by squamous epithelium throughout the whole length of the duct from the nipple to the point of junction with the fistula in five of seven cases, and the other two were lined by granulation tissue. The squamous epithelium even extended into some secondary branches of the affected duct. It is of interest that only one duct was involved. This might seem to argue against a congenital aetiology, but would explain the usual success of an operation directed towards a single duct.

Another paper which discusses the problem of squamous metaplasia is that of Habif et al.[23] and this paper is worth studying in detail for its pathological material. In contrast to Patey and Thackray, they show cases where more than one duct is lined by squamous epithelium. From their serial section studies, they dismissed the old view, still occasionally resurrected, that mammary duct fistula derives from infection of subareolar sebaceous cysts.[31]

Toker[30] argued that the metaplasia was an acquired condition (although from study of only one case) and likened it to the squamous replacement of columnar epithelium seen in the uterine cervix and other body areas.

Nipple inversion

A number of workers have noted that nipple inversion is commonly associated with both DE/PDM and mammary duct fistula. Likewise, PDM is often associated with, or followed by, the development of retracted nipple. Our experience leaves no doubt that both relationships exist. There is a high incidence of congenital nipple inversion in young girls with recurrent subareolar abscess and we have frequently documented the progressive retraction of a previously normal nipple during the evolution of severe PDM.

This association is confirmed from the observations of Schaffer et al.[32] who noted nipple retraction in 8% with a first abscess, 22% with recurrent abscesses, and 47% with a fistula. Some of this may be due to more severe cases occurring in patients with nipple inversion, but it also supports the progressive nature of nipple retraction in many cases.

Mammary duct fistula

This condition, described by Zuska et al.,[12] is seen in typical form when a young woman develops an abscess under the edge of the areola of one breast. Simple drainage of the abscess results in persisting discharge, or recurrent abscesses presenting at the same point. The condition has been likened to a perianal fistula with a sinus lined by granulation tissue leading down to a dilated sump-like duct (Figure 11.1).

It seems likely that the discrepancies are best explained by at least two separate pathologies: a congenital lining of squamous epithelium in the terminal duct and stagnation of duct contents due to DE. The first is commonest in young women, and is frequently accompanied by congenital nipple inversion. The pathology was well described by Patey and Thackray.[18] The second is seen in older patients, without nipple inversion. While some patients have a fistula always discharging from the same duct, others will have external openings communicating with different ducts. In this group, nipple retraction usually follows the inflammatory process. It is important that this dual pathology is recognized, because treatment of multiple duct disease by operation directed towards one duct will lead to recurrence, while failure to recognize the solitary congenital duct abnormality will lead to unnecessarily radical surgery.

Periductal inflammation – pathology

Histological PDM

Histological changes of periductal inflammation with periductal histiocytes and inflammatory cells are usually present with dilated ducts but may be seen whether the ducts are dilated or not. There is sometimes a granulomatous reaction, and often a lipophagic reaction with a picture similar

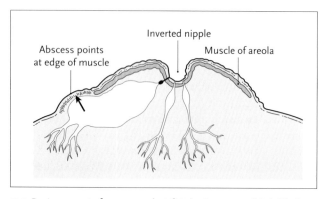

11.1 Basic concept of mammary duct fistula. Squamous debris blocks the duct leading to dilatation of the subareolar portion. Because of the tough muscle of the areola skin, an abscess will tend to burst through the skin at the edge of the areola.

to fat necrosis. Plasma cells may or may not be prominent among the infiltrate.

Davies[29] has stressed the relationship of cellular infiltration with focal ulceration, disruption of elastic tissue and subsequent fibrosis. In the presence of clinical PDM, these changes spread into the surrounding breast tissue to form an inflammatory mass.

Davies[24] has made a detailed study of periductal inflammation in both ectatic and non-ectatic ducts. In the latter group, the paradoxical aspect of this condition can be seen in the presence of narrow sclerosing ducts, which led to the old term 'mastitis obliterans' or 'mazoplasia obliterans'. He has demonstrated a striking periductal infiltration by four cell types, apparently of macrophage origin, which can lead to total obliteration of the duct. Their presence is associated with marked damage to the duct wall and epithelial lining. The lumen may be filled with the colostrum cells typical of DE, but the eventual outcome is fibrosis and obliteration of the ducts. The study shows a predominance of fibrous obliteration occurring in young women although the study was biased towards this group because it derived from biopsy material for benign breast disorders. It was present in a wide variety of benign breast conditions, including those with no clinical evidence of PDM.

It is not clear what relation this intense periductal inflammation and duct wall damage has to the ectatic form of duct disease, but both duct obliteration and duct dilatation could be seen to result in different areas of the same breast. This process probably explains the shortening of ducts leading to nipple retraction; it may be part of normal ductal involution or an aberration of that process. Hence, histological PDM can be seen as a normal process, which may contribute to DE, to duct obliteration or to duct shortening, and also as a possible precursor of clinical PDM.

The histological picture of PDM shows a further spectrum of changes from the 'normal' juxtaductal infiltration of macrophage-derived cells, through a more extensive spread of inflammation characterized by plasma cells or lymphocytes. The final stage is frank abscess formation when more acute inflammatory cells are obvious, often along with lipid-laden foreign body giant cells and granulomas. These latter changes were responsible for confusion with tuberculosis in earlier literature.

A histological grading system (grades 1–3) for severity of each of the two main pathological processes – dilated ducts and periductal inflammation – has been put forward,[26] although, confusingly, grade 1 is most severe for periductal inflammation but least severe for DE.

Clinical PDM

Abscesses from PDM are usually subareolar or juxta-areolar. They are typically single, small (1–2 cm), well localized and unilocular. (In contrast, puerperal abscesses are commonly large, poorly localized and multilocular.) In the rare case of peripheral abscess (usually multiple) associated with PDM, the ducts are macroscopically dilated to the site of the abscess. Abscesses may be sterile, or associated with a wide range of bacteria; the latter is more likely as the process increases in severity or recurrence.

In younger women PDM is often associated with congenital inverted nipple without evidence of gross DE; in the latter half of reproductive life, it is more likely to be associated with multiple ectatic ducts. These should be differentiated from the peripheral staphylococcal abscesses sometimes seen in postmenopausal women, without anaerobes. It is not clear whether these are associated with PDM or represent a random infection. The ducts are not grossly dilated, and the abscess can be expected to resolve with drainage and antibiotics, without duct surgery. This is discussed in Chapter 13.

Bacteriology

Until recently there has been remarkably little work done on the bacteriology of PDM and it is still a matter of some controversy. For many years it was believed that most cases were sterile early in the disease and that the inflammation was due to chemically irritant fatty acids leaking into the periductal tissue. The histological picture, similar to fat necrosis, supported this.

In recurrent cases a variety of bacteria have been found. Anaerobes, *Staphylococcus aureus*, *Proteus* sp. and streptococci have been reported. Many are undoubtedly secondary invaders. With the advent of techniques for reliable demonstration of anaerobic organisms, it became clear that these bacteria were sometimes present in earlier cases. Beigelman and Rantz[33] reported growth of *Bacteroides* sp. and anaerobic streptococci from a breast abscess as early as 1949.

More recently, several detailed studies of the microbiology have been reported.

Walker *et al.*[34] have carried out a prospective study in 29 patients aged 20–85 and report the detailed culture results. A total of 108 strains were recovered, anaerobes outnumbered aerobes by 2:1. Only two abscesses were sterile; both had had antibiotics. The commonest anaerobes were peptostreptococci (47%). These and the other anaerobes found are normally inhabitants of the vagina or oropharynx; gut anaerobes are rarely present. Many of their patients reported oro-nipple contact. Anaerobic cocci usually occur together with other anaerobes and facultative microorganisms in a mixed flora. The synergistic pathogenicity of anaerobic cocci in mixed infections is well documented. The commonest aerobe (60%) was *Staph. epidermidis*; *Staph. aureus* was found in only 8%. *Staph. epidermidis* adheres to the squames of the skin and nipple, so it is not surprising that it finds its way into these abscesses.

Interesting work has been conducted on enzyme production by peptostreptococci.[35] *Peptostreptococcus magnus* is an opportunist organism often found in abdominal infections (where it does not seem to cause serious problems), non-puerperal breast abscesses and diabetic foot infections.

P. magnus obtained from abdominal infections is relatively inactive enzymatically, whereas the strains grown fom non-puerperal abscess and foot infections are much more active, particularly in producing collagenase and gelatinase. This may explain the burrowing activity seen in these infections.

Leach and co-workers have reported anaerobic subareolar abscesses after vaginal manipulation,[36] suggesting bloodstream spread of bacteria to settle in the stagnant duct secretions. The same organisms found in an acute subareolar abscess have been cultured from a high vaginal swab, in this case bacteraemia from sexual activity and direct oral transfer of vaginal organisms to the nipple were possible modes of transmission.[37]

Bundred and colleagues[38] studied the bacteriology of spontaneous discharge from 51 patients and of pus from 17 patients with abscess or fistula. Bacteria were isolated from 62% of patients with discharge due to DE and only 5% from those with discharge due to other causes. (The separation of patients into 'duct ectasia' and 'other causes' was made rather arbitrarily on 'clinical and radiological' grounds.) All the patients with abscesses or fistulas grew bacteria. The bacteria included enterococci, anaerobic streptococci, *Bacteroides* sp. and *Staphylococcus aureus*.

There is clearly room for further investigation into whether all clinical PDM is bacterial since there are still some discrepancies.

The clinical, painful masses of evanescent PDM resolve without treatment and with surprising rapidity for a bacterial infection. This sequence would be far more compatible with a chemical reaction to leaking duct contents as suggested by Haagensen, as is the histological picture, which is so similar to fat necrosis.

Dixon has argued strongly that bacterial infection is primary in all cases, and DE secondary or unrelated, even though evidence from that unit is conflicting.[39] He bases his view on histological studies,[26] on the fact that they were able to grow pathogens from nipple discharge in 62% of patients with DE,[38] and on an increased incidence of wound infection in patients with DE/PDM (10%) compared with 2% with other breast conditions.

There seems to be a discrepancy between 10% wound infections and 62% growing pathogens. Furthermore, another worker in the same unit using the same bacteriological methods grew a pathogen (*Staph. aureus*) from retroareolar biopsy material from only one of 11 patients with overt and histological DE/PDM, and no biopsy grew the typical mixed aerobic and anaerobic organisms.[40] This latter study is much more in keeping with our own experience, in which careful examination with immediate bacteriological culture for aerobic and anaerobic organisms has failed to demonstrate bacteria in a significant proportion of our cases with overt inflammatory masses on initial presentation, and many such cases fail to respond to appropriate antibiotics. In contrast, we find it usual to grow bacteria in recurrent inflammatory lesions.

It is also important to distinguish between PDM diagnosed on histology, and the gross inflammatory complications seen clinically. Dixon reported 108 patients with a histological diagnosis of DE/PDM.[26] He found histological PDM to occur at a younger mean age than DE (although the difference in mean ages was small). From this he has argued that PDM is the primary cause of DE.[39] This study confirms the earlier work of Davies[24,29] that periductal inflammation is common in unselected breast biopsies, and the many earlier studies that have shown that DE is a common involutional occurrence. It is misleading to suggest that either finding is relevant to the severe inflammatory complications encountered in clinical practice.

Operative findings have been recorded prospectively in all cases in the author's series of primary and recurrent PDM. The patterns are quite clear, and fall into two main groups, although with some overlap. In young women, typically 20–30 years old, the pathology is restricted to a single sump-like duct, associated with congenital nipple inversion or squamous metaplasia. In older women, typically 40–50 years, there are obviously dilated ducts, usually three or four, sometimes many more. The degree of DE, and the recent onset of the active inflammation, leaves little doubt that the ectatic duct precedes the onset of inflammation.

Not all cases conform to these patterns; we have seen multiple grossly ectatic ducts at 26 years, and multiple typical ectatic ducts as young as 20. Conversely, some older women have a single ectatic duct, and are cured by fistulectomy directed to that single duct.

It is possible that subclinical periductal inflammation leads to ectatic ducts, but there is no direct evidence. It is more likely that it leads to duct sclerosis, the outcome clearly demonstrated by Davies. So there is no reason based on evidence to abandon the classical view that stagnation of secretion, for differing reasons in the young and old, is the primary cause of clinical PDM.

Current evidence is that in some cases, particularly early inflammatory masses or the first abscess, the inflammation is non-bacterial whereas the incidence of bacterial involvement rises with repeated abscesses and drainage. It is likely that stagnation, from any of the causes above, favours leakage of duct contents into periductal tissue to give chemical inflammation, and also provides a focus for bacterial colonization. Equally, there is no doubt that bacteria play a major role in more overt cases, even from the outset of clinical presentation, as discussed in detail later in this chapter.

PDM – pathogenesis
Is there a hormonal basis to PDM?
Unlike most breast conditions, hormonal abnormalities have not generally been associated with the DE complex, although DE itself is generally regarded as part of the perimenopausal involutional process. However, Peters has been a strong advocate of hyperprolactinaemia as an important aetiological factor in PDM.[41] His group measured serum prolactin levels in 108 patients before, during and after therapy for non-puerperal mastitis. One quarter of the patients exhibited transient rises in serum prolactin during the period of inflammation, which returned to normal levels, 22 presented with higher levels of hyperprolactinaemia, and 15 were found to have pituitary microadenomas; in 11 the inflammatory episode was the first symptom. In a second study from this unit, 83 patients known to be hyperprolactinaemic were questioned about symptoms of PDM; one in five reported such symptoms, compared with none of the controls.

Thus, established hyperprolactinaemia appears to be a cause of PDM, while this can be a cause of transient hyperprolactinaemia. However, the situation is clouded by the very wide symptom complex that these workers include within the scope of PDM. Shousa et al.[42] also reported three postmenopausal patients with prolactinomas who had an unusually florid degree of DE.

It is surprising that so little interest has been shown in these findings; it would seem to be an area requiring further investigation.

Cigarette smoking
A recent development of considerable interest is the recognition that cigarette smoking is related to the more serious inflammatory complications of DE. The association was first noted in Switzerland[32] when a case control study showed that 85% of patients with recurrent subareolar abscess were smokers compared to 37% of the controls, with relative risks of 9 for light smokers and 26 for heavy smokers. Only 10% had never smoked, most had smoked for many years, even a 15-year-old girl had smoked heavily for 3 years.

Bundred and co-workers have studied the clinical and pathological implications in greater detail.[43–45] Cigarette smoking is associated with the presence of histological evidence of PDM, development of non-puerperal breast abscess, recurrent abscess after treatment and development of mammary duct fistula. Heavy smokers are more likely to have anaerobic bacteria and severe inflammatory complications. Smokers also seem to have a greater chance of squamous metaplasia in the ducts.

Smoking was not associated with the degree of ductal dilatation, or with recurrence after lactational abscess. About 30% of patients with histological PDM are not current smokers, so smoking is more related to clinical complications than the underlying process.

Although histological changes of PDM were associated with smoking in patients with this diagnosis, the same changes were not associated with smoking in patients presenting with a duct papilloma,[46] so smoking is only one element of a multifactorial pathogenesis.

The mechanism by which smoking causes these changes is not clear at present. A number of possibilities may be relevant. Toxic products have been demonstrated in ductal secretions of smokers. These may damage the duct epithelium, facilitating extravasation of secretions.

Smoking also has an anti-oestrogenic effect, producing an early menopause, and inhibits Gram-positive bacteria *in vivo* and *in vitro*, which may facilitate overgrowth of anaerobic bacteria. The altered bacterial spectrum in the mouth of smokers may be relevant to the oro-nipple route of infection.

Of relevance to these theories is the fact that the relationship of smoking to severe inflammatory complications of PDM also holds for males. All five male patients with periareolar abscess or fistula seen in our clinic were heavy smokers.[47]

THE DEVELOPMENT OF THE DE/PDM COMPLEX

The classic view (Figure 11.2)

Each of the 15–20 ducts opening on to the nipple normally has a diameter only of 1 mm or less and the subsegmental and terminal ducts become progressively narrower.

In the sequence proposed by Haagensen[1] and developed by Ewing, (Table 11.2)[22] the first change to occur is DE, commonly restricted to the portion of the duct deep to the areola.

In a few cases dilatation extends peripherally to involve segmental and even subsegmental ducts. The dilated ducts fill with stagnant secretion, leading to nipple discharge. Persisting stagnation may lead to ulceration, resulting in blood-stained nipple discharge and in leakage of stagnant secretions into the periductal tissue; the irritant fatty acids then induce an inflammatory response, which is chemical rather than bacterial. This is usually seen beneath the edge of the areola, but where dilatation extends into the subsegmental ducts, PDM may occur more peripherally, or even form a granulomatous mass more peripheral to the obviously dilated ducts. In severe cases the inflammation progresses to abscess formation. Simple drainage is unlikely to be curative and gives an increasing likelihood of secondary bacterial infection.

Some cases may develop a chronic indurated mass stopping short of abscess formation and the clinical signs in this situation may simulate cancer exactly. The periductal inflammation leads to fibrosis and subsequent contracture leads to nipple retraction.

The current view

Any mechanisms of pathogenesis must be compatible with the findings (a) that within one breast some ducts are normal and some dilated; (b) that most workers have been able to demonstrate bacterial infection in only a proportion of cases; and (c) that obstruction must be due mainly to stagnation rather than mechanical obstruction, since most patients show no obvious duct obstruction on radiology or at surgery. In addition, the primary symptom according to the classic view, nipple discharge, is seen mainly in older women, while the supposedly secondary symptom, mastitis and abscess formation, is seen at all ages, often in quite young women.

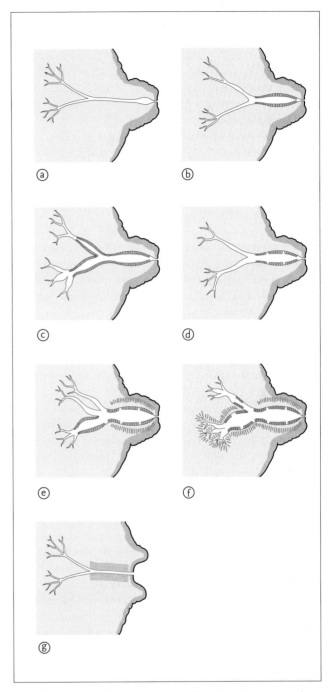

11.2 Classic view of the pathogenesis of the clinical spectrum of duct ectasia. (See text for more recent alternative theories.) (a) A normal segmental duct, uniformly narrow except for the terminal sinus, and breaking up into subsegmental and finally terminal ducts. (b) The proximal subareolar part of the duct dilates with stagnation of secretion. Intact mucosal epithelium is seen lining the dilated ducts. (c) The dilatation may extend into the subsegmental ducts. (d) The stagnant secretions lead to patchy mucosal ulceration which may give bloody discharge. (e) The contents of the duct leak through the ulcerated areas giving a chemical inflammatory response. (f) This may affect subsegmental ducts or even occur peripherally beyond the major duct system. (g) Inflammation leads to fibrosis of the duct wall, and as the fibrous tissue contracts nipple retraction is produced.

Table 11.2 The classic view of the pathology of duct ectasia/periductal mastitis

Process	Clinical manifestations
Duct ectasia (?A hormonal effect)	Stagnation of secretions
	Nipple discharge
Epithelial ulceration	Bloody nipple discharge
Leakage of secretion into periductal tissue	Evanescent painful mass
Granulomatous reaction + secondary bacterial infection	Abscess/fistula
Periductal fibrosis	Nipple retraction

The frequent occurrence of bilateral involvement must be taken into consideration in any discussion of pathogenesis, and the frequency with which the disease starts in the second breast shortly after control of that in the first breast is a striking observation.

No single mechanism which meets these requirements has yet been put forward. A clinicopathological picture consistent with evidence and experience is best based on a number of processes, which may occur individually or in combination with others, and with differing emphases in the young, the mature and the elderly. These are:

- Stagnation of secretion due to squamous metaplasia, either congenital or acquired, seen particularly in young women, and often associated with congenital nipple inversion.
- Stagnation due to dilatation of the ducts, probably due to a hormone effect or damage by periductal inflammation, possibly autoimmune, possibly an exaggeration of the normal involutional process.
- Histological periductal inflammation as is found in 1 in 5 'normal' breasts, and which leads to fibrous obliteration of ducts as well as DE. Together with simple DE, this can be considered as part of normal involution, so that nipple discharge and nipple retraction can be regarded as manifestations of ANDI.
- Exacerbation of periductal inflammation from leakage of duct contents, and further exacerbation from bacterial colonization.
- Colonization by bacteria probably from sexual contact, oro-nipple or intercourse-related bacteraemia.
- Fibrosis related to bacterial inflammation, or normal duct involution, which leads to secondary nipple retraction.
- Cigarette smoking, which plays an important role in facilitating bacterial invasion.

THE CLINICAL SPECTRUM OF DE/PDM (*SEE* TABLE 11.1)

Nipple discharge

Considering the pathology of DE, it is not surprising that it is sometimes associated with nipple discharge. The commonest complaint is a small amount of purulent discharge, which is confirmed by the patient expressing material from the nipple. Rarely it is so profuse as to cause severe social embarrassment (Figure 11.3).

The colour varies over the spectrum seen in the ducts at operation: off-white, creamy, brown, grey or green; sometimes it is as thick as toothpaste (Figure 11.4).

Blood-stained discharge is less common than these coloured discharges, although Dixon et al.[26] found positive occult blood in about half of their cases with nipple discharge. Certainly, in our experience a blood-stained discharge, even from a single duct, in the older age group (35 and over) is more commonly due to DE than to duct papilloma. Typically it comes from a number of ducts; it is then even more likely to be due to DE (Figure 11.5a,b).

Patients with nipple discharge and palpable ducts tend to be in the peri- or postmenopausal age group.

Breast masses associated with PDM (Table 11.3)

Palpable subareolar ducts were described by Bloodgood as very characteristic of this condition. He likened it to a varicocele. This degree of gross duct dilatation is rather uncommon in our experience.

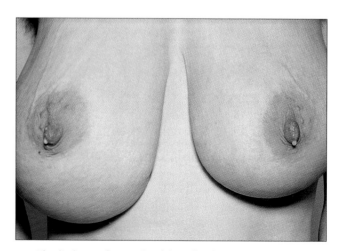

11.3 The discharge of DE is often bilateral and sometimes so severe as to be socially embarrassing.

Evanescent mass

This is a very common presentation of the disease. The patient notices a small, slightly tender mass in the subareolar region. By the time she is seen in a clinic 7–10 days later, the mass has often disappeared. Such rapid development and regression of a breast mass is uncommon in any other breast condition. These masses are typically 1–2 cm in diameter, firm, tender and not attached to surrounding tissues. The subareolar situation distinguishes evanescent PDM from the pain of leakage of fluid from a cyst which is usually a little more peripheral in the breast and is not associated with a small localized mass; in fact a palpable cyst may disappear with the onset of pain. Masses of PDM may progress to reddening of the overlying skin and still regress in a few days. As Haagensen[16] commented: 'The most remarkable thing about these episodes is the rapidity with which they develop, and, if left alone, the promptitude with which they subside.' This pattern of behaviour makes it very difficult to assess any form of medical treatment. The patients have often been given antibiotics and naturally attribute their improvement to the treatment.

Recurrent mass

While an evanescent mass may not recur, it has a tendency to do so at the same site at intervals of a few months to 10 years or more. The condition also has a tendency to become more severe with each recurrence. There is an appreciable incidence of bilateral involvement and it is not uncommon for the opposite breast to become involved shortly after successful control of one breast, although we have also seen an involvement of the contralateral breast as long as 10 years after the first one.

Persistent mass

If a mass persists for some weeks, it is usually firm and fairly well defined. Aspiration cytology is characteristic, showing foamy macrophages and inflammatory cells. Cancer cannot be excluded absolutely, but this cytological appearance (i.e. inflammatory cells without epithelial cells) is highly characteristic and justifies a short course of appropriate antibiotics. If the mass does not resolve rapidly, biopsy excision is desirable in women of cancer age group. Provided there is no overt abscess formation, a periareolar biopsy wound will heal

---

Table 11.3 Breast masses associated with duct ectasia/periductal mastitis

Palpable ducts
Subareolar or periductal mass
     evanescent
     recurrent
     persistent → subareolar abscess
     chronic   → simulating cancer
Peripheral mass
     peripheral abscess

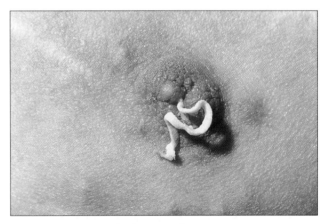

11.4 Thick grumous nipple discharge of DE.

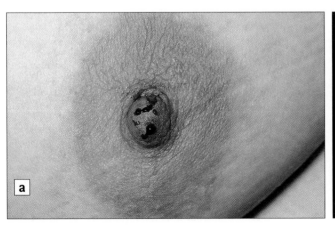

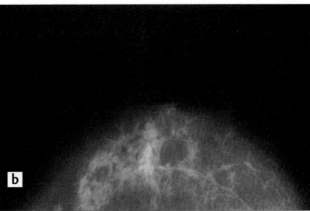

11.5 (a) Blood-stained nipple discharge from multiple ducts is usually due to DE. (b) Mammogram of postmenopausal patient with blood-stained discharge and segmental-shaped opacity. Histology of the excised segment showed DE only.

satisfactorily and there is no need to perform a formal duct excision. In fact, macroscopically dilated ducts are not particularly common in the presence of a simple PDM mass.

Some people have split off a condition which has been called granulomatous mastitis.[48] It is far from certain that this is not a variant of PDM, but it is discussed more fully in Chapter 17.

Chronic mass

This is the lesion that simulates cancer closely. It is a hard, oedematous mass fixed to the skin, with nipple retraction and sometimes with axillary node enlargement. In the past, many such cases were subjected to radical mastectomy because the lesion could show some resemblance to cancer even when cut across. It may also be impossible to distinguish the two on mammography, but aspiration cytology will allow a presumptive diagnosis to be made and a trial of antibiotics given before biopsy. In these cases, the typical large ducts with their pultaceous contents are more likely to be present. A formal duct excision procedure, together with excision of the mass, is usually indicated. This should be done under appropriate antibiotic cover. This lesion is seen less frequently than 30 years ago, probably because of the more widespread use of antibiotics effective against anaerobes.

Abscess

Any of these subareolar masses may proceed to abscess formation. The underlying mass becomes attached to the skin which first becomes reddened and then shows bluish discoloration. Nipple retraction will often develop if not already present, and nipple oedema may be marked. These abscesses are associated with discomfort which varies from mild to severe, but not usually as severe as with pyogenic abscess. Aspiration will yield creamy or dirty, watery pus and bacteriological culture may be sterile on the first occasion.

If not treated, the abscess will burst spontaneously with considerable relief, but a persistent sinus remains, or the abscess recurs sooner or later and usually at the same site. A typical disease sequence is shown in Figures 11.6–11.8.

Recurrent abscesses are more likely to grow bacteria – anaerobes or staphylococci.

While most sinuses are situated in the juxta-areolar region and are reasonably well localized, more severe abscesses may occur in association with DE, sometimes involving most of the breast (Figure 11.9).

Peripheral mass

While most masses arise in relation to major ducts near the areola, similar masses are occasionally seen in the periphery of the breast. Figure 11.10 shows a large tender mass in the mid, upper, right breast, which slowly increased in size over 2 months.

Mammography and cytology were both consistent with benign diagnosis, but the patient requested excision because of constant aching. Figure 11.11 shows the presence of multiple small abscesses and Figure 11.12 shows the typical histology of intense inflammatory infiltration around duct remnants.

The clinical pattern resembles that recorded with 'granulomatous mastitis'. It was cured by excision of the mass in continuity with duct excision, an approach we believe should be considered in cases of apparent granulomatous mastitis.

Figure 11.13 shows a 45-year-old woman who presented with recurrent abscesses involving a large area of the upper, outer quadrant of the right breast.

Each abscess was painful and discharged to leave a chronic sinus and to be followed by further abscesses. At operation the mammary ducts were grossly distended into the axillary tail and filled with thick, dark green material. The abscesses were sufficiently incapacitating for the patient to request a large segmental excision. A few further small abscesses later developed adjacent to the excision margin, but were not sufficiently incapacitating to warrant further

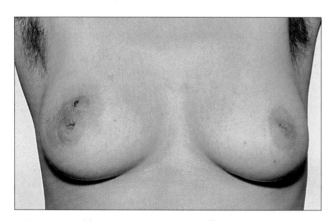

11.6 A 28-year-old woman presenting with a diffuse periareolar abscess which has burst spontaneously while she was taking antibiotics. Note the bilateral congenital nipple inversion. The patient was successfully treated by major duct excision because of the diffuse nature of the sepsis.

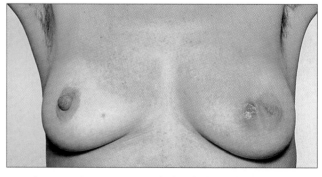

11.7 The patient (as in Figure 11.6) had no further problem with the right breast. Eight years later she presented with a similar condition of the left breast unresponsive to appropriate antibiotics. Treatment was by local drainage, followed by major duct excision 6 weeks later. (This was done in preference to fistulectomy at the patient's request, so that the inverted nipple could be corrected.)

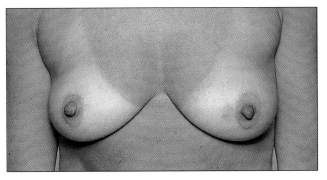

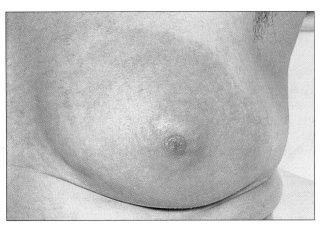

11.8 The result (patient in Figures 11.6 and 11.7) 2 years later. The small scar of conservative drainage is visible medial to the left nipple. She has had no further problems.

11.9 A diffuse breast abscess associated with DE. The patient had relatively little pain, despite the gross inflammation.

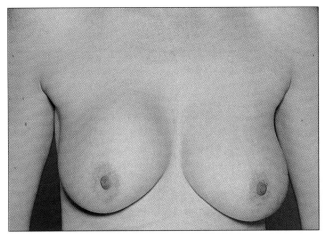

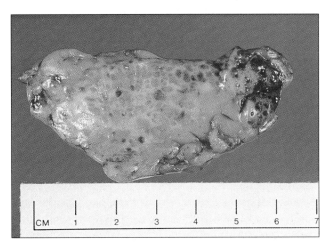

11.10 A 28-year-old woman with a peripheral mass in the upper aspect of the right breast, due to perilobular mastitis.

11.11 The cut specimen from Figure 11.10 showing multiple small abscesses, sterile on culture.

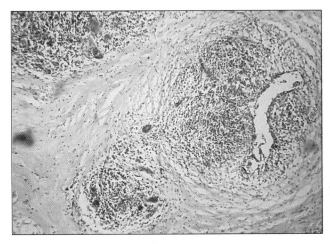

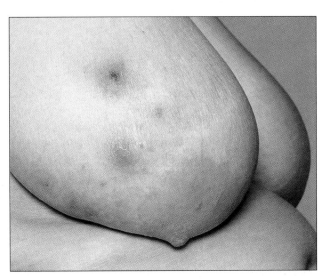

11.12 The histological picture of Figure 11.11 which shows intense focal inflammation.

11.13 Multiple peripheral sinuses following abscesses due to DE/PDM.

treatment. This clinical pattern may be confused with hidradenitis suppurativa.

Mammary duct fistula

The major papers describing this condition have been outlined in the historical survey. The typical features are classic. A young woman – of average age in the early thirties but sometimes as early as the teenage years – presents with a history of having several abscesses in one breast which had been treated by surgical drainage or have discharged spontaneously. The appearance is so typical that a spot diagnosis can usually be made (Figure 11.14).

The features are partial inversion of the nipple and a sinus or scar at the edge of the areola. In cases recurrent on many occasions, the areola is distorted, scarring having reduced the distance between the nipple and the edge of the areola in the radius of the fistula.

A majority of patients developing the condition have nipple inversion, for example 19 of 28 in Atkins' series[17] and 23 of 40 in the series by Bundred et al.[49] However, neither states the number of these in which inversion was congenital. In our experience many of the patients have always had inverted nipples, but the history is sometimes vague in patients developing abscesses in their thirties, with inversion of long standing. About one in five of patients first develop an abscess in association with pregnancy or lactation.

Bundred et al.,[49] in a retrospective case note study, reported 13 of 40 patients developing a fistula after breast biopsy, by implication in the absence of an abscess. This is an unusual finding and, in our experience, biopsy of non-suppurative PDM usually heals uneventfully.

Nipple retraction

There is a complex relationship between nipple inversion or retraction and the syndrome of DE/PDM. It occurs in about one-third of patients requiring surgery for DE/PDM but it is difficult to estimate its incidence in patients with asymptomatic DE. There are at least three aspects of this complex relationship:

- There can be little doubt that congenital inversion of the nipple predisposes to the development of subareolar abscess and fistula (see Figure 11.6 and Table 11.3), and that this is a very significant factor in the pathogenesis of the condition in teenagers and young women.
- There is frequently a close temporal relationship between overt PDM and the development of nipple retraction. The nipple inversion is characteristically transverse and of minor extent in the early stages (Figure 11.15), but subsequently progresses to more complete retraction over a period of 1 or 2 years. It not infrequently commences following a pregnancy. The initial changes may precede, coincide with, or follow the development of overt PDM.
- Nipple retraction is frequently seen as an isolated event, without other evidence of DE. These cases are usually

around or beyond the menopause. The retraction is circular (Figure 11.16) and progresses over 1 or 2 years often followed by the same process in the other breast. It seems likely that this type of retraction is due to the obliterative changes described by Davies[29] where microscopic periductal inflammation leads to disruption and periductal fibrosis without clinical ectasia or inflammation – probably more a normal involutional process than a disease.

We have previously described the clinical features of nipple retraction in this condition.[50] Thirty patients were seen in a 3.5-year period and an incidence of one case of nipple retraction due to DE per 100 new patients seen in the breast clinic was noted. The age range of the patients was 25–75 years with a mean of 52 years. The duration of retraction ranged from 3 months to 16 years. The incidence of parity and breastfeeding did not differ from that of other conditions presenting to the breast clinic. Retraction was partial in 12 cases, complete in 18. The left nipple was affected in 14, the right in 11 and was bilateral in 5. Early transverse retraction is easily withdrawn but the eversion becomes more difficult as retraction becomes more complete with the passage of time. However, eversion is still sometimes possible in advanced cases of long duration. The second nipple may show similar changes which may lag months or years behind the first in the development of retraction.

Some clinical features help in the differentiation from carcinoma. Retraction is more likely to be complete in carcinoma and to be accompanied by distortion of the areola when the breast is examined in different positions, while central and symmetrical retraction favour a diagnosis of DE. Eversion of the nipple by pressure behind the areola is more likely to be possible in DE. Pain is of little help in differential diagnosis because two-thirds of patients with nipple retraction due to DE have no pain. The presence of nipple discharge of the type typical of DE favours this diagnosis, as does a long history of a year or more, particularly when no mass is palpable.

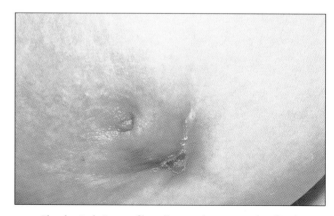

11.14 The classical picture of late diagnosed mammary duct fistula.

Bilateral retraction favours DE. However, it must be stressed that no feature is absolutely diagnostic and cancer must always be excluded with care.

Mammography will usually exclude cancer in the fatty radiolucent postmenopausal breast, but this may not be so easily achieved in the dense breast of the young patient. Typical radiological features of DE (see below) may be present.

Mastalgia

We believe that a considerable proportion of cases of non-cyclical mastalgia are associated with DE and PDM, although it is difficult to prove this except in acute episodes. It would not be surprising if the intense periductal inflammation and subsequent fibrotic process, described by Davies, was a cause of chronic pain.

The evidence associated with the two conditions is derived largely from an association of radiological signs of DE with pain.[51] Sometimes serial mammograms have shown the subsequent development of typical calcification of this disease at the site of pain.

Eczema

Bloodgood[3] described a case of eczema of the areola which was ascribed to nipple discharge. Azzopardi[25] mentioned similar cases. We have also seen this phenomenon (Figure 11.17), in a 35-year-old woman who was adamant that the eczema always followed nipple discharge.

After some hesitation, duct excision was performed and the typical changes of DE were demonstrated. The condition promptly developed on the other side, but again responded to duct excision. Several years later the patient complained of recurrent discharge and recurrent eczema in the right breast. The operation was repeated with a further period of relief. (The question of the reconnection of divided ducts is discussed later.)

While there seems to be good evidence from these cases for an association between eczema and nipple discharge, it is very difficult to exclude a factitial element. However, on balance,

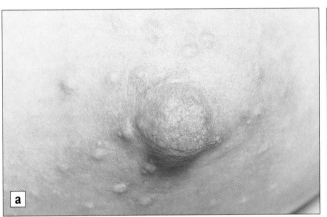
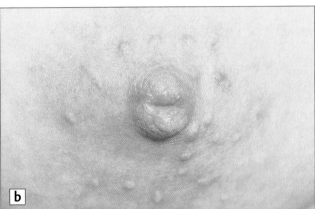

11.15 The classical transverse central retraction of early nipple involvement in DE(b). The right (a) nipple developed retraction 2 years later.

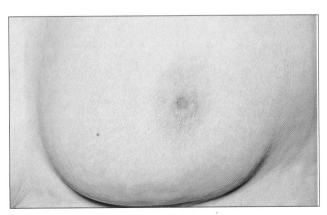

11.16 Well-advanced nipple retraction due to periductal fibrosis in a postmenopausal woman.

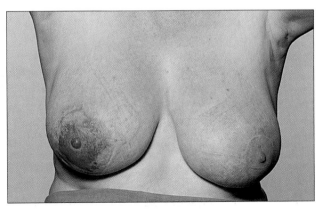

11.17 Severe, recurrent eczema of the areola and surrounding breast which the patient claimed always followed nipple discharge. Note the scar of a major duct excision on the left breast.

we accept the likelihood that some areolar eczema may be due to sensitization of the skin to some element in nipple discharge.

Neonatal DE

The hypertrophy of breast tissue seen in neonates results from the transplacental passage of maternal hormone and both males and females respond in the same way. The degree of secretory change may be sufficient to induce considerable DE. The changes regress spontaneously in most cases but have been described as a cause of bloody nipple discharge.[52]

DE in the male

The male breast may occasionally show much of the clinical spectrum of DE/PDM, including nipple discharge, nipple retraction, recurrent subareolar abscess and bilateral involvement.[53] As in women, inflammatory complications are usually associated with heavy cigarette smoking.[47] Tedeschi and McCarthy[54] reported a patient presenting with a tender lump which showed a typical histological picture of PDM. Habif et al.[23] also reported two cases. The condition is further discussed in the section on the male breast (see Chapter 16).

FREQUENCY OF DE/PDM

Simple duct ectasia is very common. Sandison[55] found 'gross DE with much dilated and thickened ducts containing grumous, yellowish green material, ramifying through the fibrofatty parenchyma of the organ' in 11% of women at autopsy, with the greatest incidence in the elderly. Clearly the great majority of these had never experienced clinical disease in relation to these ducts. One group[56] encountered 40 cases requiring surgery over a 10-year period, during which time 732 breast operations of all types were performed. The frequency of presenting features in their series and three other series are given in Table 11.4.

Dixon et al.[26] found the mean age of presentation for pain, lump and nipple discharge to be similar at about 40 years, while nipple retraction was seen at a mean age of 53 years. However, in all these series, it is difficult to assess the figures given because it is not possible to differentiate between congenital and acquired nipple retraction, and mammary duct fistula is not considered.

Non-puerperal breast abscess associated with DE is becoming more common, and now exceeds the incidence of puerperal abscess,[57] perhaps associated with the increase in cigarette smoking among young women.

The disease probably occurs in all races, although literature from developing countries is scant. It occurs with approximately equal frequency in whites, blacks and hispanics.[58]

RADIOLOGY

The changes on mammography have been described by a number of authors.[60,61] Nipple retraction will be obvious and prominent ducts will be shown as a conical opacity with the apex of the cone towards the nipple. The individual ducts may be seen leading into this opacity but it is not possible to distinguish radiologically between DE, intraductal hyperplasia and periductal collagenosis.[62] In a few cases of gross dilatation, the fatty contents may be sufficiently radiolucent to outline the ducts and confirm their ectatic nature (Figure 11.18).

DE is frequently associated with characteristic coarse calcification. This may be ring-like – the calcification lying on the duct wall – or circular or needle shaped, when the duct contents are calcified (Figure 11.19).

The ultrasound appearances have also been described.[63]

Plasma cell mastitis gives moderately dense opacities, usually in the subareolar region and often flame shaped. Overlying skin and nipple oedema or retraction are sometimes seen (Figure 11.20).

MANAGEMENT

Although there is a very large literature on this subject, many record results of retrospective case-note studies, provide no details of operative technique or long-term follow-up, and hence tend to confuse or to be misleading rather than helpful.

Table 11.4 Presenting features of mammary duct ectasia/periductal mastitis

	Cromar & Dockerty[59]	Haagensen[16]	Walker & Sandison[21]	Thomas et al.[56]
No. of patients	24	67	34	78
Mean age	40	50	–	45
Nipple discharge	21	24	47	44
Nipple inversion	42	30	8	32
Mass	100	30	8	32
Sepsis	–	–	9	9

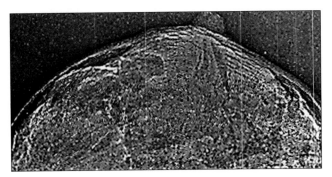

11.18 Mammogram showing negative shadows due to ducts filled with radiolucent lipoid material seen just below the nipple.

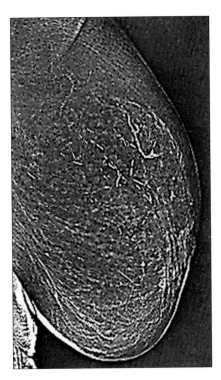

11.19 Mammogram showing the typical coarse calcification of DE, some round, some elongated and orientated in the direction of the duct. Note the retracted nipple.

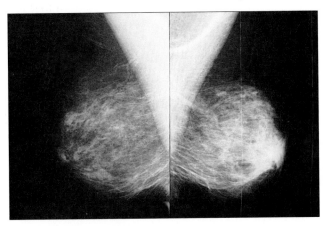

11.20 Mammogram showing the typical features of plasma cell mastitis with an associated flame-shaped subareolar opacity and oedema of skin and Cooper's ligaments (left breast).

Medical management

There can be little hope for efficacious medical management until more is known about the causes of DE and PDM, in both sterile and suppurative forms. Because simple DE with nipple discharge causes trivial symptoms, and other cases are asymptomatic, no active treatment is necessary in many cases. In the more troublesome patients with gross infective lesions, medical management is unlikely to give long-term control, while dilated ducts act as a sump with stagnant secretions forming a nidus for persisting bacterial colonization. It is difficult to assess reports of medical therapy because of the evanescent nature of early PDM and also because diagnosis is imprecise in the absence of biopsy material. These factors militate against meaningful controlled trials.

Nipple discharge

Galactorrhoea is usually readily distinguished from the nipple discharge in DE by the volume and consistency of the fluid, but, where any doubts exists, serum prolactin measurement should be performed to exclude a prolactinoma. We have not seen benefit from bromocriptine therapy in patients with profuse discharge due to DE and this drug is often poorly tolerated by patients with a normal serum prolactin.

The late Dr JP Minton of Columbus, Ohio, reported that nipple discharge may be associated with excess caffeine ingestion. He reported that exclusion of caffeine and other xanthines from the diet may result in resolution of the nipple discharge due to DE, although it took 6–9 months for an effect to be seen (personal communication). We have no experience of this approach to management.

Painful PDM

Peters and his co-workers[64] have recently reported rapid resolution of non-puerperal mastitis after prescribing bromocriptine at a dose of 7.5 mg per day for 3 days, reducing to 5 mg per day for 11 days. The group was a mixed one but included some patients with typical PDM. Symptoms relapsed on stopping treatment but responded again to a 6-month maintenance course of bromocriptine 2.5 mg daily. There is no obvious rationale for this treatment and the results take no account of spontaneous remission, related to the evanescent nature of many early attacks of PDM. We have not had such satisfactory results but further results of this approach will be watched with interest.

Antibiotics

Many patients with painful breast lumps have already been started on antibiotics before attending a breast clinic and will report that symptoms have improved. By the time the patient is seen, it is impossible to determine whether this was spontaneous resolution or the result of antibiotic therapy. However, if the work quoted earlier[35] reflects the bacteriology of mild PDM, the antibiotics generally used in general practice, such as ampicillin and erythromycin, would not be effective. This suggests that any benefit of such antibiotic therapy may be due to spontaneous resolution. Because anaerobic bacteria and staphylococci are the commonest organisms, metronidazole and flucloxacillin would be the appropriate combination with the addition of a broad-spectrum antibiotic such as erythromycin if these two are not effective. Augmentin is another option. The result of this therapy has been variable in our experience and we are not aware of any reported controlled trial.

A controlled trial would be difficult to organize because of the diagnostic uncertainty in presuppurative cases. It is likely from general principles that the efficacy of antibiotic therapy is dependent on the underlying pathology. Early bacterial PDM could be expected to respond while non-bacterial mastitis would not benefit. Advanced cases with grossly dilated ducts might be expected to be resistant because bacteria in the thick duct secretions would not be reached by the antibiotics. This variable response due to diverse pathology would be consistent with our results. In practice, we would recommend the following approach.

Mildly painful and tender masses behind the areola should be observed initially with the likelihood that they would resolve spontaneously. More painful masses should be explored with a 21-gauge needle and any fluid aspirate submitted to cytology and culture with meticulous use of transport medium appropriate to the detection of anaerobic organisms. In the absence of pus, patients are started on a combination of metronidazole and flucloxAcillin while awaiting the results of culture. Antibiotics are continued on the basis of sensitivity tests and many of these mild cases respond satisfactorily, especially in the short term. Where there is more than a minimum amount of pus, it is best to proceed to conservative surgical drainage with continuing antibiotic cover. Once a large amount of pus has formed, repeated aspiration is unlikely to lead to resolution (although some recommend it) but results in destruction of breast tissue and skin with a less satisfactory cosmetic result in the long term. Antibiotic therapy is particularly useful in recurrent inflammation after

formal duct excision and a prolonged course – at least 2 weeks and repeated once if necessary – should always be tried before resorting to further surgery.

Surgery

A striking feature of reports of surgical treatment of the DE/PDM complex is the variation in the frequency with which operations are performed and the varying indications given for surgery and for individual operations. Thus Cox et al.[65] reviewed 753 consecutive new outpatient referrals to a breast clinic. No operation was performed specifically for this condition, and only one case of mammary duct fistula and one case of DE were diagnosed, although no fewer than 332 patients in this group had some form of surgical operation. In contrast, another recent series[56] reports 78 major duct excisions in a series of 732 breast operations, 40 being for DE. Urban[20] was able to report 160 major duct excisions in 150 patients, while Hadfield[19] reported 139 similar operations.

We operated on 200 cases over 15 years, giving an average operation rate of 15 cases per 1000 new referrals to the breast clinic. However, this figure is undoubtedly higher because of the tertiary referrals to our unit, but conversely we find it necessary to operate on only a proportion of clinically significant cases. Indications for surgery in 148 cases of major duct excision in our unit are shown in Table 11.5.

Recently some workers have reported that surgery can be avoided in most cases by antibiotic therapy. Our own experience does not support this view in the longer term and suggests that the more enthusiastic reports of successful antibiotic therapy reflect cases of mild severity followed for a short time.

Surgeons reporting large series of total duct excision have tended to use this operation very freely, many being performed for simple non-bloody discharge or for an otherwise straightforward lump which lies behind the areola. Hadfield[19] and Thomas et al.[56] both used total duct excision as the procedure of choice for recurrent subareolar sepsis in preference to the operation of fistulotomy or fistulectomy favoured by other surgeons.

Table 11.5 Indications for operation in the 148 patients undergoing major duct excision					
Indication	Total	Right	Left	Bilateral (simultaneous)	Bilateral (sequential)
Nipple discharge	83	29	41	11	2
Discharge plus inflammation	9	3	3	0	3
Discharge plus mass	2	1	1	0	0
Subareolar inflammation	32	10	16	4	2
Mass	15	6	9	0	0
Other	7	4	3	0	0
Total	148	53	73	15	7

With such a diversity of thought and practice, it is not possible to give a consensus from the literature. Hence we give our own views derived from an experience of some 200 operations for DE and its complications, performed over 15 years and from a considerable experience of tertiary referrals of problem cases following earlier surgery.

Indications for surgery

Surgery may be required in the following clinical situations:

- Nipple discharge – coloured, opalescent, bloody, serous.
- Correction of nipple inversion.
- Diagnosis of a retroareolar mass.
- Subareolar abscess.
- Fistula.
- Eczema.
- Recurrence after previous surgery.

Non-bloody nipple discharge

This condition, typically from several ducts and sometimes bilateral, is a benign condition with no increased cancer risk. It is not normally an indication for surgical treatment. We do not believe that investigation or treatment is necessary except in those rare cases where discharge is so profuse as to require constant wearing of a pad and to cause significant social embarrassment. In this situation, we would exclude a prolactinoma, and then offer the patient the operation of total duct excision, bilateral if necessary.

Blood-related discharge

The management of this symptom is dealt with more fully in Chapter 12. Over the age of 40 years there is a significant risk of cancer or hyperplastic lesions and the operation of total duct excision has some advantages over more conservative procedures. It provides a good histological specimen and relieves the anxiety of the symptom. Where the cause proves to be one which is potentially multifocal, such as DE or a hyperplastic epithelial lesion, it pre-empts further discharge from other ducts.

Correction of nipple inversion

Patients are more likely to request correction of congenital nipple inversion than retraction due to DE occurring later in life, but some patients request correction of retraction for this condition. Although the results are usually satisfactory, patients seeking correction for cosmetic reasons should be aware of the possibility of nipple necrosis, of interference with sensation, of the inability to breastfeed and the possibility that postoperative fibrosis will lead to late reinversion.

Because the condition is due to shortening of the ducts, it can only be corrected permanently by a complete division of the subareolar ducts.

We usually do not encourage operative correction on cosmetic grounds alone, but when patients have had the procedure carried out for complications of PDM, the resulting correction of nipple inversion has been a much appreciated side-effect. Such patients may then press for operative correction of a contralateral inverted nipple. Accumulation of debris in an inverted nipple can be malodorous; this provides another indication for correction.

Diagnosis of a retroareolar mass

The tender acute retroareolar mass of PDM frequently resolves spontaneously, so surgery should be delayed if aspiration biopsy is suggestive of this diagnosis. Where a mass persists for several weeks, we would treat it by simple excision biopsy, even if dilated ducts filled with pultaceous material are encountered. Primary healing is the rule; only in the presence of an overt abscess is postoperative sepsis likely. If such an abscess is encountered at operation, we would either undertake simple drainage with a view to formal surgery should the problem recur, or proceed immediately to formal total duct excision under appropriate antibiotic cover. We tend to the first course in young women and to the latter in women past the child-bearing period.

Subareolar abscess

The diagnosis is confirmed by needle aspiration, which also provides a specimen for cytology and bacterial culture. In our experience, aspiration under antibiotic cover rarely leads to a satisfactory long-term result with an established abscess, which is best treated by conservative open drainage. Drainage is conservative because, unlike puerperal abscess, the infection is usually unilocular and often associated with a single duct system, and it is desirable to confine the process to a single segment. More radical drainage may spread the infection or damage adjacent normal ducts.

A majority of patients with anaerobic bacteria will develop recurrent infection and/or a fistula, so in most cases it is advisable to proceed to a definitive procedure (fistulotomy or duct excision) when the infection has settled after 6–8 weeks. The resulting wound can be managed satisfactorily by open healing by secondary intention, or by primary closure under antibiotic cover,[66] depending on the acuteness and extent of inflammation.

If the patient prefers a more conservative approach, aspiration under antibiotic cover is a reasonable alternative, and has been advocated by Dixon.[67] Aspiration is facilitated by ultrasound guidance. Repeated aspirations are often necessary, and in his series, 40% of cases with anaerobic bacteria had recurred after a short follow-up period. Scholefield *et al.*, reporting a 10-year follow-up, found that 90% of patients with anaerobes suffered recurrent infection.[57] It is not yet clear if cessation of cigarette smoking will lessen the risk of recurrence.

Recurrent abscess with fistula

This situation provides a difficult problem of surgical judgement, the decision whether a fistula with recurrent sepsis should be treated by fistulotomy or by major duct excision. Some of the factors bearing on this decision are set out in Table 11.6.

When a small localized periareolar abscess recurs at the same point, and a fistula is clearly present, the operation of choice is fistulotomy (or fistulectomy – see Chapter 20). It is a simple procedure with minimal complications and a high degree of success. Should it fail (in spite of being carried out correctly), total duct excision can still be used. Some authors are still advocating formal duct excision in all cases,[68] rather than the selective approach which allows many patients a simple effective procedure with minimal disruption to the breast.

Where subareolar sepsis is diffuse rather than localized to one segment or where more than one fistula opening is present, total duct excision is the procedure of choice. The former situation is likely to be seen in young women with squamous metaplasia of a single duct, the latter in an older woman with multiple ectatic ducts. However, age is not a reliable guide and we would recommend fistula excision as the initial procedure for localized lesions irrespective of age. One exception is where there is marked nipple inversion and the patient wishes to have this corrected. This tips the balance towards total duct excision, particularly if the patient does not wish to breastfeed in the future. Figures 11.6, 11.7 and 11.8 show a case where duct excision was considered appropriate in a young patient.

Eczema

Where there is good evidence that eczema of the areola follows nipple discharge, total duct excision is the only procedure likely to give relief. However, other forms of eczema and factitial injury should be considered carefully before resorting to surgery, since DE is a rare cause of areolar eczema.

THE CONSEQUENCES AND RESULTS OF OPERATIONS FOR DE

Patients should be aware of the consequences of these operations before undergoing surgery, particularly where this is recommended for conditions other than sepsis, because a patient is unlikely to be satisfied if a less than optimal result is obtained. With severe or recurrent sepsis, the morbidity of the disease is such that most patients happily accept the results of surgery which relieves them of their episodes.

Consequences

Cosmesis

In general, the cosmetic effect is excellent when performed for nipple discharge, but less satisfactory when done for sepsis, especially for long-standing sepsis. In the first group the nipple is not distorted and a typical result is shown in Figure 11.21.

Satisfactory results may also be obtained when operating for sepsis, provided the operation is done before gross scarring has occurred and if the cosmetic result is considered when performing operations (see Figure 11.8). Once skin destruction is allowed to occur and multiple abscesses have been drained, severe distortion of the nipple has occurred and cannot be readily corrected. The situation is even worse when recurrent sepsis occurs more peripherally in the breast after duct excision and this is discussed below in relation to operations for recurrent disease.

Although failure to lactate after the operation suggests that glandular atrophy must occur with time, there is no change in size of the breast after the operation.

Sensation

Tactile sensation is usually lost in part over the half of the nipple raised as a flap (Figure 11.22).

Multiple incisions around different segments are likely to increase the sensory loss, so should be avoided if possible. It is possible to perform the operation through small incisions, with less effect on sensation, but these carry a risk of leaving residual ducts unless performed meticulously.

Lactation

Patients cannot breastfeed after this operation and there are few reports of the consequences of pregnancy following duct excision. Urban[20] reported that four of his 150 patients

Table 11.6 Treatment of recurrent subareolar sepsis	
Suitable for fistulectomy	**Suitable for total duct excision**
Abscess small and localized to one segment	Abscess large, affecting >50% of areolar circumference
Recurrence always at the same site	Recurrence involving a different segment
Probe passes easily from fistula through nipple at interval operation	Probe may be 'lost' in cavity
Mild congenital nipple inversion or no inversion	Gross nipple inversion
Patient unconcerned about nipple inversion	Patient requests correction of nipple inversion
Younger patient	Older patient
No discharge from other ducts	Purulent discharge from other ducts between episodes
	Recurrence after fistulectomy

became pregnant after the operation. Minimal engorgement occurred following delivery but this rapidly subsided when lactation was suppressed with hormones. Hadfield[69] recommended patients to defer pregnancy for a year after the operation. He reports an unspecified number of pregnancies after the operation. Lactation occurred normally on the unoperated side, but no discharge from the operated breast. When pregnancy occurred within a year of operation, there were varying degrees of enlargement from activity in the operated breast which subsided quickly after delivery.

We also advise our patients to avoid pregnancy for 1 year after operation and have seen no problem under these circumstances. One of our patients had proximal duct excision for sepsis of the left breast, and the same procedure of the right breast 2 years later. She became pregnant 2 months after the second procedure. She had no problem with the left breast, but

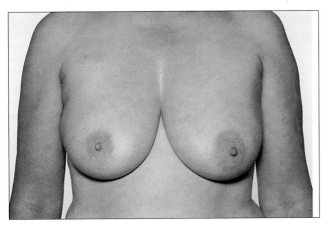

11.21 A typical long-term postoperative result of (right-sided) major duct excision of nipple discharge. Operation for sepsis often leaves a less satisfactory result.

the right became engorged, and the infection flared up. This was controlled temporarily by antibiotics and drainage, but left two fistulas requiring reoperation after suppression of lactation. The typical chronic abscess was found under the nipple.

Restoration of duct continuity

Duct discharge sometimes recurs after the operation and it must be assumed that occasionally the ducts reconnect to an aperture in the nipple. Indeed one of our patients claimed to breastfeed successfully for 9 months after this operation, but the breast at this time was involutional to palpation compared to the normal breast and we saw no milk from the operated nipple. Collection of debris in an inverted nipple can lead a patient to believe discharge has recurred.

Behaviour of residual ducts

There is a surprising lack of information about what happens to the remainder of the breast ducts after subareolar duct excision. Haagensen[16] makes no comment nor do the writers of any of the other series. In our experience, the small number of patients coming to further operation have shown that the ducts remain dilated and filled with the same material seen at the primary operation. Since most cases of reoperation have been for recurrent sepsis, this group may behave differently to the majority of patients without further trouble, but the same dilated ducts have also been encountered occasionally where reoperation has been performed for causes other than infection.

The fact that dilated ducts can remain in this state for years following major duct excision throws doubt on the suggestion that bacteria can be cultured from most cases of PDM. In contrast to the persistence of dilated collecting ducts, the minimal response of the breast to pregnancy after long-standing division of the ducts suggests that back pressure may lead to atrophy of the secretory acinar elements of the duct system.

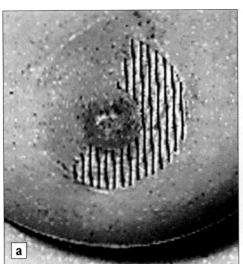
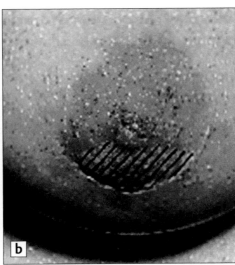

11.22 Patient following bilateral major duct excision for severe recurrent sepsis multiple on the right side. The stippled area outlines the loss of sensation.

Cancer risk

The long-standing presence of secretions stagnant in ducts completely obstructed by major duct excision would seem to provide a background for carcinogenesis. However, Haagensen[16] and Urban[20] both state that there have been no excess cases of cancer in their patients having duct excision, many of whom were followed for a long time. Our experience would support this although it must be admitted that there are inadequate data based on documented long-term follow-up to provide a definitive answer to the question.

The results of operations for DE

Major duct excision

Early authors reported excellent results from operations for DE and PDM, which are somewhat surprising, especially because many such operations were performed before the importance of anaerobic organisms and appropriate antibiotic therapy was realized. Urban[20] concludes his study of 167 major duct excisions by stating that the operation 'results in satisfactory cosmetic appearance. There have been no recurrence of symptoms and no complications in our hands'. Hadfield[69] reported equally satisfactory results. All patients were left with a normal looking breast and nipple, there was no instance of recurrent disease on the operation side, and no case of cancer developing during follow-up of 1–7 years.

More recent series have not been so encouraging. Thomas et al.[56] reported good results when the operation was performed for nipple retraction, nipple discharge and subareolar mass, although nine of their patients continued to have nipple discharge for up to 1 year after the operation. One patient required reoperation to correct nipple reinversion. However, they had 100% recurrent infection following major duct excision for abscess, and two of their patients eventually had a mastectomy.

Hartley et al.[70] also report a considerable postoperative complication rate after careful surgery (by a single operator) for all indications. This was despite operating only when sepsis was quiescent and using antibiotic cover routinely. Wound drainage was avoided in all cases.

Donegan[71] found that results deteriorate with time: 45% of 26 patients had recurrent sepsis at 1 year, 60% by 7 years. He believes that recurrence is due to downgrowth of epithelium of the nipple into the cavity, and advocates the radical approach of excision of the nipple with secondary reconstruction. In his hands this is always associated with long-term cure. While agreeing with the thesis that residual ductal epithelium facilitates recurrence, we feel that the operation of core excision of the nipple (Chapter 20) almost always achieves the same result without cosmetic deformity and avoids the need for reconstruction.

The sole dissenting recent author is Dixon,[72] who obtains excellent results with minimal recurrence. It is not clear why his results differ, or whether they will hold up in the longer term.

In our unit 122 patients have had formal examination and follow-up at 1–10 years after major duct excision. Thirty-four patients (28%) had suffered a problem affecting the breast subjected to major duct excision (Table 11.7).

Nineteen of the patients have required further surgery to the breast related to the original operation, eight drainage of an abscess, five required further duct excision, four laying open of the fistula, four biopsies and two mastectomies. Hence it is also our experience that most recurrent problems are related to surgery for subareolar sepsis.

This high problem rate falls with increasing operator experience and is also now lower because of better use of appropriate antibiotic therapy. The interval between operation and development of further problems varies from a few weeks to several years. Recent papers also report improving results, probably reflecting the recognition for the need to remove completely the affected duct(s). Passaro et al.[58] reported satisfactory results in 47 of 48 patients, although some had needed up to three operations, and some follow-up was short. They used a radial incision through areolar and nipple to ensure complete removal of the terminal ducts, reinforcing the prime importance of this element of the operation.

Fistulotomy/fistulectomy

Atkins[17] had no recurrence following his operation of fistulotomy with saucerization, although length of follow-up was not detailed. Lambert et al.[73] reported 48 fistulas: 13 were laid open, 25 were excised and allowed to granulate, 8 were excised with primary closure. One recurrence occurred 6 weeks after a primary closure. They made no attempt to correct inversion of the nipple. Like many series reporting good results, follow-up is relatively short at a mean of 25 months and the operations were performed in a specialist breast centre. Bundred et al.[66] reported results in 36 women with mammary duct fistula, 12 of whom had fistulectomy with two recurrences. Our experience of tertiary referral cases suggests that the results from less specialized centres are far from uniformly satisfactory, and surgical experience has a marked influence on the outcome.

Complications of operations

The complications of fistulectomy are slow healing and recurrent abscess and fistulas. Both are commonly due to inadequate technique.

Table 11.7 Breast problems following major duct excision	
Mastalgia	9
Infection	9
Discharge	7
Lump	6
Haematoma	3
Recurrent eczema	1
? Raynaud's disease of the nipple	1

The complications of major duct excision are haematoma, infection, flap necrosis, nipple inversion, cosmetic deformity, pain and recurrence of the original condition.

The commonest problem calling for further surgery is recurrent infection; less common is persisting nipple discharge or reinversion of the nipple.

RECURRENT INFECTION AFTER SURGERY FOR PDM

Aetiology of recurrent sepsis after duct surgery

Recurrent sepsis tends to be more common after major duct excision than after simple fistulotomy, but this probably reflects the fact that the fistulotomy operation is more appropriate to less severe degrees of sepsis, and those which are confined to a single duct. Nevertheless, the underlying cause of recurrent sepsis is basically the same for both operations. The common denominator is a chronic abscess lined by granulation tissue, under the nipple, but a number of disparate factors may contribute to the persistence of this chronic abscess (Table 11.8).

The commonest cause of persisting problems following surgery is incorrect or inappropriate surgery. Intractable disease, in spite of adequate surgery, is less common. The first approach to a patient with recurrent problems is careful inspection for evidence of inadequate surgery. If this is found, revisional surgery is usually the best approach. Where surgery appears to have been satisfactory, a trial of prolonged antibiotic therapy for recurrent sepsis is preferable to early operation. The causes of recurrence of symptoms in patients referred to us are shown in Table 11.8.

Persistent abscess cavity

Any chronic abscess with a thick rigid wall must be eradicated either by opening the cavity so widely that it granulates from its base, or by excising any rigid cavity wall back to pliant tissues so that the cavity obliterates. It may be associated with persistent proximal duct.

Persistent proximal duct

When infection recurs after laying open of a fistula, it is not uncommon to find that the incision extends only half way on to the areola; a recurrent abscess will then discharge through the proximal end of the incisional scar. Operation in such a case is likely to show a persistent segment of terminal duct which may be only 7 or 8 mm in length (Figure 11.23).

The essential feature of the fistulotomy operation is to pass a probe through the fistula and out of the opening of the duct on to the nipple, and then use a small racket-shaped incision to ensure that the whole of the terminal portion of the duct is removed. Attempts to perform this procedure by subareolar dissection of the tract invite recurrence (and make assessment more difficult), while the ultimate cosmetic appearance is more related to eradication of the infection than a transareolar incision.

The same mistake can occur with a major duct excision. It is easy to leave terminal elements of duct attached to the undersurface of the nipple after transecting the duct cone and this has been the cause of several recurrent cases in our experience (Figure 11.24).

As well as forming an entry site for bacteria, it provides a focus for epithelial downgrowth into the cavity. It can be prevented by inverting the nipple with a finger tip and removing the terminal portion of all the ducts with scissors (Chapter 20), or more certainly by central core excision of the nipple.

Residual ducts

It is also common for inexperienced operators to miss some of the breast ducts, especially those furthest from the incision, when performing major duct excision (Figure 11.25).

This must be assumed to be the case when nipple discharge persists immediately following surgery. Details of technique to avoid this are given in Chapter 20.

If the symptoms merit further treatment, operation to remove the residual ducts may be indicated. We have found

> **Table 11.8 Causes of recurrent disease following fistulectomy and major duct excision for duct ectasia/periductal mastitis.**
>
> Persisting abscess cavity
> Persistent proximal ducts
> Persistent distal ducts
> Persisting or recurrent nipple inversion
> Early pregnancy
> Contralateral disease
> Factitial disease

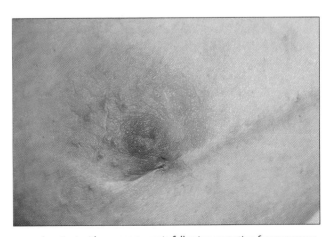

11.23 A patient with recurrent sepsis following operation for mammary duct fistula. Note that the incision does not reach the centre of the nipple. The causative pathology has not been eliminated.

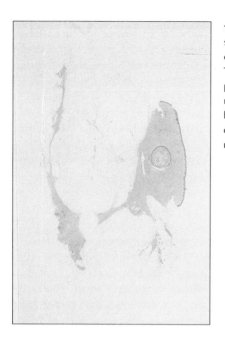

11.24 Histological section after excision of a persisting fistula. The patient had previously undergone major duct excision but a terminal portion of duct had been left under the nipple.

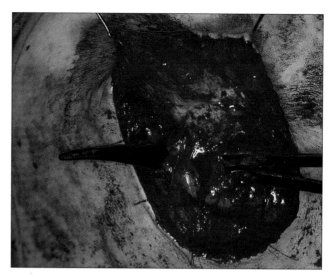

11.25 At operation for persisting nipple discharge after major duct excision; some ducts have been left at the far end of the dissection.

this necessary occasionally both for eczema of the nipple related to nipple discharge and for recurrent infection.

Residual peripheral ducts

The surprising aspect of operations on the major ducts for DE is that the residual distal ducts give so little trouble. Haagensen[1] noted this as early as 1951 and it has proved to be general experience. Even when dilated ducts are cut across and drain into the wound, late trouble from the residual breast is uncommon. Nevertheless, most authors report recurrent disease in a proportion of cases, some being sufficiently severe to lead to mastectomy. We have seen a number of similar cases. An example, and the way it was managed, is shown in Figures 11.26–11.29.

Intensive antibiotic therapy should be the first approach in such cases, but will not control all. It is of interest that some of these inflammatory attacks occurring after duct excision settle without treatment even when quite severe, resolving in 3 or 4 days in exactly the same manner as can be seen in the initial evanescent attacks of PDM. Once again this seems to be incompatible with heavy bacterial colonization of the residual ducts and suggests a 'chemical' inflammatory response to irritant materials.

Where inflammation persists and pus can be aspirated, and antibiotics have not given control, a further wedge excision is the appropriate treatment because inflammatory changes in the residual breast tend to be segmental in outline. At the same time as this wedge excision is carried out under antibiotic cover, the subareolar area should be explored to exclude persisting ducts or a hidden abscess cavity.

We have performed only two mastectomies for DE . With further experience, we now believe that local incisions under antibiotic cover will control most cases if the proximal duct excision had been correctly performed and core nipple resection may avoid mastectomy. However, there are some patients whose disease is sufficiently intractable and peripheral to warrant mastectomy. The complications are not inconsiderable because of scarring of previous operations, and any reconstructive procedure is better delayed to allow all sepsis to settle.

Persisting nipple inversion

The inverted nipple, so often associated with periareolar sepsis, becomes normally everted after total duct excision, and this is a bonus of the operation which is greatly appreciated by the patient. However, in longstanding cases with much sepsis the nipple remains fixed in the inverted position even after the terminal ducts have been excised.

Persisting nipple inversion leads to collection of grumous material in the inverted cavity which discharges periodically and leads the patient to believe that she has recurrent duct discharge. The material is sometimes offensive. Collection of material in an inverted nipple undoubtedly predisposes in some cases to further subareolar sepsis, particularly staphylococcal. Presumably organisms ingress through the old duct openings in the nipple.

For this reason, and for reasons of cosmesis, we believe that complete nipple eversion should always be ensured as part of the operation of major duct excision. If inversion, or a tendency to inversion, persists after excision of all the terminal ducts on the undersurface of the nipple, a purse-string suture is inadequate to give correction. It is necessary to excise the central dense fibrotic core of the nipple, only 5–6 mm in diameter, leaving normal supple nipple (external skin) which everts easily and shows no tendency to reinvert.

The defect in the apex of the nipple is closed loosely with a couple of fine absorbable sutures.

One of the disadvantages of the simple fistulotomy operation of Atkins is that marked nipple inversion is not corrected. This fact may tip the balance of choosing major duct excision in favour of simple fistulotomy, especially in the older woman who is not concerned with future breastfeeding.

Once nipple inversion is corrected by total duct division, it usually remains everted but a few cases will reinvert after some time, presumably due to formation of scar tissue and subsequent fibrous contraction. It does not occur after core excision of the nipple.

Contralateral disease

It is an unfortunate feature of PDM that it is frequently bilateral. It is not easy to determine the true frequency, since few series give long-term follow-up, and the incidence of bilateral disease increases with time, sometimes occurring as long as 10 years after operation on the first side. Our best estimate is that about 20% of patients will eventually develop bilateral disease. It will be interesting to see if patients can be persuaded to give up cigarette smoking with a beneficial effect.

Results of treatment are often better on the second side because the patient recognizes what is happening, and presents earlier to a surgeon who is familiar with the condition. It is our practice to treat the abscess on the second side by early drainage under antibiotic cover, proceeding to definitive operation after about 6 weeks when infection is quiescent, again under antibiotic cover. This allows primary wound closure with a good cosmetic result.

Factitial disease

The problem of self-inflicted disease is discussed in Chapter 17. This question must always be considered when recurrent sepsis becomes a problem after operation for DE. The

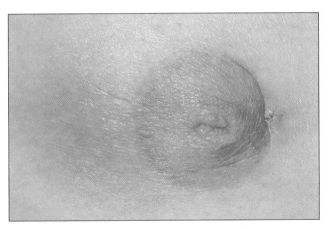

11.26 A patient with recurrent sepsis following major duct excision. Note the nipple inversion has not been corrected.

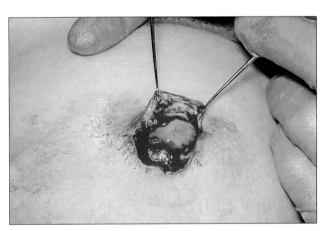

11.27 At reoperation there is a chronic abscess under the nipple with sepsis extending out into the breast. Several ducts had been missed at the original operation.

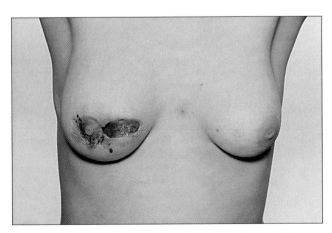

11.28 This was treated by re-excision of the ducts and segmental excision in continuity.

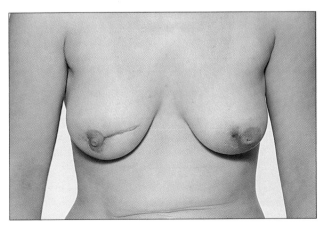

11.29 The patient one year later. The right breast has healed satisfactorily but the patient has developed the same condition in the left breast, reflecting the frequent bilateral incidence of this condition.

presence of bowel organisms, such as *Escherichia coli*, *Streptococcus faecalis* and colonic *Bacteroides* sp. (as opposed to the oral or vaginal organisms commonly found) should raise the possibility of a factitial basis. Persistent bleeding from the nipple after major duct excision, particularly if no epithelial lesion was demonstrated, is also suggestive of this condition. Ill-advised mastectomy is likely to be followed shortly by bleeding or other problems with the other nipple so the whole process is repeated.

The patients often seem rather odd, but as is the case with other chronic painful conditions, their psyche may take a turn for the better if the condition is corrected. Most of the cases we have seen where factitial disease has been suspected have been shown to have had inadequate surgery and have healed uneventfully after reoperation. In one case it has been necessary to resort to excision of nipple and areola with secondary reconstruction, with a satisfactory result.

Management of recurrent sepsis

Because of the role of mixed bacterial infection in persistent cases, the first approach to recurrent sepsis following surgery should be to give a 2-week course of antibiotics. A combination of flucloxacillin or erythromycin and metronidazole usually provides a satisfactory spectrum to cover these organisms.

Occasionally long-term control will be obtained but more commonly one of the causes set out above will underlie the recurrence and require correction. Our approach is summarized in Table 11.9.

Mastectomy should be considered only as a last resort, and reconstruction delayed for some months if prosthetic material is to be used.

Table 11.9 Management sequence for sepsis after surgery for periductal mastis

Antibiotics – two weeks
Assessment and surgical exploration, core nipple resection in appropriate cases.
Antibiotics – six weeks
Consider artefactual disease
More radical exploration, core excision of nipple, or mastectomy

REFERENCES

1. Haagensen CD. Mammary duct ectasia – A disease that may simulate cancer. *Cancer* 1951; **4**: 749–761.
2. Sandison AT & Walker JC. Inflammatory mastitis, mammary duct ectasia and mammillary fistula. *British Journal of Surgery* 1962; **50**: 57–64.
3. Bloodgood JC. The clinical picture of dilated ducts beneath the nipple frequently to be palpated as a doughy, worm-like mass ñ the varicocele tumour of the breast. *Surgery, Gynecology and Obstetrics* 1923; **36**: 486–495.
4. Birkett J. *The Diseases of the Breast and their Treatment*. London: Longman, 1850.
5. Bloodgood JC. The pathology of chronic cystic mastitis of the female breast with special consideration of the blue-domed cyst. *Archives of Surgery* 1921; **3**: 445–452.
6. Cutler M. Benign lesions of the female breast simulating cancer. *Journal of the American Medical Association* 1933; **101**: 1277–1282.
7. Cheatle GL & Cutler M. *Tumors of the Breast*. Philadelphia: Lippincott, 1931.
8. Adair FE. Plasma cell mastitis, a lesion simulating mammary carcinoma. *Archives of Surgery* 1933; **26**: 735–749.
9. Tice GI, Dockerty MB & Harrington SW. Comedomastitis. A clinical and pathological study of Data in 17 cases. *Surgery, Gynecology and Obstetrics* 1948; **87**: 525–540.
10. Rodman JG & Ingleby H. Plasma cell mastitis. *Annals of Surgery* 1939; **109**: 921–930.
11. Frantz VK, Pickren JW, Melcher GM & Auchinloss H. Incidence of chronic cystic disease in so-called normal breasts. *Cancer* 1951; **4**: 762–783.
12. Zuska JJ, Crile G Jr & Ayres WW. Fistulas of lactiferous ducts. *American Journal of Surgery* 1951; **81**: 312–17.
13. Deaver JB & McFarland J. *The Breast: Its Anomalies, its Diseases and their Treatment*. Philadelphia: Blakiston, 1917.
14. Bonnet. Memoire sur les fistules des conduits du lait. *Archives Gènèrales de Mèdècine* Paris 25 1835; **IX**: 451–464
15. Waters JJ. Mammary sinus subsequent to abscess; treatment by a listerian method; cure. *British Medical Journal* 1892; **ii**: 209.
16. Haagensen CD. *Disease of the Breast*, 3rd edn. Philadelphia: WB Saunders, 1986.
17. Atkins HJB. Mammillary fistula. *British Medical Journal* 1955; **2**: 1473–1474.
18. Patey DH & Thackray AC. Pathology and treatment of mammary duct fistula. *Lancet* 1958; **ii**: 871–873.
19. Hadfield GJ. Excision of the major duct system for benign disease of the breast. *British Journal of Surgery* 1960; **47**: 472–477.
20. Urban JA. Excision of the major duct system of the breast. *Cancer* 1963; **16**: 516–520.
21. Walker JC & Sandison AT. Mammary duct ectasia. *British Journal of Surgery* 1964; **51**: 350–355.
22. Ewing M. Stagnation in the main ducts of the breast. *Journal of the Royal College of Surgeons of Edinburgh* 1963; **8**: 134–142.
23. Habif DV, Perzin KH, Lipton R & Lattes R. Subareolar abscess associated with squamous metaplasia of lactiferous ducts. *American Journal of Surgery* 1970; **119**: 523–526.
24. Davies JD. *Periductal mastitis*. MD thesis, University of London, 1971.
25. Azzopardi JC. *Problems in Breast Pathology*. London: WB Saunders, 1979.
26. Dixon JM, Anderson TJ, Lumbsdon AB et al. Mammary duct ectasia. *British Journal of Surgery* 1983; **70**: 601–603.
27. Tedeschi LG, Ouzouman G & Byrne JJ. The role of ductal obstruction and hormonal stimulation in main duct ectasia. *Surgery, Gynecology & Obstetrics* 1962; **114**: 741–744.

28. Davies JD. Histological study of mammae in oestrogenized rats after izoimmunization. *British Journal of Experimental Pathology* 1972; 53: 406–414.

29. Davies JD. Inflammatory damage to ducts in mammary dysplasia: a cause of duct obliteration. *Journal of Pathology* 1975; 117: 47–54.

30. Toker C. Lactiferous duct fistula. *Journal of Pathology and Bacteriology* 1962; 84: 143–146.

31. Maier WP, Berger A & Derrick BM. Periareolar abscess in the non-lactating breast. *American Journal of Surgery* 1982; 144: 359–361.

32. Schaffer P, Furrer G & Mermillod B. An association of cigarette smoking with recurrent subareolar breast abscesses. *International Journal of Epidemiology* 1988; 17: 810–813.

33. Beigelman PM & Rantz LA. Clinical significance of bacteroides. *Archives of Internal Medicine* 1949; 84: 605–631.

34. Walker AP, Edmiston CE Jr, Krepel CJ & Condon RE. A prospective study of the microflora of non-puerperal breast abscess. *Archives of Surgery* 1988; 123: 908–911.

35. Krepel CJ, Gohr CM, Walker AP et al. Enzymatically active Peptostreptococcus magnus: Association with site of infection. *Journal of Clinical Microbiology* 1992; 30: 2330–2334.

36. Leach RD, Eykyn SJ & Phillips I. Vaginal manipulation and anaerobic breast abscesses. *British Medical Journal* 1981; 282: 610–611.

37. Bennett KW, Wistanley TG, Taylor AKM & Shorthouse AJ. Anaerobic curved rods in breast abscess and vagina. *Lancet* 1989; 1: 564.

38. Bundred NJ, Dixon JM, Lumsden AB et al. Are the lesions of mammary duct ectasia sterile? *British Journal of Surgery* 1985; 72: 844–845.

39. Dixon JM. Periductal mastitis/duct ectasia. *World Journal of Surgery* 1989; 13: 715–720.

40. Aitken RJ, Hood J, Going JJ et al. Bacteriology of mammary duct ectasia. *British Journal of Surgery* 1988; 75: 1040–1041.

41. Peters F & Schuth W. Hyperprolactinaemia and nonpuerperal mastitis (duct ectasia). *Journal of the American Medical Association* 1989; 261: 1618–1620.

42. Shousa S, Backhouse CM, Dawson PM & Alaghband-Zadeh J. Mammary duct ectasia and pituitary adenomas. *American Journal of Surgical Pathology* 1988; 12: 130–133.

43. Bundred NJ, Dover MS, Coley S & Morrison JM. Breast abscesses and cigarette smoking. *British Journal of Surgery* 1992; 79: 58–59.

44. Bundred NJ, Dover MS, Aluwihari N, Faragher EB & Morrison JM. Smoking and periductal mastitis. *British Medical Journal* 1993; 307: 772–773.

45. Bundred NJ. The aetiology of periductal mastitis. *The Breast* 1993; 2: 1–2.

46. Furlong AJ, Al-Nakib L, Knox WF, Parry A & Bundred NJ. Periductal inflammation and cigarette smoke. *Journal of the American College of Surgeons* 1994; 179: 417–420.

47. Thomas JA, Williamson MR & Webster DJT. The relationship of cigarette smoking to breast disease ñ the Cardiff experience. In: Mansel RE (ed.) *Recent Developments in the Study of Benign Breast Disease*, pp 221–226. Carnforth: Parthenon, 1994.

48. Kessler E & Wolloch Y. Granulomatous mastitis: a lesion clinically simulating cancer. *American Journal of Clinical Pathology* 1972; 58: 642–646.

49. Bundred NJ, Dixon JM, Chetty U & Forrest APM. Mammillary fistula. *British Journal of Surgery* 1987; 74: 466–468.

50. Rees BI, Gravelle IH & Hughes LE. Nipple retraction in duct ectasia. *British Journal of Surgery* 1977; 64: 577–580.

51. Preece PE. *A study of the aetiology, clinical patterns and treatment of mastalgia.* MD thesis, University of Wales, 1982.

52. Stringel G. Infantile mammary duct ectasia – a cause of bloody nipple discharge. *Journal of Pediatric Surgery* 1986; 21: 671–676.

53. Mansel RE & Morgan WP. Duct ectasia in the male. *British Journal of Surgery* 1979; 66: 660–662.

54. Tedeschi LG & McCarthy PE. Involutional mammary duct ectasia and periductal mastitis in the male. *Human Pathology* 1974; 5: 232–236.

55. Sandison AT. *A postmortem study of the adult breast.* MD thesis, University of St Andrews, 1957.

56. Thomas WG, Williamson RCN, Davies JD & Webb AJ. The clinical syndrome of mammary duct ectasia. *British Journal of Surgery* 1982; 69: 423–425.

57. Scholefield JM, Duncan JL & Rogers K. Review of hospital experience of breast abscess. *British Journal of Surgery* 1987; 74: 469–470.

58. Passaro ME, Broughan TA, Sebek BA & Esselstyn CB Jr. Lactiferous fistula. *Journal of the American College of Surgeons* 1994; 178: 29–32.

59. Cromar CDL & Dockerty MB. Plasma cell mastitis. *Proceedings of the Staff Meeting of the Mayo Clinic* 1941; 16: 775–782.

60. Evans KT & Gravelle IH. *Mammography, Thermography and Ultrasonography in Breast Disease.* London: Butterworths, 1973.

61. Sweeney DJ & Wylie EJ. Mammographic appearances of duct ectasia that mimic breast carcinoma in a screening programme. *Australasian Radiology* 1995; 39: 18–23.

62. Mansel RE, Gravelle IH & Hughes LE. The interpretation of mammographic ductal enlargement in cancerous breasts. *British Journal of Surgery* 1979; 66: 701–702.

63. Matricardi L & Lovati R. Ultrasonic appearance of a case of mammary duct ectasia. *Journal of Clinical Ultrasound* 1991; 19: 568–570.

64. Peters F, Hilgarth M & Breckноldt M. The use of bromocriptine in the management of non puerperal mastitis. *Archives of Gynecology* 1982; 233: 23–29.

65. Cox PJ, Li MKW & Ellis H. Spectrum of breast disease in outpatient surgical practice. *Journal of the Royal Society of Medicine* 1982; 75: 857–859.

66. Bundred NJ, Webster DJT & Mansel RE. Management of mamillary fistula. *Journal of the Royal College of Surgeons of Edinburgh* 1991; 36: 381–383.

67. Dixon JM. Outpatient treatment of non-lactational breast abscesses. *British Journal of Surgery* 1992; 79: 56–57.

68. Khoda J, Lantsberg L, Yegev Y & Sebbag G. Management of periareolar abscess and mamillary fistula. *S Gynecol Obstet.* 1992; 175: 306–308.

69. Hadfield GJ. Further experience of the operation for excision in the major duct system of the breast. *British Journal of Surgery* 1968; 55: 530–535.

70. Hartley MN, Stewart J & Benson EA. Subareolar dissection for duct ectasia and periareolar sepsis. *British Journal of Surgery* 1991; 78: 1187–1188.

71. Donegan WL. In: Donegan WL & Spratt JS (eds) *Cancer of the Breast*, 4th edn, p 98. Philadelphia: WB Saunders, 1995.

72. Dixon JM & Thomson AM. Effective surgical excision for mammary duct fistula. *British Journal of Surgery* 1991; 39: 1185–1186.

73. Lambert ME, Betts CD & Sellwood RA. Mammillary fistula. *British Journal of Surgery* 1986; 73: 367–368.

Chapter 12

Nipple discharge

CONTENTS

KEY POINTS AND NEW DEVELOPMENTS

1. The visual assessment of the discharge is still of prime importance because it correlates with clinical significance.
2. Of the three groups: milk (galactorrhoea), coloured opalescent discharge and blood-related (serous, blood-stained and watery) discharge, only the third group carries a risk of serious breast disease.
3. Galactorrhoea is most commonly due to mechanical breast stimulation or drugs, and rarely to prolactinoma.
4. Blood-related discharge is usually due to papillary lesions (duct papilloma or carcinoma) or duct ectasia (DE).
5. Duct papillomas fall into three main categories: 'solitary' papilloma, in major ducts and with little malignant risk; multiple papillomas, in peripheral ducts with risk of recurrence and malignancy; and juvenile papillomatosis, a rare but distinctive condition.
6. Galactography is gaining popularity, in spite of few data on effectiveness – cost and therapeutic – with routine use.
7. Galactography is also combined with adjunctive techniques, such as hook-wire insertion, and ultrasound-guided fine needle aspiration (FNA) or percutaneous dye injection.
8. High-resolution ultrasound, fibreoptic ductography and intravenous enhanced MRI galactography look like promising developments.
9. Ductolobular segmental resection is sometimes an alternative to the standard operations of microdochectomy or major duct excision.
10. There is some evidence of increased risk of malignancy with benign papillomas, but not sufficient to warrant routine long-term follow-up.

Nipple discharge is important when it occurs spontaneously and as the dominant symptom. Spontaneous presentation is important, because a high incidence will be recorded if milky discharge that occurs only following squeezing or expression of the breast is included in series of patients with nipple discharge. Such a discharge is common in parous women and will often be reported on direct questioning. This is not galactorrhoea and can be safely ignored.

Nipple discharge loses its significance when it is accompanied by a dominant lump. The lump then takes precedence in assessment and management.

A patient may present with discharge because she fears she may be developing malignancy, because the amount may be sufficient to cause social embarrassment, or as an incidental accompaniment of other breast symptoms. In general, the patient will delay no longer before presenting with discharge than with a lump.

Management will be directed at relieving the patient's concern regarding malignancy, and providing treatment for the minority of women who require treatment for the discharge itself. The ratio of patients falling into the two groups varies considerably in the literature because of different referral patterns and different views as to what constitutes discharge. For example, Gulay et al.[1] found that with an overall referral rate of 5%, the nipple discharge was spontaneous in only half; the other half had expressed the discharge themselves. In some African and Asian countries, nipple discharge accounts for a smaller proportion of referrals.[2]

DEFINITION

Nipple discharge is defined as spontaneous efflux of fluid from the nipple apart from the physiological function of the puerperium and lactation. Discharge can be elicited by squeezing in about 20% of patients, and application of negative suction with a pump can increase this to 50%.[3] Some patients report that nipple discharge follows mammography.

This chapter considers spontaneous nipple discharge in the absence of a dominant lump. In the latter case, the lump takes precedence in assessment and management. An associated discharge does not increase the likelihood of a mass being malignant at any age.[4]

Several conditions may simulate nipple discharge, especially skin exudate as from eczema of the nipple, and discharge from Montgomery's tubercles, seen particularly in adolescent girls.

INCIDENCE

Nipple discharge is a relatively uncommon presenting complaint in a breast clinic. Devitt[5] has reviewed the literature of nipple discharge in breast clinics. About 5% of referrals are concerned with this symptom, and of these about 5% will prove to have cancer. Haagensen[6] reported that 3% of patients referred to him complained of nipple discharge. Our own experience is analysed in Table 12.1.

Table 12.1 Diagnosis and type of discharge

Referred cases 4012	
Nipple discharge	259 (6.4%)
Cancer	14 - 57% bloody
Duct papilloma	15 - 60% bloody
Duct ectasia	87 - 17% bloody

These figures relate to the 1970s and 1980s. In the mid-1990s 8% of all referrals were for nipple discharge, although it remained an uncommon presentation of cancer.[7] Since many of these cases fall outside the guidelines produced for general practitioner referrals to hospital in the UK[7] it seems likely that many are unnecessary. The guidelines recommend referral for cases in women over 50 years, for younger women with blood-stained discharge, and for persistent single duct discharge.

Leis[8] reported that 7.4% of 8703 breast operations were performed for the indication of nipple discharge. In a study from Guy's Hospital over a 10-year period, 6.6% of referrals were for nipple discharge and of the 6000 operations performed 4.5% related to treatment of nipple discharge.[9]

Nipple discharge is rare in males. In a series where 10% of 3787 breast clinic patients complained of a nipple discharge, only 1.5% of the nipple discharge occurred in males and none were associated with cancer.[4] However, not all series agree with the lack of association with cancer, Leis[8] reports that nipple discharge in males is more likely to be associated with cancer, being the dominant symptom in 20% of his cases, while a multicentre study of male intraduct cancer in France showed nipple discharge to be the main presenting symptom.[10]

CHARACTER AND SIGNIFICANCE OF DISCHARGE

The character of the discharge should be recorded accurately, as a good correlation exists between macroscopic appearance and underlying pathology (Table 12.2). Failure to be specific has led to confusion in much of the literature, by including common coloured discharges of little surgical significance.

Nipple discharge can be assigned to one of four groups:
- Physiological galactorrhoea
- Secondary galactorrhoea
- Coloured opalescent (or grumous)
- Serosanguineous and watery.

Only the last carries a risk of serious breast disease. The commoner causes of the different types of discharge are given in Table 12.3.

Galactorrhoea
The thin, off-white, modestly opalescent quality of human milk is characteristic. There is a 'grey' area between milk

and the thicker creamy discharge of DE, but it is not commonly difficult to distinguish the two.

Physiological galactorrhoea

Galactorrhoea is defined as milk secretion unrelated to breastfeeding. Many patients complaining of milky discharge are suffering from physiological rather than pathological conditions. Pathology within the breast is so rare within this group that the cause should be sought elsewhere.

Milk production may continue long after lactation has ceased and a regular menstrual cycle has been re-established. This discharge is usually bilateral and may occasionally be copious. It is of no pathological significance and is usually due to stimulation of the breast by continued maternal attempts at expression. This is sometimes carried out in the belief that it will prevent further milk production, or that milk should not be allowed to lie in the breast. Milk discharge may result from mechanical stimulation of the breasts during sexual activity, especially in young girls. Milky discharge associated with other mechanical forms of stimulation is occasionally encountered, explaining the anecdotal reports of successful breastfeeding in the absence of prior pregnancy, and even reports of successful suckling by men!

Treatment is by reassurance and explanation of the sequence of events, that the condition is self-limiting and that cessation of expression or other mechanical stimulation will allow resolution. Occasionally, physiological milk discharge is seen at the extremes of reproductive life. At the menarche, during the period of rapid breast development, and at the menopause, squeezing of the breasts may produce small quantities of fluid. Again, explanation and reassurance are all that is required.

The appearance of 'witch's milk' in the neonate has been dealt with in Chapter 2 and is due to the transplacental transport of maternal lactogenic hormones.

Secondary galactorrhoea

The appearance of a milky discharge is occasionally seen apart from the conditions mentioned above. A careful history and examination will usually reveal the cause (Table 12.4).

These causes are mostly related to those situations in

Table 12.2 Relationship of discharge type and pathological diagnosis		
Type of discharge	Main cause	Less common cause
Blood-related		
Bloody	Hyperplastic lesions[a]	Duct ectasia, pregnancy
Serous	Hyperplastic lesions	Duct ectasia
Watery	Hyperplastic lesions	Duct ectasia
Coloured opalescent	Duct ectasia	Cyst
Milk	Physiological	Galactorrhoea of endocrine origin

[a] Hyperplastic lesions include hyperplasia, papilloma, carcinoma-in-situ and invasive ductal carcinoma.

Table 12.3 Causes of nipple discharge	Blood related			Opalescent	Milk
	Bloody	Serous	Watery		
Physiological					
Neonatal	−	−	−	−	+
Lactation	−	−	−	−	+
Pregnancy	±	−	−	−	+
Postlactational	−	−	−	−	+
Mechanical stimulation	−	−	−	−	+
Hyperprolactinaemia	−	−	−	−	+
Ductal pathology					
Duct ectasia	±	±	±	+	−
Cysts	−	−	−	+	−
Papilloma	+	+	±	−	−
Cancer	+	+	±	−	−

+, Common or likely cause; ±, rare but well defined; −, unusual or unknown.

Table 12.4 Causes of galactorrhoea

Physiological
Mechanical stimulation
Extremes of reproductive life (puberty, menopause)
Postlactational
Stress

Drugs
Association with hyperprolactinaemia
    Dopamine receptor-blocking agents
        Phenothiazines, e.g. chlorpromazine
        Haloperidol
        Metoclopramide, domperidone
    Dopamine-depleting agents
        Reserpine
        Methyldopa
Others
    Oestrogen (including the contraceptive pill)
    Opiates

Pathological
Hypothalamic and pituitary stalk lesions
Pituitary tumours
    Adenoma
    Microadenoma

Miscellaneous
    Ectopic prolactin secretion (e.g. bronchogenic carcinoma)
    Hypothyroidism
    Chronic renal failure

which there is an increase in the levels of circulating prolactin. The important causes are prolactinoma and various drugs. Vorherr[11] reviewed the literature and gives a list of 17 causes of galactorrhoea. It is likely that some of these are in reality pituitary microadenomas secreting prolactin, a condition which was unrecognized at the time of the original descriptions. The diagnosis of prolactinoma is suggested by the history of galactorrhoea, amenorrhoea and relative infertility. If the tumour is large, expansion of the pituitary fossa, and possible erosion of the floor of the sella, may be seen on radiography and help to confirm the diagnosis. More often the lesions are microadenomas and skull radiology is normal. Diagnosis is then dependent on dynamic hormonal studies of prolactin, and on imaging of the pituitary fossa. The galactorrhoea disappears following appropriate treatment with a dopamine agonist such as bromocriptine or cabergolamine.[12] Surgical removal of the adenoma may be indicated in some patients.[13]

Drug-induced galactorrhoea is not uncommon and occurs with a number of tranquillizing agents, particularly of the phenothiazine group, oral contraceptives and antihypertensives as well as drugs which have a direct action on the hypothalamic pituitary axis such as domperidone and metoclopramide.[14] The mechanism of action of some of these changes is obscure. Drugs which have been implicated in the production of galactorrhoea are listed in Table 12.4.

In clinical practice, quite gross galactorrhoea can occur for which no cause can be found on extensive investigation, or on long-term follow-up.

Coloured opalescent discharges

It is generally agreed that all coloured opalescent discharges, after sanguineous discharges and milk have been excluded, may be put into a single group in relation to significance. In particular, they are associated with no increased cancer risk. Such discharges are common in late reproductive life, often intermittent, sometimes persisting and occasionally very profuse. Multiple ducts of one or both breasts are often involved and with discharge of differing appearance from individual ducts. They show a wide range of colours and consistency from a creamy purulent appearance through yellow, brown, green and black. In general, the brown, green and black discharges tend to be of fluid consistency, the creamy discharge is more grumous, sometimes as thick as toothpaste (see figure 11.4). The coloured discharges resemble the range of appearances seen in cyst fluid (see Figure 9.3).

When a pathological entity can be defined, this is most commonly due to DE (see Chapter 11). At operation for DE, it is noticeable that some ducts are of normal calibre and others dilated, while the material in adjacent dilated ducts of the same breast will be of widely differing appearance; creamy, brown and green material may be seen in the same patient.

Nipple discharge associated with DE is dealt with further in Chapter 11.

In some cases, nipple discharge is clearly due to cysts; occasionally a ductogram for nipple discharge will show the dye entering a cyst from the duct (Figure 12.1). Other circumstantial evidence in support of this view comes from patients who relate the appearance of nipple discharge to the disappearance of a previously palpable lump.

Coloured discharges are usually readily distinguished from sanguineous ones, but where a brownish discharge causes difficulty a urine dipstick to test for blood is helpful.

Composition of coloured opalescent discharges

Ogan *et al.*[15] have studied the biochemical nature of these discharges. They found that nipple discharge fluid usually contained casein, suggesting that such discharges are derived from glandular epithelium secreting milk. Petrakis *et al.*[16] have measured nipple aspirates for the presence of GCDFP-15, a marker for apocrine metaplasia. GCDFP-15 was found in all but one of 115 women. This suggests that gross cystic disease fluid and nipple duct fluid have a similar composition and therefore a common origin. Petrakis *et al.*[17] extensively studied nipple aspirates from both asymptomatic women and those with benign breast disease. They found no difference in the constitution with respect to lactose, Na^+, K^+ and colour; they did however find changes which were age related. Lactose concentrations fell with age while the discharges became darker. In a previous study, Petrakis *et al.*[18] considered that the colour was likely to be due to pigmented products of apocrine gland secretion, lipofuscin complexes of peroxidated lipoprotein and breakdown products of haemoglobin. Interestingly they also showed a positive correlation between smoking and dark colour of discharge.

Blood and serosanguineous discharge

Serous discharge is characterized by the yellow colour and sticky quality of serum (Figure 12.2).

Serous, serosanguineous (pink) (Figure 12.3) and heavily blood-stained discharges (Figure 12.4) carry the same significance.

Such discharge is due either to a hyperplastic epithelial lesion or to DE. The epithelial hyperplasia is usually benign, one or more duct papillomas, less commonly malignant. The risk of malignancy increases with age, being much greater after 55 years than before the menopause. In Selzer's series[4] the overall incidence of cancer in patients presenting only with nipple discharge was 12%. This broke down into 3% in patients under the age of 40, 10% between 40 and 60 and 32% for patients over 60 years.

In those patients with DE, it is usually assumed that the bleeding arises from areas of ulceration within the stagnant ducts, although we are not aware of any formal study of this question.

In many series, a percentage of cases with sanguineous discharge show no clear-cut pathology, even after operations such as major duct excision. Hence, it is not surprising that conditions of low specificity in pathological terms have been invoked to explain the bloody discharge. Older series often specify cystic disease as the cause. Some seem to

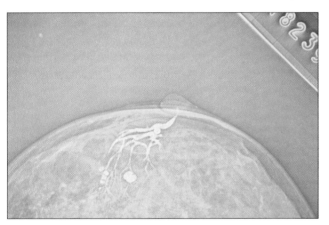

12.1 Duct injection for nipple discharge showing communication with small cysts.

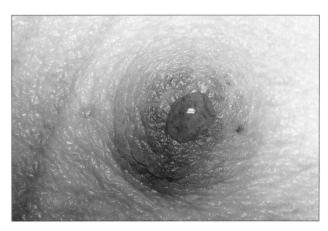

12.2 Serous discharge, showing the characteristic straw colour.

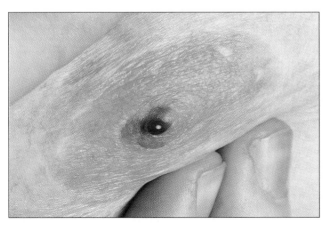

12.3 Serosanguineous discharge, due to a duct papilloma, with characteristic pink colour.

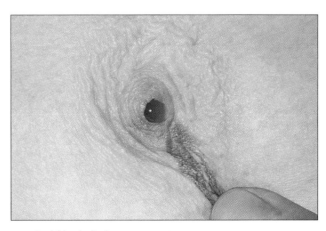

12.4 Dark bloody discharge.

refer to macroscopic cysts, others to the micropapillomatosis element which we now regard as part of ANDI. With these conditions which are part of the spectrum of normality, specificity as to the cause of bleeding is suspect, and the same must be true of a condition as common as DE, the diagnosis we believe to be most common. Hence, the cause of some serosanguineous discharges must remain uncertain, even after surgery. At least the satisfactory long-term follow-up of such cases shows that they are not associated with significant pathology which has been missed at surgery.

Haagensen's experience with serous and bloody discharge showed an identical significance for both types.[6] Duct papilloma was the cause in 70% and breast cancer in 10%, with both types of discharge. Likewise, 50% of benign papillomas presented with each type of discharge, and cancer cases with nipple discharge were divided evenly between the two. In the Philadelphia series the incidence of cancer was also the same for serous or bloody discharge.[4] Our experience is similar, although a higher proportion (29%) of our cases of serous or bloody discharge is associated with DE.

Chaudary et al.[9] have described the role of routine use of an occult blood test in patients admitted for operation for discharge from a solitary duct. In 292 microdochectomies, 215 were positive for blood. All 16 carcinomas were in this group but, in the benign conditions, the presence of blood did not usefully help to distinguish DE from benign papillomas.

Postsurgery nipple discharge

Lee et al. draw attention to spontaneous nipple discharge which appears shortly after breast surgery.[19] It can be due to communication with the operation site, or to a second undiagnosed pathology. Galactography was helpful in demonstrating a communication with the operation site, and the discharge subsequently ceased spontaneously.

Blood-stained nipple discharge of pregnancy

A little recognized problem that occurs occasionally in pregnancy is blood-stained nipple discharge due to epithelial proliferation as the breasts respond to pregnancy. At term the proliferation ceases, the cells swell and develop into secretory cells under hormonal control from prolactin and milk is produced.

This blood-stained discharge is typically bilateral, as have been the cases in our experience, but can be unilateral, when it occurs in the larger of the two breasts.[20] It usually starts in the second or third trimester of the first or second pregnancy. When bilateral, the condition carries no serious significance and requires simple explanation and reassurance that it is self-limiting. It rarely persists for more than 2 months postpartum.[21] Further investigation and treatment should be avoided because cytology may be misleading in this situation. It often shows epithelial cell clusters similar to those of intraductal papilloma and the cells may appear to be cytologically active.[22] As it is self-limiting and disappears with breastfeeding firm reassurance is all that is required.

It has been suggested recently that blood-stained discharge from a single breast during pregnancy should also be managed expectantly. Lafreniere[20] has reviewed the literature and found no example where this symptom has led to a subsequent diagnosis of cancer. This is reassuring, although clinical judgement should be exercised in a unilateral case. Breast examination and monitoring with ultrasound might be wise.

Watery discharge

This is a rare but very distinctive type of discharge (Figure 12.5) which carries the same significance as serous or blood-stained discharge.

Why a blood-related discharge should be watery rather than serous is not obvious. It is crystal clear, copious and associated in our experience in four cases with multiple papillomas of the large ducts: with macroscopic papillomas in one case and with florid microscopic papillomatosis in the others. As yet, none has developed cancer (after 5 years of follow-up). Haagensen believes the large papilloma condition to be premalignant, although he could only record one such case, which was associated with papillary intraduct cancer. We have also had a case where the only pathology on duct excision was a gross degree of DE. Lewison and Chambers[23] present evidence that this type of discharge is associated with breast cancer and Leis[8] found cancer in a third of 15 cases with watery discharge.

PATHOLOGY UNDERLYING NIPPLE DISCHARGE

Duct papilloma

Benign duct papillomas ocur in three main forms: solitary (discrete) duct papilloma, multiple duct papilloma and juvenile papilloma. These are three reasonably discrete clinico-pathological complexes, but because of overlapping features, these terms are not ideal in terms of descriptiveness or specificity. For example, 'solitary' duct papilloma is often multiple.

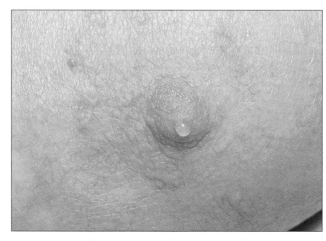

12.5 Clear watery discharge, distinct from serous and sanguineous.

However, these are the terms proposed by Haagensen, who was primarily responsible for defining the three conditions. As these are now in general use and we cannot suggest better terms, we retain them. Being familiar with, and understanding, the three clinical–pathological pictures and their implications is the priority, so that a patient can be put into the appropriate group.

It is also important to differentiate these macroscopic lesions from the microscopic papillary hyperplasia often referred to in the past as papillomatosis in American literature, and as hyperplasia or epitheliosis (without atypia) in the British literature. This latter condition, part of ANDI, is not related to the duct papillomas described here.

In summary, discrete 'solitary' papillomas are the most common of the three; they occur in a large subareolar duct, frequently cause blood-related nipple discharge, and have little malignant potential. Multiple papillomas are rare, more peripheral, less likely to cause nipple discharge and have greater malignant potential. Juvenile papillomatosis is an exceedingly rare condition with yet another clinical picture.

Solitary (discrete) duct papilloma

The commonest hyperplastic lesion causing a serous or sanguineous discharge is discrete duct papilloma: single or multiple. The defining feature is its occurrence in a large duct. In about half the cases, the discharge is bloody, in the other half it is serous. A subareolar lump is palpable in less than half of the cases. The history is sometimes a long one; the discharge may have been present for several years.

The typical ductal papilloma is just 2–3 mm in diameter (Figure 12.6), but as it grows it elongates and extends along the duct system so that it may be 1 cm or more long.

Larger papillomas tend to cause, and lie within, a local pocketing of the duct, a diverticulum which alters the normal line of the duct. Fine probes passed into the duct tend to get side-tracked into these diverticula. The papilloma has a narrow, fragile stalk and delicate fronds. The narrow stalk predisposes to torsion, which may result in infarction and this is not uncommonly seen on histology. It is presumably the reason why bloody discharge frequently remits spontaneously, particularly in young women. The sequence of events is summarized in Figure 12.7.

The delicate fronds account for the marked tendency to haemorrhage. As the papilloma elongates and grows along the ducts, torsion becomes less likely but partial ischaemia may lead to fibrosis and adhesion to the duct wall, making differentiation from papillary carcinoma more difficult. Some authorities believe this to be the origin of ductal adenoma. Typical small lesions have many fronds with a fibrovascular core and a covering of regular epithelium, although mitoses may be quite frequent (Figure 12.8).

Although a well-known lesion, solitary papilloma is relatively uncommon. There were only 15 'solitary' duct papilloma cases in the 259 nipple discharge patients in our

Cardiff study and the figure of 29% of operations for nipple discharge is similar to the 37% operations for nipple discharge described by Leis.[8] Most papillomas appear in the

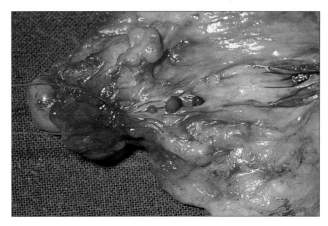

12.6 Microdochectomy specimen opened to show three small duct papillomas.

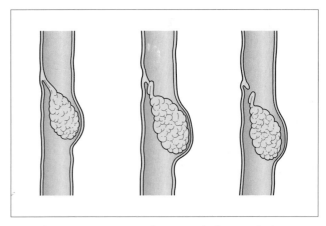

12.7 Schematic representation of torsion and infarction of a duct papilloma.

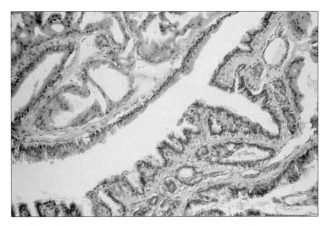

12.8 Histology of benign large duct papilloma showing the typical core vascular stroma with covering epithelium.

fourth and sixth decades with a peak age incidence in the fifth decade. However, it has a wide range of age incidence and we have seen it at the age of 16 and in an octogenarian. Sandison,[24] in his postmortem study of 800 women, found an incidence of duct papilloma of 1.6%. This suggests that many papillomas go undetected through life.

The usual location of a duct papilloma is in the subareolar major ducts, within 5 cm of the nipple. Macroscopic papillomas are usually solitary, but it is not uncommon to find two or three distinct papillomas in the one segment of duct (see Figure 12.6). In fact this is commoner than most reports suggest, and depends on the assiduousness with which the duct is dissected (and the state of the specimen presented to the pathologist!). This is also the reason why the term 'solitary' papilloma is not entirely appropriate; perhaps 'discrete' is a better term since each is a small discrete lesion as seen in Figure 12.6.

In older patients there may be 10 or more such lesions distributed throughout the larger ducts of a single segment, with the whole segmental system distended to its periphery. But the papillomas remain small, discrete and with benign histology, and so represent the extreme of the spectrum of 'solitary' papilloma. They are still better included in the 'solitary' group than the 'multiple papilloma' group, which has a different clinico-pathological picture as discussed below.

Duct papillomas are sometimes bilateral. Seven of the 173 cases reported in Haagensen's series were bilateral, and bilateral involvement was simultaneous in one case. In the remainder, the average time to presentation in the opposite breast was 8 years.

Solitary intraduct papilloma is not usually considered to be premalignant. Many recent studies have shown no increased incidence of cancer, but it must be admitted that there is a paucity of sound long-term follow-up data. The recent American College of Pathologists (ACP) consensus statement[25] puts papilloma with a fibrovascular core in the group with a slightly increased risk of cancer (see Chapter 18).

Occasionally, a papilloma develops in the terminal subareolar duct, when it may distend the nipple or prolapse through the duct orifice on to the nipple (see Chapter 14). When this occurs, usually in an elderly patient, it requires separation from a distinct entity, erosive papillomatosis (Chapter 14). The characteristic feature of a prolapsed ductal papilloma is that the surface of the nipple is unaffected. With erosive papillomatosis, the nipple itself is eroded. Haagensen[6] gives clear guidelines for distinguishing the two.

Multiple duct papillomas

The term 'multiple duct papilloma' is better reserved for the uncommon condition of papillomas occurring in small peripheral ducts. They occur in a ratio of about 1 case to 8 cases of solitary, large duct papilloma. They are more commonly palpable, more peripheral in the breast, more likely to be bilateral and less likely to give rise to nipple discharge

than the 'solitary' or discrete type. The condition is of such rarity that few have a significant experience of it, and it is difficult to be certain that the small series reported are homogeneous with regard to the type of cases included.

A distinctive group described in detail by Haagensen differed from common experience in that almost all were large enough to be palpable and clustered together with obvious multiplicity. Haagensen[6] described 53 examples of this condition and found the mean age to be slightly younger than those with solitary papilloma though with a similar age range of 20 to 70+. A tumour was usually palpable with a diameter >2 cm, only a quarter were central compared with 90% of 'solitary' lesions, while local recurrence and subsequent carcinoma were respectively 15 and 3 times as common. For this reason, Haagensen considered this lesion to be premalignant, and 15 of his 39 patients developed carcinoma. In general, both benign local recurrrence and subsequent malignancy occurred in the same segment of the breast as the original lesion, but this was not always the case. Nevertheless, Haagensen advises a conservative approach, reserving mastectomy (somewhat reluctantly) for multiple recurrences.

In more recent reports, cases have been diagnosed earlier, when tumours are smaller and less likely to be palpable than cases reported by Haagensen, but the implications are similar. Thus a subclinical variant where tumours are less likely to be palpable may be a halfway house between intraduct cancer and Haagensen's palpable benign tumours. The smaller lesions have common features with the larger ones: multiplicity, peripheral location (often in continuity with the terminal ductal lobular unit, TDLU), and a distinct association with cancer. Because these lesions are uncommon, and reported series are retrospective or of few cases, it is difficult to put together a coherent picture. However, there is a general uniformity regarding a high recurrence rate after local excision, the presence of atypical hyperplasia in association with the lesions,[26-28] and a considerable subsequent incidence of cancer. Haagensen's series probably included cases of juvenile papillomatosis, which was a less well-defined entity before Rosen's publication.

In our small experience this syndrome was associated with a watery discharge, and the tumours involved multiple breast segments. It seems likely that this is often a multisegmental system, in contrast to the unisegmental single duct system involved by 'solitary' papillomas, and this is at least part of the reason for the high local recurrence rate. For this reason it has seemed appropriate to us to advise local mastectomy, with immediate reconstruction where desired, but a more conservative approach as recommended by Haagensen seems reasonable where the pathology appears to be well localized.

Juvenile papillomatosis

In this very rare condition, multiple papillary lesions are found in young women at an average age of 23. Nipple discharge has been described in 15%, but because the dominant presentation is as a lump rather than nipple discharge, it is described in greater detail in Chapter 17. Recurrence after excision and associated breast cancer is a considerable problem, particularly in those with a strong family history of breast cancer. The clinical diagnosis is often fibroadenoma, because of the age of the patient, and the first suggestion of the diagnosis may come when FNA produces watery fluid.

Papillary carcinoma

Papillary carcinoma is the usual type of malignancy associated with nipple discharge. However, most papillary carcinomas do not present in this way. Only 26% of Haagensen's cases presented with a nipple discharge; in 80% it was sanguineous or serosanguineous, and in the remaining 20% the discharge was serous. This diagnosis becomes much more likely over the age of 50 than in younger patients, and forms a continuum with the second type of multiple papilloma described above. This condition is outside the scope of this book, and an excellent description can be found in Haagensen's textbook.[6]

DE

DE may give rise to blood-related discharges as well as the typical cream/brown/green black colours. It is uncommon for more than a few of the 15–20 ducts to be affected. The ducts are usually about 2–5 mm in diameter, often very thin walled but sometimes become thick walled. The discharge varies in consistency from thin to thick to grumous (tooth-paste-like), which has to be squeezed out, and the colour is usually creamy coloured but is often brown or greenish. Analysis of the discharge shows fatty crystals and large foamy macrophages and much amorphous cell debris. Pigmented cells termed 'ochrocytes' by Davies[29] are also presumed to be macrophages which have ingested the ceroids produced by degeneration of the fatty material in the ducts which gives this type of discharge its wide variety of colour.

It is not always realized that DE is also a common cause of blood-related discharge, both serous and blood-stained. It is presumed that this arises from small ulcerated areas of duct mucosa. We have also had a case with profuse watery discharge which required major duct excision, and no pathology was found in the specimen except markedly dilated ducts.

The pathology is dealt with in detail in Chapter 11.

Cysts and 'fibrocystic disease'

It is uncertain how commonly cysts are the cause of nipple discharge. They are undoubtedly responsible in some cases, because injection for nipple discharge may show the duct communicating with the cyst (see Figure 12.1). Sometimes aspiration of the cyst will be followed immediately by discharge of similar material through the nipple; presumably release of intracystic tension allows the draining duct to open. The frequency of multiple duct involvement with coloured opalescent discharge suggests that DE is a more common cause than cyst, as does the frequency of ectatic ducts at operation where this type of discharge has been seen.

The situation is confused by the fact that cysts have often been regarded in the past as a variant of DE, with both being merely a part of the spectrum of 'fibrocystic disease', especially in the American literature. It is now well demonstrated that cysts arise from lobules, and have a different pathogenesis to DE.

Many series also describe 'fibrocystic disease' as the cause of up to 25% of blood-related discharge. There is no obvious explanation as to the underlying pathogenesis, and since this is no more than part of the spectrum of normality, the possibility that a conservative microdochectomy may have missed the true cause should be considered.

Nipple discharge in children and adolescents

Duct papilloma is occasionally seen in the later teenage years, but 'nipple' discharge in the earlier years is more likely to come from the surface of the nipple. The commonest cause is probably related to Montgomery's tubercles.[30,31] The discharge may be clear to brown or bloody, with an associated lump. The discharge usually resolves spontaneously over a few weeks, but the lump may take several months to resolve. The cause is not obvious, but may be related to trauma to the duct orifice, since irritating clothing is another cause of nipple discharge in this age group.[32] We have also seen bloody discharge from Montgomery's tubercle in an adolescent with no underlying pathology. Again, the probable cause was trauma.

In children under the age of 5, DE is well recognized and probably the most common cause of bloody discharge in this age group.[33] It is associated with a mass, the histology of which shows cystically dilated ducts with thickened walls and containing acellular material with cholesterol clefts, and blood. The duct lining shows focal ulceration and granulation tissue. Most settle spontaneously, although this may take months. It is particularly important to avoid surgery in young girls, otherwise breast development may be compromised.

ASSESSMENT

History

The history will cover duration, frequency, associated symptoms (pain, lump and nipple inversion) and precipitating causes. Careful questioning will usually reveal the nature of the discharge, its spontaneity and whether single or multiple duct openings are involved. Note should be made of menstrual irregularities and medication, particularly oral contraception in young women and hormone replacement therapy in older women. In women with a milky discharge, particular attention needs to be paid to previous lactation, breastfeeding and history of mechanical stimulation of the breast.

Physical examination

A useful sequence is as follows:

- Inspection: This should reveal whether discharge is from a solitary duct (and, if so, which duct) or from multiple ducts, and the colour and nature of the fluid. It is usually most convenient for the patient to express a little fluid herself while the physician watches. Where discharge is scant, a magnifying glass may be useful. Where no discharge is produced, inspection of the brassière may reveal sufficient staining to determine whether or not it is sanguineous.
- Palpate slowly and systematically around the areola to determine where pressure will produce discharge and which duct is involved. If this is successful, a smear may be taken for cytology. When the segment has been localized, feel carefully for a palpable mass or dilated duct, especially under the areola. By pinching the areola between finger and thumb an assessment of the bulk of the ductal tissue can be made and the two sides compared.
- Careful standard examination of both breasts and axillae.

Investigations

Mammography

Mammography is advisable in all patients over 35 years with nipple discharge, and particularly so where the discharge is serous, bloody or watery. The most important finding is microcalcification along the line of ducts as it may draw attention to an otherwise unsuspected intraduct carcinoma. Prominent ducts may be noted together with the coarse, large calcifications which are typical of DE (see Figure 11.19).

Galactography

Small papillomas may be demonstrated by cannulation of the duct and injection with contrast material (Figure 12.9) (or by a percutaneous, ultrasound-guided technique if the duct cannot be cannulated[34]) but false positives and false negatives are not uncommon, in spite of some series reporting a strong correlation between radiological and pathological findings.

Debris or blood clot may masquerade as papillomas, while others may be missed in dilated ducts. Baker et al.[35] found that 20% of lesions seen on galactography could not be found in the pathology specimen. Equally, surgical series often report a high proportion of blood-related discharges as due to 'fibrocystic disease', with no evidence that this is the cause.[36] Duct injection is distinctly uncomfortable for the patient and, for this combination of reasons, we do not use the procedure as a routine investigation. It rarely alters management, but it does have a role in unusual or difficult cases. Ultrasound-guided FNA can be used to obtain cytology of a lesion demonstrated on galactography, and Sardanelli et al. found this twice as accurate as nipple discharge cytology.[37]

An extension of the technique is to insert a Kopan's spring-hookwire into the duct at galactography, to facilitate locating a lesion at surgery.[38] These authors found the technique satisfactory in 29 of 34 patients; in the other five the wire was dislodged.

Another alternative is to inject methylene blue into the duct at the time of galactography, to aid the identification of the affected duct system.[39] This requires galactography to be scheduled on the day of surgery to give maximum effectiveness. A bloody discharge will outline the duct without methylene blue, which can also cause problems if accidental damage to the duct leads to extravasation of the dye into the wound.

Those who advocate routine use of galactography[40] recommend it for all spontaneous discharges, both for diagnosis and to facilitate surgery, and if no pathology is demonstrated, will use it repeatedly until something is found or the patient refuses further examination. Cardenosa et al.[41] state that preoperative galactography can demonstrate an abnormal course of a duct, and 'preoperative mapping of the abnormal duct can expedite surgery and facilitate accurate minimal volume breast biopsies'. However, they give no documentation to support this statement, nor evidence that minimal volume surgery based on ductography will reliably remove all pathology. They concede that the description of normal duct anatomy in the literature is deficient, while abnormal variations of duct anatomy, or whether duct systems interconnect is still unknown.

It would appear that definitive work on the anatomy of the duct system, and the effectiveness of routine galactography, is still needed.

Ultrasound

In our experience ultrasound has a limited role in assessment of nipple discharge. It may be used to amplify information about palpable or radiological abnormalities defined during initial assessment. Ultrasound can demonstrate

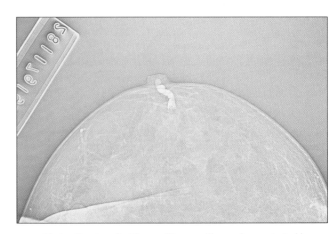

12.9 Obstruction to a duct by a solitary papilloma, demonstrated by galactography. We do not recommend its routine use (see text).

dilated subareolar ducts. Chung et al.[42] have found that ultrasound is more effective than galactography in the detection of lesions smaller than 0.5 cm but as their series was of only 15 patients this may not apply more generally. With the continuing improvements in the quality and resolution of ultrasound hardware, an open mind is appropriate regarding its use in the immediate future.

A recent report[43] claims that high-resolution ultrasound should be the first line investigation of nipple discharge. In this study, 75% of lesions were visualized with 85% diagnostic accuracy, and this is now the pattern in our clinic.

Fibreoptic ductography
A recent development has been the description of a silica fibrescope of 0.48 mm diameter with which the breast ducts can be directly visualized. Small intraduct carcinomas, intraduct papillomas and other benign lesions can be seen. Apparently, this procedure does not require anaesthesia, although the description of the original Japanese series suggests that this might not be acceptable to a Western population. Confirmation of the original reports[44,45] is awaited with interest. Love and Barsky[46] attempted duct endoscopy in nine patients known to have intraduct cancer and were successful in seven, obtaining epithelial cells in five. We have no experience of this technique.

Exfoliative cytology
Cytological examination of nipple discharge has been used for a long time: the first report of diagnosing a carcinoma by this technique was in 1914.[47] This investigation will sometimes indicate intraduct carcinoma as the cause of the discharge. However, there are too many false negatives for it to be regarded as a completely reliable investigation. For example, Kjellogren[48] found a 16% false-negative and a 4% false-positive rate. Aspiration cytology of any associated mass is obviously appropriate (see Chapter 6) and is considered more reliable.[49]

Groves et al.[50] have carried out an audit of nipple discharge cytology and found that although the test has a low sensitivity for carcinoma (46.5%) it does have a high specificity (99.5%). They conclude that this approach is of limited value but in view of the ease with which it may be performed it should not be discarded completely. Dunn et al.[51] reviewed a 12-year experience in Bristol and found similar sensitivity (55%) and specificity (100%) rates. Two cancers in this series were diagnosed by cytology alone. This investigation is particularly appropriate for patients with blood-related discharge.

An expanded approach to exfoliative cytology is directed at samples obtained by suction rather than those of spontaneous discharge. Wrensch et al. have studied the factors affecting ability to obtain cytological specimens by suction.[52] Specimens are more likely to be obtained during age 35–50 years, from women with an early menarche, non-Asian patients (versus Asian) and those with a history of lactation (parity alone has no effect). King et al.[3] have shown that it is possible to identify atypical cells as well as those which are unequivocally malignant. However, satisfactory specimens were obtained in less than half of the patients they studied so the value of this technique in routine practice is limited. Because of the very active epithelium in pregnancy, false positives are particularly likely at that time.

Cytology may be helpful in confirming DE, especially when it is associated with periductal mastitis. Large foamy macrophages with few, if any, epithelial cells are typically seen.

We regard cytology of the discharge as useful in those over 35 years old, but as with other tests for malignancy, negative results should be ignored. Sometimes a positive cytology is the sole positive investigation in the assessment of a patient with serosanguineous discharge.

Occult blood testing
In most cases it is easy to determine from the fluid whether it is blood stained or not. Where there is doubt, use of a Clinistix paper applied to the discharge will give a rapid answer.

Other biochemical tests
Tests for various enzymes and biological markers in the discharge have been described, but cannot yet be regarded as sufficiently discriminatory to enter routine clinical use. An example is that of Inaji et al,.[53] who used the combination of Erb-2 and CEA levels to detect cancer, though with some false-positive results with benign proliferative lesions.

MANAGEMENT

The importance of accurate assessment of the nature of the discharge cannot be overestimated, since most patients will have benign disease and can be reassured – some with, and some without, investigation. Coloured, opalescent discharges are very common, and can be treated expectantly, as can any discharge which cannot be reproduced in a young woman. Similarly most galactorrhoea can be ignored if a specific endocrine cause is excluded. Most such discharges will stop spontaneously, and firm reassurance that cancer has been excluded will be satisfactory for most patients. A minority will dislike the discharge so much that they wish to have it stopped even though it carries no serious import. The only reliable method of achieving this is complete division of the duct system, and this procedure is described in Chapter 20. We have no experience of blocking the offending ducts with fibrin as described by Hockel and Klose.[54]

The management of the blood-related group of discharges is more contentious. If cancer can be confidently excluded then an expectant management policy can be followed. Several series have now shown that if the diagnostic workup is effective enough, not all patients will require surgery to establish a diagnosis. Treatment can thus be aimed at securing symptomatic relief.

This is a far cry from recent conventional practice and it is useful to consider the approach to management of nipple discharge from an historical perspective as the philosophy of management of serous or serosanguineous discharge has changed radically in the last 50 years. Opinion regarding the likelihood of it being due to cancer was sharply divided early in this century. Judd,[55] in 1917, reported a 57% incidence of cancer in 100 cases at the Mayo Clinic. At about the same time, Bloodgood[56] regarded it as an innocuous symptom due to duct papilloma and not duct carcinoma. Two papers in the 1930s played an important role in influencing the vogue for mastectomy which dominated the mid-decades of this century. In 1930, Adair reported 108 cases from the Memorial Hospital, with 47% malignant. In 1931, Cheatle and Cutler[57] argued strongly from pathological evidence that benign papillomas could progress to papillary carcinoma. This led to simple mastectomy being the standard treatment for blood-related discharge in many clinics.

However, in the last 30 years, a more conservative approach has become accepted, resulting particularly from the studies of Haagensen in the USA and Atkins and Wolff[58] in the UK, who all recognized that those patients whose discharge was due to duct papilloma were cured by removing the papilloma. Both groups recommended conservative operations, Atkins developed the operation of microdochectomy and Haagensen[6] used a procedure intermediate between the microdochectomy of Atkins and the major duct excision operation of Urban.[59]

More recent series have given a better indication of the likely pathology of these blood-related discharges. Leis's study of 560 patients undergoing breast surgery for discharge showed that only 20% of those with blood-related discharge had cancer or a premalignant condition.[8] Funderbunk and Syphax[40] give a clear breakdown of the causes of 167 cases of nipple discharge. Of 46 which were opalescent or green, none had cancer or hyperplasia; but of 121 patients with a clear, serous or bloody discharge, 11 had cancer, 11 had 'papillomatosis' (hyperplasia) and 59 had a duct papilloma. All series show a marked relationship between the incidence of cancer and increase in age, as discussed below.

More recently, non-sanguineous discharges have also become better recognized and management of nipple discharge is now related to a number of factors, particularly the type of discharge, the age of the patient, and whether a blood-related discharge can be localized to a single duct.

General principles of management
Nature of the discharge
If the discharge is milk, look for a cause outside the breast, such as an endocrine cause or continuing mechanical stimulation.

Coloured, opalescent discharges have no serious significance. They should only be treated if causing social embarrassment. In doubtful cases, blood should be excluded by a chemical test.

Blood-related discharges cause much more concern to the patient and are associated with cancer risk. The risk is minimal in young patients but more significant with increasing age.

Age of the patient
This is important only in blood-related discharges, because of the cancer risk. No active treatment is necessary in young patients if the discharge ceases spontaneously. Wilson et al.[60] followed 74 young women and adolescents and found that none of them developed cancer before the age of 30. The threshold for advising surgical biopsy is clearly lower in older women but even then most women can be assessed preoperatively and be treated conservatively if they so wish. The adoption of a conservative approach to blood-related discharge is dependent on the availability of high-quality imaging and cytological assessment.

Localization
If the discharge can be localized to a single duct, microdochectomy gives satisfactory results in younger patients with minimal interference to the breast. In older patients where breastfeeding is not required, major duct excision may be preferable irrespective of whether the discharge is localized to one duct, both to avoid the inconvenience of further discharge from a different duct and to provide more comprehensive histology.

Specific details of management
The management of nipple discharge is summarized in Table 12.5 and Figure 12.10.

Blood-related discharge –
serous, serosanguineous, sanguineous, watery
Under the age of 30, risk of malignancy is low so the patient may be safely observed after full assessment as above. If discharge persists, and a solitary duct can be identified, the

---

Table 12.5 Management of milky and opalescent discharge

Milk discharge (galactorrhoea)
Eliminate mechanical stimulation
Stop or change medication
Measure serum prolactin
Reassure

Coloured opalescent discharge
Exclude blood
Mammogram to exclude other pathology
(over age 35 only)
Reassure
Major duct excision if socially embarrassing

procedure of choice is microdochectomy (see Chapter 20). While standard descriptions of this operation suggest removing approximately 2 cm of duct, the duct excision should be extended into the breast if the duct remains distended at this level. If the discharge ceases and does not recur within a year, no further follow-up is indicated.

When surgery is indicated for patients over 45 our preferred operation is a formal excision of the major duct system (2.5 cm or as far as dilated ducts contain blood/serum) on the affected side (see Chapter 20), with urgent paraffin section. It is important to remember to mark the terminal part of the ducts immediately behind the nipple so that the pathologist can orientate the specimen. The advantages of this approach are that it is not essential to isolate a solitary offending duct, it deals with multiple papillomas if these are present and gives maximum histological information, and it deals with DE if this proves to be the cause. With well-performed surgery (and in the absence of

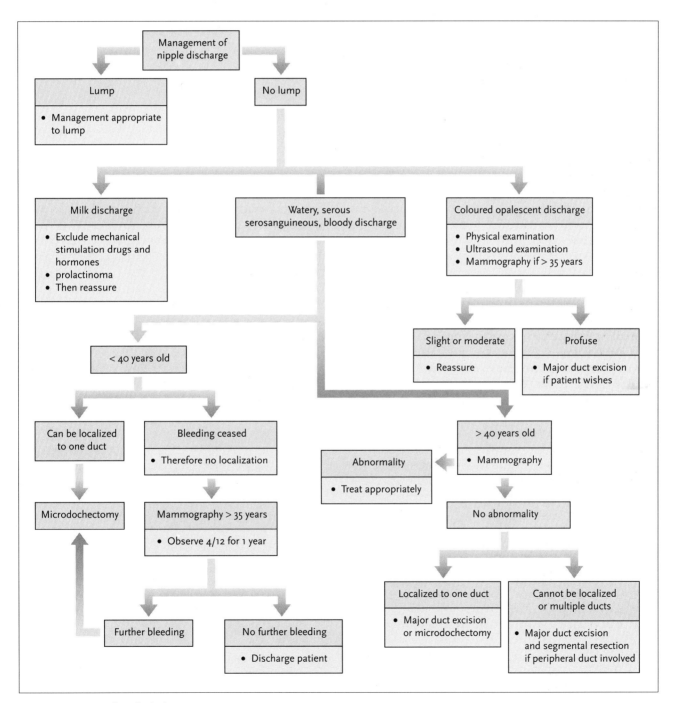

12.10 Management of nipple discharge.

chronic infection) there is no significant difference in the cosmesis following single or multiple duct excision.

If dilated blood-filled ducts are found extending into the periphery of the breast, the excision should be extended to a segmental resection with a clear margin of normal tissue (see Chapter 20). This is particularly important in elderly women who sometimes have multiple discrete intraductal papillary lesions of low malignancy in a single duct system, when planned segmental excision can be adequate treatment. In fact, a sound case can be made for including a full segmental resection (if appropriate in conjunction with total duct excision) in all cases where a blood-related discharge can be localized to a single duct, in older patients where there is a significant risk of cancer. If subsequent histology shows a ductal cancer of low malignancy (i.e. no comedo component) and adequate margin, careful segmental excision can be adequate treatment.

Ito *et al.*[61] reported a series which provides support for this approach in selected cases of non-palpable cancer presenting with nipple discharge. It is also in keeping with increasing evidence that some cancers have a segmental localization.

However, frank intraductal cancer found on histology, particularly of comedo type or with extensive intraductal spread (as opposed to discrete lesions), increases the likelihood of residual disease in the breast.[62]

Patients between 30 and 45 are suitable for either approach. In general, they may be treated as for the under-30 age group, but may be moved towards major duct excision by additional factors, e.g. strong family history of breast cancer, a particularly worried patient, or coexisting nipple inversion which the patient wants corrected.

Is it acceptable to avoid surgery in older patients with normal mammograms and no palpable mass? One group[63] has advocated this because only two patients were found to have ductal carcinoma-in-situ (DCIS) in a retrospective analysis of their experience. However, their excisions included non-blood-related discharge, which is not usually managed surgically, so the risk of DCIS in their blood-related discharges is understated. Furthermore, their high degree of accuracy in diagnosing minor degrees of DCIS on mammography are not necessarily experienced in all centres. A more representative experience is that from another major oncology centre, where only one-third of invasive and in-situ cancers presenting with nipple discharge were detected on mammography.[36]

Leis[8] found a false-negative rate of 9.5% for mammography and 17.8% for cytology in 84 patients with cancers. Hence we believe the emphasis should remain on surgical exploration for those judged to be at risk of cancer on the above criteria. We still recommend surgery in all blood-related cases defined by our criteria set out above. The operation is a minor one, and DCIS, at the very least, is an important indicator of cancer risk in that breast. For example Bauer *et al.*[64] reviewed the pathological findings in 277 women following surgery for spontaneous blood-related discharge; 15.5% were found to have DCIS. The discharge was bloody in 29, clear in 8 and brown in 6. Very occasionally a benign papilloma becomes so large that a mastectomy is justified.[65]

Coloured opalescent discharge

This only requires treatment if the amount of discharge is personally embarrassing with the need to wear pads constantly. The only effective procedure is a total duct excision, and in well-selected cases is welcomed by the patient.

Galactorrhoea

The management is that of the underlying cause. Prolactinomas are treated by bromocriptine or carbergolamine, or surgical excision. For drug-induced galactorrhoea, an alternative medication is usually available if the galactorrhoea remains unacceptable. In cases of physiological discharge, reassurance and cessation of mechanical stimulation should prove sufficient.

Follow-up

Patients who prove to have solitary duct papilloma have insufficient increase in the risk of subsequent malignancy to justify routine follow-up (see Chapter 4). Patients with multiple papillomas do have an increased risk[65] and should be kept under annual review with biennial mammography. Because the risk is small, long-term and affecting both breasts, long-term follow-up is more appropriate than prophylactic mastectomy.

Carty *et al.*[66] followed a small mixed series of patients with mainly non-blood-related discharge for 5 years and showed that the discharge had resolved spontaneously in three-quarters of the women in that period.

REFERENCES

1. Gulay H, Bora S, Kilicturgay S et al. Management of nipple discharge. *Journal of American College of Surgeons* 1994; **178**: 472–474.

2. Cheung KL & Alagaratnam TT. A review of nipple discharge in Chinese women. *Journal of Royal College of Surgeons of Edinburgh* 1997; **62**: 179–181.

3. King EB, Chew KC, Petrakis NL & Ernster VL. Nipple aspirate cytology for the study of breast cancer precursors. *Journal of National Cancer Institute* 1983; **71**: 1115–1121.

4. Selzer MH, Perloff LJ, Kelley RI & Fitts WT. The significance of age in patients with nipple discharge. *Surgery, Gynecology and Obstetrics* 1970; **131**: 519–522.

5. Devitt JE. Management of nipple discharge by clinical findings. *American Journal of Surgery* 1985; **149**: 789–792.

6. Haagensen CD. *Diseases of the Breast*, 3rd edn. Philadelphia: WB Saunders, 1986.

7. Cochrane RA, Singhal H, Moneypenny IJ et al. Evaluation of general practitioner referrals to a specialist clinic according to the UK national guidelines. *European Journal of Surgical Oncology* 1997; **23**: 198–201.

8. Leis HP. Management of nipple discharge. *World Journal of Surgery* 1989; **13**: 736–742.

9. Chaudary MA, Millis RR, Davies GC & Hayward JL. Nipple discharge. The diagnostic value of testing for occult blood. *Annals of Surgery* 1982; **196**: 651–655.

10. Cutuli B, Dilhuydy JM, DeLaFontan B et al. Ductal carcinoma in-situ in the male breast. Analysis of 31 cases. *European Journal of Cancer* 1997; **33**: 35–38.

11. Vorherr H. *The Breast, Morphology, Physiology and Lactation*. New York: Academic Press, 1974.

12. Webster J, Piscitelli G, Polli A et al. A comparison of carbergolamine and bromocriptine in the treatment of hyperprolactinaemic amenorrhoea. *New England Journal of Medicine* 1994; **331**: 904–909.

13. Scanlon MT, Peters JR, Picton-Thomas J et al. The management of selected patients with hyper-prolactinaemia by partial hypophysectomy. *British Medical Journal* 1986; **291**: 1547–1550.

14. Hall R, Anderson J, Smart GA & Besser M. *Fundamentals of Clinical Endocrinology*, 3rd edn. Tunbridge Wells: Pitman Medical, 1980.

15. Ogan A, Yanardag R, Colgar U et al. Lipid composition of nipple discharges of women with galactorrhoea. *Gynecology and Endocrinology* 1994; **8**: 109–114.

16. Petrakis NL, Lowenstein JM, Wiencke JK et al. Gross cystic disease fluid protein in nipple aspirates of breast fluid in Asian and non-Asian women. *Cancer, Epidemiology, Biomarkers and Prevention* 1993; **2**: 573–579.

17. Petrakis NL, Lim MI, Miike R et al. Nipple aspirate fluids in adult non-lactating women – lactose content, cationic Na$^+$, K$^+$, Na$^+$/K$^+$ ratio and coloration. *Breast Cancer Research and Treatment* 1989; **13**: 71–78.

18. Petrakis NL, Miike R, King EB et al. Association of breast fluid colouration with age, ethnicity and cigarette smoking. *Breast Cancer Research and Treatment* 1988; **11**: 255–262.

19. Lee EH, Venta LA, Morrow M & Dawes L. The role of galactography in patients with post-operative nipple discharge. *Breast Journal* 1997; **3**: 74–76.

20. Lafreniere R. Bloody nipple discharge during pregnancy: a rationale for conservative treatment. *Journal of Surgical Oncology* 1990; **43**: 228–230.

21. O'Callaghan MA. Atypical discharge from the breast during pregnancy and/or lactation. *Australian and New Zealand Journal of Obstetrics and Gynaecology* 1981; **21**: 214–216.

22. Kline TS & Lash SR. The bleeding nipple of pregnancy and the post-partum period. *Acta Cytologica Philadelphia* 1964; **8**: 336.

23. Lewison EF & Chambers RG. Clinical significance of nipple discharge. *Journal of the American Medical Association* 1951; **147**: 295–299.

24. Sandison AT. An autopsy study of the human breast. *National Cancer Institute Monograph No. 8*, US Dept Health, Education and Welfare, 1962.

25. Winchester DP. ACP consensus statement. The relationship of fibrocystic disease to breast cancer. *American College of Surgeons Bulletin* 1986; **71**: 29–31.

26. Cardenosa G & Eklund G. Benign papillary neoplasms of the breast – mammographic findings. *Radiology* 1991; **181**: 751.

27. Ohuchi N, Abe R & Kasai M. Possible cancerous change of intraductal papilloma of the breast: a 3-D reconstruction study of 25 cases. *Cancer* 1984; **54**: 605–611.

28. Murad T, Contesso G & Mouriesse H. Papillary tumours of the large lactiferous ducts. *Cancer* 1981; **48**: 122–133.

29. Davies JD. Pigmented periductal cells (ochrocytes) in mammary dysplasias: their nature and significance. *Journal of Pathology* 1974; **114**: 205–216.

30. Heyman RB & Rauth JL. Areolar gland discharge in adolescent females. *Journal of Adolescent Health Care* 1983; **4**: 285–292.

31. Watkins F, Giacomantonio M & Salisbury F. Nipple discharge and breast lump related to Montgomery's tubercles in adolescent females. *Journal of Paediatric Surgery* 1988; **23**: 718–720.

32. Casteels-Van Daele M, Wijndaele L, Eeckels R et al. Nipple discharge in children and adolescents: an irritating cause. *Clinical Pediatrics* 1990; **29**: 53.

33. Miller JD, Brownell MP & Shaw A. Bilateral breast masses and bloody nipple discharge in a 4 year old boy. *Journal of Paediatrics* 1990; **116**: 744–747.

34. Hussain S & Lui DM. Ultrasound guided percutaneous galactography. *European Journal of Radiology* 1997; **24**: 163–165.

35. Baker KS, Davey DD & Stelling CB. Ductal abnormalities detected with galactography: frequency of adequate excisional biopsy. *American Journal of Roentgenology* 1994; **162**: 821–824.

36. Welch M, Durrans D, Gonzales J et al. Michrodochectomy for discharge from a single lactiferous duct. *British Journal of Surgery* 1990; **77**: 1213–1214.

37. Sardanelli F, Imperiale A, Zandrino F et al. Breast intraductal masses. US-guided fine-needle-aspiration after galactography. *Radiology* 1997; **204**: 143–148.

38. Vega BA, Landeras AR & Ortega GE. Intraductal placement of a Kopan's spring-hookwire guide to localise non-palpable breast lesions detected by galactography. *Acta Radiologica* 1997; **38**: 240–242.

39. Saarela AO, Kiviniemi HO & Rissanen TJ. Preoperative methylene blue staining of galactographically suspicious breast lesions. *International Surgery* 1997; **82**: 403–405.

40. Funderbunk WW & Syphax B. Evaluation of nipple discharge in benign and malignant disease. *Cancer* 1969; **24**: 1290–1296.

41. Cardenosa G, Doudna C & Eklund GW. Ductography of the breast: technique and findings. *American Journal of Roentgenology* 1994; **162**: 1081–1087.

42. Chung SY, Lee KW, Park KS et al. Breast tumours associated with nipple discharge. Correlation of findings on galactography and sonography. *Clinical Imaging* 1995; **19**: 165–171.

43. Cilotti A, Campassi C, Bagnlesi P *et al.* Pathological nipple discharge. High resolution versus conventional ultrasound in the evaluation of ductal disease. *Breast Disease* 1996; **9**: 1–13.

44. Ozaki A, Ozaki M & Asaishi K. Fibreoptic ductography of the breast. *Japanese Journal of Clinical Oncology* 1991; **21**: 188–193.

45. Makiti M, Sakamoto G, Akiyama F *et al.* Duct endoscopy and endoscopic biopsy in the evaluation of nipple discharge. *Breast Cancer Research and Treatment* 1991; **18**: 179–181.

46. Love SM & Barsky SH. Breast duct endoscopy to study stages of cancerous breast disease. *Lancet* 1996; **348**: 997–999.

47. Nathan M. Diagnostic precoce d'un neoplasme du sein par l'examen de son suintement hemmorragique. *Clinique, Paris* 1914; **60**: 38–39.

48. Kjellogren O. The cytologic diagnosis of cancer of the breast. *Acta Cytologica* 1964; **8**: 216–223.

49. Rimsten A, Skoog V & Stenkvist B. On the significance of nipple discharge in the diagnosis of breast disease. *Acta Chirugica Scandinavica* 1976; **142**: 513–518.

50. Groves AM, Carr M, Wadhera V & Lennard TWJ. An audit of cytology in the evaluation of nipple discharge. A retrospective study of 10 years experience. *Breast* 1996; **5**: 96–99.

51. Dunn JM, Lucarotti ME, Wood SJ *et al.* Exfoliative cytology in the diagnosis of breast disease. *British Journal of Surgery* 1995; **82**: 789–791.

52. Wrensch MR, Petrakis NL, Gruenke LD *et al.* Factors associated with obtaining nipple fluid: Analysis of 1428 women and literature review. *Breast Cancer Research and Treatment* 1990; **15**: 39–51.

53. Inaji H, Koyama H, Motomura K *et al.* Erb-2 protein levels in nipple discharge: role in diagnosis of early breast cancer. *Tumour Biology* 1993; **14**: 271–278.

54. Hockel M & Klose KJ. Treatment of non-neoplastic nipple discharge with fibrin adhesive. *Lancet* 1987; **ii**: 331–332.

55. Judd ES. Intracanalicular papilloma of the breast. *Journal Lancet* 1917; **37**: 141.

56. Bloodgood JC. Benign lesions of female breast for which operation is not indicated. *Journal of American Medical Association* 1922; **78**: 859–863.

57. Cheatle GL & Cutler M. *Tumours of the Breast*. Philadelphia: JB Lippincott Co., 1931.

58. Atkins H & Wolff B. Discharges from the nipple. *British Journal of Surgery* 1964; **51**: 602–606.

59. Urban JA. Excision of the major duct system of the breast. *Cancer* 1963; **16**: 516–520.

60. Wilson M, Craner ML & Rosen PP. Papillary duct hyperplasia of the breast in children and young women. *Modern Pathology* 1993; **6**: 570–574.

61. Ito Y, Tamaki Y, Nakano Y *et al.* Non-palpable breast cancer with nipple discharge. How should it be treated? *Anticancer Research* 1997; **17**(1B): **791–794**.

62. Ohuchi N, Furuta A & Mori S. Management of ductal carcinoma in situ with nipple discharge. *Cancer* 1994; **74**: 1294–1302.

63. Locker AP, Galea MH, Ellis IO *et al.* Michrodochectomy for single duct discharge from the nipple. *British Journal of Surgery* 1988; **75**: 700–701.

64. Bauer RL, Eckhert KH & Nemoto T. Ductal carcinoma in situ-associated nipple discharge: a marker for locally extensive disease. *Annals of Surgical Oncology* 1998; **5**: 452–455.

65. Carter D. Intraductal papillary tumours of the breast – A study of 78 cases. *Cancer* 1977; **39**: 1689–1692.

66. Carty NJ, Mudan SS, Ravichandran D *et al.* Prospective study of outcome in women presenting with nipple discharge. *Annals of the Royal College of Surgeons of England* 1994; **76**: 387–389.

Chapter 13

Infections of the breast

CONTENTS

KEY POINTS AND NEW DEVELOPMENTS

1. In hospital practice non-lactational infections are now more common than lactational infections; the reverse is still true in the community.
2. Lactational abscesses are nearly always due to *Staphylococcus aureus*; non-lactational abscesses have a variable microbiology.
3. Initial assessment should be by ultrasound and/or needling; treatment with ultrasound controlled aspiration and antibiotics gives satisfactory resolution in many cases.
4. In most cases breastfeeding can be continued.
5. Non-puerperal infections fall into two main groups:

periareolar associated with duct ectasia/periductal mastitis (DE/PDM) and sterile or with mixed aerobic and anaerobic bacteria; and peripheral, often in older women and usually due to staphylococcus.
6. Many specific infections can occur in the breast, particularly associated with tropical diseases, but also seen in immunocompromised patients.
7. The finding that bacteria may be cultured from deep in the normal breast may help explain the origin of some iatrogenic infections.
8. Beware the occasional case of inflammatory cancer presenting as a surgical emergency.

Infection of the breast may occur as a localized phenomenon or as part of a systemic illness. The common acute infective conditions are usually easy to diagnose; the importance of the rarer infections of the breast lies in the similarity of their presentation to a carcinoma, a painless indurated mass. There are a number of specific infective conditions which are now uncommon in the UK but are of historical interest. Tuberculosis remains important in British practice with respect to immunocompromised patients and immigrant populations, particularly from the Indian subcontinent. The other infections are mainly interesting curiosities.

Studies based on hospital experience are likely to give a distorted picture of the true incidence of breast infection. In hospital practice, non-puerperal abscess is more common than lactational abscess,[1,2] but in general practice a survey showed 80% of infective episodes were puerperal.[3]

LACTATIONAL BREAST INFECTION

Epidemiology

Lactational mastitis is a common condition which has been described as occurring in up to 9% of puerperal women[4] but seems far less common today, an opinion shared by Benson.[5] Our experience (Figure 13.1) gives an indication that puerperal breast infection remains a significant problem.

In a review of 966 lactating women, Kaufmann and Foxman[6] reported an incidence of 2.9% in the first 7 postpartum weeks. Newton and Newton[7] halved the incidence of breast abscess during postnatal hospitalization from 0.82%

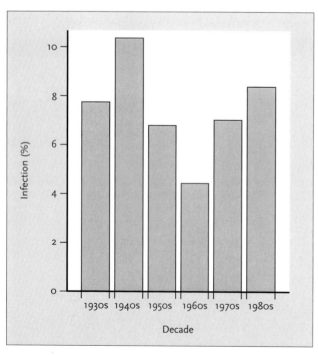

13.1 Incidence of puerperal infection, reported retrospectively by 425 patients undergoing 1000 pregnancies between 1930 and 1988.

to 0.47% by routine administration of penicillin. Although puerperal breast infection is sometimes described in sporadic and epidemic forms, the pathological processes within the breast are identical. The epidemic form is seen in institutional outbreaks in which the organism is transmitted from infant to infant by cross-infection and thence to its mother.

Prophylaxis

Attention to detail in the care of the breast during pregnancy and lactation can do much to reduce the chances of developing infection. Good hygiene and avoidance of breast engorgement or cracked nipple are important. During pregnancy, daily washing will remove the dried secretions that will otherwise collect on the nipple. After feeding the infant, the nipples should be dried and any segments of the breast that have not been adequately emptied during feeding expressed. A bland moisturizing cream can then be applied.

Pathology

The organism most commonly implicated is *Staph. aureus*, which presumably gains entry via a cracked nipple. Occasionally, the infection is haematogenous. Milk provides an ideal culture medium, so bacterial dispersion in the vascular and distended segment is easy. In the early stages, the infection tends to be confined to a single segment of the breast and it is relatively late that extension to other segments may occur. The pathological process is identical to acute inflammation occurring elsewhere in the body, although the loose parenchyma of the lactating breast and the stagnant milk of an engorged segment allow the infection to spread rapidly if unchecked. Because this is an infection of breast parenchyma, the bacteria are excreted in the milk.

Bacteriology of lactational abscess

The vast majority of lactational breast abscesses are caused by *Staph. aureus*. In the early, commonest type of abscess, this is most likely to be hospital acquired. The antibiotic resistance of the organisms will reflect this. Many hospital staphylococci are now penicillinase producing. In the study of Goodman and Benson,[8] all the hospital-acquired infections were *Staph. aureus* and, of the 98 hospital-acquired infections, only 50% had penicillin-sensitive organisms. A wide variety of organisms may occasionally be encountered. Typhoid is a well-recognized cause of breast abscess in countries where this disease is common. This is a particularly important diagnosis to make because the organism is secreted in the milk.

Clinical features

Nursing mothers are most vulnerable to breast abscess at two stages:
- During the first month of lactation following the first pregnancy when, due to inexperience, the nipples are more likely to be damaged and hygiene inadequate. Eighty-five per cent of lactational breast abscesses occur during the first month after delivery.[7]

- At weaning, when the breasts are more likely to become engorged. An additional factor after about 6 months is that the baby's teeth increase the likelihood of nipple trauma.

The patient complains of a painful red swollen breast associated with constitutional upset and fever. The local signs of infection vary greatly with the stage of infection. In early cases, a little cellulitis or nothing at all is found; in neglected cases a fluctuant abscess with overlying skin necrosis may be observed (Figure 13.2).

In patients who have already had treatment, the signs may have been masked by antibiotics leading to a mass without the classic signs of infection, and which may or may not be tender.

Figure 13.3 shows the sites of breast abscesses. Most lie in the parenchyma. Abscesses in the less common sites, such as the retromammary space, periareolar region or subcutaneous tissue, should alert the clinician to the possibility of an underlying pathology.

Assessment

The clinical problem may be resolved into three categories: cellulitis without pus formation; uncertain; and abscess. The importance of an accurate assessment of the situation cannot be overemphasized. Surgery in the early cellulitic phase is meddlesome and unnecessarily destructive; continued antibiotic therapy in the presence of an abscess may lead to unnecessary tissue destruction by the disease process. Test needle aspiration of the cellulitic area, preferably with ultrasound examination, should be performed.[9] It is wrong to wait for the development of fluctuation and pointing before proceeding to drainage, because further destruction of breast tissue will occur. The aspiration of pus will indicate that an abscess has formed; the absence of pus indicates that the condition is still in the cellulitic phase. In either event the opportunity should be used to carry out bacteriological examination of the aspirated material.

A useful bonus of this approach is that the rare case of inflammatory carcinoma may be diagnosed on the smear, thus avoiding operation in this difficult condition (Figure 13.4).

Needle aspiration can have a high degree of accuracy in diagnosis of inflammatory lesions of the breast.[10]

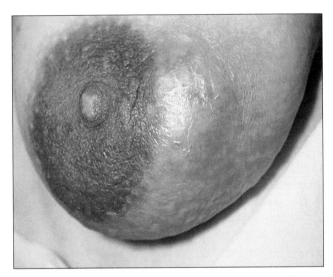

13.2 Late typical lactational breast abscess with compromised skin.

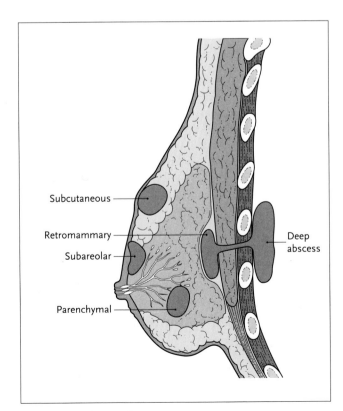

13.3 The sites of breast abscesses.

Subcutaneous

Retromammary

Subareolar

Deep abscess

Parenchymal

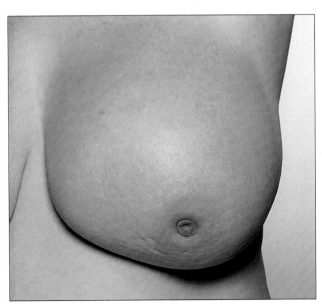

13.4 Inflammatory carcinoma of the breast.

Treatment

Taylor and Way[11] clearly enunciated the principles of treatment: curtail infection and empty the breast. The methods of achieving this differ in the cellulitic and abscess stages.

Curtailing infection – cellulitic phase

During the cellulitic phase, treatment with antibiotics may be expected to give rapid resolution. The predominance of *Staph. aureus* allows a rational choice of antibiotic without having to wait for the results of bacteriological culture. A penicillinase-resistant antibacterial should be given; flucloxacillin 250 mg four times daily will prove satisfactory but, if the patient has a penicillin sensitivity, erythromycin is a satisfactory alternative. If rapid improvement does not occur, repeated aspiration will usually reveal the presence of pus. After 24 hours, the results of culture should give guidance to a possible change in antibiotic therapy if the lesion is not improving and no pus is found on repeat aspiration. If resolution is proceeding satisfactorily, no further action is required.

Antibiotics are secreted in milk so tetracyclines, aminoglycosides, sulphonamides and metronidazole should be avoided because of their possible ill-effects on the child. Penicillin, cephalosporins and erythromycin, however, are considered safe. Such a regimen will prove adequate in most cases but in 5–10% an abscess will develop,[12,13] although Bates et al.[3] found that 24% failed to respond to antibiotics and progressed to abscess formation.

Curtailing infection – abscess phase

Once abscess formation has occurred, which is likely after 48 hours, use of antibiotics may cause a temporary regression of the symptoms without sterilizing the abscess and lead to a protracted illness. Newton and Newton[7] observed in the 1950s that the introduction of antibiotics led to delayed resolution of the abscess. At that time, opposition to the use of antibiotics was often vehement, on the basis that it led to chronic, thick-walled abscesses which could simulate cancer, as well as being difficult to eradicate. This view is still sometimes put forward in a number of surgical situations. Such chronic indurated abscesses undoubtedly occurred at that time, but are not seen today. In retrospect, they probably arose from the treatment of subareolar abscesses, and abscesses elsewhere, with antibiotics innefective against anaerobic organisms, at a time when the importance of these bacteria was not fully appreciated, and when effective antibiotics were not available.

In cases where the development of an abscess is uncertain, aspiration should resolve the point. The routine use of ultrasound in the evaluation of breast abscesses allows a rational approach to be developed. O'Hara et al.[14] studied 53 suspected cases of abscess, in 18 no abscess was seen and antibiotics caused complete resolution in 16; one of these developed an abscess which required drainage, the other had an inflammatory cancer.

Where an abscess has formed, surgical intervention is required, with antibiotic cover to reduce systemic infection and local cellulitis. The traditional method is to use open drainage but a number of reports now suggest that a successful outcome may be achieved by aspiration of the pus. For example, O'Hara et al.[14] treated 22 abscesses with aspiration, 19 of which settled without surgical intervention. Eight patients were treated with open drainage and five discharged spontaneously. Dixon[15] reports a rather similar experience selecting patients without skin thinning over the abscess for aspiration. It seems to us that repeated drainage by aspiration is preferable to the placement of percutaneous drainage catheters advocated by some.[16,17] The series of O'Hara et al.[14] supports this policy of repeated aspiration.

Whichever method is used, ultrasound should be used to detect any undrained loculi. When open drainage is indicated our preference is for open drainage and packing but Benson and Goodman[18] have argued for a policy of immediate closure under antibiotic cover. The results they describe suggest that this approach is as good as the conventional approach. Unfortunately, their study was uncontrolled and gave no indication as to how patients were allocated to the different treatment groups. Overall, patients required a longer course of antibiotics than if open drainage is instituted, when antibiotics may be avoided altogether in some patients. We still prefer conventional open drainage, but accept the case that primary closure may have a role.

The selection of antibiotics should follow the guidelines given in the cellulitic phase. In the absence of systemic symptoms, a well-localized abscess should be drained and antibiotics withheld.

Emptying the breast

This important aspect of the management of puerperal breast infection is sometimes ignored. The breast may be emptied either by suckling or by expression. Rowley[19] in 1772 described and illustrated the use of a breast pump which is similar to some still in use today. Although bacteria are present in the milk, no harm appears to be done to the infant if breastfeeding is continued.[13]

After draining an abscess, suckling may be difficult for a few days for mechanical reasons on the affected side, but the mother should be encouraged to feed on the unaffected side. The infected breast, however, should be emptied either by manual expression or by a pump.

Suppression of lactation

Following development of a breast abscess, patients are often advised to abandon breastfeeding.[20] This advice is given on the grounds that the bacteria are excreted in the milk and may then infect the infant, and that continued pain makes it difficult to empty the affected breast satisfactorily, thus causing further engorgement and stasis leading to rapid spread of the infecting organisms. There is no real basis for these views, and with skilled nursing assistance the infant may be safely fed on the contralateral breast and the affected breast may be expressed by pump until such time as feeding can be recommenced.[21] Indeed, except when the presence of the cavity makes suckling impossible, there is no indication to remove the child from the affected breast. The bacteria in the milk do not appear to harm the child. A leading article in the *British Medical Journal*[22] reviewed the evidence and concluded that mothers with breast abscesses should be encouraged to continue breastfeeding.

If it is decided to abandon breastfeeding, lactation should be suppressed as quickly as possible. The most effective suppressant currently available is probably cabergolamine which is effective as a single dose and so is preferable to bromocriptine 2.5 mg twice daily for 14 days.[23] The engorged breast should be emptied as far as possible mechanically. Fluid restriction and firm binding are not necessary.

NON-LACTATIONAL BREAST ABSCESS

Non-lactational abscess is more common than lactational abscess in hospital practice, but as pointed out earlier, is less common in family practice. The average age of the patients tends to be older than that for patients with lactational infections (Figure 13.5).

It falls naturally into two main groups, subareolar and peripheral, which differ in many respects. The microbiological profile of non-lactational abscess is far more variable than that of lactational breast abscess; this is particularly true of the subareolar group. In addition there are several specific groups of abscesses which need to be treated separately, those in immunocompromised patients, iatrogenic abscesses, factitial abscess and those in neonates.

Subareolar abscess

Subareolar abscess is seen mainly in women in their reproductive years, is mainly due to the DE/PDM complex and associated with a mixed bacterial spectrum. It is associated with cigarette smoking[2,24] and is likely to recur unless the underlying pathology is dealt with. This very important group of infections is dealt with fully in Chapter 11, and is not considered further here.

In contrast, peripheral abscesses usually (but not always) occur as an isolated phenomenon, and are due to *Staph. aureus* in older women, or to less pathogenic bacteria in patients with other disease, such as diabetes or steroid therapy. They are cured by simple drainage with or without antibiotics. Rarely they are due to the DE/PDM complex.

Peripheral abscess

This is much less common than subareolar abscess. The most typical presentation is in a postmenopausal woman who presents with a recent-onset, typical breast abscess with no underlying pathology. Aspiration will produce non-offensive pus from which *Staph. aureus* is cultured. Standard management is effective.[14] The pathogenesis of these

abscesses is uncertain. In view of the age group, it is possible that they are associated with a degree of the involutional form of DE, where mildly dilated ducts provide a focus for the proliferation of organisms frequently present in low numbers in the normal breast. Whether or not this is the basis, no treatment of any underlying disorder is necessary, in contrast to subareolar abscess.

Similar abscesses are seen with less pathogenic bacteria in patients with other disease, such as diabetes, or those on steroids. An example is the occurrence of an abscess due to coagulase-negative staphylococcus in a diabetic patient.[25] In general they respond to simple drainage, but these probably represent an overlap with the group discussed below, those in immunocompromised patients.

Peripheral abscesses are occasionally seen arising on the basis of gross DE (in older patients) or conspicuous histological PDM (in younger women). In such cases the underlying disease requires excision, and examples of both types are given in Chapter 11. We believe that some of these are examples of the condition also called granulomatous lobular mastitis. Whether this is a specific condition – there are many causes of granulomatous histology in the breast including PDM – is arguable. The main problem is failure to heal or recurrence after numerous excisions. In our experience, they heal if excision is carried out in continuity with the retroareolar ducts.

Treatment

Treatment of non-lactational abscesses should follow general principles. Dixon[15] has shown that the majority of such abscesses can be managed as outpatients either aspirating the pus or draining it under a local anaesthetic. If an aspiration approach is used, multiple attempts are to be expected. The overall management is much more complex than that needed for lactational abscess with a high incidence of recurrence. Management is discussed in detail in Chapter

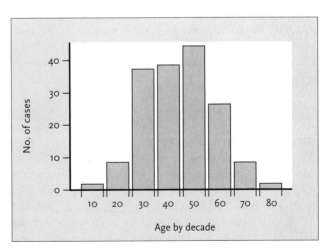

13.5 The age distribution of 160 non-lactational abscesses in Cardiff series.

11. In view of the likelihood of finding anaerobic bacteria[26,27] it would seem advisable to add an agent such as metronidazole to the antibiotic regimen used in the treatment of non-puerperal breast infection.

INFECTIONS IN IMMUNOCOMPROMISED PATIENTS

These have classically occurred in patients on immunosuppressive drugs, and were sufficiently uncommon to escape detailed attention. With the advent of AIDS as a major problem, opportunistic infections have become more obtrusive, and the abscesses are found to have similar features in both groups: unusual organisms, poor host resistance and often fulminant progression.

HIV infection
Breast abscess in these patients is increasing in incidence, and presents a bewildering variety of organisms. In Zimbabwe 30% of breast abscesses in young women are non-lactational, and 77% of these are associated with HIV.[28]

Tuberculosis is also seen as a cause of breast abscess in these patients, and may present as an apparently normal pyogenic abscess, and even be the first manifestation of HIV infection.[29] This emphasizes the need for full bacteriological, and where possible, histological assessment of all non-lactational abscesses.

In patients with established AIDS, infections may progress rapidly in spite of treatment, as reported in a young women who died following a *Pseudomonas aeroginosa* breast abscess.[30] Breast abscesses are also being seen in male HIV-positive patients (see Chapter 16).

Immunosuppressive drugs
Immunosuppressed patients provide similar problems. An example is an abscess due to *Nocardia asteroides* in a patient with systemic lupus erythematosus (SLE).[31] Nocardia infections are well recognized in immunocompromised patients, so it is not surprising that it should be found in a breast abscess. This patient was a 57-year-old woman treated with azathiaprine and cyclophosphamide for SLE. She developed a 9 x 5-cm abscess from which nocardia was isolated. It responded to appropriate antibiotics and drainage.

IATROGENIC ABSCESS

Bacteriology of the normal breast
It has always been recognized that skin flora can often be isolated from the terminal centimetre or so of the mammary ducts, but generally considered that the central area of the breast is sterile. Recent work by Thornton and colleagues[32] questions this assumption. They took multiple tissue samples from the breast during plastic surgical procedures and submitted them to stringent culture. Fifty-three per cent of the cultures grew *Staph. epidermidis*, and the presence of these,

and the other organisms grown, did not vary with the depth of the biopsy from the surface. Other common aerobic organisms were haemolytic streptococcus, diptheroids, lactobacillus and enterococci. Anaerobic organisms cultured included *Propionobacterium acne*, peptostreptococcus and *Clostridium sporogenes*. They also found some correlation between organisms grown from biopsies and subsequent postoperative infection. If this work is confirmed, it may explain some of the infections after elective surgery, but does not explain why they are not much more common.

Breast abscesses following surgical treatment are not rare, and are diverse in origin and clinical features.

Abscess following lumpectomy and radiotherapy
This is more common than may be realized, and occurred in 6% of patients in one series.[33] The abscesses occurred between one and 8 months following treatment, at a median of 5 months. The incidence was not related to prophylactic antibiotic use, adjuvant radiotherapy or individual surgeons, but was related to large biopsy cavities, prior biopsy infection, skin necrosis and repeated seroma aspiration. Six of seven abscesses grew staphylococci, but three were coagulase negative, suggesting introduction of skin organisms into an area of reduced resistance following radiotherapy. All abscesses occurred in patients whose operation included axillary dissection, although few of the patients were not in this group. All abscesses resolved with drainage and antibiotics, but with impaired cosmesis.

Periprosthetic breast infections
Infection around a silicone prosthesis occurs in about 1% of placements, more in subcutaneous than subpectoral. The commonest organism is *Staph. aureus*, but a wide variety can be responsible, including *Pseudomonas*, *Staphy. epidermidis* and mycobacteria. The *Mycobacterium fortuitum* group is particularly associated with prostheses,[34] but unless special precautions are taken in culturing the fluid, the organism is unlikely to be identified. The mammographic and CT findings in infected prosthesis have been described by Walsh *et al.*[35] Such infections may present in the classical way with redness, swelling and pain, others may be relatively quiescent.

Periprosthetic infection is likely to occur more frequently than 1% in patients who have primary reconstruction in association with some other procedure on the breast. Careful aseptic technique is particularly necessary in these cases. Generous lavage with a solution of tetracycline (1 g/L saline) during as well as at the end of the procedure, is particularly effective in preventing infection. Once infection has occurred, the prosthesis is usually removed, and reinserted some months later when the infection has subsided. Even then, it is difficult to guarantee that reinfection will not occur, particularly if *Staph. aureus* was the organism. Some surgeons have recommended conservative management with antibiotics and drainage of the pus, leaving the prosthesis *in situ*, but this is best reserved for special situations.

Retained foreign bodies

Many different surgical foreign bodies have been reported as the cause of delayed abscess, including a piece of drainage tube left at an operation for an abscess 35 years earlier, and presenting as a dense mass suggestive of cancer.[36]

A similar case was due to migration of plombage material through the chest wall after 40 years; it was demonstrated on CT scan.

Following central venous catheterization

A number of reports have demonstrated that the breast may be affected if a central venous catheter leaves its intended path. In one report[37] a late perforation of the right internal mammary vein by a catheter inserted via the left subclavian vein led to extravasion of parenteral nutrition fluid and a breast abscess. They describe three cases, all with good early function of the catheter, then chest pain and signs of inflammation in the contralateral breast. They stress the importance of promptly investigating this combination of symptoms if the complication is to be diagnosed early.

Factitial abscess

This condition should always be considered with abscesses which do not seem to fit the normal pattern, but confident diagnosis is notoriously difficult.[38] It is seen most commonly in nurses and members of other paramedical disciplines. Abscess may follow self-injection or insertion of foreign bodies. The condition is discusssed more fully in Chapter 17.

Toxic shock syndrome

This has been reported a number of times in association with breast infections. It is usually mild, and especially related to periprosthesis infections or minor postoperative collections. The sudden deterioration occurs, usually in a young woman, when an apparently innocuous collection is drained.[39] It is rare, does not seem to differ significantly from the more common occurrence with tampon use, and is managed in the same way.

Neonatal breast abscess (Figure 13.6)

This is uncommon, Efrat et al.[40] reported 21 cases of neonatal mastitis over 8 years. Half presented with mastitis and half with an established abscess. Staphylococcus was present in 85% of cases, and 50% resolved on antibiotics alone, usually intravenous orbenin or augmentin. Abscess was treated by needle drainage or incision, and both were effective.

The detailed bacteriology has been reported in a series of 14 cases over a 10-year period.[41] In this series there were ten girls and four boys, with a mean age of 13 days, range 12–28.

A wide variety of organisms were recovered, more reminiscent of non-puerperal abscess in adults than of lactational abscess. Aerobic organisms were found in 57%, anaerobic in 21% and mixed organisms in 21%. The commonest isolates were *Staph. aureus* (7), bacteroides (5), streptococcus group

B (2), *Escherichia coli* (2) and peptostreptococcus (2). No clinical differences were seen among abscesses harbouring different organisms, and no recurrence was seen after management with antibiotics and conservative drainage. A neonatal abscess due to group B streptococcus has followed 5 days after a maternal breast abscess due to the same organism.[42] Streptococcal abscess is very rare, but this organism may show a greater propensity to spread via the milk.

If neonatal mastitis is encountered, care needs to be taken to ensure that as little tissue damage as possible is caused either by disease or surgery. It is easy to remove the whole breast disc at this stage leading to secondary amastia. The incision should avoid the breast bud behind the nipple and no tissue should be excised.

SPECIFIC INFECTIONS OF THE BREAST

Tuberculosis

Experience with tuberculosis of the breast is changing rapidly, so that the subject needs to be discussed from two points of view: the classical disease is rarely seen in Western countries but still commonly occurs in developing countries; and the new disease pattern is seen in immunocompromised patients, especially those with HIV infection.

Tuberculosis is an uncommon condition in the UK today, but was more frequent in the earlier part of this century. Scott in 1904[43] reported that 1.5% of the breast cases seen at St Bartholomew's Hospital in London were due to tuberculosis. This represented one case for every 40 new cancers seen. In India it is still a relatively common condition: Rangabashyam et al.[44] reviewed 215 cases of breast disease over a 5-year period in Madras and recorded seven cases of tuberculous disease (3%), while Banerjee et al.[45] found 1.06% of all breast lesions were due to tuberculous mastitis. Murthy et al.[46] reported tuberculosis in 10 of 302 benign breast biopsies performed over a 10-year period in Papua New Guinea. Alagaratnam and Ong[47] reported that they still found one case per year in Hong Kong.

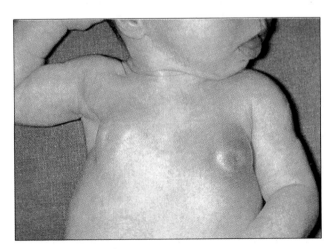

13.6 Neonatal breast abscess.

In a mammographic survey Makanjuola et al.[48] reported that 0.52% of 1152 consecutive examinations showed evidence of tuberculosis. Shinde et al.[49] have reported 100 cases referred with a diagnosis to the Tata Memorial Hospital in Bombay. Although tuberculosis is now seen mainly in developing countries, it is still not uncommon in recent immigrants to the UK.[50] Newly diagnosed breast tuberculosis in Western populations has been reported as the first manifestation of AIDS.[29] However, not all granulomatous lesions of the breast prove to be tuberculosis. In the past, the foreign body granulomas of PDM were frequently confused with tuberculosis.

In most patients, the diagnosis is relatively straightforward as they have evidence of tuberculosis elsewhere. However, in a few patients breast disease is the first manifestation and since on clinical grounds it can be difficult to differentiate between tuberculosis and cancer a high index of suspicion needs to be maintained. Tuberculosis in the breast may appear as one of three types: nodular, disseminated and sclerosing.[49] Each of these may be difficult to differentiate from cancer. The nodular form may appear as a painless mass which later involves the skin, forming sinuses and ulcers. In the disseminated form multiple foci become confluent and caseate with skin ulceration and associated with axillary lymphadenopathy. In sclerosing tuberculosis there is more fibrosis than caseation and nipple retraction is a common consequence. It may also be secondary to retromammary abscess, spreading through the chest wall from pleural disease. Since mammography may not show underlying chest wall disease, CT scanning should be used when mammary disease reaches the posterior aspect of the breast.[51]

The condition appears to occur more frequently during pregnancy.[52,53] Pathological examination of the tissue shows granulomatous reactions which are indistinguishable from those seen in other granulomatous diseases. Diagnosis is dependent on identifying the organism either in the sections or on culture. Shinde et al.,[49] however, were able to culture only 12 of their 100 patients successfully. It follows that the clinician needs to be aware of this disease and to plan the appropriate bacteriological investigations in suspected cases.

Treatment should follow general principles. The infection is controlled by a prolonged course of antituberculosis chemotherapy. The scarred and deformed breast may require surgical revision or even mastectomy. Shinde et al.[49] gave 18 months of antituberculous chemotherapy although 14 patients had to have mastectomy. Wilson and MacGregor[53] claim that even with chemotherapy, lesions tend to persist and recur if pregnancy ensues; they advise simple mastectomy, a view echoed by Rangabashyam et al.[44] However, Alagaratnam and Ong[47] were able to treat all but four of their 16 cases without resorting to this procedure. Banerjee et al.[45] obtained good results from chemotherapy in their 18 patients, only 2 of whom required mastectomy. Certainly the long-term results of surgery are good, as they were even in the days before effective chemotherapy,[54] but it would seem reasonable to pursue a course of modern antituberculosis therapy before resorting to surgery. If mastectomy is required, it would seem appropriate to consider a reconstructive procedure at a later date.

Other mycobacteria

Mycobacterial species other than tuberculosis also occasionally cause problems in the breast. Leprosy has been described and is usually accompanied by other manifestations of the disease.[55] Clegg et al.[34] have described atypical mycobacterial infection occurring around prostheses used in augmentation mammoplasty.

Syphilis

This disease is now very rare but deserves a mention if only for historical reasons. The breast used to be regarded as a common site of extragenital chancres. Fitzwilliams[54] quoted the findings of Buckley, who described 1148 examples of nipple chancre.

Tertiary syphilis may effect the breast either as a diffuse fibrotic reaction or as a gumma. The gumma usually appears as a discrete lump which disappears when appropriate antisyphilitic treatment is instituted.

Today, these conditions are a medical curiosity, but awareness of the possibility of a primary chancre needs to be considered because early treatment is curative.

Actinomycosis and brucellosis

Actinomycosis occasionally occurs in the breast. It is not different to actinomycosis elsewhere in the body and is characterized by induration, sinus formation and excretion of sulphur granules. There is usually actinomycosis elsewhere, but sometimes the breast is the first or only part afflicted.[56] Both breast abscess and granulomatous mastitis due to brucellosis has been reported.[57]

Mycotic infections

Mycotic infections occasionally occur and have been reviewed by Symmers.[58] Salfelder and Schwartz[59] speculated on the rarity of mycotic infection of the breast and considered that many cases were overlooked. A number of fungi have been demonstrated in the breast. Blastomycosis has been most commonly described and may be diagnosed on fine needle aspiration cytology.[60] The usual mode of presentation is of a breast mass clinically suspicious for carcinoma. Other fungi causing similar problems are Pityrosporum,[61] Cryptococcus,[62] Aspergillus[63] and Histoplasma.[60] Appropriate antifungal treatment is successful in many cases although excision may also be required. Three cases of fungal infection complicating augmentation mammoplasty have been reported.[64]

Painful nipple during breastfeeding may be associated with thrush infection. Candida may also be a problem in the inframammary fold, particularly in those with pendulous breasts.

Protozoan infections

These are extremely rare in the Western world. In developing countries where the appropriate conditions are common, they are met from time to time when they presumably represent metastatic septic foci. Marsden *et al.*[65] have, however, described two cases of leishmaniasis of the nipple which they considered to have been directly infected – one from the mouth of her suckling child.

Helminthic infection

Filaria

This is relatively common in Asia and is clinically easily confused with carcinoma. In Madras, there were five cases in the 215 cases of benign disease described by Rangabashyam *et al.*[44] The pathological process appears to be confined to the superficial dermal layers and lymphatics, the glandular tissue being spared. In the early stages, appropriate antifilarial therapy is effective although, when secondary damage has occurred, simple mastectomy may be indicated in occasional patients.

Filaria is the most frequently reported infestation of the breast and may take a variety of forms. The adult worm may appear at the nipple,[66] or a granulomatous reaction may present as a mass.[67,68] Most of the reports emanate from south-east Asia but Periar[68] records examples occurring in France. The diagnosis may be made on fine needle aspirates. Kapila and Verma[69] recorded nine cases in 4714 benign breast cytological examinations reported over a 15-year period. Among the cases of filariae in breast aspirates, gravid adult females of *Wuchereria bancrofti* were seen in three cases and microfilarial larvae in four. In the remaining two cases, an intense, eosinophilic infiltrate was seen in breast aspirates, while microfilariae were identified in aspirates from draining axillary lymph nodes. Living *W. bancrofti* have been demonstrated on ultrasound.[70]

Other infestations

Hydatid disease may rarely occur in the breast in parts of the world where this is common. It was known as an entity to Sir Astley Cooper,[71] who clearly described a case in his work. Such an event occurs in less than 0.5% of patients with hydatid cysts.[72] The lesion is usually cystic and the diagnosis made on aspiration. If the possibility is considered prior to this, full appropriate precautions for dealing with hydatid cysts should be taken. Excision of the cyst should prove curative for the local disease, although it should always be assumed that it is secondary to internal hydatid disease, usually of the liver.

Cysts due to cysticercosis have also been reported.[73] The diagnosis may be made on cytological examination.[69] Guinea-worm infection has also been reported. The adult worms may be seen on mammography.[74] Similarly schistosomiasis may affect the breast.[75,76]

Viral infections

Mastitis is frequently described as a complication of mumps. The incidence is uncertain because the only symptom, swelling and tenderness of the breast, is such a common one that recognition that this is a separate condition may be difficult. Philip *et al.*,[77] in their study of a mumps epidemic in an isolated Eskimo population, reported that 15% of 158 women had mastitis. The ages of the affected patients ranged from 12 to 61; the incidence of mastitis was 31% of women over 15 years old. As the majority of women in this age group would be menstrually active, it is difficult to be certain that the symptoms were not related to cyclical discomfort rather than mumps-specific mastitis. We have never seen a case which could be attributed to mumps.

INFECTIONS OF ASSOCIATED STRUCTURES

Skin lesions

The breast is covered by normal skin and any cutaneous infection may occur on the breast. Perhaps the commonest of these is an infected sebaceous cyst. Furuncles and carbuncles may also occur occasionally. There is not usually any problem with diagnosis because they are clearly dermal in origin, or involving the subcutaneous tissue in the case of carbuncle.

Hidradenitis suppurativa may occur. When it occurs in association with axillary disease, diagnosis is not a problem. Isolated hidradenitis, particularly in the intermammary cleft or the inframammary fold, may cause difficulty. When this condition occurs in the skin overlying the breast, differentiation from an underlying peripheral DE with PDM may be difficult. It is dealt with more fully in Chapter 17.

Pilonidal abscess

In the series of mammary duct fistula described by Patey and Thackray,[78] it is recorded that loose hairs were found in a lactiferous sinus of one of their patients. They also record that they found loose hairs in a normal lactiferous sinus. Because there are no hair follicles in the nipple, it seems that this event is analogous to the classic pilonidal sinus. A case which appears to be pilonidal abscess occurring in the breast has been reported in the UK.[79] Bowers[80] has described three cases of periareolar pilonidal abscess acquired as work-related disease in sheep shearers and barbers. Gannon *et al.*[81] have described a patient with recurrent periareolar abscesses. Hairs from her male patients were seen to protrude from the nipple ducts and were also found within the abscess cavity. Routine questioning of hairdressers in the clinic suggests that they at least recognize this as a common problem.

REFERENCES

1. Scholefield JM, Duncan JL & Rogers K. Review of hospital experience of breast abscess. *British Journal of Surgery* 1987; **74**: 469–470.

2. Bundred NJ, Dover MS, Coley S & Morrison JM. Breast abscesses and cigarette smoking. *British Journal of Surgery* 1992; **79**: 58–59.

3. Bates T, Down RHL, Tant DR & Fiddian RV. The current treatment of breast abscess in hospital and in general practice. *Practitioner* 1973; **211**: 541–547.

4. Fulton AA. Incidence of puerperal and lactational mastitis in an industrial town of some 43,000 inhabitants. *British Medical Journal* 1945; **1**: 693–696.

5. Benson EA. Breast abscesses and breast cysts. *Practitioner* 1982; **226**: 1397–1401.

6. Kaufmann R & Foxman B. Mastitis among lactating women: occurrence and risk factors. *Social Science and Medicine* 1991; **33**: 701–705.

7. Newton M & Newton NR. Breast abscess. A result of lactation failure. *Surgery, Gynecology and Obstetrics* 1950; **91**: 651–655.

8. Goodman MA & Benson EA. An evaluation of current trends in the management of breast abscesses. *Medical Journal of Australia* 1970; **1**: 1034–1039.

9. Hayes R, Michell M & Nunnerly HB. Acute inflammation of the breast – the role of breast ultrasound in diagnosis and management. *Clinical Radiology* 1991; **44**: 253–256.

10. Das DK, Sodham P, Kashyap V *et al.* Inflammatory lesions of the breast: diagnosis by fine needle aspiration. *Cytopathology* 1992; **3**: 281–289.

11. Taylor MD & Way S. Penicillin in treatment of acute puerperal mastitis. *British Medical Journal* 1946; **2**: 731–732.

12. Devereux WP. Acute puerperal mastitis. Evaluation of its management. *American Journal of Obstetrics and Gynecology* 1970; **108**: 78–81.

13. Marshall BR, Hepper JK & Zirbell CC. Sporadic puerperal mastitis: an infection that need not interrupt lactation. *Journal of the American Medical Association* 1975; **233**: 1377–1379.

14. O'Hara RJ, Dexter SPL & Fox JN. Conservative management of infective mastitis and breast abscesses after ultrasonographic assessment. *British Journal of Surgery* 1996; **83**: 1413–1414.

15. Dixon JM. Outpatient treatment of non-lactational breast abscesses. *British Journal of Surgery* 1992; **79**: 56–57.

16. Pluchinotta AM & Catania S. Percutaneous drainage of peripheral nonlactational breast abscesses. *Breast Disease* 1996; **9**: 223–227.

17. Berna JD, Garcia Medina V, Madrigal M *et al.* Percutaneous drainage of breast abscesses. *European Journal of Radiology* 1996; **21**: 217–219.

18. Benson EA & Goodman MA. Incision with primary suture in the treatment of acute puerperal breast abscess. *British Journal of Surgery* 1970; **57**: 55–58.

19. Rowley WA. *Practical Treatise on Diseases of the Breast of Women.* London: Newberry & Ridley, 1772.

20. Vorherr H. Contraindications to breast feeding. *Journal of the American Medical Association* 1974; **227**: 676.

21. Applebaum RM. The modern management of successful breast feeding. *Pediatric Clinics of North America* 1970; **17**: 203–225.

22. Editorial. Puerperal mastitis. *British Medical Journal* 1976; **1**: 920–921.

23. European Multicentre Group for Cabergoline in Lactation Inhibition. Single dose cabergoline versus bromocriptine in inhibition of puerperal lactation: randomised double blind multicentre study. *British Medical Journal* 1991; **302**: 1367–1371.

24. Schafer P, Furrer C & Merillod B. An association of cigarette smoking with recurrent subareolar breast abscess. *International Journal of Epidemiology* 1988; **17**: 810–813.

25. Surani S, Chandna H & Weistein RA. Breast abscess: coagulase negative staphylococcus as a sole pathogen. *Clinical Infectious Diseases* 1993; **17**: 701–704.

26. Leach RD, Eykyn SJ, Phillips I & Corrin B. Anaerobic subareolar breast abscess. *Lancet* 1979; **i**: 35–37.

27. Hale JE, Perinpanayagam RM & Smith G. Bacteroides: An unusual cause of breast abscess. *Lancet* 1976; **ii**: 70–71.

28. Cotton MH. Breast abscesses in Nigeria. Lactational versus non-lactational. *Journal of the Royal College of Surgeons of Edinburgh* 1997; **42**: 61.

29. Hartstein M & Leaf HL. Tuberculosis of the breast as a presenting manifestation of AIDS. *Clinical Infectious Diseases* 1992; **15**: 692–693.

30. Roca B, Vilar C, Perez EV *et al.* Breast abscess with lethal septicaemia due to *Pseudomonas aeroginosa* in a patient with Aids. *Presse Medicale* 1996; **25**: 803–804.

31. Simpson AJH, Juma A & Das SS. Breast abscess caused by *Nocardia asteroides. Journal of Infection* 1995; **30**: 266–267.

32. Thornton JW, Argenta LC, McClatchy KD & Marks MW. Studies on the endogenous flora of the human breast. *Annals of Plastic Surgery* 1988; **20**: 39–42.

33. Keidan RD, Hoffman JP, Weese JL *et al.* Delayed breast abscess after lumpectomy and radiotherapy. *American Surgeon* 1990; **56**: 440–444.

34. Clegg HW, Foster MT, Sanders WE & Baine WB. Infections due to organisms of the *Mycobacterium fortuitum* complex after augmentation mammaplasty: clinical and epidemiological features. *Journal of Infectious Diseases* 1983; **147**: 427–433.

35. Walsh R, Kliewer MA, Sullivan DC *et al.* Periprosthetic mycobacterial infection – CT and mammographic findings. *Clinical Imaging* 1995; **19**: 193–196.

36. Hoda SA, Borgen P & Rosen PP. Unanticipated presentation of unusual foreign body in the breast. *Breast Disease* 1994; **7**: 227–230.

37. Clark KR & Higgs MJ. Breast abscess following central venous catheterisation. *Intensive Care Medicine* 1991; **17**: 123–124.

38. Rosenberg MW & Hughes LE. Artefactual breast disease: a report of three cases. *British Journal of Surgery* 1985; **72**: 539–540.

39. Tobin G, Shaw RC & Goodpasture HC. Toxic shock syndrome following breast and nasal operations. *Plastic and Reconstructive Surgery* 1987; **80**: 111–114.

40. Efrat M, Mogilner JG, Iutjman M *et al.* Neonatal mastitis – Diagnosis and treatment. *Israel Journal of Medical Sciences* 1995; **31**: 558–560.

41. Brooke I. The aerobic and anaerobic microbiology of neonatal breast abscess. *Pediatric Infectious Disease Journal* 1991; **10**: 785–786.

42. Rench MA & Baker CJ. Group B streptococcal breast abscess in a mother and mastitis in her infant. *Obstetrics and Gynecology* 1989; **73**: 875–877.

43. Scott SR. Tuberculosis of the female breast. *St Bartholomew's Hospital Reports* 1904; **40**: 97–122.

44. Rangabashyam N, Gnanaprakasam D, Krishnaraj B *et al.* Spectrum of benign breast lesions in Madras. *Journal of the Royal College of Surgeons of Edinburgh* 1983; **28**: 369–373.

45. Banerjee SN, Ananthakrishnan N, Mehth RB & Parkash S. Tuberculous mastitis: A continuing problem. *World Journal of Surgery* 1986; **11**: 105–109.

46. Murthy DP, Sengupta SK & Muthaiah AC. Benign breast disease in Papua New Guinea Papua. *New Guinea Medical Journal* 1992; **35**: 101–105.

47. Alagaratnam TJ & Ong GB. Tuberculosis of the breast. *British Journal of Surgery* 1980; **67**: 125–126.

48. Makanjuola D, Murshid K, Al Sulaimani S & Al Saleh M. Mammographic features of breast tuberculosis: the skin bulge and sinus tract sign. *Clinical Radiology* 1996; **51**: 354–358.

49. Shinde SR, Chandawarkar RY & Deshmukh SP. Tuberculosis of the breast masquerading as carcinoma: a study of 100 patients. *World Journal of Surgery* 1995; **19**: 379–381.

50. Apps MCP, Harrison NK & Blauth CIA. Tuberculosis of the breast. *British Medical Journal* 1984; **288**: 1874–1875.

51. Chung SY, Yang I, Bae SH *et al.* Tuberculous abscess in the retromammary region – CT findings. *Journal of Computor Assisted Tomography* 1996; **20**: 766–769.

52. McKeown KC & Wilkinson KW. Tuberculous disease of the breast. *British Journal of Surgery* 1952; **39**: 409–429.

53. Wilson TS & MacGregor JW. Tuberculosis of the breast. *Canadian Medical Association Journal* 1963; **89**: 1118.

54. Fitzwilliams DSL. *On the Breast*. London: William Heinmann, 1924.

55. Furniss AL. Leproma occurring in a female breast presenting as a carcinoma. *Indian Medical Gazette* 1952; **87**: 304.

56. Jain BK, Schgal VN, Jagdish S *et al.* Primary actinomycosis of the breast: clinical review and a case report. *Journal of Dermatology* 1994; **2**: 497–500.

57. Al Abdely HM & Amin TM. Breast abscess caused by brucellosis mellitensis. *Journal of Infection* 1996; **33**: 219–220.

58. Symmers WS. The breasts. In: Payling Wright G (ed.) *Systemic Pathology*, Vol 1, pp 953–955. London: Longman Green, 1966.

59. Salfelder K & Schwartz J. Mycotic 'pseudotumours' of the breast. *Archives of Surgery* 1975; **110**: 751–754.

60. Farmer C, Stanley MW, Bardales RH *et al.* Mycoses of the breast: diagnosis by fine-needle aspiration. *Diagnostic Cytopathology* 1995; **12**: 51–55.

61. Bertini B. Cytopathology of nipple discharge due to pityrosporum orbiculare and cocci in an elderly woman. *Acta Cytologica* 1975; **19**: 38–42.

62. Goldman M & Pottage JC. Cryptococcal infection of the breast. *Clinical Infectious Diseases* 1995; **21**: 1166–1167.

63. Govindarajan M, Verghese S & Kuruvilla S. Primary aspergillosis of the breast. Report of a case with fine needle aspiration cytology diagnosis. *Acta Cytologica* 1993; **37**: 234–236.

64. Williams K, Walton RL & Bunkis J. Aspergillus colonisation associated with bilateral silicone mammary implants. *Plastic and Reconstructive Surgery* 1983; **71**: 260–261.

65. Marsden PD, Almeida EA, Llanos Cuentas EA *et al.* *Leishmania braziliensis* infection of the nipple. *British Medical Journal* 1985; **290**: 433–434.

66. Lahiri VL. Microfilariae in nipple secretion. *Acta Cytologica* 1975; **19**: 154.

67. Chen Y. Filarial granuloma of the female breast. A histopathologic study of 131 cases. *American Journal of Tropical Medicine and Hygiene* 1981; **30**: 1206–1210.

68. Periar JM. Dirofilariasis of the breast in France. *American Journal of Tropical Medicine and Hygiene* 1980; **29**: 1018–1019.

69. Kapila K & Verma K. Diagnosis of parasites in fine needle breast aspirates. *Acta Cytologica* 1996; **40**: 653–656.

70. Dreyer G, Branda AC, Amaral F *et al.* Detection by ultrasound of living adult *Wuchereria bancrofti* in the female breast. *Memorias do Instituto Oswaldo Cruz* 1996; **91**: 95–96.

71. Cooper A. *Illustrations of the Diseases of the Breast*. London: Longman, 1829.

72. Dew HR. *Hydatid Disease*. Sydney: Australia Medical Publishing, 1928.

73. Leggat CAC. Cysticercosis of the breast. *Australian and New Zealand Journal of Surgery* 1983; **53**: 281.

74. Stelling CB. Dracunculiasis presenting as a sterile abscess. *American Journal of Roentgenology* 1982; **138**: 1159–1161.

75. Gorman JD, Champaign JL, Suinida FK & Canavan L. Schistosomiasis involving the breast. *Radiology* 1992; **185**: 423–424.

76. Sloan BS, Rickman LS, Blau EM & Davis CE. Schistosomiasis masquerading as carcinoma of the breast. *Southern Medical Journal* 1996; **89**: 345–347.

77. Philip RN, Reinhard KR & Lackman DB. Observations on a mumps epidemic in a 'virgin' population. *American Journal of Hygiene* 1959; **69**: 91–111.

78. Patey DH & Thackray AC. Pathology and treatment of mammary duct fistula. *Lancet* 1958; **ii**: 871–874.

79. Goepel JP. Trichogranulomatous mastopathy: an unusual cause of nipple bleeding. *Postgraduate Medical Journal* 1980; **56**: 850–851.

80. Bowers PW. Roustabouts' and Barber's breasts. *Clinical and Experimental Dermatology* 1982; **7**: 445–448.

81. Gannon MX, Crowson MC & Fielding JWL. Periareolar pilonidal abscesses in a hairdresser. *British Medical Journal* 1988; **297**: 1641–1642.

Chapter 14.

Disorders of the nipple and areola

CONTENTS

KEY POINTS AND NEW DEVELOPMENTS

1. Nipple inversion occurs in about 10% of women but self-correcting changes often occur during pregnancy and nursing, allowing breastfeeding.
2. Nipple retraction is more commonly due to duct ectasia/periductal mastitis (DE/PDM) than cancer, although exclusion of the latter is the prime consideration.
3. PDM causes progressive retraction (initially a transverse slit) in young women; DE is associated with circular retraction in the perimenopausal period.
4. Erosive adenomatosis of the nipple has a distinct appearance, which usually allows clinical differentia-

tion from prolapsing duct papilloma and Paget's disease. It is not premalignant, but is associated with an increase in cancer elsewhere in the breast.
5. Nipple pain associated with breastfeeding may be associated with candida or staphylococcal infection.
6. Raynaud's phenomenon and CRPS (complex regional pain syndrome) are rare causes of nipple pain, sometimes occurring after surgery.
7. Secretions from Montgomery's glands, milk-like, serous or blood-stained, are easily mistaken for nipple discharge, especially in younger patients.

The nipple and the areola constitute an area of skin modified by the underlying breast tissue and ducts. In addition, the nipple has an extensive network of smooth muscle whose fibres are mainly arranged in circular fashion. The areola surrounds the nipple, both having more pigment than the surrounding skin, and contains the glands of Montgomery which provide a protective lubrication during lactation. The areola also has circular smooth muscle fibres and may contain auxiliary breast tissue which secretes milk during lactation.

In the past there has been debate regarding the number of lactiferous ducts opening on to the nipple. Haagensen[1] stated that there were about 20, but others have put the number at seven. The difference of opinion arose from the fact that 20 ducts are seen in cross-section at the nipple, but experience with lobar excision shows that a single duct system occupies much more than one-twentieth of the breast parenchyma. The discrepancy is due to the fact that the lobular systems extending from individual ducts vary greatly in extent. Some of the ducts are rudimentary, only about seven developing to form fully functional lobes.

Koernecke[2] found that the functional ducts are arranged around the periphery of the nipple, the rudimentary ducts opening on to the centre of the nipple. More light has been thrown on the subject from another detailed study of a single breast, where the extent of individual ductolobular segments is very variable, confirming the view that some ducts lead to small glandular systems.[3] This is discussed more fully in Chapter 2.

Further confusion arises from failure to appreciate the sebaceous glands and tiny milk-producing glands that also open directly on to the nipple.

NIPPLE INVERSION AND RETRACTION

The failure of full nipple eversion during breast development is common. It is termed 'inversion' and is dealt with other congenital conditions of the nipple in Chapter 15. Alexander and Campbell[4] have reviewed the prevalence of nipple inversion and non-protractility. They found that such changes occurred in almost 10% of 3006 women. The prevalence was lower in those who had previously breastfed and they attributed this to changes occurring during pregnancy and lactation. In a longitudinal study, 238 women were investigated and it was found that protractility increased during gestation. In most cases the changes were bilateral, but they were unilateral in a significant minority.

It is clear that in most cases nipple inversion is a self-limiting condition that does not preclude breastfeeding. Attempts to increase the effectiveness of breastfeeding by using nipple shells or Hoffman's exercises does not seem to be helpful.[5] For those who find the changes unacceptable a plastic procedure is required. The range of available options suggests that none is entirely effective, as discussed in Chapter 20.

Nipple retraction is an acquired condition and occurs after previous normal nipple development. The patients will give a clear history that a previously normal nipple has changed shape, and become retracted.

Bryant[6] made an appeal for careful assessment of nipple retraction over a hundred years ago, pointing out that many cases were not due to malignancy. Nevertheless, the erroneous view that most cases of recent nipple retraction are due to malignancy is still sometimes held. Recent changes in the appearance of the nipple do portend an underlying pathological process which requires evaluation. The principal diagnoses to be considered are malignancy and DE. The presence of a clinical lump associated with nipple changes increases the likelihood of an underlying carcinoma, but is also seen with PDM. In the absence of clinical or mammographic malignancy, nipple retraction is likely to be due to some aspect of the DE/PDM syndrome.

The relation between nipple inversion and retraction and DE/PDM is complex. In younger women, congenital inversion predisposes to overt inflammatory complications of PDM, while the same process may cause progressive retraction of a previously normal nipple. We have observed this progression over a period of 2 years or so in many patients. In this situation, the retraction is typically transverse, especially in the early stages.

In older, peri- or postmenopausal women, recent nipple retraction (circular in outline) is frequently seen in the absence of inflammation. This appears to be due to the periductal fibrosis element of the DE syndrome, and as such is considered to be an aberration of normal mammary involution (ANDI).

Few women are sufficiently concerned to wish to undergo surgery for retraction alone. For those cases due to DE, a formal excision of the major ducts is necessary (for details, see Chapter 20).

Assessment of nipple retraction

Although the early retraction of DE typically produces a transverse crease (see Figure 11.15), in established cases the appearance is not sufficiently clear-cut to allow reliable distinction from cancer. If the changes are bilateral the diagnosis is more likely to be DE. Carcinoma is uncommon when the retraction has been present for more than one year, but even in DE the signs may be of recent onset. Associated masses may be difficult to assess clinically, but aspiration cytology is usually diagnostic. Cancer will give atypical epithelial cells while typical inflammatory cells (including macrophages and foam cells) occur in patients with DE and PDM. Similarly, cytology of any associated discharge may provide helpful information. Mammography is helpful because it will usually show the typical features of cancer, or a notable absence of these features in patients with DE.

In the rare event where doubt as to the underlying diagnosis remains, core biopsy of the associated mass or open biopsy of the duct system will provide the definitive diagnosis. Excision of the major duct system has the added advantage that the inverted nipple can be corrected by duct excision. The pathology, differential diagnosis and management of nipple retraction due to the DE complex are considered more fully in Chapter 11.

CRACKED NIPPLES

Cracked nipples are the bane of nursing mothers, for these are the source of entry of bacteria in lactational breast infection. Pain in the nipple on suckling is a common event in the first few days of breastfeeding and may occur in up to 17% of nursing mothers.[7] In most of these, careful examination, using a magnifying lens if necessary, will reveal a small erosive lesion.[8] The mechanism suggested is that during vigorous suckling the skin of the nipple exposed between tongue and hard palate is subjected to a high negative pressure – if the milk does not flow easily the infant will suck harder – which produces a small blood blister. This lesion usually regresses spontaneously but, if the trauma is repeated, especially if the nipple skin becomes macerated due to the moist environment that often occurs, the lesion may progress to the typical fissure often referred to as a cracked nipple, seen about one week postpartum. This is often infected with bacteria or with *Candida* sp.

As in many such conditions, prevention is better than cure, and recognition of the predisposing factors is important. Good hygiene and a pattern of cleansing in the pre-confinement period are helpful. The nipples should be washed gently in water and dried secretions removed. The breasts are then dried by dabbing rather than rubbing. Care needs to be taken in establishing suckling; the infant will find an overengorged breast difficult to empty and short or inverted nipples may also lead to overvigorous suckling. If one breast is painful, feeding should commence on the unaffected side, so that by the time the infant is applied to the affected breast, the draught reflex will allow easy flow of milk. After feeding the breasts should be cleaned and dried carefully, and then kept as dry as possible until the next feed.

In the established case, correct feeding habits need reinforcing and in addition an antibiotic-based cream should be applied to the nipple. If candidal infection is suspected a nystatin-containing cream should be used. With care, the fissure will heal and breastfeeding can be maintained, although manual expression for a few days may be necessary. Neglect at this stage may lead to the development of an abscess as described in Chapter 13. If nipple inversion is the problem, leading to difficulty with suckling, the use of nipple shields may be tried,[9] although the evidence for benefit is conflicting.

NIPPLE CRUSTING

This symptom (Figure 14.1) usually represents dried up secretions which may accumulate, particularly in association with inverted or retracted nipples.

Sometimes it hides an underlying nipple lesion such as Paget's disease, eczema or erosive adenomatosis. Beyond reassurance, having excluded the conditions mentioned above, no action is required other than advice about cleaning the nipple.

Verrucous nipple

The nipple and areola may be affected by verrucous change, a benign condition in which the nipple and areola show hyperkeratotic thickening with dark pigmentation. This rare condition is seen in women of child-bearing age, when it is thought to be related to oestrogens or their metabolites. (A similar condition may arise in males having oestrogen treatment for prostatic cancer.) It also takes a naevoid form appearing in young women after puberty.[10]

A verrucous nipple may cause itching, malodour and interference with breastfeeding. A number of dermatological measures have been used, but treatment is difficult.

EROSIVE ADENOMATOSIS

This is a rare condition which is also described as papillary adenoma, florid papillomatosis of the nipple, subareolar papillomatosis and erosive adenomatosis of the nipple.[11] While usually seen in the middle aged to elderly, it can occur at any age and has been reported as early as 9 years. It has been described in an accessory nipple.[12]

Erosive adenomatosis is termed 'adenoma' by Haagensen,[1] who points out the difficulties of diagnosis and records that many of the early cases were treated by radical mastectomy in the belief that the lesion was a carcinoma. It usually presents as a papilliferous lesion of the nipple, often

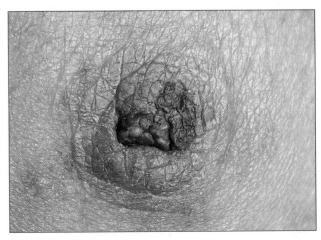

14.1 Crusting of the nipple.

with ulceration which may be concealed under a crust[13] (Figure 14.2).

The condition is sometimes painful, the commonest descriptions being burning or itching,[14] although Perzin and Lattes[13] only recorded pain in one of their 51 cases. Our own experience with this condition would favour the latter view that it is relatively painless.

On examination, the whole nipple may be indurated, has an expanded appearance and may be ulcerated. The main differential diagnoses are prolapsing intraductal papilloma, Paget's disease of the nipple, artefactual disease and eczema. The differential diagnosis from Paget's disease can only be made with certainty by biopsy, although the characteristic clinical features are different. Pinto and Mandreker[15] have described a case in which the diagnosis was made on fine needle cytology. Erosive adenomatosis does not extend on to the areola like established Paget's disease, and it has the appearance of a deeper lesion eroding through the nipple; early Paget's disease is superficial in appearance. When a papilliferous lesion erodes through the nipple duct, it is more likely to represent this condition than an intraductal papilloma (Figure 14.3).

An intraductal papilloma tends to expand the nipple rather than erode it, but if a papilloma prolapses through the opening of a duct, the nipple remains normal; it is not ulcerated.

Azzopardi[11] describes this lesion as being an extensive ramifying proliferation of two-layered tubules: an outer layer of myoepithelial cells and an inner layer of cuboidal cells. Although associated malignant breast disease has been described in about 8% of 200 collected cases, the lesion is not itself usually regarded as premalignant.[13] Associated benign duct papilloma has also been reported to occur more commonly than would be expected by chance. This incidence of associated breast cancer calls for careful assessment of both breasts. Erosive adenomatosis is adequately treated by local excision of the affected part of the nipple; there is no need to remove the whole nipple as advocated by some.[16]

SYRINGOMATOUS ADENOMA

Rosen[17] has described a benign infiltrating lesion of adnexal skin origin which he differentiates from erosive adenomatosis, in four women and one man. It is more likely to recur than erosive adenomatosis so adequate treatment may require nipple resection. We have no experience of this condition.

SIMPLE FIBROEPITHELIAL POLYP

This not uncommon condition was first described by Hutchinson,[18] who thought it arose from Montgomery's tubercles, although the polyps are found more frequently on the nipple than the areola. They are pedunculated dry lesions resembling the skin tags seen elsewhere in the body (Figure 14.4).

Neurofibromas occurring at this site may also be pedunculated. They are readily treated by local excision and do not recur.

ECZEMA

There are many causes of red, oozing and crusted nipples recognized by dermatologists, including psoriasis, seborrhoeic dermatitis, contact dermatitis, neurodermatitis and atopic dermatitis. It is particularly common in atopic patients. Scabies and chronic friction require exclusion. Chronic infection, e.g. with *Staphylococcus aureus* or candida, can persist in the moist, traumatized conditions of breastfeeding and can give rise to unusual clinical and histological appearances.[19]

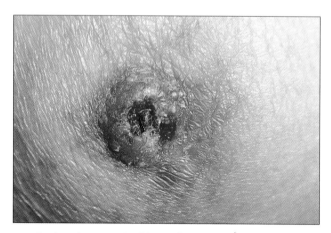

14.2 Erosive adenomatosis of the nipple.

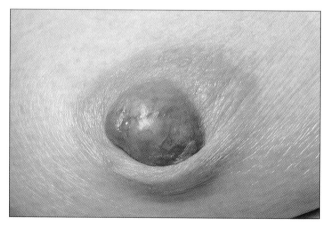

14.3 A large benign papilloma of the terminal duct, distending the nipple of an elderly woman.

Eczema may occur in a form localized mainly or completely to the nipple and areola (Figures 14.5 and 14.6) and requires to be distinguished from the non-eczema conditions of Paget's disease and erosive adenomatosis which also have an eczematous appearance.

Paget's disease and eczema can usually be differentiated on clinical grounds (Table 14.1).

In spite of this, Paget's disease is still often neglected because of an erroneous diagnosis of eczema. It is important to think of Paget's disease in every inflammatory condition of the nipple and areola and to be aware of the range of appearances of Paget's disease (Figures 14.7 and 14.8).

Even so, biopsy in all cases is the safest course to follow. The typical Paget cells (Figure 14.9) usually allow the pathologist to make the diagnosis without difficulty.

Table 14.1 Clinical features of eczema of the nipple and Paget's disease

Eczema	Paget's disease
Usually bilateral	Unilateral
Intermittent history, with rapid evolution	Continuous history with slow steady progression
Moist	Moist or dry
Indefinite edge	Irregular but definite edge
Nipple may be spared	Nipple always involved and disappears in advanced cases
Itching common	Itching common

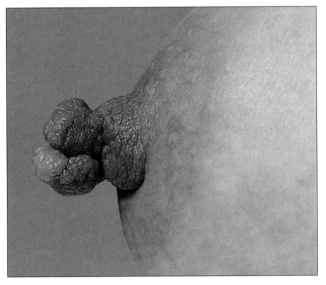

14.4 Benign pedunculated fibroepithelial polyp.

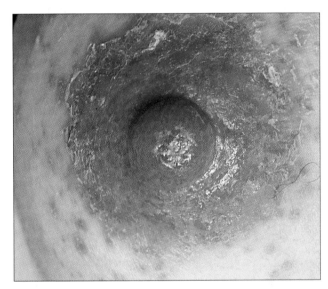

14.5 Eczema of the nipple and areola – note the uniform involvement.

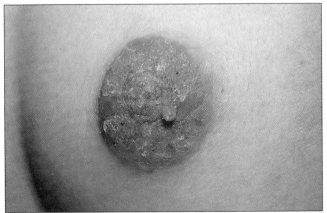

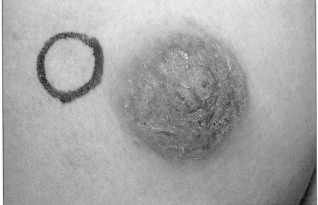

14.6 Eczema of both areolae, with an unrelated benign cyst in the right breast.

In patients with eczema of the nipple and areola, the condition is bilateral and in many patients there is evidence of eczema elsewhere. When this is not the case, eczema is usually symmetrical and does not extend beyond the areola (see Figure 14.6). The possibility of an artefactual syndrome (see Chapter 17) should not be overlooked.

Treatment in cases of eczema follows the same guidelines as eczema elsewhere in the body.

Other general skin conditions may cause concern when the first, or only, manifestation of the condition occurs on the nipple or areola. Figure 14.10 shows a patient with vitiligo confined to the areola who showed such concern.

LEIOMYOMA

Leiomyoma of the nipple is surprisingly uncommon in view of the large quantities of smooth muscle present. When it occurs it appears as a smooth round lump, obviously within the skin of the areola or nipple. It can occur at any age, is usually about 6–7 mm in diameter and may have been present for some years. Haagensen[1] distinguishes between this superficial leiomyoma, arising in the smooth muscle of the nipple and areola, and deep leiomyoma which arises from smooth muscle associated with blood vessels. Both are adequately treated by local excision.

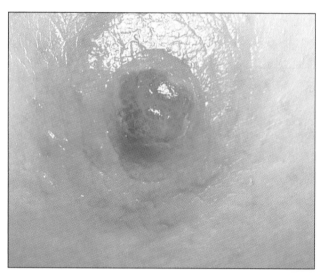

14.7 The moist, erosive form of early Paget's disease.

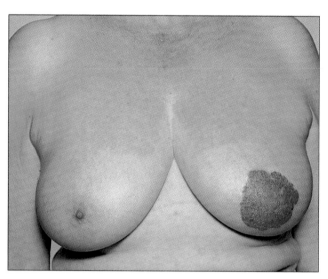

14.8 More advanced, 'dry' form of Paget's disease. The nipple is disappearing.

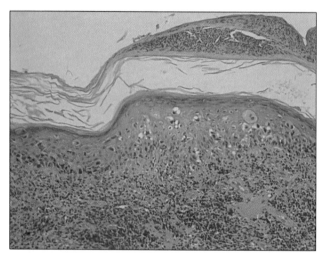

14.9 Typical Paget cells, large pale vacuolated cells distributed along the squamous epithelium of the nipple.

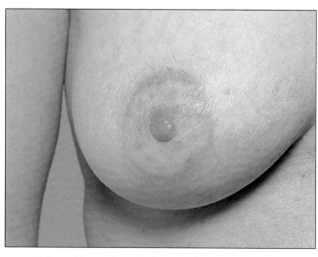

14.10 Vitiligo of the nipple as the first manifestation of the condition.

TRAUMATIC LESIONS

The nipple is occasionally the site of trauma and the condition of jogger's nipple is well recognized.[20] This lesion is presumably the result of constant friction of an unprotected warm and moist nipple on ill-fitting clothing. It is sometimes severe enough to produce bleeding. Related conditions are cyclist's nipple[21] which appears to be a cold injury with the subsequent pain lasting for several days, and tassle dancer's nipple;[22] the rings placed in the nipple may produce unusual radiological artefacts.[23] Artefactual trauma of the nipple is also seen occasionally (see Chapter 17).

NIPPLE PAIN

Patients around the menopause often describe various sensations of irritation, pricking and burning in the nipple region. They are usually irritating rather than of greater severity. No clear aetiological basis has been put forward; the most likely explanation relates to the histological periductal inflammatory changes regarded as part of the normal involutional process. In favour of this explanation is the fact that these sensations may accompany the circular nipple retraction also seen in the perimenopausal period. Another possible explanation is hormonal imbalance associated with declining ovarian function, since similar nipple sensations may be experienced with hormone administration. Paget's disease must also be carefully excluded, since itch, pricking and irritation are commonly experienced in the early phase of this condition.

Raynaud's phenomenon

Raynaud's phenomenon has also been described in the breast. It is probably more common than is usually recognized. In one series from New Zealand, it was thought that up to 1 in 20 pregnant women had symptoms suggestive of Raynaud's phenomenon during cold weather.[24] The changes typically occur in lactating women after or between feeding.[25]

Lawlor-Smith and Lawlor-Smith[26] have described five patients with Raynaud's phenomenon affecting the nipple presenting to an Australian general practice in a 2-year period. All patients experienced severe pain and nipple changes; in three the classical triphasic response of colour change was exhibited. In two patients symptoms antedated their first pregnancy. Strangely, affection of the nipples does not seem to be associated with the typical changes in the extremities, questioning whether or not it is the same condition.

The nipple necrosis described after vasopressin is also presumably due to vascular spasm.[27]

Professor N O'Higgins (personal communication, Dublin) has provided details of a 53-year-old patient who had Raynaud-like changes that were subsequently shown to be due to pagetoid infiltration by intraduct cancer. The patient described sudden episodic pain in the nipple associated with sequential white and bluish-purple colour changes. The areolar glands usually became prominent and the nipple partially inverted. The symptoms recurred randomly day or night, and were not related to ambient temperature.

Postsurgical pain

It is now well recognized that CRPS may affect parts of the body other than the limbs, where it has long been recognized as a reflex sympathetic dystrophy of the causalgia type. Similar changes have been reported in the breast, especially the nipple area after surgery.

We have seen such a case after major duct excision, which was related to cold. Even though the patient was warmly clothed, the nipples were subjectively intensely cold and objectively so to examination. The attacks gradually abated over a period of 4–5 years.

A case following breast reduction surgery has recently been reported.[28] The 27-year-old patient had pain, swelling, epidermal scaling and temperature changes persisting for a year. Liquid crystal thermography scanning confirmed a hypothermic region in the breast. Intravenous phentolamine gave temporary relief, with long-term relief provided by stellate ganglion blockade.

Recent interest in this condition has led to consensus statements on classification and taxonomy.[29]

Pain during breastfeeding

Pain is common during breastfeeding, especially following the first pregnancy. The various causes are well recognized, but the importance of candida infection as a cause is not always appreciated. The relationship of candida infection to persistent nipple pain (burning in nature and radiating to the breast) has recently been investigated by Amir et al.[30] Microbiological assessment (culture of nipple and baby's mouth, and of expressed breast milk) was carried out in 61 lactating women with breast pain, 64 women without breast pain and 31 non-lactating women. Candida was grown from 19% of women with breast pain, but only 3% of those without. Nipples affected by candida did not have the usual appearance of thrush elsewhere, but looked mildly inflamed and were tender to touch. Candida infection was associated with recent use of antibiotics (usually for mastitis), with candida in the baby's mouth, and with use of a dummy. Treatment was with topical miconazole oral gel to nipple and baby's mouth and oral nystatin.

Staph. aureus was associated with breast pain, and independently with cracked nipple. Neither organism was grown from non-lactating women.

NIPPLE DISEASE AND HIV INFECTION

Nipple disease is very common among African HIV-positive women suckling HIV-positive infants, and the status of the infant is the most important determinant of nipple disease in the mother.[31] Kambarami and Kowo reported that

31% of such mothers had nipple disease, 22% eczema, 11% cracked nipples and 11% painful nipples.[31]

MONTGOMERY'S GLANDS

Montgomery, an Irish obstetrician, in 1837 gave a classic description of the changes in the areolar tubercles occurring during pregnancy. These structures, which now bear his name, had in fact been described by Morgagni in 1719. There are three types of gland in the areola: (1) apocrine sweat glands; (2) modified sebaceous glands; and (3) rudimentary mammary glands.

There is clear evidence that aprocrine sweat glands are a normal finding in the areolar skin.[32] The modified sebaceous glands which lie under the tubercles of Montgomery are similar to sebaceous glands elsewhere, except that they are associated with a lactiferous duct extending from a more deeply placed mammary gland.[33] The rudimentary mammary glands and the sebaceous glands both undergo changes during pregnancy which lead to typical changes in the tubercle described by Montgomery. The position and relative sizes of these glands are depicted in Figure 14.11.

In addition to the areolar glands, there are dermal sebaceous glands of the nipple and occasional deep ectopic sebaceous glands which open into the main breast ducts. These are discussed below and in Chapter 11 in relation to the aetiology of mammary duct fistula.

When the detailed anatomy of the glandular components of Montgomery's tubercles is considered, the clinical problems of retention cysts (Figure 14.12) and milk-like discharge are not surprising.

It is perhaps more surprising that discharge from the tubercles is as rare as it seems to be in the literature.[34] Infection of the tubercles may mimic subareolar abscess associated with DE and the persisting lesion suggests a mammary duct fistula, although it will present on the areola rather than at the periphery of the areola as occurs with mammary duct fistula.

Histological sectioning of the areola in mature females shows that the mammary elements of Montgomery's glands are subject to many of the conditions affecting the mamma, including hyperplasia, cyst formation, periductal fibrosis and apocrine metaplasia.[33]

Bleeding from Montgomery glands is occasionally seen in young girls (Figure 14.13) and may be confused with bleeding from the nipple.

No obvious cause is usually found on biopsy and the bleeding may be due to trauma.

SEBACEOUS CYST OF THE NIPPLE

This rare condition presents as a painless lump palpable immediately below and attached to the nipple (Figure 14.14).

Because this lies deeper than the dermal sebaceous glands

of the nipple, its origin can be explained by the findings of Patey and Thackray[35] that ectopic sebaceous glands may occasionally be found deep in the nipple, opening into the terminal portion of the duct. It is satisfactorily treated by excision. However, this is obviously a more extensive operation than that necessary for a retention cyst of the dermal sebaceous glands. Some authors have considered that all mammary duct fistulas arise on the basis of infection of these

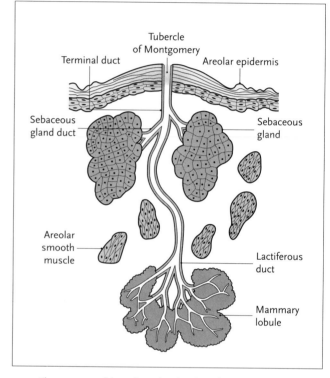

14.11 The anatomy of the subareolar glands. (After Smith *et al.*[13])

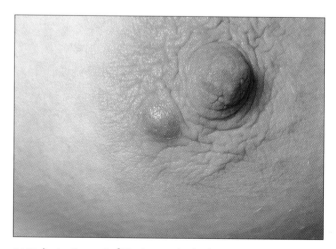

14.12 A retention cyst of Montgomery's gland.

deep sebaceous glands. However, in our experience, the two conditions are quite separate. Sebaceous glands lie more centrally and when infected give a local juxta-nipple mass, not a mass at the edge of the areola, as is seen with recurrent subareolar abscess secondary to mammary duct fistula.

The increasing use of nipple rings is likely to be associated with occasional complications such as dermoid inclusion cysts and infection.[36]

VIRAL INFECTIONS

Molluscum contagiosum occasionally occurs in the skin of the nipple. It produces a discrete lump which may ulcerate,[1]

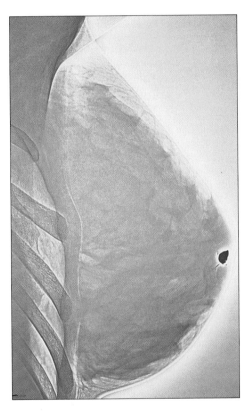

14.13 Microinjection of a subareolar gland which presented with bleeding from the areola.

and is readily recognized on histopathology. It is uncommon,[37] which is perhaps surprising as this pox virus is usually transmitted sexually. Herpes virus lesions[38] and genital warts of the nipple (condyloma acuminatum)[39] are also seen occasionally.

HIDRADENITIS SUPPURATIVA OF THE AREOLA

The areola is one of the classical sites for hidradenitis in most descriptions of the disease, presumably because apocrine-like sweat glands are found there. Despite a very large experience of hidradenitis, including many cases involving the breast, we have not seen a single case involving the areola, nor have we seen a credible description of one. If it occurs, it must be exceedingly rare. It is likely that this is one of those conditions copied faithfully from text to text, with no one noticing that they have not seen a case. The original description probably derives from misdiagnosis of a mammary duct fistula. Mammary hidradenitis suppurativa is described in Chapter 17.

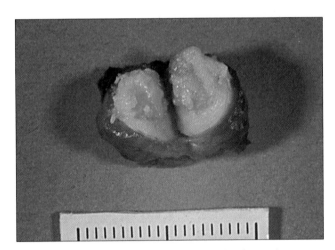

14.14 A sebaceous cyst presenting as a lump within the nipple – treated by conservative enucleation.

REFERENCES

1. Haagensen CD. *Disease of the Breast*, 3rd edn. Philadelphia: WB Saunders, 1986.

2. Koernecke IA. An anatomical study of the mammary gland twenty four hours post-partum. *American Journal of Obstetric Gynecology* 1934; **27**: 584–592.

3. Moffatt DF & Going JJ. Three dimensional anatomy of complete duct systems in human breast – pathological and developmental implications. *Journal of Clinical Pathology* 1996; **49**: 48–52.

4. Alexander JM & Campbell MJ. Prevalence of inverted and non-protractile nipples in antenatal women who intend to breast feed. *Breast* 1997; **5**: 88–89.

5. Alexander JM, Grant AM & Campbell MJ. Randomised controlled trial of breast shells and Hoffman's exercises for inverted and non-protractile nipples. *British Medical Journal* 1992; **304**: 1030–1032.

6. Bryant T. On the diagnostic value of the retracted nipple as a symptom of breast disease. *British Medical Journal* 1866; **2**: 635–637.

7. Gans B. Breast and nipple pain in early stages of lactation. *British Medical Journal* 1958; **2**: 830–832.

8. Gunther M. Sore nipples. Causes and prevention. *Lancet* 1945; **ii**: 590–593.

9. Waller H. The early failure of breast feeding. A clinical study of its causes and their prevention. *Archives of Disease in Childhood* 1946; **21**: 1–12.

10. Alpsoy E, Yilmaz E & Aykol A. Hyperkeratosis of the nipple: report of two cases. *Journal of Dermatology* 1997; **24**: 43–45.

11. Azzopardi JG. *Problems in Breast Pathology*. London: WB Saunders, 1979.

12. Civatte J, Restout S & Delomenie D-C. Adenomatose erosive sur mamelon surnumeraire. *Annals Dermatologie et Venerologie* 1977; **104**: 777–779.

13. Perzin KH & Lattes R. Papillary adenoma of the nipple (florid papillomatosis, adenoma, adenomatosis). *Cancer* 1972; **29**: 996–1009.

14. Taylor HB & Robertson AG. Adenomas of the nipple. *Cancer* 1965; **18**: 995–1002.

15. Pinto RGW & Mandreker S. Fine needle aspiration cytology of adenoma of the nipple: a case report. *Acta Cytologica* 1996; **40**: 789–791.

16. Blamey RW (ed.) *Complications of Breast Surgery*. London: Baillière Tindall, 1986.

17. Rosen PP. Syringomatous adenoma of the nipple. *American Journal of Surgical Pathology* 1983; **7**: 739–745.

18. Hutchinson J. Polypoid outgrowths of the nipple areola. *Archives of Surgery, London* 1897; 37–39.

19. Paslin D. *Staphylococcus aureus* induction of inflammatory plaques of nipples and areolae. *American Academy of Dermatology* 1989; **20**: 932–934.

20. Levit F. Jogger's nipples. *New England Journal of Medicine* 1977; **297**: 1197.

21. Powell B. Bicyclist's nipples. *Journal of the American Medical Association* 1982; **249**: 2457.

22. Collins REC. Breast disease associated with tassle dancing. *British Medical Journal* 1981; **283**: 1660.

23. Healey T. Nipple piercings – unusual artefacts. *Radiography* 1979; **45**: 164–165.

24. Hood L. Raynaud's phenomenon of the nipple. *New Zealand Medical Journal* 1983; **84**: 294–295.

25. Gunther M. *Infant Feeding*. London: Methuen, 1972.

26. Lawlor-Smith L & Lawlor-Smith C. Vasospasm of the nipple – a manifestation of Raynaud's phenomenon: case reports. *British Medical Journal* 1997; **314**: 644–645.

27. Reddy KR, Iskandarani M, Jeffers L & Schiff FR. Bilateral nipple necrosis after vasopressin therapy. *Archives of Internal Medicine* 1984; **144**: 835–836.

28. Papay FA, Verghese A, Stanton-Hicks M & Zins T. Complex regional pain syndrome of the breast in a patient after breast reduction. *Annals of Plastic Surgery* 1997; **39**: 347–352.

29. Stanton-Hicks M, Janig W, Hassenbusch S *et al.* Reflex sympathetic dystrophy: changing concepts and taxonomy. *Pain* 1995; **63**: 127–133.

30. Amir LH, Garland SM, Dennerstein L & Farish SJ. *Candida albicans*: Is it associated with nipple pain in lactating women? *Gynecologic and Obstetric Investigation* 1996; **41**: 30–34.

31. Kambarami RA & Kowo H. The prevalence of nipple disease among breast feeding mothers of HIV sero-positive infants. *Central African Journal of Medicine* 1997; **43**: 20–22.

32. Craigmyle MBL. *The Aprocrine Glands and the Breast*. Chichester: John Wiley & Sons, 1984.

33. Smith DM, Peters TG & Donegan WL. Montgomery's areolar tubercle. A light microscopic study. *Archives of Pathology and Laboratory Medicine* 1982; **106**: 60–63.

34. Heyman RB & Rauch JL. Areolar gland discharge in adolescent females. *Journal of Adolescent Health Care* 1983; **4**: 285–286.

35. Patey DH & Thackray AC. Pathology and the treatment of mammary duct fistula. *Lancet* 1958; **ii**: 871–873.

36. Fiumara NJ & Capek M. The brustwarze, or nipple ring. *Sexually Transmitted Disease* 1983; **9**: 138–139.

37. Carrahlo G. Molluscum contagiosum in a lesion adjacent to the nipple. Report of a case. *Acta Cytologica (Baltimore)* 1974; **18**: 532–534.

38. Quinn PT & Lofberg JV. Maternal herpetic breast infection: Another hazard of neonatal Herpes Simplex. *Medical Journal of Australia* 1978; **2**: 411–412.

39. Wood C. Condyloma accuminatum of the nipple. *Journal of Cutaneous Pathology* 1978; **5**: 88–89.

Chapter 15

Congenital and growth disorders

KEY POINTS AND NEW DEVELOPMENTS

1. Congenital abnormalities of the breast, relating mainly to absence, hypoplasia or ectopia, are sometimes part of wider congenital syndromes, with particular tendency to affect the urinary tract or limb girdles.
2. It is now recognized that the fetal 'milk line' is not as extensive in humans as in some animals, so most ectopic tissue is found between the axilla and epigastrium.
3. Axillary accessory breasts can be subject to all varieties of pathology seen in the breast proper, so axillary masses should be assessed individually, as well as in association with any breast mass.

4. Breast hypertrophy conforms to the ANDI concept, and can be loosely categorized as normal (the larger end of the normal spectrum), aberration (when breast weight is sufficient to cause physical symptoms as well as embarrassment) and disease (the rapid and extreme enlargement of gigantomastia, requiring urgent intervention).
5. Gigantomastia shows characteristic pathology, including excess ducts and stroma with a paucity of lobules, oestrogen receptor negative but progesterone receptor positive, but the aetiology remains obscure and treatment unsatisfactory.

The breast, like other physical features, exhibits a wide range of appearances. There is variation in size, shape and, to some extent, position. The borderline of what is socially and cosmetically acceptable is one of perception because most variants retain normal function. Other conditions show a greater deviation from normal, arising on a congenital basis, or as an aberration of development of the breast during reproductive life. Those aspects of these conditions related to general principles of breast development, aetiology and pathophysiology are dealt with in this chapter. The details of management, particularly those involving reconstructive and cosmetic surgery, are dealt with in Chapter 21.

DEVELOPMENTAL ANOMALIES

These may be unilateral or bilateral, involve either nipple or breast or both, and be seen as absent, hypoplastic, supernumerary or ectopic structures. They may occur as isolated abnormalities, but may also be associated with a variety of other developmental abnormalities, particularly of the upper limb and urinary tract. Hypertrophy of the breast is also considered in this chapter, as an aberration of growth of uncertain aetiology, with only a few known to have an underlying genetic component.

The development of the breast has been described in Chapter 2. The fetal mammalian milk line has classically been considered to run from the base of the upper limb bud to the base of the lower limb bud, but the validity of this theory in humans is now challenged (see Chapter 2). In most adult mammals, breast tissue is confined to this milk line but, in some, breast tissue is found in other sites: either the milk line is more extensive or breast tissue migrates. Examples of these ectopic sites are the labia in whales and dolphins, the scapular region in nutria, abdominal midline in the possum, dorsal thigh in the viscaccia, and the acromium in a species of lemur. The occurrence of breast-like structures or pathology in these areas, along or outwith the milk line, has been regarded as evidence of embryological remnants of a human axilla–groin milk line. However, true congenital lesions in the human are overwhelmingly confined to the axillo-pectoral region.

Polythelia and supernumerary nipples
Some authors use these terms synonymously; others reserve polythelia for those examples of more than one nipple appearing on the same breast mound.[1] We see no benefit in the distinction and regard the terms as interchangeable.

Supernumerary nipples may occur in association with accessory glandular breast tissue or more commonly occur alone. This condition is as common in men as in women, the extra nipples usually appearing along the upper part of the 'milk line'.

The reported incidence of supernumerary nipples varies greatly in the literature. The condition is usually considered to be more common in Oriental populations.[2] Méhes[3] screened 4000 neonates in Hungary and found an incidence

of polythelia of only 0.2% and described an association with renal abnormalities. This association is supported by the findings of another study which found an incidence of supernumerary nipples in 16% of patients with end-stage renal failure, but only 2% of control patients.[4] Two other studies have failed to confirm the findings. In one study of 1691 births, an incidence of 2.5% supernumerary nipples was found.[5] Robertson *et al.*[6] found an incidence of 1.2% in 2875 black children with no evidence of associated renal anomalies.

The balance of evidence suggests that supernumerary nipples are common (1–2%) and associated congenital abnormalities rare.[7] However, the associations and classifications of congenital abnormalities linking breast/nipple, urinary tract and limbs are becoming more complex, and should be borne in mind when any of the abnormalities are found in the newborn. The subject has recently been reviewed.[8]

Extra nipples are most commonly found on the lower part of the breast, chest wall and upper abdomen just below the rib margin and are often mistaken for naevi (Figure 15.1).

No treatment is required for this condition except when it is accompanied by active breast tissue or if the patient finds it cosmetically unacceptable.

Athelia
Absence of the nipple is an extremely rare event and usually is associated with absence of the breast. Occasional examples of imperforate nipple have been reported as a cause of failure to lactate with an engorged breast. It is difficult to be certain that these obstructed nipples were not secondary to trauma such as burns.

Nipple inversion
Nipple inversion is a common finding. There are three main causes: congenital, periductal inflammation and tumour infiltration. The last of these is beyond the scope of this book but in our series represents only a small percentage of observed nipple retraction.

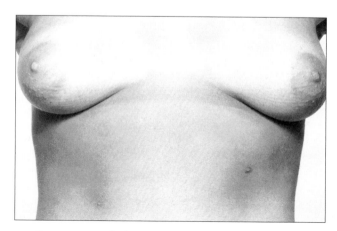

15.1 Supernumerary nipples.

The distinction between inversion and retraction is rather arbitrary: we use inversion to describe the nipple that did not protrude at the time of adolescent development and retraction for those cases in which a previously everted nipple is affected by an underlying pathological process.

Congenital

During fetal life, the nipple is represented by a central depression which persists after birth until development of the underlying breast produces elevation of the areola. Subsequent retraction of the surrounding smooth muscle leads to flattening of the mound and protrusion of the nipple.[9]

Schwager et al.,[10] in their study of 339 breasts, found six with inversion of the nipple (a prevalence of 1.8%). There was no qualitative difference in the constituents of the areola, mammary ducts, smooth muscle or collagen, but there was a deficiency in the supporting stroma immediately behind the nipple. An alternative view is to regard the inversion as due to the failure of the smooth muscle bundles of Sappy (circular) and Myerholtz (radial) to relax.[11] In any event it appears that inversion is best regarded as failure of normal eversion to occur. In the established case, the ducts are shortened and deeply attached, while the normally tough musculo-fibro-collagenous tissue behind the nipple is replaced by a potential hollow cavity into which the nipple retracts.

The findings are usually bilateral, but often to different degrees, and it is not rare to find one side completely inverted and the other normal. The true incidence of congenital nipple inversion is hard to determine because such women are more disposed to periductal inflammation, the second most common cause of nipple inversion.

Problems related to inverted nipples are functional (associated with breastfeeding) and cosmetic.

Inverted nipples and breastfeeding

The problems associated with breastfeeding have been reviewed by Inch.[12] Waller[13] found that nearly 40% of young women in their first pregnancy had at least a minor degree of failure of normal protrusion of the nipple, but maintained that this should not be considered a contraindication to breastfeeding, as so many maintain. He recommended a 'pinch test' to assess protrusion, and patients failing this test were given a glass (Woolwich) shield to wear during pregnancy, the purpose of which was gradually to stretch and loosen the non-protractile nipple. Of patients with poorly protractile nipples treated in this way, only 44% were deemed to have breastfed successfully.

In contrast, Hytten[14] found that only 14% of 2461 primiparae had unsatisfactory nipples, and only 16% of these had breastfeeding problems as a direct result. Of those with normal nipples, 3.5% had similar problems. Thus, although antenatal examination of the nipples might have some predictive value, most patients with poor nipples will have no related problems with breastfeeding.[15]

These findings may be explained by cineradiographic[16] and ultrasound studies[17] of breastfeeding, which show that the nipple itself plays a relatively small part in the anatomical aspects of suckling. The infant makes a 'teat' from the surrounding breast tissue as well as the nipple, in a ratio of about 3:1. Thus mothers with inverted nipples should be encouraged to ensure that the baby has an adequate mouthful of breast to form the teat, and be reassured that the contribution of the nipple is relatively small. Correct positioning during feeding is perhaps the most important factor and the patient should be given skilled help from a midwife before starting to breastfeed.

Inverted nipples and cosmesis

Treatment consists of reassurance that there is no serious underlying disease and, when the cosmetic defect is severe (or the patient very concerned about it), consideration of surgical correction. An added problem can arise with malodour, if the inversion interferes with cleansing, giving retained secretions, although this is more commonly seen in retraction due to duct ectasia (DE) in older women.

It is said that inversion can be improved by repeated massage, although there are few data from controlled studies to support this. In severe cases surgical correction may be requested. In general, a procedure involving excision of the shortened ducts, with core nipple excision if there is a persisting tendency to reinversion (as described for DE in Chapter 20), gives good long-term results, but is much too radical a procedure to be appropriate for most young girls.

Pitangay[11] has described a procedure of dividing the muscle bundles without damaging the lactiferous tissues – an important consideration in young women who may still wish to feed their children. However, the large number of procedures described for congenital inverted nipple suggest that none of them is ideal. There is considerable doubt about the efficacy of procedures which do not divide the ducts, although new procedures continue to be recommended. A recent technique using a cartilage graft claims to give no recurrence at 5 years.[18] Strombeck reported a 23% recurrence rate in his own unit, even after completely dividing the ducts.[19] The uncertain long-term outcome of any lesser procedure should be explained to the patient if surgery is advised. Our own views on surgical management are given in Chapter 20.

Retracted nipples following periductal inflammation

Periductal inflammation is discussed more fully elsewhere. While congenital inversion predisposes to inflammatory complications of periductal mastitis, and the associated secondary nipple retraction may give rise to problems of cosmesis, management needs to be directed towards the inflammatory process, and so is dealt with in Chapters 11, 14 and 20.

Supernumerary breasts (accessory breasts, axillary breasts)

The incidence of supernumerary breasts, defined as structures which produce milk under appropriate hormonal influences, remains uncertain although the condition has been recorded since antiquity. Statues of both Artemesia and Diana of Ephesus represent these ancients as having supernumerary breasts. Fitzwilliams[1] gave a good account of many of the earlier, and often colourful, descriptions. Darwin was clearly aware of the existence of polymastia and used the condition as an illustration of an atavistic phenomenon.[2] Most accessory breasts develop along the milk line, and of these the great majority occur in the axilla. Indeed, we have not seen one occurring outside the axillo-pectoral area.

Ectopic milk-producing structures have been described at all the ectopic sites that occur in the mammals described above, but the commoner examples used to justify an extensive milk line in humans, such as mammary-like tumours of the groin and labia, are now recognized to arise in glands (mammary-like glands) related to eccrine sweat glands occurring in that region. Thus the widely quoted concept of a milk line extending to the groin in humans is now questioned.[20] Supernumerary breasts may rarely be found anywhere on the body, outside the so-called milk line. An example has been reported in the perineum,[21] and similar examples have been found in the middle of the back.

The commonest site of accessory breasts is the axilla. It is remarkable how often these remain unnoticed until the second or third pregnancy (Figure 15.2).

These accessory glands do not always have nipples and may be quite troublesome during pregnancy and lactation. It is presumably because of hormonal stimulation that accessory breasts are more frequently recorded in women than in men (there being no embryological reason to suppose a difference).

The most important aspect of axillary breasts, apart from the discomfort associated with pregnancy and lactation, arises from the fact that axillary breasts are subject to all the pathological processes seen in the breast, and as such can give rise to diagnostic errors. An example is the occurrence of nodularity of ANDI (fibroadenosis) in an accessory breast suggesting metastatic lymph nodes in a patient with breast cancer.[22] Conditions as diverse as fibromatosis, phyllodes tumour and primary cancer have been described. This reinforces the need for histological diagnosis of axillary as well as breast lesions and considerable accuracy can be achieved in cytological assessment of lesions in axillary breast tissue.[23]

Treatment is only indicated if the accessory breast proves troublesome to the patient, the treatment then being surgical excision. Many examples of accessory breast remain undiagnosed until removed with a clinical diagnosis of lipoma which is found to contain mammary tissue.

Accessory breast tissue may be isolated or may be connected to an accessory nipple. In the former case, the breast will involute soon after parturition, in the latter an active secreting gland may produce sufficient milk to sustain the infant.

Amastia and hypoplasia

Amastia is a rare condition and is presumably due to failure of the milk line to develop, or to complete its involution. It is not surprising that such an obvious abnormality was recorded in biblical times (Song of Solomon, viii 8). The condition is quite uncommon, however, and is usually unilateral. The rare bilateral cases may show an autosomal dominant pattern of inheritance.[24] Some of the cases have absence of the pectoral muscles and associated syndactyly (a condition known as Poland's syndrome following his description in 1841). In spite of its popular eponym, this condition was apparently first described in 1839 by Floriep. The terminology has been challenged and, although Ravitch[25] has argued that the term should be abandoned, descriptions of Poland's syndrome persist. The familial nature of this condition was first remarked upon in 1894 by Whyte and, more recently, it has been established that it is transmitted as an autosomal dominant feature.[24]

Mild, partial forms of Poland's syndrome are commoner than the full picture, and frequently go undiagnosed when they consist only of breast asymmetry and a horizontal anterior axillary fold due to partial absence of the pectoralis muscle (Figure 15.3).[26]

Poland's syndrome is the best known of a number of inherited disorders of breast development, most of which are extremely rare. The Pallister ulnar-mammary syndrome (UMS) is an example; the common manifestations of a very varied clinical picture include limb deficiencies and failure of breast development. A description of 33 members from a six-generation kindred has recently been published, and the associated gene defect mapped.[27]

Congenital absence of the breast is as common in boys as in girls but its exact incidence is unknown.

Hypoplastic breasts of a lesser degree are not uncommon and there is some evidence of an association with mitral valve prolapse. Patients attending for breast augmentation have a higher incidence of mitral valve prolapse; patients with a diagnosis of mitral valve prolapse have been found to have smaller breasts than controls, the putative defect occurring during a time of mesenchymal development in the sixth week.[28]

Asymmetry

Minor degrees of breast asymmetry are very common and the patient may be reassured. When the discrepancy is great (Figure 15.4), surgical correction may be indicated to equalize the breasts.

Augmentation of the smaller breast, reduction of the larger breast, or both procedures, may be required to obtain a satisfactory result.

More severe cases may be partially expressed examples of Poland's syndrome or follow trauma (usually burns or surgery) in childhood when the breast bud is damaged.

Thoracotomy by the anterolateral or posterolateral route in prepubertal girls may result in ipsilateral hypoplasia of moderate degree and the thoracotomy technique should be modified appropriately to avoid this.[29]

Tubular breasts (trunk breast)

This is a distressing developmental abnormality where the areola is of excessive size relative to the rest of the breast.[30] Most of the spectrum lies within a normal or acceptable degree, but in severe examples the breast is elongated from a narrow base to take a sausage-shaped contour, with a disproportionately large and protuberant areola and nipple. The breast parenchyma may herniate into the large areola. Management requires skilled plastic surgery; a standard augmentation procedure merely accentuates the protrusion of the narrow breast (see Chapter 21). Ribiero and colleagues have recently reported a new approach.[31]

Fusion of the breasts

There is a wide variation of normality in the placing of the breasts on the chest wall. With one extreme, the breasts are fused in the midline (Figure 15.5). This can cause difficulty and discomfort with clothing, and we have found it worth while separating the breasts by the simple plastic procedure shown in Figure 15.6.

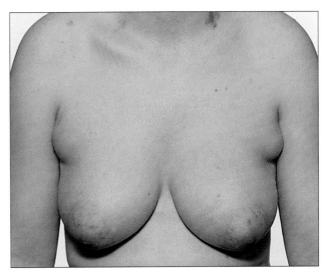

15.2 Accessory (axillary) breasts. First noticed at time of lactation following first pregnancy.

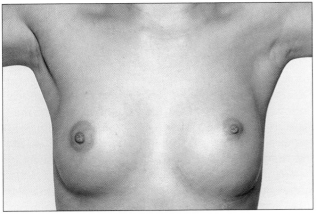

15.3 Partial degree of Poland's syndrome (left), with a horizontal axillary fold due to hypoplasia of pectoral muscles, and asymmetry of nipple and areola.

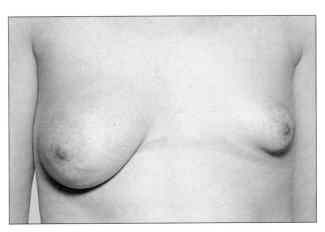

15.4 Marked asymmetry of breasts for which plastic surgery is indicated.

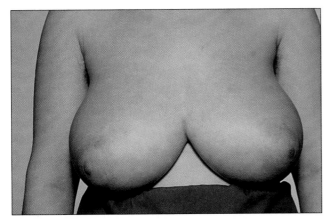

15.5 Fused breasts.

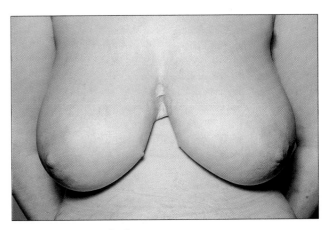

5.6 Postoperative result of patient in Figure 15.5.

PREMATURE BREAST DEVELOPMENT

An otherwise normal breast may enlarge for no discernible reason at several stages in childhood and adolescence. This excludes those cases due to excessive hormone production in childhood, e.g. from tumours, and in none of the conditions described below has any abnormality of circulating hormones been demonstrated.

Neonatal enlargement

Reference has already been made to neonatal hyperplasia in Chapter 2. It is normal to have some palpable breast tissue at birth and for this to disappear by the age of 6 months, although it tends to remain longer in girls than boys.[32]

Prepubertal (premature) thelarche

Premature breast development (thelarche) may occur as an isolated occurrence, usually a constitutional deviation from normal, or as a part of precocious puberty. This is defined as occurring before the age of 8 years in girls, since it is not uncommon to see breast development at about this age. This is often unilateral. It is of no significance in the absence of other signs of precocious puberty and in 50% of cases it is the first sign of early puberty.[33]

The clinical appearances are of a firm discoid lesion behind the nipple, not unlike that found in the pubertal boy with gynaecomastia. The importance of the lesion is in recognizing it for what it is – normal breast tissue! Surgical removal of the mass is a disaster because it represents the whole of the developing breast. Removal will result in secondary amastia on the affected side. In a review of the natural history of this condition in 46 cases, 32% regressed completely over a 2-year period, 57% remained unchanged and 11% underwent progressive enlargement.[34]

Breast development before the age of 8 years requires full endocrine assessment, although in most cases no cause can be discovered and the prognosis is benign.[35]

Verroti reported a long-term follow-up of 46 girls to see if those with isolated thelarche could be differentiated from those who would develop the full process of precocious puberty.[36] Endocrine assessment gave similar results in the two groups, but the age of onset was important; those showing thelarche between the age of 2 and 8 years were more likely to develop precocious puberty, while breast development before the age of 2 was more likely to regress.

Precocious breast development is one of the greatest causes of psychological upset in these girls. However, one-third can expect to have reversion of breast development to normal or near normal with treatment such as the long-acting GnRH agonist triptorelin.[37]

Pubertal asymmetry

The breasts do not always develop synchronously and parents sometimes seek advice about a unilateral lump. The same considerations apply to this condition as to the prepubertal variety – biopsy and excision must be avoided. Asynchronous development is not uncommon in normal pubescent girls.

HYPERTROPHIC ABNORMALITIES OF THE BREAST

Large breasts range across a wide spectrum, from the 'well-endowed' who may consider their breasts a boon or an embarrassment depending on their individual outlook, through a size where discomfort, back and neck pain and interference with normal activities are added to embarrassment, to extreme enlargement (usually of sudden onset and rapid progression) where breast size may be life-threatening through ulceration and bleeding. This division fits well into the ANDI concept, the first being normal, the second an aberration and the third, disease (see Chapter 4).

The three degrees are also useful with regard to management, following the general approach to benign processes fitting the ANDI concept. Surgery should be approached with reluctance in the first group, where there is a high chance that the patient will consider the scarring and any complications as a poor exchange; in the second surgery may be welcomed because of improvement in physical symptoms as well as relief from embarrassment; and surgery is imperative in the third group, at least until an effective pharmacological control becomes available.

Equally, it is useful to use precise nomenclature for the three groups, even though they merge and overlap: large breasts for the first, hypertrophy (virginal, gravid or involutional) for the second, and gigantomastia for the third. The retention of such an inelegant term as gigantomastia is justified by the necessity to recognize this as a specific condition which may require urgent and radical treatment.

Division into the three groups is a subjective exercise, although objective guidelines have been proposed by Lalardrie and Jouglard, based on frontal projection and height of the breast (Table 15.1).[38]

Clearly such measurements must be assessed in relation to general habitus, obesity and the patient's own perception. Changes in body weight tend to be reflected in the breasts. Strombeck has calculated that a gain of 1 kg of body weight gives 20 g enlargement of each breast, so

Table 15.1 Objective assessment of breast size	
1. Ideal	250–300 cc
2. Moderate hypertrophy	400–600 cc
3. Rather significant	600–800 cc
4. Significant	800–1000 cc
5. Gigantomastia	> 1500 cc
Adapted from Lalardrie and Jouglard.[38]	

that a weight gain of 7–8 kg is equivalent to prostheses of 150 g.[19]

The grosser degrees of hypertrophy occur most commonly in young adolescents, less commonly during pregnancy, and least commonly as an involutional phenomenon. The latter is probably a different condition, with a greater proportion of fat to stroma than in younger women, although the proportion of fat to parenchyma varies considerably in all groups. Because of the rarity of extreme cases, histological and endocrine analysis using recent techniques is based mainly on individual cases, but adolescent and pregnancy cases appear to have common features. In one series of 41 cases, 32 were juvenile, 7 gravid and 2 involutional.[39] A family history was frequent, and two cases in monozygotic twins were recorded.

Macroscopically, the tissue is pale grey with a uniform rubbery consistency, and a variable amount of fat. The histology is distinctive, with abundant, large ducts and stroma contrasting with the lack of lobules; the atrophy or destruction of lobular units is associated with extensive fibrosis. The stroma is often of the loose connective tissue type seen in gynaecomastia. 'Juvenile units', consisting of ramified new ducts proceeding to atrophy, are sometimes seen in all types, and when seen in association with atrophic lobular units, are diagnostic of this condition.[39]

Equally characteristic is the absence of oestrogen receptors but presence of progesterone receptors, found also in reduction mammoplasties for less severe degrees of hypertrophy. It is difficult to explain this finding when there is much clinical evidence for a local hyper-responsiveness to oestrogen; the most plausible suggestion is that oestrogen acts through an intermediary substance, not directly on the ER.[40]

The pathology of the 'second degree group', the average patient seeking reduction mammoplasty, is similar, with relatively more ductal tissue and stroma than lobular tissue. The relative amounts of fat and parenchyma, relevant to the use of suction lipectomy as an adjuvant to reduction, varies greatly.[41] It can be assessed preoperatively more accurately by MRI than by mammography.[42] The amount of 'abnormal' pathology found in reduction mammoplasty does not vary from what would be expected in the general population.[43] The majority of findings are manifestations of ANDI. In 295 specimens 69 cases of 'fibroadenosis', 10 of DE, 3 of fibrosis and 3 fibroadenomas were found.[43]

There have been a number of studies of the psychological factors motivating women to seek breast reduction surgery. In general they are more concerned with physical limitations and discomfort (and increasing confidence) than the concern for femininity and womanliness which motivate many women seeking breast augmentation. Symptoms complained about most frequently include body discomfort 97%, and difficulty buying clothes 96%, while more than three-quarters complain of local, back and neck pain. There is an excess of single and cohabiting women among those seeking reduction compared with a control obstetric population.[44]

Outcome studies have shown that patients report a high degree of satisfaction with competently performed reduction surgery. In a study of 363 consecutive patients treated at the Mayo Clinic, 90% responded to a questionnaire, and of these 90% regarded the procedure as very or completely successful, against 1.5% taking the opposite view.[45] Miller and colleagues found similar results, but were unable to find a formula for predicting which patients would, or would not, benefit from surgery.[46]

There has been much interest in whether breast reduction surgery might reduce the incidence of subsequent breast cancer. It has been hypothesized that reducing the mass of glandular tissue at risk would provide a corresponding reduction, or that a decreased epithelial mass might be at risk of greater stimulation by circulating hormones etc. Observational studies have given conflicting results, but a recent study from Denmark gives some support to both concepts.[47] In a long-term study of 7720 women undergoing breast reduction surgery, breast cancer incidence was reduced overall by 50%, but only in women over 40 years of age at the time of surgery, and particularly those over 50.

Adolescent (virginal) hypertrophy

The normal development of the breast occasionally continues unchecked so that huge breasts result (Figure 15.7).

Gigantomastia is the most acute and extreme end of the spectrum. This condition, first reported in 1669,[48] is almost invariably bilateral but occurs as a unilateral disease sufficiently often to imply that it is due, at least in some cases, to local factors rather than a hormonal imbalance. No hormonal problem has been identified in these patients except possibly a rather high rate of infertility.[2] However, episodes of epidemic breast enlargement which seem to be caused by exogenous steroids rather militate against the view that hypertrophy is not a hormonal event. Epidemics of breast

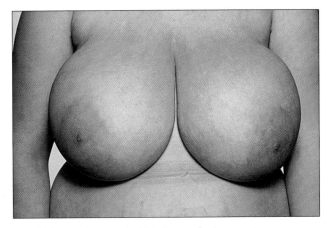

15.7 Adolescent hypertrophy. This degree of enlargement causes great psychological and physical embarrassment. It may be more severe and acute than shown here.

enlargement attributed to steroids present in chicken meat have been reported from Italy[49] and Puerto Rico.[50] Gigantomastia may also occasionally be induced by drugs such as D-penicillamine,[51] or occur immediately after starting the contraceptive pill,[40] presumably in a patient who was constitutionally predisposed to the condition.

As the breasts enlarge and become pendulous, the nipple and areola may stretch to an extent where they are recognized with difficulty. The superficial veins enlarge and palpation reveals general firmness with a varying degree of nodularity, sometimes minimal, sometimes very marked. The weight results in back pain, the characteristic grooving of the shoulders by the brassière straps, and even orthopnoea. Once a significant degree of hypertrophy has become established, regression does not seem to occur.[2]

Multiple giant fibroadenomas can enlarge rapidly in adolescent girls and cause confusion with virginal hypertrophy (see Chapter 7).

When the enlargement of the breast occurs rapidly, medical treatment with danazol[51] and bromocriptine[52,53] may be tried but insufficient data exist to give clear guidelines as to their use. Dihydrogesterone has also been recommended, both before and for 6 months after surgery.[54] On general principles, danazol is probably the drug whose pharmacology is best documented, and is the first choice on the basis of safety and lack of side-effects. Tamoxifen has been used as an adjuvant after reduction mammoplasty for gross cases. On the whole, surgery is at present the only reliable method of control. It is usually advised that the operation is deferred to the age of 17, but this is purely arbitrary and in the most severe forms surgery cannot be delayed.

Modest degrees of hypertrophy are much more common than the gross examples, and in this age group psychological reactions are particularly distressing. Taunts and ridicule from peers may take the situation out of perspective, increasing the difficulty of making a decision about reduction mammoplasty.

Patient selection and management are discussed further in Chapter 21.

Hypertrophy in pregnancy (gravid hypertrophy)

Very occasionally, bilateral or unilateral gross hypertrophy occurs in relation to pregnancy, usually the former. The aetiology is uncertain, but there is an increased incidence of a maternal family history, and in some cases there appears to be a paternal element, in that it has occurred in the first pregnancy following remarriage. Beischer et al. report three cases and give a helpful review of the literature.[55] It occurs in about 1:100 000 pregnancies. It may not occur in the first or second pregnancy, but once it occurs it is very likely to recur with subsequent pregnancies. It may arise very early, becoming obvious before the first period is missed. The breasts always lose the ability to produce milk, as would be expected with the defective lobular formation.

Treatment of this condition should follow the same guidelines as adolescent hypertrophy, although it may progress to the stage where ulceration or infarction may occur. Medical treatment is not usually effective; in one case reported tamoxifen, bromocriptine and steroids were ineffective.[56] In some of the more extreme cases occurring in pregnancy, more than one resection may be needed if further progression occurs.[2] Usually a combination of anti-hormone therapy and surgery is required to curtail the problem and the patient should be warned that a similar event may occur in subsequent pregnancies. Some authors suggest that the appropriate treatment is bilateral total mastectomy with reconstruction.[57] In such a case occurring in the first 12 weeks of the third pregnancy, bilateral total mastectomy was performed (removing 6.5 and 7 kg respectively) and the pregnancy carried to a successful conclusion.[58]

In less severe cases, regression can be expected postpartum, although not necessarily complete. There is a high probability of recurrence (perhaps more severe) in subsequent pregnancies.

Elevation of parathyroid-related protein and hypercalcaemia have been reported in association with mammary hypertrophy.[59]

EXCESSIVE POSTLACTATIONAL INVOLUTION

Women not uncommonly complain that after pregnancy and lactation, their breasts involute excessively and are much smaller than before. This is to be regarded as physiological. If the involution is marked and the psychological distress is great, augmentation mammoplasty is well justified. It is usually performed by submammary or subpectoral silicone implants.

GENETIC ABNORMALITIES INVOLVING THE BREAST

A number of genetic abnormalities involve the breast in addition to those arising as disorders of development. They may cause clinical and imaging problems, and lead to unnecessary or inappropriate biopsy if not recognized. An example is the Carney syndrome, where multiple breast fibroadenomas or ductal adenomas may be part of a multisystem disorder.[60] They are dealt with in parts of this book appropriate to the individual condition.

REFERENCES

1. Fitzwilliams DCL. *On the Breast*. London: William Heinemann, 1924.

2. Haagensen CD. *Disease of the Breast*, 3rd edn. Philadelphia: WB Saunders, 1986.

3. Méhes K. Association of supernumerary nipples with other anomalies. *Journal of Pediatrics* 1979; **95**: 274–275.

4. Matesanz R, Teniel JL, Garcia-Martin F *et al.* High incidence of supernumerary nipples in end stage renal failure. *Nephron* 1986; **44**: 385–386.

5. Mimoumi F, Merlob P & Reisner SH. Occurrence of supernumerary nipples in newborns. *American Journal of Diseases of Children* 1983; **137**: 952–953.

6. Robertson A, Sale P & Sathyanarayan. Lack of association of supernumerary nipples with renal anomalies in black infants. *Journal of Pediatrics* 1986; **109**: 502–503.

7. Lewis EJ & Crutchfield CE. Accessory nipples and associated conditions. *Pediatric Dermatology* 1997; **14**: 333–334.

8. Urbani CE & Betti R. Mammo-renal and acro-renal syndromes. A nosologic approach, synopsis and update. *European Journal of Dermatology* 1997; **7**: 251–256.

9. McFarland J. Residual lactation acini in the female breast. Their relation to chronic cystic mastitis and malignant disease. *Archives of Surgery* 1922; **5**: 1–12.

10. Schwager RG, Smith JW, Gray GF & Goulan D. Inversion of the human female nipple, with a simple method of treatment. *Plastic and Reconstructive Surgery* 1974; **54**: 564–569.

11. Pitangay I. Reconstruction of congenital nipple deformities. In: Chang WHJ. & Petry JJ (eds) *The Breast, an Atlas of Reconstruction*, pp 355–361. Baltimore: Williams and Wilkins, 1984.

12. Inch S. Inverted nipples and breast feeding. In: Chalmers I, Enkin M & Kierse M (eds) *Effective Care in Pregnancy and Childbirth*. Oxford: Oxford University Press, 1989.

13. Waller H. The early failure of breast feeding. A clinical study of its causes and their prevention. *Archives of Disease in Childhood* 1946; **21**: 1–12.

14. Hytten F. Clinical and chemical studies in human lactation: IX Breast feeding in hospital. *British Medical Journal* 1954; **2**: 1447–1452.

15. L'Esperance CM. Pain or pleasure. The dilemma of early breast feeding. *Birth and the Family Journal* 1980; **7**: 21–26.

16. Ardran GM, Kemp FH & Lind J. A cineradiographic study of breast feeding. *British Journal of Radiology* 1958; **31**: 156–162.

17. Weber F, Woolridge MW & Baum JD. An ultrasonographic analysis of suckling and swallowing in new born infants. *Pediatric Research* 1984; **18**: 806.

18. Pribaz JJ & Pousti T. Correction of recurrent nipple inversion with a cartilage graft. *Annals of Plastic Surgery* 1998; **40**: 14–17.

19. Strombeck JO. In: Strombeck JO & Rosato FE (eds) *Surgery of the Breast*. Stuttgart: Verlag, 1986.

20. Vanderputte SC. Mammary-like glands of the vulva and their disorders. *International Journal of Gynecological Pathology* 1994; **13**: 150–160.

21. Leung W, Heaton JPW & Mormes A. Uncommon urologic presentation of a supernumerary breast. *Urology* 1997; **50**: 122–124.

22. Kitamura K, Kuwano H, Kiyomatsu K *et al.* Mastopathy of the accessory breast in the bilateral axillary regions occurring concurrently with advanced breast cancer. *Breast Cancer Research and Treatment* 1995; **35**: 221–224.

23. Das DK, Matthew SU, Sheikh ZA & Al-Rubah NAR. Fine needle aspiration cytologic diagnosis of axillary accessory breast tissue, including its physiological changes and pathologic lesions. *Acta Cytologica* 1994; **38**: 130–135.

24. Nelson MM & Cooper CKN. Congenital defects of the breast – an autosomal dominant trait. *South African Medical Journal* 1982; **61**: 434–436.

25. Ravitch MM. Poland's syndrome – a study of an eponym. *Plastic and Reconstructive Surgery* 1977; **59**: 508–512.

26. Aznar JMP, Urbano J, Laborda EG *et al.* Breast and pectoralis muscle hypoplasia – a mild degree of Poland syndrome. *Acta Radiologica* 1996; **37**: 759–762.

27. Bamshad M, Root S & Carey JC. Clinical analysis of a large kindred with the Pallister Ulnar-Mammary syndrome. *American Journal of Medical Genetics* 1966; **65**: 325–331.

28. Rosenberg CA, Derman GH, Grubb WC & Buder AJ. Hypomastia and mitral valve prolapse. Evidence of a linked embryologic and mesenchymal dysplasia. *New England Journal of Medicine* 1983; **309**: 1230–1232.

29. Cherup LL, Siewers RD & Futrell JW. Breast and pectoral muscle maldevelopment after anterolateral or posterolateral thoracotomies in children. *Annals of Thoracic Surgery* 1986; **41**: 492–497.

30. Seitler D & Beller FK. The trunk breast (protrusion of the breast). *Breast Disease* 1988; **1**: 121–127.

31. Ribiero L, Canzi W, Buss A *et al.* Tuberous breast: a new approach. *Plastic and Reconstructive Surgery* 1998; **101**: 42–52.

32. McKiernan JK & Hull D. Breast development in the newborn. *Archives of Diseases of Childhood* 1981; **56**: 525–529.

33. Marshall WA & Tanner JM. Variations in pubertal changes in girls. *Archives of Diseases of Childhood* 1969; **44**: 291–303.

34. Mills JL, Stolley PD, Davies J & Moshang T. Premature thelarche. Natural history and etiologic investigation. *American Journal of Diseases of Children* 1981; **135**: 743–745.

35. Hall R, Anderson J, Smart GA, Besser M (eds) *Fundamentals of Clinical Endocrinology*, 3rd edn, p 414. Tunbridge Wells: Pitman Medical, 1980.

36. Verrotti A, Ferrarri M, Morgese G *et al.* Premature thelarche: a longterm follow-up. *Gynecological Endocrinology* 1996; **10**: 214–217.

37. Xhrouet-Heinrichs D, Lagrou K, Heinrichs C *et al.* Longitudinal study of behavioural and affective patterns in girls with central precocious puberty during long-acting triptorelin therapy. *Acta Paediatrica* 1997; **86**: 808–815.

38. Lalardrie JP & Jouglard JP. *Plasties mammaires pour hypertrophie et ptose*. Paris: Masson, 1973.

39. Anastassiades OT, Choreftaki T, Ioannovich J *et al.* Megalomastia: histological, histochemical and immunohistochemical study. *Virchows Archiv – A, Pathological Anatomy and Histopathology* 1992; **420**: 337–344.

40. Hugh JC, Friedman MH, Danyluk JM *et al.* Absence of oestrogen receptors in a case of virginal hypertrophy of the breasts related to oral contraception. *Breast Disease* 1993; **6**: 143–148.

41. Lejour M. Evaluation of fat in breast tissue removed by vertical mammaplasty. *Plastic and Reconstructive Surgery* 1997; **99**: 386–393.

42. Lee NA, Rusinek H, Weinreb J *et al.* Fatty and fibroglandular tissue volumes in the breasts of women 20–83 years old: comparison of X-ray mammography and computer-assisted MR imaging. *American Journal of Radiology* 1997; **168**: 501–506.

43. Titley OG, Armstrong AP, Christie JL & Fatah MFT. Pathological findings in breast reduction surgery. *British*

Journal of Plastic Surgery 1996; **49**: 447–451.

44. Birtchnell S, Whitfield P & Lacey JH. Motivational factors in women requesting augmentation and reduction surgery. *Journal of Psychosomatic Research* 1990; **34**: 509–514.

45. Schnur PL, Schnur DP, Petty PM *et al.* Reduction mammoplasty: an outcome study. *Plastic and Reconstructive Surgery* 1997; **100**: 875–883.

46. Miller AP, Zacher JB, Berggren RB *et al.* Breast reduction for symptomatic macromastia: can objective predictors for operative success be identified? *Plastic and Reconstructive Surgery* 1995; **95**: 77–83.

47. Boice JD Jr, Friis S, McLaughlin JK *et al.* Cancer following breast reduction surgery in Denmark. *Cancer Causes and Control* 1997; **8**: 253–258.

48. Durston W. Concerning a very sudden excessive swelling of a woman's breasts. *Philosophical Transactions for Anno 1669.* London Royal Society, 1670.

49. Fara GM, Del Corvo G, Bernuzzi S *et al.* Epidemic of breast enlargement in an Italian school. *Lancet* 1979; **ii**: 295–297.

50. Bongiovanni AM. An epidemic of premature thelache in Puerto Rico. *Journal of Pediatrics* 1983; **103**: 245–246.

51. Taylor PJ. Successful treatment of D-penicillamine induced breast gigantism with danazol. *British Medical Journal* 1981; **282**: 362–363.

52. Kullander S. Effect of 2Br alpha ergocryptin (CB134) on serum prolactin and clinical picture in a case of gigantomastia in pregnancy. *Annales Chirugiae et Gynaecologie Fenniae* 1976; **65**: 227–233.

53. Hedberg K, Karlsson K & Lindstedt A. Gigantomastia during pregnancy: effect of a dopamine agonist. *American Journal of Obstetrics and Gynecology* 1979; **133**: 928–931.

54. Mayl N, Vasconez LO & Jurkiewicz MJ. Treatment of macromastia in the actively enlarging breast. *Plastic and Reconstructive Surgery* 1974; **54**: 6–12.

55. Beischer NA, Hueston JH & Peperell RJ. Massive hypertrophy of the breast in pregnancy – report of 3 cases and review of literature. *Obstetrical and Gynecological Survey* 1989; **44**: 234–243.

56. Abid SU, Gutman M, Herman O *et al.* Massive breast hypertrophy during pregnancy: failure of medical treatment. *The Breast* 1995; **4**: 153–155.

57. Stavides S, Hacking A, Tiltman A & Dent DM. Gigantomastia in pregnancy. *British Journal of Surgery* 1987; **74**: 585–586.

58. Gogas JC, Markopovlos M, Gogas HJ *et al.* Gigantomastia developing in post-partum period and exacerbated by subsequent therapy. *Breast Disease* 1994; **7**: 231–234.

59. Khosa LS, van Heerden JA, Charib H. Parathyroid related protein and hypercalcaemia secondary to mammary hyperplasia. *New England Journal of Medicine* 1990; **322**: 1157.

60. Courcoutsakis NA, Chow CK, Shawker TH *et al.* Syndromes of spotty pigmentation, myxomas, endocrine overactivity and schwannomas (Carney complex). Breast imaging findings. *Radiology* 1997, **205**: 221–227.

Chapter 16

The male breast

CONTENTS

KEY POINTS AND NEW DEVELOPMENTS

1. Primary gynaecomastia is so common at the commencement and senescence of male sexual life that minor degrees are best regarded as part of the spectrum of normality.
2. Most cases of secondary gynaecomastia are related to drug therapy. However, the number of conditions associated with gynaecomastia is so great that it is almost impossible to give a comprehensive list.
3. True gynaecomastia needs to be differentiated from pseudogynaecomastia and pectoral muscle hypertrophy; all three may contribute in patients on steroids, as is seen particularly among weightlifters.
4. Most cases can be treated expectantly but drug therapy is reasonably successful in more severe cases, especially where pain and tenderness are obtrusive.
5. Surgery for gynaecomastia should now be regarded as a complex procedure. The cosmetic results achieved from simple excision in the past may no longer be acceptable to many patients.
6. Carcinoma-in-situ in males is a rare but curable condition, analogous to that in women. Most cases present as nipple discharge or a mass.
7. Most breast conditions seen in females may rarely occur in males, including duct ectasia, phyllodes tumour and fibroadenoma.
8. Infective conditions are an increasing problem in males immunocompromised by HIV infection.

Before puberty, breast development is similar in males and females. In neonates the incidence of mastitis neonatorum is similar. The incidence of absent breast or nipple and presence of supernumerary nipples is similar to that found in the female. At puberty, the male breast develops ductal structures but, in the absence of oestrogenic stimulation, lobular structures are not formed. It follows that most of male breast pathology relates to ductal structures but in the presence of long-term oestrogen stimulation pathology related to lobular structures may occur.

GYNAECOMASTIA

Gynaecomastia is defined as an enlargement of the ductal and stromal tissue of the male breast which is palpably and histologically different from the surrounding subcutaneous fat. It may range in size from a small retroareolar button of tissue to enlargement indistinguishable from the normal female breast.[1]

Gynaecomastia is the commonest condition affecting the male breast. The term was used by Galen to describe the changes that would now be described as pseudogynaecomastia. The term appears to have been reintroduced in the 1860s.[2,3] The alternative form of gynaecomazia is now regarded as obsolete.

Gynaecomastia may be either primary (physiological) or secondary (to a defined extramammary stimulus). It requires careful distinction from pseudogynaecomastia in which the external appearance suggests the presence of breast tissue, but palpation (and histology) reveals that the swelling is all fat with no increase in breast tissue.

Clinical presentation
The patient usually presents with a swelling of the breast, often unilateral (Figure 16.1), which is frequently tender.

He may be concerned about the tenderness itself, cosmetic appearance or the possibility of underlying malignancy. In many cases, especially in secondary gynaecomastia, changes are asymptomatic and are noted by the attending physician. Examination reveals a firm disc of retroareolar tissue which is mobile and often tender. There is usually a clear, but not sharp, demarcation of the firm, often slightly tender, breast tissue from softer surrounding fat. It needs to be distinguished from carcinoma of the male breast and pseudogynaecomastia, retroareolar fat deposition in obesity.

The hallmark of gynaecomastia is its concentricity, if an eccentric mass is found an alternative diagnosis should be considered and fine needle aspiration (FNA) or biopsy performed. At the initial assessment careful examination is needed to decide whether the enlarged breast is due to breast tissue, fat or muscle. In cases where clinical examination leaves doubt, mammography will allow quantification of the amount of fat and breast parenchyma. Hypertrophy of the pectoral muscles may simulate or accentuate gynaecomastia. Such changes are particularly likely in weightlifters who may have gynaecomastia from steroid use, so the pectoral contribution should be assessed separately.

Histology
The histological pattern of gynaecomastia progresses from an early, active phase to, eventually, an inactive senescent phase (Figure 16.2).

This progression occurs no matter what the aetiology, and is even seen when the hormonal stimulus continues. In the active phase there is proliferation of ducts with active epithelial proliferation and hyperplasia of the loose, cellular intralobular stromal tissue. The ductal proliferation may be accompanied by multiplication, branching and elongation of the ducts. There is also periductal, or more widespread, infiltration by plasma cells, lymphocytes, and large mononuclear cells.[4] When the inactive stage has been reached there is atrophy of the ductal epithelium with prominent stromal fibrosis. As the process passes into the inactive phase, breast enlargement may diminish, although persisting dense fibrous tissue means that the gynaecomastia is unlikely to regress completely.

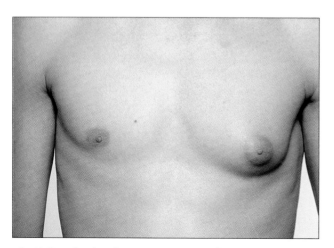

16.1 Unilateral, pubertal gynaecomastia in a male.

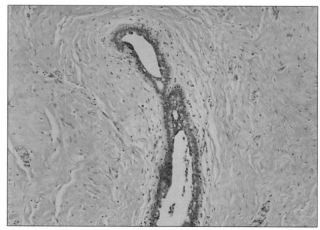

16.2 Typical histological features of gynaecomastia.

Lobular formation seems to occur only after long-term oestrogen treatment or in Klinefelter's syndrome,[5] although Andersen and Gram[6] described six cases of focal lobular formation in a series of 76 surgical resections in whom they failed to identify a source of oestrogens and so concluded that oestrogenic stimulation was unnecessary for acinar formation. In view of the obscure source of some exogenous oestrogens,[7] this view must remain unproven. Azzopardi[8] has commented on the lack of periductal elastic tissue in these patients in comparison to the female.

Incidence

The histological incidence of gynaecomastia at autopsy has been estimated by Sandison[5] as 4% and by Andersen and Gram[9] as 55%. However, Andersen and Gram[9] described three phases of gynaecomastia: active, inactive and intermediate. However, only a few (7%) of the cases were active or intermediate, so there is less discrepancy than is immediately apparent.

A review of the literature will reveal conflicting information on the incidence and significance of clinical gynaecomastia. Specialist endocrinologists who see a selected group of patients may consider the development of gynaecomastia to be of sinister significance.[10] In one series it was considered that 27 out of 46 cases had endocrine causes susceptible to, or curable by, endocrine therapy.[11] It is unusual to find a defined endocrinological cause in patients referred to a surgical clinic.

Mild forms of gynaecomastia are very common although presentation as a clinical complaint is far less frequent. Nydick et al.[12] showed in their study of 1855 boy scouts, that the overall incidence between the ages of 10 and 16 was 38%; this reached a maximum of 65% in the 14-year-old boys which had dropped to 14% in those of 16 years. Nuttall[13] in his study of 306 men showed that an incidence of 17% in youths in their late teens gradually increased in the following decades so that the incidence was 57% in those over 50 years. The overall incidence was 36% and in the vast majority bilateral disease existed. Figure 16.3 combines the findings of Nydick et al.[12] and Nuttall.[13]

Georgiadis et al.[14] found 40.5% of 954 healthy men aged 18–26 to have gynaecomastia. The majority of these were bilateral but 14% were unilateral. They also established a relationship between obesity and hirsutism in this age group.

The literature, however, provides conflicting information on the laterality of gynaecomastia; for example, in his study of the radiology of this condition Dershaw[15] found 28 had unilateral disease, four had symmetrical involvement and eight had bilateral but asymmetrical involvement. In another radiological study, 63% of 94 patients had bilateral but usually asymmetrical involvement.[16] The variations in these reports probably reflect referral patterns as diagnostic doubt is likely to be increased when the condition is unilateral.

Primary gynaecomastia is usually considered under the headings neonatal, pubertal and senescent, although, as can be seen from the foregoing, it would be better to regard it as a continuum with a peak at puberty, which falls in the late teens to be followed by steadily increasing incidence with age, as illustrated in Figure 16.3.

Aetiology

Because of the clear relationship between the incidence of gynaecomastia and hormonal events, the role of an endocrine abnormality in gynaecomastia needs to be seriously considered.

Androgen physiology

The major androgen in the adult human male is testosterone produced by the testes; the adrenal gland produces an insignificant amount of this hormone. The active hormones are dihydrotestosterone, produced peripherally from testosterone at its site of action, and androstenedione, which is derived from the adrenal cortex. Both testosterone and androstenedione may be converted to oestrogens by peripheral aromatization.

Hormonal defects in gynaecomastia

The putative hormonal defects in gynaecomastia have been well studied. Prolactin appears to have no influence on the development of gynaecomastia,[17,18] although Lee[19] recorded a transient rise in prolactin levels just prior to the development of gynaecomastia. Most patients with gynaecomastia have normal prolactin levels; few men with hyperprolactinaemia and/or galactorrhoea develop gynaecomastia. Leggett[20] has reported such a case in which the cause of the hyperprolactinaemia was unclear. A number of studies have shown a relative alteration in circulating sex steroids in patients with gynaecomastia.

Lee[19] prospectively studied 29 boys, 20 of whom subsequently developed gynaecomastia. Those who did so had a transient increase in oestrogen levels before the gynaecomastia became clinically apparent. Moore et al.[18] studied 30 pubertal boys with gynaecomastia and 20 without and

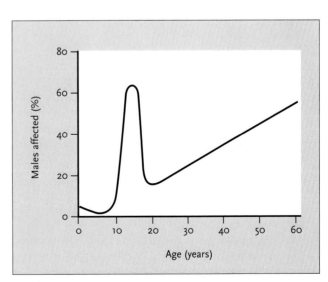

16.3 The age incidence of gynaecomastia found on routine examination. (Derived from Nydick et al.[12] and Nuttall.[13])

demonstrated a lower (^{4}-androstenedione/oestrone and oestradiol ratio (the testosterone/oestrone ratio remaining normal) in the affected boys and postulated that the cause was peripheral conversion of adrenal androgens to oestrone and oestradiol. Pirke and Doerr[21] have shown that the androgen/oestrogen ratio falls with increasing age: an observation that fits well with the observation of increasing incidence of gynaecomastia with age.[13]

Despite these somewhat inconsistent results, it seems likely that the development of gynaecomastia is the result of a relative increase in the levels of circulating oestrogens with respect to androgens and that in most cases of primary gynaecomastia, this is the operative mechanism. It seems likely that examples of secondary gynaecomastia are due to a similar perturbation of hormonal equilibrium.

The mechanisms by which these changes may occur have been reviewed by Wilson et al.[22] Unilateral gynaecomastia presumes a local factor – presumably related to hormone receptors or local hormone conversion – but remains an endocrinological enigma.

Physiological gynaecomastia
Infantile
A small percentage of male neonates have noticeable breast enlargement due to circulating maternal hormones. This resolves by the age of 4 months. It is usually bilateral but may be unilateral. No treatment beyond reassurance of the mother is required.

Adolescence
This is a common age to develop gynaecomastia. Nydick et al.[12] in their study of 1855 boy scouts aged between 10 and 16, found a 38% incidence of gynaecomastia. They have shown that the majority resolved within 6 months, although 27% of cases persisted for 2 years and 8% for 3 years. In 25% of cases the disease was unilateral, but when bilateral the sides were usually affected to different degrees and the onset was usually asynchronous.

Adult
Asymptomatic gynaecomastia in the adult usually persists unless a reversible underlying cause is found. When symptomatic it runs a variable course and often undergoes spontaneous remission, although examination will reveal persisting enlargement of the breast disc. Psychological stress has been postulated as a possible cause of intermittent gynaecomastia.[23]

Secondary gynaecomastia
A number of disparate conditions are associated with gynaecomastia as summarized in Table 16.1.

In fact, the range of conditions that can be associated with gynaecomastia is much greater than can be given in a table such as this, and endocrinology textbooks should be consulted for a more comprehensive list. When the clinical sign of gynaecomastia is so common in healthy men, care needs to be taken in ascribing such findings to underlying pathology or medication. A number of well-described associations do, however, merit some discussion.

Tumours
A number of tumours which secrete hormones may be associated with gynaecomastia. Both teratomas and seminomas of the testis may secrete sufficient oestrogens to produce gynaecomastia. In a study of 636 patients with testicular tumour, 10% presented with extratesticular complaints and gynaecomastia or mastalgia was the second most common of these. Many of these patients had inappropriate treatment, although the correct diagnosis should have been suggested by abnormal testicular findings, raised serum markers or cryptorchidism.[24] Bronchogenic carcinoma is a well-recognized source of ectopic hormone production and may also produce hormones with oestrogenic activity. Tumours of the pituitary and hypothalamus may also produce gynaecomastia, presumably mediated via the testis by gonadotropic hormones. Oestrogenic precursors produced by adrenal tumours are considered an exceedingly rare cause of gynaecomastia.[1]

Testicular failure – Klinefelter's syndrome
This chromosomal anomaly, when an apparent male has an XXY karyotype, is due to non-disjunction of the parental

Table 16.1 Causes of secondary gynaecomastia
Decreased androgens
Reduced production
Congenital anorchia
Chromosomal abnormalities, e.g.
Klinefelter's syndrome
Bilateral cryptorchidism
Viral orchitis
Bilateral torsion
Granulomatous disease
Renal failure
Androgen resistance
Testicular feminization
Increased oestrogens
Increased secretion
Testicular tumours
Carcinoma lung
Increased peripheral aromatization
Adrenal disease
Liver disease
Starvation refeeding
Thyrotoxicosis
Drug induced
see Table 16.2

sex chromosomes. The clinical features of the syndrome are testicular atrophy, eunuchoid habitus with female hair distribution and gynaecomastia. Confirmation of the diagnosis depends on chromosomal examination. The gynaecomastia in this condition is unusual in that the patient may develop lobular structures,[5] and is associated with an increased incidence of carcinoma.[25]

Secondary testicular failure

Testicular damage from any cause may result in decreased testosterone production and a change in the androgen/oestrogen ratio. The absolute levels of oestrogen do not need to be raised for gynaecomastia to occur. Viral orchitis, most commonly due to mumps, is the most frequent cause of testicular atrophy but a variety of causes should be considered. Leprosy is a common cause in relevant geographical areas. One in five cases of lepromatous leprosy have gynaecomastia due to testicular invovement which in turn is due to the preference of the organism for cooler parts of the body.[26]

Liver disease

With the exception of drug-induced changes, this is probably the commonest cause of secondary gynaecomastia. The failing liver fails to eliminate androstenedione, which is then available for peripheral conversion to oestrogens by aromatization.[27]

Starvation refeeding

The mechanism by which this occurs is probably related to the fatty liver change that occurs in such patients. Originally described in liberated prisoners of war,[28] it may also be seen in patients who have been severely ill on intensive care units.

Drugs

A large number of drugs have been implicated in the development of gynaecomastia (Table 16.2).

When the finding of gynaecomastia is as common as it appears to be, isolated case reports need to be treated with scepticism. Thompson and Carter[29] have reviewed the literature on drug-induced gynaecomastia. They conclude that calcium channel blockers, cancer chemotherapeutic agents, H_2 receptor blockers, ketoconazole and spironolactone may cause gynaecomastia. They consider the evidence regarding digitalis, neuroleptic agents and marijuana as inconclusive. However, a number of clear associations can be accepted. These changes are produced either by a relative increase in oestrogenic activity or inhibition of androgenic activity. Administration of female sex hormones, for example stilboestrol in treatment of prostatic cancer, not surprisingly leads to increased breast development. Perhaps more surprising is that enough oestrogen may be absorbed from topical preparations to cause gynaecomastia.[30,31] Some other drugs may have oestrogenic effects; well-known examples of this group are digitalis and marijuana.

Some drugs have antiandrogenic effects either as part of their intended therapeutic action, e.g. cyproterone used for prostatic cancer, or as an unwanted and unexpected effect, as seen with cimetidine or spironolactone (Figure 16.4).

Although it is usual to ascribe the cause to the drug administered, it is sometimes due to metabolites, e.g. it is tetrahydrocannabinol rather than its parent that is

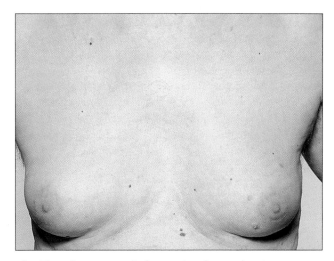

16.4 Bilateral gynaecomastia due to spironolactone therapy.

Table 16.2 Drugs associated with gynaecomastia

Drug	Mechanism
Androgens	? Peripheral aromatization
Cyproterone	Antiandrogens
Spironolactone	
Stilboestrol	
Digitalis	Bind to oestrogen receptors and oestrogenic activity
Calcium channel blockers	
Cannabis	
Griseofulvin	
Ketaconazole	
Phenothiazines	Disturbance of gonadotrophin control
Reserpine	
Tricyclics	
Cimetidine	
Methyldopa	
Isoniazid	
Metoclopramide	
Cancer chemotherapy agents	

After Hall *et al.*[1] and Thompson and Carter.[29]

responsible for marijuana-induced gynaecomastia. Conversely, the gynaecomastia of spironolactone, almost universal when used for treating hepatic ascites, may be avoided by administration of its active metabolite potassium canrenoate.[32]

Rodriguez and Jick[33] studied a population of 81,000 men receiving anti-ulcer drugs to quantify the incidence of gynaecomastia. Cimetidine carried a relative risk of some seven times. The risk was dose related, so that current users on a dose of 1000 mg had a risk of 40 times non-users, and was highest 7–12 months after starting cimetidine. Misoprostol, omeprazole and ranitidine carried no significant risk. Spironolactone and verapamil carried an equivalent risk to cimetidine.

A current fashion among weightlifters to take anabolic steroids with tamoxifen to counteract the resulting gynaecomastia can produce histological changes suggestive of pre-malignancy, though we have not yet seen a case of invasive cancer from this combination.

Diabetic mastopathy

Diabetic mastopathy is well recognized in young women with longstanding insulin-dependent diabetes (discussed in Chapter 17) and a similar picture may be seen in male diabetics with apparent gynaecomastia. The histological picture is one of marked perivascular and periductal round cell infiltration with a predominance of B lymphocytes, together with focal fibrosis. This picture of diabetic mastopathy is different to gynaecomastia, with which it is likely to be confused clinically.[34]

Assessment of gynaecomastia
Clinical

In the majority of patients, history and examination will reveal the likely cause of the gynaecomastia. The age of onset, relation to drug ingestion and underlying ill-health are the main pointers from the history. Examination of the liver, testes and chest as well as the gynaecomastia itself is clearly important.

Investigation

Investigation should be confined to liver function tests and a chest radiograph in the older patient, unless there is reason to think that there is an underlying endocrine abnormality, when more sophisticated investigations may be indicated. Serum markers for testicular tumours should be measured where appropriate, especially in patients with testicular swelling or maldescent.

Exclusion of malignancy

In addition to clinical and endocrinological studies of male patients with breast disease, aspiration, cytology and radiology should be used to exclude malignant disease in the older patient. This is particularly important in the absence of a well-defined cause, in unilateral disease and

when the palpable mass is eccentric instead of having the usual concentricity.

Mammography images gynaecomastia well (Figure 16.5) and its role in the male breast has been reviewed by Dershaw.[15]

Gynaecomastia appears as a flame-shaped opacity extending into the surrounding fat. It is possible to distinguish those patients on oestrogens when the breast takes on the appearance of the female. Cases of pseudogynaecomastia can be readily identified by the absence of breast tissue. Malignancy can usually be diagnosed by mammography. The value of ultrasound is less well established but may provide guidance for FNA cytology.[35]

FNA cytology

FNA cytology of the male breast has been regarded as problematic because the hyperplastic epithelial cells associated with gynaecomastia have erroneously been reported as malignant.[36,37] Now that the cytological features of gynaecomastia are well described this test can be approached with considerable confidence.[38–40]

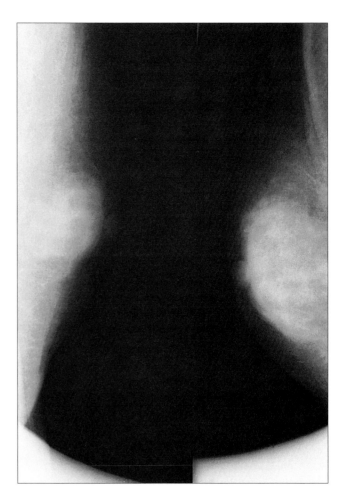

16.5 Mammograms of bilateral, asymmetric gynaecomastia.

Treatment

The management of gynaecomastia is governed by two premises. First, the majority are due to minor hormonal imbalances or to drugs and carry no serious significance. Secondly, a serious cause should be considered in each case and, in the older patient, breast cancer excluded. In the majority of cases reassurance that this is a benign self-limiting condition which is not premalignant will suffice. A minority of patients will require treatment either for tenderness or for cosmesis.

For the minority of patients in whom firm reassurance proves inadequate, a number of options are open.

Drug therapy

A hormonal basis for gynaecomastia is widely accepted[21] so it is not surprising that attempts have been made to correct the putative abnormality. What is surprising is that no agent has been studied in a systematic manner. Testosterone has been reported to be of variable value but occasionally produces a dramatic effect.[41] Eberle et al.[42] treated four pubertal patients with dihydrotestosterone heptanoate, which does not undergo peripheral aromatization, and claimed good results. The clinical improvement was associated with falls in circulating oestradiol, luteinizing hormone, follicle-stimulating hormone and free testosterone. There had been no return of symptoms during a follow-up period ranging between 5 and 15 months.

Other drugs whose use has been reported are clomiphene[43,44] and tamoxifen[45,46] which act as antioestrogens, and danazol, an antigonadotrophin which has a weak androgenic effect. These reports are of a few patients only with a number of heterogeneous causes and the results are variable from one report to another. For example, Stephanas et al.[43] reported that 18 of 19 patients responded to clomiphene 50 mg daily, whereas Plourde et al.[44] found a similar dose unsatisfactory in a group of 12 patients.

Tamoxifen 10 mg twice daily has been reported to be beneficial in both secondary[45,46] and primary gynaecomastia[47] but, as with clomiphene, small uncontrolled studies are reported. Parker et al.[48] reported a crossover study of 10 men between the ages of 54 and 80. Seven regressed, one of whom recurred after cessation of treatment. No patient responded to the placebo. McDermott et al.[49] reported a crossover trial in six men with painful gynaecomastia; 5 of 6 men responded to the tamoxifen and 1 of 6 during the placebo phase. There was a significant rise in luteinizing hormone and total oestrodiol during tamoxifen treatment.

The largest series reported is that of Alagaratnam,[50] who treated 61 Chinese men with idiopathic gynaecomastia with an 80% complete regression. Dosage was 40 mg tamoxifen daily for 2 months, and sometimes to 4 months. He noticed no untoward side-effects with follow-up in excess of 3 years. Symptomatic response

was seen in 2 weeks, although swelling took longer to resolve. This series is very positive, although further well-documented studies are desirable before recommending its routine use.

Buckle[51] reported the results of danazol treatment in 42 patients: 25 had marked regression of the gynaecomastia and 10 moderate regression. The dosage used in adults was 100 mg three times daily increased to 200 mg three times daily if no response was seen, continued for between 4 and 6 months followed by maintenance at the lower dose for 4 months. In adolescents the dosage used was 100 mg twice daily. Side-effects were acceptable and no patient stopped treatment on account of these. The levels of testosterone fell during treatment as did the levels of gonadotrophins; oestrogen levels were not measured.

Jones et al.[52] have reported a randomized study of danazol which confirms its safety and the therapeutic benefit. Our own experience is that about half of the patients obtain useful relief of symptoms. Tenderness disappears rapidly in those who are going to respond but there has been slower change in the patients whose main complaint is cosmetic. We have used varying doses between 100 mg and 200 mg three times daily with no definable side-effects. A typical course is 100 mg three times daily for 4 weeks then 100 mg twice daily for 8 weeks. Age of onset and duration of symptoms were not predictive of those who were going to respond although a good response would not be expected in longstanding fibrotic cases.

We reviewed experience in our clinic of danazol in 18 patients with a median age of onset of 21 years (range 12–54). It was unilateral in 11, painful in 14, focal in 5 and diffuse in 13. Seven patients had a complete response and three a partial response. Treatment failed in six patients and two failed to take the tablets. There were no side-effects. The time to response was 6–12 weeks, and there was no recurrence at a median follow-up of 8 months, extending to 18 months.

Surgery

When reassurance is inadequate, and drug treatment either inappropriate or unsatisfactory, surgical removal of the breast tissue is indicated. Although the operation is usually described as a subcutaneous mastectomy, it is important to leave a small area of subareolar breast tissue as overzealous resection will replace the cosmetic deformity of a swelling with one of a hollow. In obese patients particularly the cosmetic benefit may be marginal, and the patient should appreciate the difficulty in judging the right amount of tissue. Too much or too little removed from the obese is likely to leave a dissatisfied patient. In other cases, the gynaecomastia may merge with firm subcutaneous fat rather than form a localized protrusion (Figure 16.6) and these cases are also unlikely to get a satisfactory cosmetic result from surgery.

Recurrence arising from ductal tissue under the areola is well recognized; tamoxifen has been suggested as a possible treatment of such recurrence.

It is useful to be able to grade the degree of gynaeco-mastia in assessment and planning treatment, as well as for comparing results. A three-stage grading was proposed by Simon and colleagues (Table 16.3).[53]

With grades I, IIa and IIb, treatment will leave the nipple approximately in its correct position. With grade III, mas-tectomy will leave unsightly skin folds and the nipple much lower than normal. To overcome this, Ward and Khalid[54] have proposed an operation in which the nipple–areolar complex is left mounted on a vertical de-epithelialized pedi-cle, which can be folded on itself to leave the nipple at its correct position.

Beckenstein *et al.* studied 100 normal males to identify the ideal parameters of nipple position and areolar diame-ter to assist the cosmetic outcome in these grade III patients.[55] They found that the nipple lies 20 cm from the sternal notch and 18 cm from the midclavicular line with an ideal nipple-to-nipple distance of 21 cm. The average areolar diameter is 2.8 cm.[55]

Liposuction has established a place in the management of gynaecomastia, and is particularly useful when there is much fatty tissue. When there is dense glandular tissue this approach will need to be combined with sharp dissection. Samdal *et al.*[56] recommend that the liposuction is used first as this allows better definition of the glandular area to be resected. Details of the surgical procedures will be found in Chapter 20.

Radiotherapy

Prophylactic irradiation therapy of breast tissue to pre-vent the gynaecomastia which regularly accompanies the use of oestrogens in the management of prostatic cancer is now only of historical interest but does appear to have been effective.[57]

Treatment of secondary gynaecomastia

If a cause for the gynaecomastia is identified, it will resolve with treatment of the underlying abnormality or withdrawal of the offending drug. If the disease is not amenable to treat-ment, or if continuation of a drug is essential and treatment of gynaecomastia is still considered necessary, the plan for treatment of primary gynaecomastia may be followed with advantage. Three injections of nandrolone 25 mg at 3-week intervals have been recommended for gynaecomastia of the elderly, but we have no experience of this treatment and are not aware of any formal report in the literature.

OTHER MALE BREAST DISEASE

Any other disease of the male breast is uncommon. However, most diseases of the breast that afflict women have also been reported in men from time to time. Not surpris-ingly, lesions that have their origin in lobular tissue are excessively rare but may occur in XXY phenotypes and in patients with longstanding raised oestrogen levels.

It has been estimated that of all male breast lesions, 65%

are gynaecomastia, 25% malignant neoplasms, leaving 10% for miscellaneous benign disease.[5] However, this autopsy study greatly underestimates the frequency of pubertal gynaecomastia.

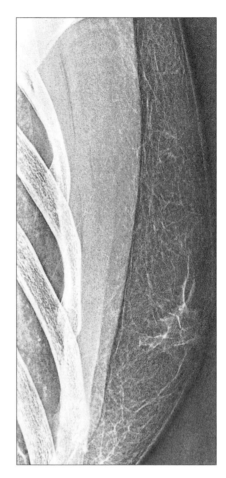

16.6 Xerograph of juvenile gynaecomastia without local protrusion.

Table 16.3 Classification of gynaecomastia proposed by Simon *et al.*[53]	
Grade I	Minor but visible breast enlargement without skin redundancy
Grade IIa	Moderate breast enlargement without skin redundancy
Grade IIb	Moderate breast enlargement with minor skin redundancy
Grade III	Gross breast enlargement with skin redundancy and ptosis so as to simulate a pendulous female breast

Fibroadenoma

In his postmortem study Sandison[5] records that one of his subjects had a localized fibroadenoma – a surprising finding in view of the absence of lobular activity in the male. Fibroadenomas require oestrogen stimulation so it is not surprising that most examples in males have occurred in patients receiving oestrogen treatment for prostatic cancer; and even then the doses used have been in excess of those normally recommended.[58] Phyllodes tumours have also been described in men with gynaecomastia,[59,60] indeed most recorded cases of male fibroadenomas are associated with gynaecomastia.[61] Ansahboatene and Tavassoli[62] have reviewed the experiences of the US armed forces and described five cases, all of whom also had gynaecomastia. A condition equivalent to fibroadenomatoid hyperplasia of the female breast has also been described in a 69-year-old man on spironolactone.[63]

Duct ectasia (DE)

This is a rare clinical entity, but Sandison[5] in his postmortem study of 500 men found that 6% of the specimens had histological evidence of DE. Andersen and Gram[6,9] found 30 examples of ectatic ducts in 100 consecutive male autopsies but in only seven of these was it diffuse. In none of these patients was there periductal inflammation; there were no clinical associations and they considered that the findings were different from DE of the female breast.

Tedeschi and McCarthy[64] described periductal mastitis in a male. Haagensen[65] describes a patient with nipple discharge which was attributed to androgens, although the description of the pathological findings in this case suggests that he had at least some degree of DE with periductal inflammation. The patient was clearly endocrinologically hypogonadal, following mumps orchitis at the age of four. We have seen a number of cases in the male, some of which have been previously reported.[66] The patients have shown all the features of the condition as seen in women with nipple inversion, nipple discharge, abscess and fistula formation (Figures 16.7 and 16.8).

More commonly, inflammatory masses around the nipple in men are due to retention cysts or infection in adjacent skin structures (Figure 16.9).

HIV-associated lesions

The incidence of DE is increased in HIV-positive males, who have a propensity to develop subareolar abscesses.[67] Whatever the underlying cause treatment is by excision of the duct system as performed in postmenopausal women.

Breast infections and abscesses are being seen more commonly in HIV-positive and otherwise immunocompromised males. In one case a 33-year-old, HIV-positive bisexual male presented with a breast abscess which grew *Pseudomonas aeroginosa* only.[68] Treatment with antibiotics, aspiration and

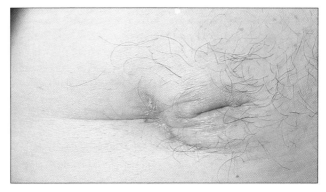

16.7 DE/periductal mastitis in a male with transverse nipple retraction and a mammary duct fistula following drainage of several subareolar abscesses.

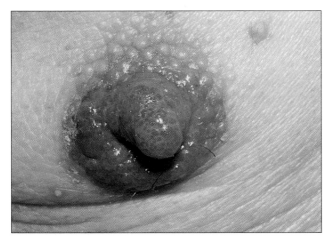

16.8 A male patient with nipple discharge due to DE resulting in inflammation of the areolar skin.

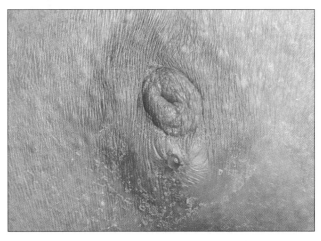

16.9 Young male with discharge from a retention cyst of an areolar gland – treated by local excision.

conservative drainage led to a prolonged course over 6 months, with healing only after wide drainage and packing. A recent series reports four breast abscesses in HIV-positive males[69] and other case reports include a tuberculous abscess, and a gonococcal infection in a homosexual patient with a nipple ring. In general, wide drainage and excision of necrotic material has been needed to obtain resolution.

Epithelial hyperplasia and carcinoma-in-situ

Sandison[5] in his review of 500 post-mortems in men records that 11 had significant epithelial hyperplasia, in three of whom it was associated with ectatic ducts. The clinical significance of this finding is uncertain. Andersen and Gram[9] found seven cases of epithelial hyperplasia in their post-mortem series. Waldo et al.[70] reported a case of florid papillomatosis, a recognized premalignant condition in women, in a man taking diethylstilboestrol.

Carcinoma-in-situ is rare in the male breast. Cutuli et al.[71] reported 31 cases treated in 19 French Regional Cancer Centres over 21 years, but this represented 5% of all male breast cancers treated. Eleven patients had gynaecomastia and three had a family history of breast cancer. Forty per cent presented with a bloody discharge, 48% with a mass and 12% with both. The left breast was affected twice as commonly as the right. One case was bilateral, and several patients had received long-term treatment for gynaecomastia. Half the patients had axillary node dissection and none were positive, so total mastectomy seems appropriate if it is clear that there is no invasion.

Local excision was followed by recurrence and sometimes invasive cancer, so this approach is to be condemned.

Nipple discharge

Detraux et al.[72] performed galactography in seven males with unilateral nipple discharge. The lesions causing discharge were two papillomas, two carcinomas, two cases of DE and one breast abscess.

Treves et al.[73] collected 42 male patients with a serosanguineous discharge in 23 years and estimated that about 2% of male breast disease had nipple discharge as a symptom. Of their 42 cases 18 were found to have benign disease and in many cases the discharge had been present for several years. The underlying cause in these cases was duct papilloma or gynaecomastia, all instances of blood-stained nipple discharge occurring with papilloma. An unusual case of blood-stained nipple discharge in an infant associated with gynaecomastia[74] is probably a variant of mastitis neonatorum; the case described by Miller et al.[75] is harder to categorize.

The galactocele described by Boyle et al.[76] is also probably a variant of mastitis neonatorum.

Fat necrosis

As with many other conditions this is occasionally recorded in men.[77]

Adenoma of the nipple

Azzopardi[8] mentions seven male patients with this condition in the world literature, and records a case of his own. It behaves identically to the same lesion in women.

Mondor's disease

We have seen but one example of this condition (Figure 16.10)[78] although Oldfield[79] considers that at least a third of the cases occur in men.

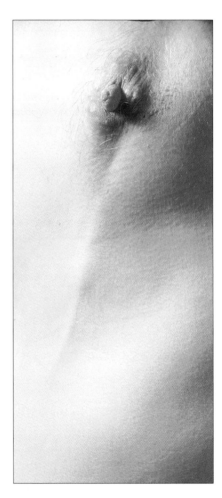

16.10 A case of Mondor's disease in a male – the appearance is similar to that seen in women.

REFERENCES

1. Hall R, Anderson J, Smart GA & Besser M. *Fundamentals of Clinical Endocrinology*. London: Pitman Medical, 1980.
2. Foot H. Remarks on gynaecomazia. *Dublin Quarterly Journal of Medical Sciences* 1866; **XLI**: 451–453.
3. Gruber F. Uber die gynaecomastie. *Memoires de l'academi du Science de St Petersburg* 7th series t 10, 1866.
4. Karsner HT. Gynaecomastia. *American Journal of Pathology* 1946; **22**: 235–315.
5. Sandison AT. An autopsy study of the human breast. *National Cancer Institute Monograph No. 8*, US Dept Health, Education and Welfare, 1962.
6. Andersen JA & Gram JB. Gynecomasty: Histological aspects in a surgical material. *Acta Pathologica et Microbiologica Scandinavica Section A: Pathologica* 1982; **90**: 185–190.
7. Smith TCG. The breast and its disorders. *Practitioner* 1982; **226**: 1454–1455.
8. Azzopardi J. *Problems in Breast Pathology*, p 14. Philadelphia: WB Saunders, 1979.
9. Andersen JA & Gram JB. Male breast at autopsy. *Acta Pathologica et Microbiologica Scandinavica Section A: Pathologica* 1982; **90**: 191–197.
10. Carlson HE. Gynecomastia. *New England Journal of Medicine* 1980; **303**: 795–799.
11. Burke CW. Gynaecomastia. *Practitioner* 1982; **226**: 1403–1410.
12. Nydick M, Bustos J, Dale JH & Rawson RW. Gynaecomastia in adolescent boys. *Journal of American Medical Association* 1961; **178**: 449–457.
13. Nuttall FQ. Gynaecomastia as a physical finding in normal men. *Journal of Clinical Endocrinology and Metabolism* 1979; **48**: 338–340.
14. Georgiadis E, Papandreou L, Evanglopoulou C *et al*. Incidence of gynaecomastia in 954 young males and its relationship to somatometric parameters. *Annals of Human Biology* 1994; **21**: 579–587.
15. Dershaw DD. Male mammography. *American Journal of Roentgenology* 1986; **146**: 127–131.
16. Kapdi CC & Parekh NJ. The male breast. *Radiological Clinics of North America* 1983; **21**: 137–148.
17. Turkington RW. Serum prolactin levels in patients with gynaecomastia. *Journal of Clinical Endocrinology and Metabolism* 1972; **34**: 62–66.
18. Moore DC, Schlaepfer LV, Paunier L & Sizonenko PC. Hormonal changes during puberty vs transient pubertal gynaecomastia and abnormal androgen estrogen ratios. *Journal of Clinical Endocrinology and Metabolism* 1984; **58**: 492–499.
19. Lee PA. The relationship of concentrations of serum hormones to pubertal gynaecomastia. *Journal of Pediatrics* 1975; **86**: 212–215.
20. Leggett CAC. Galactorrhoea. Report of a case in a male patient. *Australian and New Zealand Journal of Surgery* 1991; **61**: 540–541.
21. Pirke KM & Doerr P. Age related changes and interrelationships between plasma testosterone, oestradiol and testosterone-binding globulin in normal adult males. *Acta Endocrinologica* 1973; **74**: 792–800.
22. Wilson JD, Aiman J & MacDonald PC. The pathogenesis of gynecomastia. *Advances in Internal Medicine* 1980; **25**: 1–32.
23. Gooren LJG & Daantje CRE. Psychological stress as a cause of intermittent gynaecomastia. *Hormone and Metabolic Research* 1986; **18**: 424.
24. Cespedes RD, Caballero RL, Peretsman SJ *et al*. Cryptic presentation of germ cell tumors. *Journal of the American College of Surgeons* 1994; **178**: 261–265.
25. Cole EW. Klinefelter syndrome and breast cancer. *Johns Hopkins Medical Journal* 1976; **125**: 25–43.
26. Stacey-Clear A. Gynaecomastia. *British Journal of Surgery* 1992; **79**: 182–183.
27. Gordon GG, Olivo J, Rafii F & Southern AL. Conversion of androgens to estrogens in cirrhosis of the liver. *Journal of Clinical Endocrinology and Metabolism* 1975; **40**: 1018–1026.
28. Jacobs EC. Effects of starvation on sex hormones in the male. *Journal of Clinical Endocrinology* 1948; **8**: 227–232.
29. Thompson DF & Carter JR. Drug induced gynaecomastia. *Pharmacotherapy* 1993; **13**: 37–45.
30. Gabrilove JL & Luria M. Persistent gynaecomastia resulting from scalp inunction of estradiol: A model for persistent gynecomastia. *Archives of Dermatology* 1978; **114**: 1672–1673.
31. Edidin DV & Levitsky LL. Prepubertal gynecomastia associated with estrogen containing hair cream. *American Journal of Diseases of Children* 1982; **136**: 587–588.
32. Bellati G & Ideo G. Gynaecomastia after spironolactone and potassium canrenoate. *Lancet* 1986; **i**: 626.
33. Rodriguez LA & Jick H. Risk of gynaecomastia associated with cimetidine, omeprazole and other anti-ulcer drugs. *British Medical Journal* 1994; **308**: 503–506.
34. Hunfeld KP, Bassler R & Kronsbein H. 'Diabetic mastopathy' in the male breast – A special type of gynecomastia. *Pathology Research and Practice* 1997; **193**: 197–201.
35. Rissanen TJ, Makarainen HP, Kallioinen MJ *et al*. Radiography of the breast in gynecomastia. *Acta Radiologica* 1992; **33**: 110–114.
36. Russin VL, Lachowicz C & Kline TS. Male breast lesions: gynecomastia and its distinction from carcinoma by aspiration biopsy cytology. *Diagnostic Cytopathology* 1989; **5**: 243–247.
37. Martin-Bates E, Krausz T & Phillips I. Evaluation of fine needle aspiration of the male breast for the diagnosis of gynaecomastia. *Cytopathology* 1990; **1**: 79–80.
38. Das DK, Junaid TA, Mathews SB *et al*. Fine needle aspiration cytology diagnosis of male breast lesions. a study of 185 cases. *Acta Cytologica* 1995; **39**: 870–876.
39. Sneige N, Holder PD, Katz RL *et al*. Fine needle aspiration cytology of the male breast in a cancer centre. *Diagnostic Cytopathology* 1993; **9**: 691–697.
40. Gupta RK, Naran S, Dowle CS & Simpson J. The diagnostic impact of needle aspiration cytology of the breast on clinical decision making with an emphasis on the aspiration cytodiagnosis of male breast masses. *Diagnostic Cytopathology* 1991; **7**: 637–639.
41. Myhre SA, Ruvalcaba RHA, Johnson HR *et al*. The effects of testosterone treatment in Klinefelter's syndrome. *Journal of Pediatrics* 1970; **76**: 267–276.
42. Eberle AJ, Sparrow T & Keenan BS. Treatment of persistent pubertal gynaecomastia with dihydrotestosterone heptanoate. *Journal of Pediatrics* 1986; **109**: 144–149.
43. Stephanas AV, Burnet RB, Harding PE & Wise PH. Clomiphene in the treatment of pubertal adolescent gynaecomastia: a preliminary report. *Journal of Pediatrics* 1977; **90**: 651–653.
44. Plourde PV, Kulin HE & Santner SJ. Clomiphene in the treatment of adolescent gynecomastia. *American Journal of Diseases of Children* 1983; **137**: 1080–1082.
45. Fusco FD & Rosen SW. Gonadotropin-producing anaplastic large-cell carcinomas of the lung. *New England Journal of Medicine* 1966; **275**: 507–515.
46. Jeffreys DB. Painful gynaecomastia treated with tamoxifen. *British Medical Journal* 1979; **i**: 1119–1120.

47. Hooper PD. Puberty gynaecomastia. *Journal of the Royal College of General Practitioners* 1985; **35**: 142.

48. Parker LN, Gray DR, Lai MK & Levin ER. Treatment of gynecomastia with tamoxifen: A double blind cross-over study. *Metabolism* 1986; **35**: 705–708.

49. McDermott MT, Hofeldt FD & Kidd GS. Tamoxifen therapy for painful idiopathic gynecomastia. *Southern Medical Journal* 1990; **83**: 1283–1285.

50. Alagaratnam TT. Idiopathic gynaecomastia treated with tamoxifen. A preliminary report. *Clinical Therapeutics* 1987; **9**: 483–487.

51. Buckle R. Danazol therapy in gynaecomastia; recent experience and indications for therapy. *Postgraduate Medical Journal* 1979; **55**(Suppl 5): 71–78.

52. Jones DJ, Holt SD, Surtees P *et al.* A comparison of danazol and placebo in the treatment of adult idiopathic gynaecomastia: results of a prospecive study in 55 patients. *Annals of the Royal College of Surgeons of England* 1990; **72**: 296–298.

53. Simon BE, Hoffman S & Khan S. Classification and surgical management of gynaecomastia. *Plastic and Reconstructive Surgery* 1973; **51**: 48–52.

54. Ward CM & Khalid K. Surgical treatment of Grade III gynaecomastia. *Annals of the Royal College of Surgeons of England* 1989; **71**: 226–228.

55. Beckenstein MS, Windle BH & Stroup Jr RT. Anatomical parameters for nipple position and areolar diameter in males. *Annals of Plastic Surgery* 1996; **36**: 33–36.

56. Samdal F, Kleppe G, Amland PF & Abyholm F. Surgical treatment of gynaecomastia. Five years' experience with liposuction. *Scandinavian Journal of Plastic and Reconstructive Surgery and Hand Surgery* 1994; **28**: 123–130.

57. Malis I, Cooper JF & Wolever THS. Breast radiation in patients with carcinoma of the prostate. *Journal of Urology* 1969; **102**: 336–340.

58. Soonso IN, Rashid A & Skidmore FD. Fibroadenoma arising in the axilla of a male patient. Effect of high dose diethylstilboestrol. *The Breast* 1996; **5**: 265–266.

59. Hilton DA, Jameson JS & Furness PN. A cellular fibroadenoma resembling a benign phyllodes tumour in a young male with gynaecomastia. *Histopathology* 1991; **18**: 476–477.

60. Bartoli C, Zurrida SM & Clemente C. Phyllodes tumour in a male patient with bilateral gynaecomastia induced by oestrogen therapy for prostatic cancer. *European Journal of Surgical Oncology* 1991; **17**: 215–217.

61. Uchida T, Ischii M & Motomiya Y. Fibroadenoma associated with gynaecomastia in an adult man. *Scandinavian Journal of Plastic and Reconstructive Surgery and Hand Surgery* 1993; **27**: 327–329.

62. Ansahboatene Y & Tavassoli FA. Fibroadenoma and cystosarcoma phyllodes of the male breast. *Modern Pathology* 1992; **5**: 114–116.

63. Nielsen BB. Fibroadenomatoid hyperplasia of the male breast. *American Journal of Surgical Pathology* 1990; **14**: 774–777.

64. Tedeschi LG & McCarthy PE. Involutional mammary duct ectasia and periductal mastitis in a male. *Human Pathology* 1974; **5**: 232–236.

65. Haagensen CD. *Diseases of the Breast*. Philadelphia: WB Saunders, 1986.

66. Mansel RE & Morgan WP. Duct ectasia in the male. *British Journal of Surgery* 1979; **66**: 660–662.

67. Downs AMR, Fisher M, Tomlinson D *et al.* Male duct ectasia associated with HIV infection. *Genitourinary Medicine* 1996; **72**: 65–66.

68. Higgins SP, Stedman YF, Bundred NJ *et al.* Periareolar breast abscess due to *Pseudomonas aeroginosa* in an HIV antibody positive male. *Genitourinary Medicine* 1994; **70**: 147–148.

69. Keshtgar M, Davidson T, Soundy V *et al.* Breast disease in HIV positive males. *The Breast* 1997; **6**: 281–283.

70. Waldo ED, Sidhu GS & Hu AW. Florid papillomatosis of the male breast after diethyl stilboestrol therapy. *Archives of Pathology and Laboratory Medicine* 1975; **99**: 364–366.

71. Cutuli B, Dilhuydi JM, DeLaFontan B *et al.* Ductal carcinoma in situ in the male breast. Analysis of 31 cases. *European Journal of Cancer* 1997; **33**: 35–38.

72. Detraux P, Benmussa M, Tristant H & Garel L. Breast disease in the male: galactographic evaluation. *Radiology* 1985; **154**: 605–606.

73. Treves N, Robbins GF & Amoroso WL. Serous and serosanguineous discharge from the male nipple. *Archives of Surgery* 1956; **90**: 319–329.

74. Olcay I & Gokoz A. Infantile gynecomastia with bloody nipple discharge. *Journal of Pediatric Surgery* 1992; **27**: 103–104.

75. Miller JD, Brownell MD & Shaw A. Bilateral breast masses and bloody nipple discharge in a 4-year-old boy. *Journal of Paediatrics* 1990; **116**: 744–747.

76. Boyle M, Lakhoo K & Ramani P. Galactocoele in a male infant: case report and review of the literature. *Pediatric Pathology* 1993; **13**: 305–308.

77. Steinbach BG, Steinbach JJ & Zander DS. Bilateral breast masses in a man. *Military Medicine* 1993; **158**: 356–357.

78. Bahal V & Mansel RE. Mondor's disease secondary to breast abscess in a male. *British Journal of Surgery* 1986; **73**: 931.

79. Oldfield MC. Mondor's disease. A superficial thrombophlebitis of the breast. *Lancet* 1962; **i**: 994–996.

Chapter
17

Miscellaneous conditions

CONTENTS

This chapter brings together a number of conditions that do not conveniently fit elsewhere. They may be classified either as true breast disease or as local manifestations of systemic disease. Some are important in their own right as a source of morbidity, with others the main importance lies in a presentation which often clinically mimics carcinoma. When the breast lesion occurs as part of a widespread process, diagnosis is usually straightforward; when the breast is the first or dominant site of symptoms, diagnosis is less easy. In the past, many such diagnoses have only been made on histological sectioning of the mastectomy specimen; the more rational approach to presurgery diagnosis that now appertains means the diagnosis should be made before such a tragedy occurs.

Apart from glandular elements and supporting fibrous stroma, lesions may arise from blood vessels, nerves, fat and lymphatics.

TRAUMA

The breast is relatively infrequently damaged in trauma. Burns of the chest wall are not uncommon in children, usually as a result of scalds.[1] The resulting scars are unsightly and, if the nipple is involved, there may be subsequent problems with breastfeeding. Partial thickness burns may be disturbing but are otherwise of little importance. Full thickness burns may lead to failure of breast development. If the scarring is severe, plastic surgery may play a useful role in management,[2] and pressure garments may help to minimize scarring.

Seatbelt injury
In adult life blunt trauma is the most usual form. Even a clear history of injury, such as that obtained in car accidents, with bruising does not exclude the possibility of an underlying carcinoma. The introduction of seatbelt legislation has led to a number of reports of breast injury due to seatbelts, sometimes sufficient to cause complete disruption of the breast.[3] The injury is caused by a combination of compression between the seatbelt and the rib cage, and shearing stresses associated with torsion of the body.

The typical injury in a severe case is a furrowed deformity in the line of the seatbelt. This may be masked initially by haematoma and soft tissue oedema, but as this resolves the defect in the breast may be seen and palpated. The architectural disturbance may be revealed on mammography and ultrasonography, in particular lipid cysts and parenchymal calcification occurring in a band-like distribution.[4] In less severe cases, the clinical features of fat necrosis are evident, but beware the possibility that the accident may only have served to draw attention to a pre-existing carcinoma.

FAT NECROSIS

The most common sequel to trauma that gives rise to clinical problems is fat necrosis. This is one of those uncommon lesions which is perversely known to all medical students as a condition that simulates cancer. In spite of the universal teaching that fat necrosis may simulate cancer, procrastination with cancer still occurs because doctors accept a history of trauma from the patient and accept the possibility of a condition so familiar to them.

It would be better if the condition were unknown, for it is sufficiently rare in its classic form that no one would be disadvantaged if the condition were unrecognized without formal cytological or histological diagnosis. Breast cancer is 40 times more common than fat necrosis in Haagensen's experience.[5] We would put the figure even higher. The situation would have been very different in 1920 when Lee and Adair[6] first reported it, for radical mastectomy was then commonly performed on clinical appearance alone. Sandison[7] found evidence of fat necrosis in only two of his 800 autopsies.

Fat necrosis may appear as a complication of surgery on the breast. Mandrekas et al.[8] reported an incidence of 1% in reduction mammoplasties. A more worrying scenario for the patient is the appearance of painful lumps in the region of scars following treatment for breast cancer. We have seen this in TRAM flaps used for postmastectomy reconstruction[9] and after breast conserving surgery with postoperative radiotherapy. A number of reports now exist of fat necrosis developing in a breast treated by local excision and radiotherapy. When microcalcification with or without a palpable nodule appears in a postconservation mammogram it is wise to re-evaluate the breast formally before assuming that this represents recurrent cancer.[10,11]

Clinical features
It is not widely recognized that there are two distinct forms of fat necrosis: one simulates cancer, the other simulates simple cysts, although differing from uncomplicated cysts in having an added symptom of a dull aching pain.

The first form is more common in elderly patients, perhaps because they injure themselves more frequently and the involuted breast tissue is less able to absorb a sudden blow. The diagnosis is aided by the presence of bruising or redness of the skin, although this is not always present. The actual lump is usually small and attached to surrounding tissue. Later a more florid, inflammatory picture may produce skin fixity and oedema, resembling both cancer and the chronic form of periductal mastitis (PDM). Mammography in this group may show features consistent with carcinoma with spiculation and linear calcification, but usually with a radiolucent centre.

Ultrasound appearances of this type of fat necrosis are quite variable. Ultrasound-guided biopsy is indicated when the typical findings are of necrotic fat cells associated with macrophages. In these cases, section shows a small cavity with thick necrotic material and often white fat necrosis on the edge of the cavity. Other cases merge into a picture of haematoma with some fat necrosis around the edge.

The pathology is that of a chronic inflammatory reaction with marked histiocytic reaction and peripheral fibrosis which increases with time. The diagnosis cannot be made safely without biopsy for we have seen several cases where fat necrosis and cancer have been adjacent to each other. Mammography and cytology may both be helpful but needle biopsy is mandatory.

If there is a good history of trauma accompanied by bruising and typical fat necrosis seen on needle biopsy, an expectant treatment plan may be pursued. If the lesion resolves no further action is required. If the lesion persists or enlarges, operative intervention may be indicated to confirm the diagnosis and to remove necrotic material. Because the necrosis is usually sterile, the wound may be closed primarily with suction drainage but in case of doubt the surgeon need have no hesitancy in packing the wound and allowing it to granulate. The technique of managing the granulating wound with silicone foam dressings is particularly satisfactory, allowing rapid, painless and convenient convalescence.

The second type of fat necrosis has been seen in our experience in younger women in their forties who re-present with tender swellings after quite severe trauma such as a car accident. Nothing is noted on inspection, but palpation reveals one or more tender cystic structures which feel like ordinary cysts but with a sensation of slight thickening around the wall. Mammography may show striking cystic translucent areas (Figure 17.1).

Aspiration produces a typical oily fluid (Figure 17.2) and is curative.

Occasionally the cysts may be multiple.

The mammographic features of this type of fat necrosis have been reviewed by Hogge et al.[12] In general, the mammographic picture is sufficiently specific to allow diagnosis of oil cysts, but this is not true of ultrasound, which can give a variety of appearances, even mimicking intracystic tumours on occasions.[13]

The breast may also be involved in the relapsing, nodular panniculitis of Weber–Christian disease.

PARAFFINOMA AND SILICONE REACTIONS

Early attempts at augmentation using injections of silicone and paraffin had disastrous results with chronic discharging lesions which may appear at sites remote from the breast.[14,15] The diagnosis is not always immediately apparent because an interval of up to 35 years may occur between the injection and re-presentation.[14] Alagaratnam and Ong[14] recognized two modes of presentation: a painless hard mass clinically resembling cancer and hard masses with ulceration or sinus formation usually associated with lymphadenopathy. A further aid to diagnosis is the mammographic finding of a characteristic honeycomb appearance.

In the first group, treatment is by local excision without entering the paraffin; this remains liquid and if spilt, will lead to recurrence of the problem. The cosmetic deformity may be considerable but is preferable to a simple mastectomy. When the skin ulceration is extensive, simple mastectomy may become necessary although, in less severe cases, excision of the secondarily infected mass may be sufficient. In one series from Hong Kong, Alagaratnam and Ng[16] had to perform a mastectomy in 30 of 43 patients. Migratory masses should be removed in continuity with the breast mass. Some patients will request further reconstructive surgery. Those who have experience of this problem

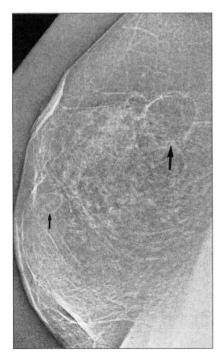

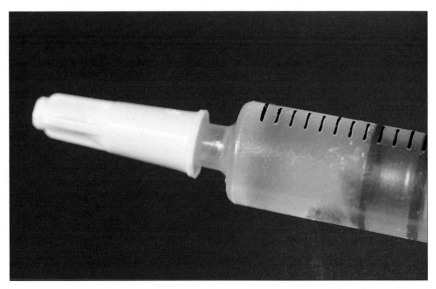

17.1 A mammogram showing oily cysts following traumatic fat necrosis.

17.2 The oily fluid aspirated from the cyst shown in Figure 17.1.

advise that reconstruction should be delayed until it is clear that the original problem will not recur.

The use of paraffin has been superseded by the use of silicone gel-filled envelopes. The two main problems of such prostheses are capsule formation and rupture of the envelope. If when the envelope ruptures the silicone remains confined within the capsule it causes little tissue reaction occurs. If it leaks outside the capsule silicone granulomas occur and silicone migrates to the lymph nodes. The clinical awareness of these events causes considerable concern to the patient. Evaluation of breast disease may be difficult as needle biopsy carries with it the risk of breaking the envelope of a prosthesis that is still intact. MRI may be helpful in elucidating difficult cases of painful breasts in patients with previous augmentation mammoplasty. If a combination of MRI, CT scan and ultrasound fails to elucidate the problem, exploration of the pocket and direct visualization of the prosthesis are indicated.

The problems of rupture of silicone gel breast implants has been well reviewed by Brown *et al.*[17] The main conclusions of their review of the published literature are that envelope rupture is more common than generally supposed, and that trauma is a rare cause of rupture which is more often associated with the age of the prosthesis. Prostheses that have been *in situ* for over 8 years have a higher incidence of rupture. This is due to a combination of maturing of the material and a fold flaw. In many cases the rupture remains asymptomatic but may cause pain. If the capsule as well as the envelope is breached, migration of the silicone may cause granuloma formation in the surrounding tissues and lymph nodes. Occasionally, the silicone may be discharged through the nipple.

Investigation should be confined to symptomatic patients; best specificity and sensitivity is obtained using MRI with a dedicated breast coil. Symptomatic ruptured prostheses should be removed but there is debate about optimal management of localized leaks retained within the capsule.

RADIATION DAMAGE

Radiotherapy is often used in the management of malignant breast disease. There was, however, a vogue for treating mastalgia with radiation between the 1920s and the 1950s.[18] The doses used are unlikely to produce local tissue damage but there are obvious implications for the induction of malignant change. Most ulcerating lesions that subsequently occur after radiotherapy for breast cancer will prove to be due to recurrent disease, but this requires histological confirmation because some of these will be due to radionecrosis. The patient has usually had radical surgery and radiotherapy, often some years previously.

The presentation is of a clinically discharging ulcer, most frequently on the medial half of the chest wall (Figure 17.3).

Examination will usually reveal necrotic underlying costal cartilage. Occasionally, severe bleeding will occur from the internal mammary artery.

The only satisfactory treatment is surgical with debridement of the ulcer and removal of the underlying necrotic costal cartilage. It is impracticable to excise the whole of the irradiated area, so skin and subcutaneous tissue need only be excised until good bleeding is seen. Because of their poor blood supply, the whole of the involved, and infected, costal cartilage will need to be removed. The underlying pleura is usually markedly thickened and the pathology lends itself to excisional surgery and reconstruction.[19] Any form of reconstruction should be with unirradiated tissue and bring with it a new blood supply. The defect may be covered by a variety of means but, if available, a latissimus dorsi myocutaneous flap will provide not only skin cover but an excellent new blood supply to facilitate healing.

LIPOMA

It is not surprising that lipomas are sometimes found in the breast. Haagensen[5] describes a series of 186 patients with a mean age of 45. The clinical features are those of lipoma elsewhere: a smooth, slightly lobulated mobile mass. Their main importance lies in distinguishing them from a clinical variant of carcinoma: the pseudolipoma. This condition is produced by shortening of Cooper's ligaments as a carcinoma infiltrates. The intervening fat lobules are compressed and 'bunched up', so that they take on a lobulated form as seen in lipoma, at the same time concealing the small underlying cancer. As lipomas occur in the cancer age group they require careful evaluation to exclude this possibility. The mammographic and ultrasound features are typical, producing a circumscribed translucent area compressing the surrounding structures. If there is any doubt about the diagnosis, the lesion is better removed.

HAMARTOMA (ADENOLIPOMA)

Haagensen[5] and Azzopardi[20] both regard this as a variant of lipoma which has incorporated epithelial elements. It tends to occur at an earlier age group than lipoma, usually in the fifth decade, but can occur over a very wide age group. Mammographically they have a typical appearance of a smooth mass with a fat halo,[21] although in detail the appearances can be very variable. With larger masses, the trite description is 'a breast within a breast'. A wide variety of appearances can be seen on sonogram.[22]

These lesions are uncommon; Crothers *et al.*[21] recorded only eight cases in 20 000 mammograms. At operation they appear well encapsulated although no capsule is found on histology (Figure 17.4).

An alternative view is to regard these lesions as hamartomas, as argued by Arrigoni *et al.*,[23] since they meet the criteria for this condition: the presence of normal components of a tissue but abnormal in proportions and arrangement. This assumes that they arise from embryonic rests, the most widely accepted theory now.

The clinicopathological features have recently been summarized by Daya *et al.* from a series of 25 cases.[22] Clinically they resemble lipomas, appearing as soft, circumscribed, mobile masses, which feel harder if there is a large proportion of fibrous tissue. They are usually a few centimetres in diameter, but may reach 10 cm, and growth may vary with pregnancy or lactation.

Greater problems can arise with pathological diagnosis, since the normal appearance of the tissues may lead a pathologist to report a biopsy as 'normal breast tissue' or 'no pathological diagnosis' or a fibroadenoma. A useful feature is the presence of both ducts and lobules, since lobules are absent or rare in a fibroadenoma. The epithelial elements may contain the whole spectrum of ductal and lobular involution. One case even contained brown fat and so was designated as an adenohibroma.[24]

Davies *et al.* have carried out a detailed dissecting microscope study of thick sections, together with conventional study of thin sections.[25] This has led them to define a distinctive combination of features to allow a precise histological diagnosis, without relying on clinical and radiological features for confirmation.

Although they usually carry no serious portent, hamartomas are removed because they grow progressively (if sometimes very slowly), and because lobular carcinoma and phyllodes tumour have been reported in them very rarely. They usually shell out easily, but recurrence is not unknown. Two of 25 cases in Daya's series recurred, presumably due to inadequate excision.

MONDOR'S DISEASE

Superficial thrombophlebitis over an area of the breast was described several times before Mondor's paper in 1939[26]; the earliest appears to be that of Fagge in 1869,[27] but Mondor's name is now firmly attached to the condition.[28] It is one of those rather rare conditions that every doctor has heard about as a medical student, and this carries two risks. The rarity of the condition may lead to unnecessary biopsy to avoid missing cancer or in the desire to recognize a condition long known about but never encountered; alternatively an atypical cancer may be described as Mondor's disease. The latter is much the more serious error, for cancer is common but Mondor's disease is rare. Haagensen[5] reported that 1 in 125 consultations were for Mondor's disease, although our experience would suggest a lower incidence.

Clinical features
Females are affected considerably more commonly than males.[29] The patient develops a dull aching pain over the breast or hypochondrium and notices a tender, elongated mass in the region (Figure 17.5).

Palpation reveals a tender narrow cord just below the skin. This is the thrombosed vein attached to the skin so that elevation of the arm produces a narrow furrow over

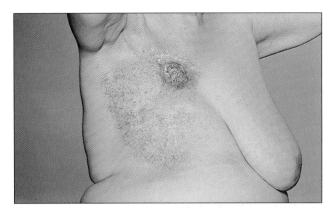

17.3 Radiation necrosis of the chest wall. There is no recurrent tumour in this case, in spite of the malignant appearance of the ulcer.

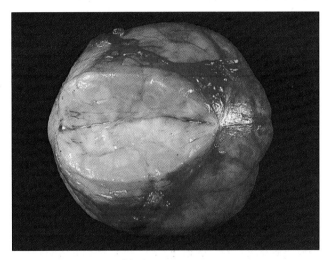

17.4 Fibroadenolipoma of the breast.

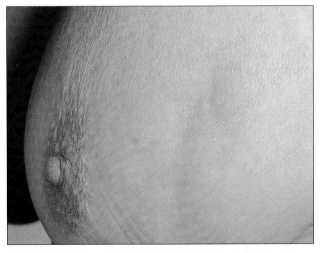

17.5 Mondor's disease, with skin retraction simulating dimpling due to cancer.

the vein, accentuated by traction from either end. The furrow is more obvious over the breast. It contracts to a bowstring if the thrombosed vein extends across the sub-mammary fold to the epigastrium. The vein usually affected is the thoraco-epigastric vein which runs from the hypochondrium up across the lateral aspect of the breast to the anterior axillary fold, although Bejanga[29] reported that it occurred more frequently in the lateral thoracic vein.

As with spontaneous thrombophlebitis elsewhere, any vein may be affected; less rare examples are a vein from the epigastrium over the lower medial quadrant of the breast and one extending vertically down from the nipple.

The thrombophlebitis follows a similar pattern to that elsewhere. The pain settles over 10 days or so, a process accentuated by rest. The tender cord resolves more slowly, taking from 2 to 12 weeks until finally no evidence remains of the lesion.

An important variant is when a short segment of vein is affected, giving local dimpling which may suggest a cancer. Of greater importance is the fact that a wedge-shaped area of ductal cancer may suggest the diagnosis of Mondor's disease to an inexperienced observer.

Pathology and pathogenesis

The pathology has been illustrated by Hughes.[30] It shows the typical stages of thrombophlebitis: a thrombosed thickened area with surrounding thrombosis.

Many cases appear to be spontaneous, a situation analogous to thrombophlebitis elsewhere. A variety of aetiological factors have been described. Unusual exercise usually involving the arms above the head is commonest. There also appears to be a trend for the condition to be associated with

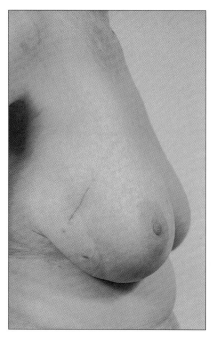

17.6 Mondor's disease following excision of a breast mass.

high parity and large breasts.[29] Operative trauma is well recognized (Figure 17.6), the condition developing distal to the scar 2 or 3 weeks after biopsy of a benign condition.

Direct trauma is of greater importance in males.[31]

Treatment

Provided the clinician is familiar with the condition and the clinical features are classic, the patient may be treated conservatively. If there is the slightest doubt, mammography should be performed.

The condition will resolve spontaneously without treatment, but symptomatic relief can be obtained with general measures appropriate to the management of thrombophlebitis: rest to the arm and support for the breast. Simple analgesics are inadequate; phenylbutazone is effective. Anticoagulants are not necessary.

Some authors have recommended introducing active approaches to management. Abramson[32] recommended disruption of the cord by forcible distraction from the ends. Millar[33] divided the cords under local anaesthesia and found symptoms relieved immediately. We have no experience of such methods but they are worth consideration in particularly painful cases.

OEDEMA OF THE BREAST

The breast may become oedematous due to heart failure and inanition. The changes in the skin of the breast are those of peau d'orange, which may progress to ulceration, so a provisional diagnosis of carcinoma is made even though no mass is palpable. General examination usually reveals evidence of generalized oedema due to either heart failure[34] or the nephrotic syndrome.[35] The so-called nursing home breast represents another variant of this problem,[36] where the unilateral localization of the oedema results from the patient being left on one side, with that breast continually dependent. A history from the attendants will usually reveal that the patient nearly always lies on the same side.

We have seen a case in which the cardiac failure went unrecognized, a clinical diagnosis of carcinoma was made and the patient treated with tamoxifen in spite of negative biopsies. Mammography revealed skin oedema but no focal lesion. The clinical and radiographic signs of malignancy resolved upon appropriate treatment of her heart failure.

The mammographic findings of this condition differ from diffuse inflammatory carcinoma. The skin oedema is thicker, there is a prominent reticular parenchymal pattern and nipple retraction is absent.[37] Nipple retraction is present in 50% of inflammatory carcinomas.

The commonest situation in which an oedemous breast is now seen is following breast-conserving surgery for breast cancer. Most often this occurs after both axillary surgery and radiotherapy. In large breasts it may pose a significant discomfort but its real anxiety lies in the difficulty of ensuring that the changes do not represent a recurrence of the carcinoma.

FIBROUS DISEASE OF THE BREAST

This is a rarely recognized clinical entity without a clear pathological basis. In this way it resembles painful nodularity and indeed parallels this condition in a number of ways. It is a reflection of exaggerated normal physiological processes proceeding to excess, in this case, the involutional replacement of lobules by dense fibrous tissue (see Chapters 1 and 3). This proceeds to an excessive degree in one area of the breast, presenting clinically as a mass, yet the pathological changes are no different to those occurring during involution in a clinically inconsequential breast.

The clearest description is that of Haagensen[5] and we have a small parallel experience of this as a clinical entity. It is uncommon; in Haagensen's experience, one case for every 10 carcinomas. We recognize it considerably less commonly. All but a few of Haagensen's patients were premenopausal although ranging in age from 24 to 72 (average 42). Our experience is mainly of patients in the fifth and sixth decades. It is difficult to explain its occurrence in the young patients, yet involutional changes are normally evident by the age of 35 and can sometimes occur earlier. One can only speculate that such changes occur earlier than usual in a particular part of the breast, perhaps a further putative example of local idiosyncratic end-organ response to hormonal stimulation, which may ultimately prove to be the cause of much obscure breast disease.

Haagensen described marked lymphocytic infiltration of the mammary lobule associated with the lobular sclerosis and atrophy. More recently, Schwartz and Strauchen highlighted this feature, categorized the lymphocytes as predominantly B cells, and suggested this might be an autoimmune disease of the breast analogous to that seen in the thyroid and salivary glands.[38]

It presents as a painless, well-defined mass but without a clear edge; it merges into surrounding breast tissue. It is usually in the upper, outer quadrant and firm rather than hard. This consistency (there is no suggestion of cragginess at all) does not raise an expectation of cancer in an experienced examiner. The modest degree of fixity to the breast tissue and the absence of skin retraction also help in the differentiation. Aspiration is possible, but an attempt at Trucut needle biopsy produces a characteristic result – bending of the cutting obturator, although the newer spring-loaded needles may do better. If resected, the tissue is dense white with an abnormally tough consistency; in fact, exactly the finding in involutional nodularity but to a more marked degree. Like this condition, it is diffuse, merging gradually with surrounding breast tissue. Hence, excision, if carried out, must be based on preoperative palpatory assessment of the extent of the disease and not on the macroscopic appearance of the breast tissue. Ignoring this will lead to a subcutaneous mastectomy.

The clinical management of this condition raises a problem, for clearly it is best if excision can be avoided. Our approach is to leave the condition if mammography convincingly excludes malignancy, as is often the case in the older patient. Where malignancy cannot be excluded, biopsy must be carried out, and the decision between incisional and excisional biopsy is made according to individual circumstances.

FIBROMATOSIS (DESMOID TUMOUR)

Fibromatosis of the breast needs to be considered in the differential diagnosis of fibrous disease. Rosen and Ernsberger[39] collected 22 cases. The condition is analogous to desmoid tumour of the abdominal wall and, like that condition, can be seen in association with colonic polyps in cases of Gardner's syndrome, although this is unusual. The disease process is much more extensive than in fibrous disease and fixes the breast to underlying tissues, such as the pectoral muscle. It can be recognized on mammography[40] but the stellate picture seen can also resemble that of cancer.

A useful study is that of Wargotz et al.[41] They describe the clinical and pathological findings of 28 examples of fibromatosis of the breast not involving the deep fascia or chest wall. This condition can occur in all age groups. Patients often give a history of surgery or trauma at the site. Five of the 20 lesions treated by local excision recurred, usually within a few months but in one case after 6 years. Rosen and Ernsberger[39] had a similar recurrence rate in their patients. The lesions that recurred had been inadequately excised initially because surgical margins showed fibromatosis. Histological features such as cellularity, atypia and mitotic figures did not help in predicting recurrence. Wide local excision appeared to have been adequate in the majority of patients, stressing the importance of documentation of free tissue margins. This is best assessed with paraffin sections since frozen section can be unreliable.[42]

DIABETIC MASTOPATHY

This condition was first described as recently as 1984 by Soler and Khardori as a variant of fibrosis in the breast associated with autoimmune thyroiditis and arthropathy of the hands.[43] Their incidence was 13% in patients with insulin-dependent diabetes mellitus (IDDM), but overall it constitutes less than 1% of all benign breast disorders. Byrd et al.[44] reported eight such patients who presented with a firm to hard discrete nodule suggestive of cancer, with mammographic changes in some also consistent with cancer. One patient had three biopsies for the same condition over 13 years.

The criteria suggested for making the diagnosis are: early onset, longstanding (usually >10 years), insulin-dependent diabetes in a premenopausal patient.[45] There is usually a hard, painless, irregular discrete mobile mass, usually multiple and often bilateral (synchronous or metachronous) but sometimes solitary. The lesions are markedly resistant to fine needle aspiration (FNA) because of the dense fibrous tissue; a specimen can be obtained in only 50%, but cells obtained will be benign. Unlike the first reports, the patients need not have autoimmune disease or arthropathy.

The mass may be found clinically or on mammogram; the latter shows dense glandular tissue, and there is marked acoustic shadowing on ultrasound.

If all the above criteria are met, it is now suggested that the condition can be managed conservatively to prevent multiple and repeated biopsies.

Formal histology shows dense, keloid-like fibrosis, B-lymphocytic infiltrates around ducts and lobules, lymphocytic vasculitis and epithelioid fibroblasts in the stroma. Perivascular lymphocytes may be confused with lobular carcinoma or lymphoma.

The most recent study[46] reports eight females and two males and provides a recent review. These workers consider that the lymphocytic infiltration is sufficient for this condition to have prelymphomatous potential, although whether or not this is so is not clear at present.

Tomaszewski et al.[47] studied eight patients and compared them with short-term insulin diabetic patients with 'fibrosis and chronic mastitis'. They described cells, which they designated 'epithelioid fibroblasts', that did not appear in other situations. These cells were found in a keloid-like matrix and were accompanied by a B cell lymphocytic infiltration around the lobules and ductules. They concluded that diabetic mastopathy may be an immune reaction to abnormal matrix. When lymphocytic mastitis occurs in non-IDDM patients, it shows a more heterogeneous pattern with less inflammation and fibrosis.

In males the condition simulates gynaecomastia.

SARCOID

Sarcoid is rarely recorded in the breast. Its importance lies not in the disease itself but because, like many other unusual conditions in the breast, it mimics carcinoma in its presentation. Haagensen[5] documents three cases from the literature, two from the UK and one from Denmark, and mentions two further cases, one his own and another from Australia. Fourteen cases had been reported up to 1985.[48,49] In all but two of the cases, there was evidence of systemic sarcoid at the time of diagnosis; in one the diagnosis became apparent 5 years later; in the other no further disease has yet appeared so that this may be an example of non-specific granulomatous mastitis. More cases have since been reported and the mammographic, ultrasound and MR findings were reviewed in 1997.[50]

AMYLOID

Amyloid deposits, mimicking the clinical presentation of cancer, have been recorded on several occasions.[51–54] The cases usually present with a lump clinically and mammographically diagnosed as a carcinoma. Extensive amyloid deposits may be found elsewhere and usually antedate the breast lesion. A case of amyloid of the nipple which presented with pruritis has also been reported.[55] We have seen a case in which an isolated deposit of amyloid mimicked a local recurrence of carcinoma following mastectomy where there was no evidence of systemic sarcoid.

GRANULAR CELL TUMOUR (MYOBLASTOMA)

This rare tumour occurs in both men and women, and approximately 6% are found over or in the breast. The granules giving its name are believed to be intracellular myelin, and it is considered most likely that the tumour is of Schwann cell origin.

Clinically and mammographically it can mimic malignancy very closely, in fact more so than any other benign condition. It occurs as a solitary (usually), progressively growing lump, hard and painless, fixed to the skin, or in the case of the breast, the underlying pectoral fascia. Size can vary from very small to 10 cm in diameter, and larger ones can ulcerate, while occasionally adjacent similar nodules may also suggest malignancy, in spite of the young age of the patient. The fixity is due to gross fibrosis and an infiltrative margin, both features also seen on histology. Pseudo-epitheliomatous hyperplasia of the overlying skin can further cloud the clinical picture.

Diagnosis is difficult on cytology so biopsy is preferred; again the hard, white cut surface can suggest malignancy. The histology is the same as with those tumours occurring more commonly in the skin. Immunocytochemistry may be helpful; the cells stain positive for S100, negative for cytokeratin, epithelial membrane antigen and myoglobin. Complete local excision is necessary to avoid local recurrence, taking any attached fascia, and confirming clearance margins.

Azzopardi[20] and McCracken et al.[56] both reviewed the literature in 1979.

VASCULITIS

It is not surprising that multifocal arteritis should occasionally afflict the breast, but it is perhaps surprising that it seems to be such a rare occurrence. The clinical manifestations mimic carcinoma, which is a particular problem if the breast is the first site of disease to present. Giant cell arteritis,[57] polyarteritis nodosa[58,59] and Wegener's granulomatosis[60] have all been reported, but even together there are less than 20 cases reported in the literature.

Gateley and Foster[61] reported two cases of pyoderma gangrenosum. In one case the diagnosis was straightforward because the patient had a known underlying disease which predisposed to pyoderma gangrenosum. In the second case, with no known predisposing cause, diagnosis was delayed and artefactual disease was considered during a prolonged period of failed wound healing. Considerable deformity remained after healing had been induced by steroid therapy. The histological features are non-specific, making clinical consideration of the diagnosis important. The marked degree of pain experienced, often apparently out of proportion to the appearance, should raise the possibility of pyoderma. Steroids are often most effective if given in very high dosage, reducing rapidly as the symptoms come under control. Selva *et al.*[62] described a case in which the only evidence of systemic disease was the presence of lupus anticoagulant.

ATHEROSCLEROSIS AND ANEURYSM

Artherosclerotic changes are often seen as incidental findings on mammograms. Kemmeren *et al.*[63] reviewed 12239 women in a screening programme. Nine per cent had evidence of arterial calcification which was associated with an increased risk of cardiovascular death of 40%. The risks were even greater in diabetic patients and the calcification was also more common in such patients. These authors conclude that mammographically demonstrated arterial calcification is an independant prognostic variable for heart disease.

A single case of an aneurysm of a vessel within the breast has been reported.[64] The diagnosis was made by auscultation and confirmed by Doppler flowmetry of the lump. It was successfully treated by local excision. Microaneurysms are not uncommonly found (histologically) after FNA examination.

INFARCTION

The breast may occasionally undergo infarction, an event first described in 1894.[65] An important review of this subject is that of Robitaille *et al.*,[66] who divide such events into those that mimic carcinoma and those that do not. Infarction of fibroadenoma has been previously described in Chapter 7, and infarction of duct papilloma in Chapter 12.

Spontaneous mammary infarction is a rare event usually occurring in pregnant (third trimester) or lactating women.[67] The clinical finding is of a tender nodule in the breast rather suspicious of lactational cancer, a diagnosis which may appear to be confirmed on frozen section.[20] It is treated by local excision, with milk fistula a possible complication.

When infarcts occur in the elderly, cancer is even more likely to be diagnosed. Infarcts have also beeen reported in association with diabetes and carbon monoxide poisoning.

Haemorrhagic necrosis complicating anticoagulant therapy
Since the first report by Flood *et al.*[68] in 1943, there has been a steady flow of papers reporting single cases of this syndrome. It may occur with any of the oral anticoagulants of the coumarin group. The sequence of events is obscure. It usually starts within a few days of commencing therapy, as a markedly painful erythematous patch with petechiae, soon turning black (sometimes within hours) with a surrounding erythematous blush. The final picture is of aseptic ischaemic necrosis with local venous and arterial thrombosis of small and medium-sized vessels, and evidence of vasculitis. The sharply demarcated necrosis is established by 48 hours, and if untreated, separates around 2 weeks later.

Extensive calcification may later develop in the breast, giving a dramatic mammogram.

Haematological consultation is urgent, both in relation to stopping coumarin therapy and replacing it with heparin to maintain control of the underlying thrombotic condition, and also because it has been suggested that prompt administration of heparin may lessen the amount of necrosis. Treatment is by debridement of the affected tissue; if the subsequent cosmetic defect is severe, secondary plastic surgery may be indicated if the underlying condition permits.

Recently an association with protein C or protein S deficiency has been recognized.[69]

Spontaneous haematoma
Although concealed trauma or factitial disease cannot be excluded with certainty, there is no reason to question a patient's claim that a haematoma has appeared spontaneously (Figure 17.7).

Our cases have been followed by slow but uneventful resolution. Mammography is always performed to exclude an underlying carcinoma.

IDIOPATHIC GRANULOMATOUS MASTITIS (NON-SPECIFIC GRANULOMATOUS DISEASE)

Granulomatous mastitis is a diagnosis of exclusion. A histological appearance of an inflammatory process with granuloma formation may be seen with a number of specific conditions, infections such as TB, leprosy and fungi; with systemic granulomatous diseases such as sarcoid; and as a reaction to lipid material, as occurs with fat necrosis and duct ectasia/periductal mastitis (DE/PDM).

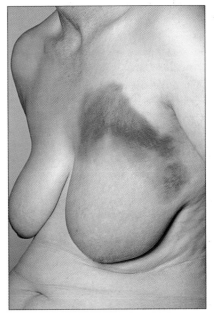

17.7 Spontaneous haematoma of the breast – no cause found.

In 1972 Kessler and Wolloch described a granulomatous condition of the breast which appeared to be unassociated with any infective process or specific granulomatous disease.[70] Fletcher et al.[71] reported a further seven cases and gave a description of the clinical features and histology. The condition was seen in young parous women within 6 years of the last pregnancy and presented as a painful, peripheral mass which could simulate malignancy. Axillary lymphadenopathy may be found. Histologically, a granulomatous inflammation closely related to the lobules was seen. They speculated on the aetiology, and came down in favour of an immunological process analogous to autoimmune thyroiditis. A report of nine cases[72] confirmed the above features, and confirmed management problems reported in other series with a protracted course after excision, and a high incidence of wound infection, delayed healing and recurrence.

Most authors recommend high-dose steroid therapy, although evidence for efficacy is not convincing. Jorgensen and Nielsen recommended 60 mg prednisone daily for 6 months and reported improvement after 3 weeks to 4 months.[73] Another group found no response in three patients.[74] Thus steroid response may not be better than natural resolution.

Is the condition related to DE/PDM? Most authors (e.g. Going et al.[72]) admit an overlap between this condition and PDM, but still believe granulomatous mastitis to be a specific entity, usually stating that PDM has been excluded 'on clinical and histological grounds'. What constitutes these grounds is not spelt out, but appears to be the peripheral location of the mass, the tendency to persistence and recurrence, and the perilobular location of the inflammation.

Going et al.[72] specifically addressed this question, comparing nine cases of granulomatous mastitis with 10 cases of DE/PDM. In most respects the cases were identical: all the DE/PDM cases were granulomatous in the sense that histological granulomas were present. The only two differences were age – the DE patients were older – and histological location of inflammation – predominantly perilobular rather than periductal. The first difference must be due to selection, and while the 'secretory disease' aspect of DE is seen in older patients, the periareolar inflammation is seen over a wide age range. The perilobular distribution of the inflammation is encompassed by the broader spectrum of the DE/PDM complex that we have always put forward on the basis of our experience. It would appear that none of these patients had the surgical procedure that we recommend, and which has been successful in our practice (Chapter 11).

Another recent paper gives further evidence of confusion, where it is believed that granulomatous mastitis can be diagnosed cytologically, without consideration of the cytological similarities of PDM.[75] In fact, this author describes duct dilatation with central suppuration in the confirmatory histology. The fallibility of cytodiagnosis in granulomatous mastitis is confirmed in another recent paper.[76]

We have seen patients with a clinical and histological picture identical to that described above which recurred after local excision but resolved completely and permanently when re-excised in continuity with the central (but clinically silent) ectatic ducts (see Figures 11.10, 11.11 and 11.12). There is an erroneous belief that PDM is only found in a juxta-areolar position, whereas it can extend from the nipple to the periphery of the breast segment, as described in Chapter 11.

Azzopardi[20] described the centrifugal progression of this condition within a segment, and also pointed out that as the process extends, the more central ducts may lose their obvious ectasia by a process of sclerosis. He made the interesting observation 'Duct ectasia is the prime example of a truly segmental disease.'

With a condition as rare as this it is not possible to be dogmatic regarding all cases. Hence we cannot claim that all non-specific granulomatous mastitis is unrecognized peripheral PDM, but we believe this to be the case sufficiently frequently that the mass should be locally excised in continuity with a central duct excision under appropriate antibiotic control, before patients are put on prolonged high-dose steroid medication, or subjected to ever wider surgical excision because of repeated recurrence. In the past, some cases of PDM were misdiagnosed as tuberculosis. Now, at least some are being misdiagnosed as 'idiopathic granulomatous mastitis'.

COLLAGENOUS SPHERULOSIS OF THE BREAST

This is a histological finding in breast biopsies with intraluminal clusters of eosinophilic spherules within areas of benign epithelial hyperplasia.[77] The condition is mainly of interest to histopathologists, because it may lead to a mistaken diagnosis of malignancy. The histological details are given in the above paper.

ARTEFACTUAL DISEASE OF THE BREAST

Artefactual or factitial disorders are ones which are created by the patient, often through complicated and repetitive actions. All reviews in the literature refer only to hospitalized patients. It is impossible for us to estimate the number of patients who have artefactual illnesses who are never suspected or who are treated as outpatients. Such disorders involving the female breast have only rarely been reported even though recognized by Hippocrates: 'It is a sign of madness when blood congeals on a woman's nipples.'[78] Sampson[79] described a case of dermatitis artefacta in which the woman had her left nipple excised for intermittent profuse bleeding. One month later she had a large tender hard mass above the incision which was found to be a pocket containing multiple small stones, gravel and sand.

General reviews of dermatitis artefacta sometimes include cases affecting the nipple.[80-82] We have reported three patients with this condition[83] and have seen others since. One complained of intermittent bleeding from her right nipple which eventually led to simple mastectomy. She was then referred to us because of bleeding which soon started from the opposite breast (Figure 17.8).

A second case was one of persistent eczema of the nipple and a third was a woman who had recurrent breast abscesses resistant to all the standard methods of treatment for DE and PDM (Figure 17.9).

The organisms grown were faecal in nature, suggesting deliberate infection. After a number of years a period in hospital with occlusion of the breast led to healing, only to be followed after discharge by a similar problem appearing on the opposite side. The patient was discharged with the advice that no active therapy would be effective, but that the lesions would eventually heal. Her local physician confirmed that this occurred, with no further problem during the following 5 years.

Such patients have usually had many investigations and operations before the nature of the underlying mechanism is recognized. Even so, establishing the diagnosis may be difficult and time consuming. Although the self-induced nature of the problem may be suspected, it is usually difficult to prove. The disorders may extend over a long period of time, may be recurrent and may result in long-term disability or cosmetic problems from tissue destruction; they are occasionally life threatening. The patients are usually young to middle-aged women, often in medically related employment.[81] They are often pleasant and cooperative and do not appear to be bizarre or psychologically disturbed, but they tend to be immature and to have problems with their sexuality. A husband who appears to be unusually (excessively) concerned may hide underlying marital stress, but this is hardly specific to artefactual disease.

Sometimes, as in two of our cases, patients will actively and without appropriate affect seek mastectomy. This should alert the clinician to the possibility of artefactual disease. The diagnosis is difficult to establish but artefactual disease should be considered where the clinical situation does not conform to common appearances or pathological processes. Unusual infections need to be considered such as tuberculosis, fungal infection or chronic subareolar abscess. A number of cases where self-injury has been suspected have cleared satisfactorily when appropriate attention was paid to this latter diagnosis.

It is difficult to give specific recommendations regarding treatment. Psychiatric consultation is often helpful in elucidating a personality disorder consistent with a diagnosis of artefactual breast disease. Direct confrontation of the patient is probably not worth while but may be considered in association with psychiatric help. These problems are difficult to manage and may extend over a long period of time. They tend to resolve if the patient is strongly reassured and attention withdrawn. Unnecessary and repetitive surgery must be avoided.

In the longer term, most factitious disorders are self-limiting and have an excellent prognosis.[84]

FOREIGN BODIES

Occasionally foreign bodies are found in the breast. Often they are found as incidental findings on mammography; less commonly they are responsible for ongoing infective episodes.

Iatrogenic materials such as catheters, localization wires and sponges have all been described and have been reviewed by Barzilai *et al.*[85] The advent of MRI scanning of the breast has revealed that small metal fragments from biopsy needles cause considerable artefacts.

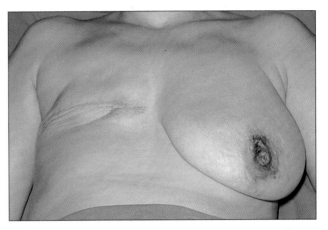

17.8 Artefactual disease: the patient had multiple operations on the right breast for recurrent severe bleeding from the right nipple, culminating in a simple mastectomy. The condition promptly occurred on the left side and has all the hallmarks of artefactual injury.

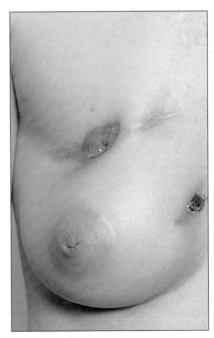

17.9 Artefactual disease: this nursing assistant had multiple operations for recurrent persistent sepsis in the right breast. Typical bowel organisms were grown from the discharge.

Consideration has to be given to the possibility of non-accidental injury and deliberate introduction of such materials, a specific type of factitious disease as described above.

MAMMALITHIASIS

In his post-mortem series, Sandison[7] noted four examples (0.5%) of laminated concretions in the breast which were either intramammary or intraductal. The nature of this rare condition is obscure, and we have not seen an example.

PSEUDOANGIOMATOUS HYPERPLASIA (PASH)

This is a benign stromal condition that simulates a vascular lesion and must be differentiated histologically from an angiosarcoma. It is seen most often as an incidental histological lesion at one end of its spectrum, but at the other end can present as a clinical lump.

Powell *et al.* have recently reviewed 40 cases, palpable clinically in 39, with an age range from 14 to 67, and a mean in the fourth decade.[86] The mass is well-circumscribed with a firm greyish-white cut surface so that it resembles a fibroadenoma. Histologically it shows a fibrotic stroma with interconnecting slit-like spaces. The cytology of the accompanying spindle cells varies from bland to plump, proliferative looking cells.

Simple excision is adequate for the lesions, as well as for the uncommon recurrences, which may occur in the same or contralateral breast. One incompletely excised lesion regressed spontaneously.

At the other end of the spectrum, a careful study of 200 consecutive breast specimens showed that 23% had at least one microscopic focus of PASH, none suspected clinically.[87]

Rosen believes the lesions most probably arise from the effect of endogenous or exogenous hormones on myofibroblasts.

NODULAR FASCIITIS

This may occur in the breast as a primary lesion, when it will behave in the same way as those in the more commonly situated soft tissue locations. It is typically a small lesion with a history of rapid growth over a few weeks, important because it may simulate malignancy, although prolonged follow-up has demonstrated it to be benign.

Cytogenetic abnormalities have recently been reported in a single case.[88]

PHANTOM BREAST SYNDROME

The presence of sensations related to a removed breast – phantom breast – has long been recognized, although it has not received nearly so much attention as the similar condition after limb amputation.

A recent useful study has looked at 97 patients who had undergone mastectomy, and found some phantom sensations in 29, with symptoms persisting more than 4 years in about half. The sensation was sited in the nipple in half, with total breast involvement in only four. The intensity was usually mild, being described as a pain in only three; the rest described the sensation as no more than discomfort.[89]

MAMMARY MUCOCELE-LIKE LESION (MML)

This lesion, which is analogous to similar lesions in the minor salivary glands, consists of a mass of cystic spaces filled with mucin and requires differentiation from a mucinous carcinoma. It also needs differentiation from cystic hypersecretory hyperplasia. Rosen described six cases in 1986,[90] and at that time they were considered always to be benign. It is now recognized that a wider spectrum occurs, with malignant forms being perhaps as common as the benign.[91] Recently, cases have been reported associated with atypical ductal hyperplasia.[92]

In its benign form, the lesion consists of a mass of mucus-containing cysts, 1–4 cm in diameter. It occurs across a wide age group, and can simulate cancer clinically and radiologically. The cystic spaces are lined by benign epithelium with some focal hyperplasia, so that diagnosis can be difficult on cytology or frozen section, and is best made on paraffin section.

Complete local excision is adequate for the benign lesions, and at present there is no evidence that the malignant ones should be treated differently to other cancers.

HIDRADENITIS SUPPURATIVA OF THE BREAST

Aprocrine sweat glands are found predominantly in the axilla and inguinoperineal regions but are described in a number of other sites. In relation to the breast, they are described in the areola and in the chest wall, particularly in the inter- and inframammary folds.[93] Hidradenitis has been described as involving the breast, in most series only one or two cases, but in a series from the Mayo Clinic it was reported in 8% of 177 women with the disease.[94] We have not been able to find a paper which details the site of the disease, but most papers suggest it is the areola. Our experience is different. We have seen it mainly in the inter- and inframammary folds, usually in obese patients. In an experience of over 150 patients requiring surgery for hidradenitis, and many more with mild disease, we have not seen a single case involving the areola. We suspect that the reported cases reflect misdiagnosis of recurrent subareolar abscesses (Chapter 11) because these reports arose at a time when this condition was not widely recognized.

Patients with extensive hidradenitis elsewhere will sometimes have an individual or a few lesions scattered on the lower part of the breast (Figure 17.10).

However, severe and extensive disease in the inter- and particularly the inframammary folds is not uncommon in obese patients, and especially in those who are also cigarette smokers. These patients often have scattered lesions on the lower half of the breast, although it is sometimes difficult to differentiate these from cystic acne – the two conditions frequently coexist. The distribution of the true hidradenitis lesion suggests that pressure is an aetiological factor. The worst lesions are seen under the strap of the brassière and on the skin surfaces where the undersurface of the breast and the chest wall are in contact and rub together.

Treatment is unsatisfactory, in contrast to surgical excision of hidradenitis in other sites.[95] Patients are urged to lose weight and cease smoking, but in our experience are rarely willing to act on such advice. We recommend conservative excision for local areas of disease, recognizing that recurrence is very likely (Figure 17.11).

Local recurrence has been seen in 50% of our cases, even after radical excision (Figure 17.12).

Even though wounds such as this will granulate to give a very satisfactory linear scar (Figure 17.13), local recurrence is usual (Figure 17.14).

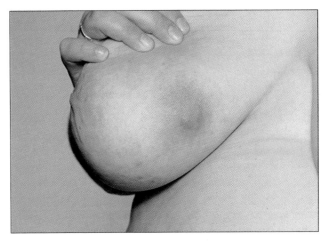

17.10 Localized lesion of hidradenitis suppurativa of the breast, in a patient with the disease elsewhere.

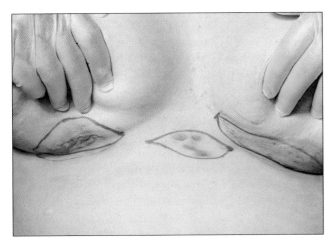

17.11 Local clusters of lesions are best treated by local excision, followed by conservative therapy for recurrence.

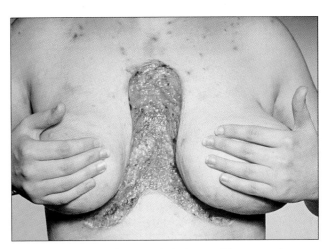

17.12 Radical excision of extensive hidradenitis of the inter- and inframammary fold.

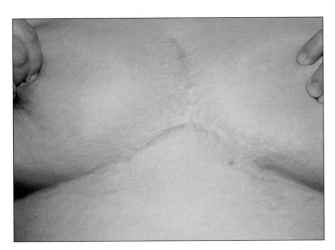

17.13 The wound was allowed to heal by granulation and gave a satisfactory scar.

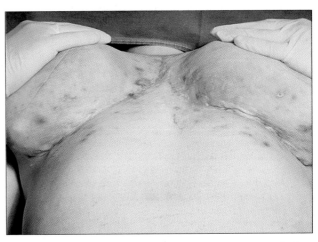

17.14 Same patient as Figure 17.13. Within 2 years there were multiple recurrent lesions of hidradenitis.

Since local pressure and sweating play a role in hidradenitis, it is possible that reduction mammoplasty might help in those who are particularly obese and have pendulous breasts. Reduction mammoplasty can be tailored to excise the area of skin in the inframammary fold most commonly involved by hidradenitis, at the same time as reducing the effects of obesity. This approach has been used in this unit on five patients, with good short-term results.

Some patients with recurrent disease benefit from conservative therapy with an antiandrogen/oestrogen combination, such as cyproterone acetate and ethinyloestradiol, as used for severe acne. There are no reports as yet of properly controlled trials of this combination in hidradenitis with adequate follow-up. In our experience, about half the patients benefit but are more likely to do so if they have mild disease, or the worst affected areas are first excised surgically.

JUVENILE PAPILLOMATOSIS (SWISS CHEESE DISEASE)

Haagensen first described eight patients with multiple intraductal papillomas which were unusual in that they were palpable, occurred in young women (age 14–24) and in which the epithelium was entirely apocrine in nature. He treated all cases by local excision without recurrence.[5]

Rosen and colleagues reported a collected series of 32 cases, and applied the term 'Swiss cheese disease' because of the multicystic nature of the masses.[96] They started a registry for these cases, and in 1985 gave a further report.[97] The patients were a little older than Haagensen's group (mean age 23 years) and typically presented with multiple small masses (1–3 cm) in the upper outer quadrant, sometimes bilateral, and because of the age group, were usually diagnosed as having fibroadenomas. The first suggestion that this might not be so was the finding of watery fluid on FNA. There was a family history of breast cancer in 25% of cases.

Macroscopically, the tumours are firm, cystic swellings with a circumscribed margin, but not enough to shell out at operation. Histology showed benign proliferative epithelium with half the cases showing a degree of histological atypia which would be regarded as precancerous in an older patient. The term papillomatosis is used in the American sense of 'epitheliosis'; it does not show a papillomatous structure with a central stromal core. A third paper reported follow-up of 41 patients after a mean period of 14 years.[98] In this group 58% had a family history (usually mother or maternal aunt) and six of 41 were bilateral. Ten per cent had developed breast cancer, and all of these had bilateral and recurrent papillomas, and a family history of breast cancer. So those without these features seem to be at low risk.

Complete excision with a small margin is recommended management at present, although recurrence does not seem to show a close relationship to clearance margins. Annual surveillance and breast self-examination are recommended for most cases, with perhaps more intensive follow-up for the high-risk cases (bilateral/recurrent/family history).

BREAST TUMOUR OF PREGNANCY (LACTATING ADENOMA)

This uncommon tumour is customarily called lactating adenoma, in spite of the fact that it is usually discovered during pregnancy, rather than lactation. Equally there is no good evidence that it is an adenoma, in the tumour sense. Hence James et al. make a plea that it be called 'breast tumour of pregnancy'.[99]

Patients usually present with a 2–4-cm mass in the second or third trimester, and are typically young, in the third decade. On histology the mass shows the normal constituents of the pregnant breast, but varies in the degree of 'pregnant' change, and is out of step with the stage of pregnancy.

Because of the rarity of this tumour, the mass is likely to be excised for histology, and carries no increased risk of cancer.

HAEMANGIOMA

Clinically significant haemangiomas of the breast are rare. Most are incidental, perilobular structures seen only on histology in biopsies for unrelated conditions. Most haemangiomas over 2 cm in diameter prove to be angiosarcomas.[100]

REFERENCES

1. Burvin R, Robinpour M, Milo Y et al. Female breast burns: conservative treatment with a reconstructive aim. Israel Journal of Medical Sciences 1996; 32: 1297–1301.
2. Neale HW, Smith GL, Gregory RO & McMillan BG. Breast reconstruction in the burned adolescent female. An 11 year, 157 patient experience. Plastic and Reconstructive Surgery 1982; 70: 718.
3. Dawes RFH, Smallwood JA & Taylor I. Seat belt injury to the female breast. British Journal of Surgery 1986; 73: 106–107.
4. Dipiro DJ, Meyer JE, Frenna TH & Denison CM. Seat belt injuries of the breast. Findings on mammography and sonography. American Journal of Roentgenology 1995; 164: 317–332.
5. Haagensen CD. Disease of the Breast, 3rd edn. Philadelphia: WB Saunders, 1986.
6. Lee BJ & Adair FE. Traumatic fat necrosis of the female breast and its differentiation from carcinoma. Annals of Surgery 1920; 37: 189.
7. Sandison AT. An autopsy study of the human breast. National Cancer Institute Monograph No. 8, US Dept Health, Education and Welfare, 1962.
8. Mandrekas AD, Assimakoloulos GI, Mastorakos DP & Pantzalis K. Fat necrosis following breast reduction. British Journal of Plastic Surgery 1994; 47: 560–562.

9. Patel RT, Webster DJT, Mansel RE & Hughes LE. Is immediate reconstruction safe in the long term? *European Journal of Surgical Oncology* 1993; **19**: 372–275.

10. El-Deeb NA. Fat necrosis of the breast: an unusual complication of lumpectomy and radiotherapy in breast cancer. Review of the literature and report of four new cases. *European Journal of Surgical Oncology* 1990; **16**: 248–250.

11. Rostom AY & El-Sayed ME. Fat necrosis of the breast: an unusual complication of lumpectomy and radiotherapy in breast cancer. *Clinical Radiology* 1987; **38**: 31.

12. Hogge JP, Robinson RE, Magnant CM & Zuurbier RA. The mammographic spectrum of fat necrosis of the breast. *Radiographics* 1995; **15**: 1347–1356.

13. Harvey JA, Moran RE, Maurer EJ & DiAngelo GA. Sonographic features of mammographic oil cysts. *Journal of Ultrasound Medicine* 1997; **16**: 719–724.

14. Alagaratnam TT & Ong GB. Paraffinoma of the breast. *Journal of the Royal College of Surgeons of Edinburgh* 1983; **28**: 260–263.

15. Raven RW. Paraffinoma of the breast. *Clinical Oncology* 1981; **7**: 157–161.

16. Alagaratnam TT & Ng WF. Paraffinomas of the breast: an oriental curiosity. *Australian and New Zealand Journal of Surgery* 1996; **66**: 138–140.

17. Brown SL, Silverman BG & Berg WA. Rupture of silicone-gel implants: causes, sequelae and diagnosis. *Lancet* 1997; **350**: 1531–1537.

18. Mattsson A, Ruden BI, Palmgren J & Rutqvist LE. Dose- and time-response for breast cancer risk after radiation therapy for benign breast disease. *British Journal of Cancer* 1995; **72**: 1054–1061.

19. Hughes LE. Repair of the chest wall defects after irradiation for breast cancer. *Annals of the Royal College of Surgeons of England* 1976; **58**: 140–143.

20. Azzopardi J. *Problems in Breast Pathology*. London: WB Saunders, 1979.

21. Crothers JG, Butler NF, Fortt RW & Gravelle IH. Fibroadenolipoma of the breast. *British Journal of Radiology* 1985; **58**: 191–120.

22. Daya D, Trus T, Dzousa JJ *et al*. Hamartoma of the breast. Clinicopathological and radiological study of 25 cases. *American Journal of Clinical Pathology* 1995; **103**: 185–189.

23. Arrigoni MG, Docherty MB & Judd ES. The identification and treatment of mammary hamartoma. *Surgery, Gynecology and Obstetrics* 1971; **133**: 577–582.

24. Damiain S & Panarelli M. Mammary adenolipoma. *Histopathology* 1996; **28**: 554–555.

25. Davies JD, Kulke J & Mumford AD. Hamartomas of the breast – six novel diagnostic features in 3-dimensional thick sections. *Histopathology* 1994; **24**: 161–168.

26. Mondor H. Tronculite sous-cutanee subaigue de la paroi thoracique antero-laterale. *Memoires Academies de Chirurgie* 1939; **65**: 1271.

27. Fagge CH. Remarks on certain cutaneous affections. *Guys Hospital Reports* 1869; **15**: 295–364.

28. Thomford NR & Holadya WJ. Mondor's disease (phlebitis of the thoraco epigastric vein). *Annals of Surgery* 1969; **170**: 1035–1037.

29. Bejanga BI. Mondor's disease: analysis of 30 cases. *Journal of the Royal College of Surgeons of Edinburgh* 1992; **37**: 322–324.

30. Hughes ESR. Sclerosing peri-angiitis of the lateral thoracic wall. *Australian and New Zealand Journal of Surgery* 1952; **22**: 17–24.

31. Oldfield MC. Mondors disease. A superficial phlebitis of the breast. *Lancet* 1962; **i**: 994–996.

32. Abramson DJ. Mondor's disease and string phlebitis. *Journal of the American Medical Association* 1966; **196**: 1087.

33. Millar DM. Treatment of Mondor's disease. *British Journal of Surgery* 1967; **54**: 76–77.

34. McElligott G & Harrington MG. Heart failure and breast enlargement suggesting cancer. *British Medical Journal* 1986; **292**: 446.

35. Muller JWT & Koehler PR. Cardiac failure simulating inflammatory cancer of the breast. *Fortschrift beb Rontgenstr Nuklearmedizin, Erganzeousband* 1984; **140**: 441–444.

36. Kaufman SA. Nursing home breast. *Archives of Surgery* 1984; **119**: 615.

37. Keller RJ & Hermann G. Unilateral edema simulating inflammatory carcinoma of the breast. *Breast Disease* 1990; **3**: 61–74.

38. Schwartz IS & Strauchen JA. Lymphocytic mastopathy. An autoimmune disease of the breast? *American Journal of Clinical Pathology* 1990; **93**: 725–730.

39. Rosen PP & Ernsberger D. Mammary fibrosis. A benign spindle cell tumour with a significant risk for local recurrence. *Cancer* 1989; **63**: 1363–1369.

40. Hermann G & Schwartz IS. Focal fibrous disease of the breast: Mammographic detection of an unappreciated condition. *American Journal of Roentgenology* 1983; **140**: 1245–1246.

41. Wargotz ESM, Norris HJ, Austin RM & Enzinger FM. Fibromatosis of the breast. A clinical and pathological study of 28 cases. *American Journal of Surgical Pathology* 1987; **11**: 38–45.

42. Yiangou C, Fadl H, Sinnett HD & Shousha S. Fibromatosis of the breast or carcinoma? *Journal of the Royal Society of Medicine* 1996; **89**: 638–640.

43. Soler NG & Khardori R. Fibrous disease of the breast, thyroiditis, and cheiro arthropathy in type I diabetes mellitus. *Lancet* 1984; **i**: 193–194.

44. Byrd BF, Hartmann WH, Graham LS & Hogle HH. Mastopathy in insulin dependent diabetes. *Annals of Surgery* 1987; **205**: 529–532.

45. Morgan MC, Weaver MG, Crowe JP & Abdul-Karim FW. Diabetic mastopathy: a clinicopathologic study in palpable and nonpalpable breast lesions. *Modern Pathology* 1995; **8**: 349–354.

46. Hunfeld KP & Bassler R. Lymphocytic mastitis and fibrosis of the breast in long-standing insulin-dependent diabetics. A histopathologic study on diabetic mastopathy and report of ten cases. *General & Diagnostic Pathology* 1997; **143**: 49–58.

47. Tomaszewski JE, Brooks JS, Hicks D & Livolsi VA. Diabetic mastopathy: a distinctive clinicopathological entity. *Human Pathology* 1992; **23**: 780–786.

48. Ross MJ & Merino MJ. Sarcoidosis of the breast. *Human Pathology* 1985; **16**: 185–187.

49. Fitzgibbons PL, Smiley DF & Kern WH. Sarcoidosis presenting initially as breast mass: report of two cases. *Human Pathology* 1985; **16**: 851–852.

50. Kenzel PP, Hadijuana J, Hosten N *et al*. Boeck sarcoidosis of the breast: Mammographic, ultrasound, and MR findings. *Journal of Computer Assisted Tomography* 1997; **21**: 439–441.

51. Fernandez BB & Hernandez FJ. Amyloid tumour of the breast. *Archives of Pathology* 1973; **95**: 102–105.

52. Sadeghee SA & Moore SW. Rheumatoid arthritis, bilateral amyloid tumours of the breast and multiple cutaneous amyloid nodules. *American Journal of Clinical Pathology* 1974; **62**: 472–476.

53. Hardy TJ. Diffuse parenchymal amyloidosis of lungs and breast. *Archives of Pathology and Laboratory Medicine* 1979; **103**: 583–585.

54. Lew W & Seymour AE. Primary amyloid of the breast. Case

report and literature review. *Acta Cytologica* 1985; **29**: 7–11.

55. Ganor S. Amyloidosis of the nipple presenting as pruritis. *Cutis* 1983; **31**: 318.

56. McCracken M, Hamal PB & Benson EA. Granular cell myoblastoma of the breast: a report of two cases. *British Journal of Surgery* 1979; **66**: 819–821.

57. Stephenson TJ & Underwood JCE. Giant cell arteritis: an unusual cause of palpable masses in the breast. *British Journal of Surgery* 1986; **73**: 105.

58. McCarthy DJ, Imbrigia J & Hung JK. Vasculitis of the breasts. *Arthritis and Rheumatism* 1968; **11**: 796–801.

59. Ng WF, Chow LT & Lam PW. Localized polyarteritis nodosa of breast – report of two cases and a review of the literature. *Histopathology* 1993; **23**: 535–539.

60. Paterson AG, Fortt RW & Webster DJT. Wegener's granulomatosis. An unusual cause of a breast lump. *Journal of the Royal College of Surgeons of Edinburgh* 1985; **30**: 332–335.

61. Gateley CA & Foster ME. Pyoderma gangrenosum of the breast. *British Journal of Clinical Practice* 1990; **44**: 713–714.

62. Selva A, Ordi J, Roca M *et al.* Pyoderma-gangrenosum-like ulcers associated with lupus anticoagulant. *Dermatology* 1994; **189**: 182–184.

63. Kemmeren JM, Beijerinck D, van Noord PA *et al.* Breast arterial calcifications: association with diabetes mellitus and cardiovascular mortality. *Radiology* 1996; **201**: 75–78.

64. Dehn RB & Lee ECG. Aneurysm presenting as a breast mass. *British Medical Journal* 1986; **292**: 140.

65. Schneck J. A case of grangenous necrosis of the mammary gland. *Journal of the American Medical Association* 1894; **23**: 181.

66. Robitaille Y, See Mayer TA, Thelmo WL & Cumberlidge MC. Infarction of the mammary region mimicking carcinoma of the brcast. *Cancer* 1974; **33**: 1183–1189.

67. Hasson J & Pope C. Mammary infarcts associated with pregnancy presenting as breast tumours. *Surgery* 1961; **49**: 313–316.

68. Flood EP, Redish MH, Bociek SJ & Shapiro S. Thrombophlebitis migrans disseminata: report of a case in which gangrene of a breast occurred. *New York State Journal of Medicine* 1943; **43**: 1124.

69. Cham CW, Chan D, Copplestone JA *et al.* Necrosis of the female breast: a complication of oral anticoagulation in patients with protein S deficiency. *The Breast* 1994; **3**: 116–118.

70. Kessler E & Wolloch Y. Granulomatous mastitis: a lesion clinically simulating carcinoma. *American Journal of Clinical Pathology* 1972; **58**: 642–646.

71. Fletcher A, McGrath IM, Riddell RH & Talbot IC. Granulomatous mastitis: a report of seven cases. *Journal of Clinical Pathology* 1982; **35**: 941–945.

72. Going JJ, Anderson TJ, Wilkinson S & Chetty U. Granulomatous lobular mastitis. *Journal of Clinical Pathology* 1987; **40**: 535–540.

73. Jorgensen MB & Nielsen DM. Diagnosis and treatment of granulomatous mastitis. *American Journal of Medicine* 1992; **93**: 97–101.

74. Salam IMA, Alhausi MF, Daniel MF & Sim AWJ. Diagnosis and treatment of granulomatous mastitis. *British Journal of Surgery* 1995; **82**: 214.

75. Kumarasinghe MP. Cytology of granulomatous mastitis. *Acta Cytologica* 1997; **41**: 727–730.

76. Martinez-Parr AD, Nevado-Santis M, Melendez-Guerrero B *et al.* Utility of FNA in the diagnosis of granulomatous lesions of the breast. *Diagnostic Cytopathology* 1997; **17**: 108–114.

77. Clement PB, Young RH & Azzopardi JG. Collagenous spherulosis of the breast. *American Journal of Surgical Pathology* 1987; **11**: 411–417.

78. Radice B (ed.) *Hippocractic Writings*, p 225. Harmondsworth: Penguin Classics, 1983.

79. Sampson D. An unusual self inflicted injury of the breast. *Postgraduate Medical Journal* 1975; **51**: 116–118.

80. Carney MWP & Brown JP. Clinical features and motives among 42 artefactual illness patients. *British Journal of Medical Psychology* 1983; **56**: 57–66.

81. Reich P & Gottfried LA. Factitious disorders in a teaching hospital. *Annals of Internal Medicine* 1983; **99**: 240–247.

82. Sneddon I & Sneddon J. Self-inflicted injury. A follow up study of 43 patients. *British Medical Journal* 1975; **3**: 527–530.

83. Rosenberg MW & Hughes LE. Artefactual breast disease: a report of three cases. *British Journal of Surgery* 1986; **72**: 539–541.

84. Masterton G. Factitious disorders and the surgeon. *British Journal of Surgery* 1995; **82**: 1588–1589.

85. Barzilai M & Roisman I. Foreign bodies in the breast. *Breast Disease* 1995; **8**: 179–183.

86. Powell CM, Cranor ML & Rosen PP. Pseudoangiomatous stromal hyperplasia (PASH). A mammary stromal tumor with myofibroblastic differentiation. *American Journal of Surgical Pathology* 1995; **19**: 270–277.

87. Ibrahim RE, Sciotto RC & Weidner N. Pseudoangiomatous hyperplasia of mammary stroma. *Cancer* 1989; **63**: 1154–1160.

88. Birdshall SA, Shipley JM, Summersgill BM *et al.* Cytogenetic findings in a case of nodular fasciitis of the breast. *Cancer, Genetics and Cytogenetics* 1995; **81**: 166–168.

89. Poma S, Varenna R, Bordin G *et al.* Phantom breast syndrome. *Revista Clinica Espanola* 1996; **196**: 299–301.

90. Rosen PP. Mucocele like tumors of the breast. *American Journal of Surgical Pathology* 1986; **10**: 87–101.

91. Hamela-Bena D, Cranor ML & Rosen PP. Mammary mucocele-like lesions. *American Journal of Surgical Pathology* 1996; **20**: 1081–1085.

92. Duun S & Rank F. Mucocele like tumours of the breast associated with atypical ductal hyperplasia. *Breast Disease* 1996; **9**: 71–73.

93. Craigmyle MBL. *The Apocrine Glands and the Breast.* Chichester: John Wiley & Sons, 1984.

94. Jackman RJ & McQuarrie HB. Hidradenitis suppurativa: its confusion with pilonidal disease and anal fistula. *American Journal of Surgery* 1949; **77**: 349–351.

95. Harrison BJ, Mudge M & Hughes LE. Recurrence after surgical treatment of hidradenitis suppurativa. *British Medical Journal* 1987; **294**: 487–489.

96. Rosen P, Cantrell B, Mullen D *et al.* Juvenile papillomatosis (Swiss cheese disease) of the breast. *American Journal of Surgical Pathology* 1980; **4**: 3–12.

97. Rosen PP, Holmes P, Lesser ML *et al.* Juvenile papillomatosis and breast carcinoma. *Cancer* 1985; **55**: 1345–1352.

98. Rosen PP & Kimel M. Juvenile papillomatosis of the breast – a follow-up study of 41 patients diagnosed before 1979. *American Journal of Clinical Pathology* 1990; **93**: 599–603.

99. James K, Bridger J & Anthony PP. Breast tumours of pregnancy ('Lactating adenoma'). *Journal of Pathology* 1988; **156**: 37–44.

100. Mitnick JS, Waisman J & Roses DF. Haemangioma of the breast. *Breast Disease* 1990; **3**: 29–33.

Epidemiology and cancer risk

KEY POINTS AND NEW DEVELOPMENTS

1. The epidemiology of benign breast disorders has been neglected in comparison with cancer. Most studies are flawed by failure to be specific regarding the conditions being studied.
2. Benign breast disorders are very common in the general population: two-thirds of women suffer mastalgia; one-third will consult their physician about it, and 10% of women will have a biopsy.
3. Studies suggest a diet high in red meat and fats and a high total food intake favour benign breast disorders; cereals and fruit appear to be beneficial.
4. Oral contraceptive use reduces the risk of benign breast disorders, including biopsy rates for fibroadenoma and histological cystic disease.
5. Hormone replacement therapy (HRT) increases mammographic density, mastalgia, and new fibroadenoma and cysts, although the incidence of the latter two is low.
6. The American Cancer Society consensus document has had a profound influence on the understanding and quantification of cancer risk related to benign disorders. However, the consensus document was not written on tablets of stone and already significant, although relatively minor, changes have evolved from new studies.
7. Histological patterns and family history are the two most important risk factors.
8. Breast cysts and fibroadenomas are two common conditions considered in the document to carry no risk, but now accepted as carrying a small risk.
9. Finding effective biochemical and molecular prognostic markers is proving elusive, with the possible exception of the breast cyst protein GCDFP-15.

The epidemiological aspects of breast cancer have been widely studied and a large number of epidemiological associations, such as age, race and age at first pregnancy are well recognized. In contrast, there has been little study of the epidemiology of benign breast conditions, although there have been some attempts to correct this deficiency recently.

Previous efforts have concentrated on the relationship between 'fibrocystic disease' and cancer, and studies have been carried out for many decades, but until recently no consensus has emerged. Because different studies report widely varying estimates of the cancer risk of benign breast disorders, it is no surprise that the confusion felt by the individual clinician is eventually transmitted to the patient, who is all too often left without clear advice regarding prognosis and follow-up. Many of the contradictions in the literature are due to badly designed studies, performed on selected populations with poorly defined diagnostic groups, as discussed in Chapter 1.

The seemingly random results are thus understandable. There are many different aspects of risk for each individual patient, such as family history, personal reproductive history and, if the patient has undergone biopsy, histology. All of these need to be taken into account in the light of studies to quantitate these risks which have been carried out over the last two decades. First the studies of Page and colleagues over the 1980s were of immense importance, as individual histological patterns were defined precisely and the cancer risk of individual elements assessed. The last decade has seen greater concentration on epidemiological and case control studies to redefine the risk of clinical entities such as cysts, fibroadenomas and duct papillomas, together with the modulating effect of family history. Most recently, all three are being integrated to give the best assessment of risk currently available from conventional parameters. The next phase is developing rapidly, as biochemical factors and molecular biology findings are explored in greater depth.

Every piece of information available will be required, because changes in clinical practice over the past decade will influence current assessments. Since these are based heavily on histological changes in benign biopsies, the dramatic fall in biopsy rate with improved diagnostic measures will remove this data in many patients, as will the widespread use of the contraceptive pill, with its effect in decreasing the number of benign breast presentations and biopsies.

EPIDEMIOLOGICAL STUDIES OF BENIGN BREAST DISORDERS

General population incidence

One of the most valuable studies in this area has come from Vancouver.[1] A 23-year prospective study of 726 nurses showed that 215 (30%) had reported breast symptoms requiring medical advice and 107 (14%) had had a biopsy with a histological report of benign breast disease during the follow-up period. The likelihood of having a benign biopsy was associated with a history of premenstrual pain or swelling, lack of oral contraceptive use and a family history of both benign and malignant breast disease. The high awareness of breast cancer among nurses would almost certainly influence these results.

Fewer biopsies for benign breast disease were performed in long-term oral contraceptive users in the large prospective Oxford-FPA study,[2] particularly for fibroadenoma and histologically confirmed cystic disease. This study also provides data on other risk factors for biopsy. It showed that the risk of having a breast biopsy was much lower in obese women. It was suggested that this was due to the greater difficulty of feeling a small dominant lump in a large breast. Several factors were found to be associated with increased risk of biopsy, including history of breast symptoms and family history. However, these would tend to sway the clinician towards biopsy of a doubtful lump and this in part may explain the observed association.

A prospective study carried out from our department of the prevalence of breast symptoms in a South Wales working population of 820 women, showed that two-thirds experienced at least mild mastalgia and 10% had had a previous benign biopsy. This study was important because it was not related to clinic populations, as has usually been the case.

Such a study of 1171 patients attending a general obstetrics and gynaecology clinic in the USA provides more general data than breast clinic attendees, although not a general population study.[3] It shows that benign breast disorders affect a similar high proportion of women in America, where two-thirds had suffered mastalgia, and one-third had consulted a doctor about it.

A number of other epidemiological studies of benign breast disorder, both descriptive and analytical, have been reviewed in a paper by Cooke and Rohan.[4] Unfortunately, these studies tend to rely on clinical diagnosis or use non-specific terms such as 'fibrocystic disease', so their value is limited.

Epidemiological studies of histological patterns have come largely from autopsy series.[5] These have clear limitations from an epidemiological viewpoint, but provide some useful guidelines.[4] They confirm the high incidence of simple hyperplasias in non-selected hospital death populations, with figures reported as high as 69%.

Incidence in high- and low-risk countries

In a collaborative study, benign breast patterns in the extratumoral tissue of breast cancer patients has been compared in three high-incidence and six low-risk countries.[6] No significant difference was found for ductal hyperplasia and sclerosing adenosis between low- and high-risk countries, but low-risk countries had a significantly lower incidence of apocrine metaplasia, apocrine hyperplasia and cysts. This gives some support to the current view that apocrine change and macroscopic cysts may be associated with a small increase in cancer risk.

The contraceptive pill and benign breast disorders

The widespread use of oral contraceptives among modern women has prompted numerous detailed studies of possible effects on benign and malignant breast disease. Worries of thromboembolic complications have prompted the use of pills with lower doses of both the oestrogen and progestogen component of the formulation, so that earlier studies are not necessarily relevant to the pills in current common use. Nevertheless, most results of large epidemiological surveys have shown that benign breast disorders are reduced in long-term pill users. The Oxford-FPA study[2] and the Royal College of General Practitioners study[7] both clearly show a reduction in the risk of biopsy for benign breast disorder in long-term pill users. These findings have been confirmed in other studies[8] and the protective effects appear to relate to the progestogen component of the pill.

Because women taking a modern oral contraceptive pill appear to have a lower incidence of benign breast disorders (of the ANDI group), patients with such disorders need not discontinue their current oral contraceptive.

One aspect causing controversy is the effect of the oral contraceptives on different types of hyperplasias. Some workers have reported that all types are reduced by oral contraceptive usage, others have suggested that benign hyperplasias are decreased but the atypical hyperplasias are unchanged or increased. Anderson et al.[9] studied the mitosis and apoptosis (cell death) rates in women taking oral contraceptives and non-users and found no significant differences between the two groups. This subject is reviewed in the paper by Cooke and Rohan[4] and clearly further work is required.

Some concern has been expressed regarding breast cancer risk in women who start taking oral contraceptives before their first full-term pregnancy. Large case-control studies suggest a small increase of 2.5 times in early contraceptive pill users, but the formulations studied were of the high-dose type and are probably not relevant to modern users.[10] The Committee on Safety of Medicines reviewed the literature and concluded in 1987 that no change in current policy is indicated.[11]

Recent reviews confirm the differential effect on benign breast disorders (reduced – particularly with high doses of progestogens) and cancer (none or slight increase), but restate the many difficulties inherent in studying this problem: differing formulations and dosages, timing and length of exposure, lack of histological specificity of many studies.[8,12]

HRT and benign breast disorders

It is not surprising that HRT has a considerable effect on the breast, reversing many of the normal involutional changes. This is reflected in persistence of clinical conditions normally not seen after the menopause, such as fibroadenoma, cysts and mastalgia, though the incidence overall is low.

Greater changes are seen radiologically, with premenopausal patterns often developing on mammography. For instance, 24% of 50 patients on HRT developed increased parenchymal density on mammography, diffuse in seven, multifocal in two and cysts in three cases.[13] Similar effects were seen with oestrogen alone or combined therapy. There is a close correlation between developing mammographic densities and mastalgia.[14] This effect results in patients on HRT having a one-third higher recall rate for incidence screening, with consequent cost and anxiety.[15] New or enlarging fibroadenomas in postmenopausal women are seen exclusively in women on HRT, although the incidence is low, about 1:10,000 women undergoing screening.[16]

New cysts are seen in about 1% of women at mammographic screening, and in those past the age of 50, 50% are associated with HRT.[17]

Along with the clear increase in benign breast disorders, there has been much interest in the question of whether HRT is also associated with an increased incidence of breast cancer. This is outside the remit of this book, and so is not dealt with in detail. In general, it is considered that there is a small increase in risk with prolonged use. However, the reviews leading to this opinion cover data with widely differing results, from clear increased incidence to equally clear protection. For instance, a prospective study of 422,373 women having oestrogen replacement therapy showed a 16% decrease in risk of fatal breast cancer at 9 years.[18] With so many types of HRT, and so many confounding factors, it will probably be many years before any increased cancer risk (if any) is clearly established.

The effect of public health education on referral rates

In the UK, a general practitioner will see an average of 13 patients with breast problems each year[19]; an overwhelming majority will be benign. Pain is the commonest presentation (47%) followed by lump (35%). Similar results were obtained in the study from Southampton[20] and the results did not differ from a study 10 years earlier.[21] In the Edinburgh study,[19] these rates were not influenced by a local health education campaign, which might have been expected to result in a large increase. Likewise, the percentage of patients requiring referral by the GP for specialist consultation did not change during the education period.

Other epidemiological factors affecting the incidence of benign breast disorders

These have been discussed in the review by Ernster.[22] Women of high socioeconomic class and those with a maternal history of cancer are liable to an increased risk of biopsy for benign disorder, although this may involve factors related to concern or awareness. Some cancer risk factors, such as age of menarche, age at first childbirth, nulliparity etc., have been reported by some workers as showing no relation to benign breast disorders, and by others to be positively associated. The balance of evidence seems to be in favour of no association, and this has also been the case for relationship between age at first birth and risk of benign breast disorder subclassified by the degree of histological atypia.

There has been much interest in the effect of diet on the incidence of benign breast disorders. Much of this is related to mastalgia (dealt with in Chapter 8) and 'fibrocystic disease'. Because of the non-specific nature of the latter, it is difficult to draw valid conclusions from most studies, while those dealing with specific entities such as epithelial hyperplasia come to different conclusions. In general, epithelial hyperplasia, and in particular atypical hyperplasia, has been associated with increased total food intake, increased fats and red meat, and increased saturated fatty acids. Cereal and fruit intake has been considered to be beneficial.[23,24]

THE CANCER RISK OF BENIGN BREAST DISORDERS

With such a high incidence in unselected hospital autopsy series of histological abnormalities in the breast, it will clearly be difficult to assign a cancer risk to many of these histological patterns, although recent work has clarified the situation.

The first important paper in this field, by Wellings et al.,[25] looked at the incidence of benign histological lesions in cancerous breasts. It suggested that the coexistence of benign and malignant is probably significant, although a concurrent study of this nature cannot give definitive data of value equal to that obtained from prospective studies. The particular significance of this work was the careful description and definition of histological patterns. Using a detailed, subgross slicing technique, Wellings et al. suggested that most hyperplastic lesions seen in the breast originate from the terminal ductal lobular unit (TDLU; see Figure 2.5) and procede to either a lobular or ductal type of hyperplasia, which they designated type A and B, respectively.

This was followed shortly by a similar study by Page et al.,[26] who also produced a detailed descriptive classification of proliferative lesions of the breast. This study was much more powerful in having a prospective element. A second publication[27] reports a series of over 10,000 biopsies with a follow-up rate greater than 90%. Their detailed findings are discussed below in relation to the American College of Pathologists (ACP) document.

A third study, from Cardiff,[28] followed 778 patients with symptomatic benign breast disorders for a minimum of 14 years. It illustrates some of the problems of translating risk factors of benign breast disorders into practical terms. Only 22 of their 770 symptomatic patients developed breast cancer, considered to be three times the background risk (although the control cancer incidence was taken from national statistics which may not be fully validated). Only 1 in 30 of the 326 patients from the series undergoing biopsy developed cancer, so a totally predictive histological marker would have only a low power of prediction of cancer arising within 14 years of follow-up. This study also indicates the difficulties of follow-up by clinical examination in an unselected series of symptomatic benign breast cases, as about 11,000 clinic visits would have been required to see each patient annually and pick up two cancers. Indeed this paper concludes that regular follow-up of patients with benign breast disease is not worth while.

The American Cancer Society consensus statement

This statement, produced for the American Cancer Society by the College of American Pathologists[29] (Table 18.1), draws heavily on the findings of Page's group[27] and is careful to assign specific terminology to the histological categories.

However, it must be accepted that assessment of these patterns embraces a considerable subjective element so that even experienced pathologists may differ in their assessment of individual lesions. The questions of assessment and definition are discussed more fully at the end of this chapter.

This consensus statement is based solely on histological findings on biopsy and stresses the importance of specifying the component elements of benign breast disorders we have included under the umbrella of ANDI (Chapter 3). However, there is no reason to believe that their relative risk assessment may not be applied to clinical conditions,

---

Table 18.1 Relative risk for invasive breast carcinoma based on pathological examination of benign breast tissue (American College of Pathologists consensus statement)[29]

No increased risk
- Adenosis, sclerosing or florid
- Apocrine metaplasia[a]
- Cysts macro[a] and/or micro
- Duct ectasia
- Fibroadenoma
- Fibrosis
- Hyperplasia (mild 2–4 epithelial cells in depth)
- Mastitis (inflammation)
- Periductal mastitis
- Squamous metaplasia

Slightly increased risk (1.5–2 times)
- Hyperplasia, moderate or florid, solid or papillary
- Papilloma with a fibrovascular core[a]

Moderately increased risk (5 times)
- Atypical hyperplasia
  - Ductal
  - Lobular

Insufficient data to assign a risk
- Solitary papilloma of lactiferous sinus
- Radial scar lesion

[a] The risk of these conditions is more controversial than suggested by this statement (for details see text).

---

provided this is limited to those conditions where the gross and histological diagnosis are clearly related, e.g. macroscopic cysts, duct ectasia (DE) or lactational mastitis. With other conditions, risk must be assessed on biopsy material.

The simplest approach to the discussion of subsequent cancer risk of benign breast disorders is a pragmatic one, discussing the risks and management of individual patients in relation to the diagnostic groups listed in Chapter 3 and described in succeeding chapters, dealing with them as they present in clinical practice. Non-histological risk factors, in particular family history of breast cancer, must also be taken into consideration.

One problem relates to the fact that the diagnosis of some conditions, e.g. fibroadenoma in young girls and macroscopic cysts, is often made clinically and the conditions managed without obtaining biopsy material for histological study. Similarly, a patient with mastalgia or cyclical nodularity will not need a biopsy, but may still wish to have an assessment of cancer risk. The incidental finding of a specific hyperplasia in a biopsy performed for a dominant lump also requires assessment. Thus, in practice, both clinical and histological aspects must be taken into consideration, although histological findings have the greatest predictive power when available. Conditions are discussed in three risk groups according to the ACP consensus statement: no increased risk, slight and moderate increase. However, the risk of individual lesions is sometimes more controversial than the statement suggests and our own assessment is given in some detail in each section.

Conditions without increased risk

There is general agreement that the malignant potential of most conditions in the galaxy of benign breast disorders is very low (less than 1.5 times normal) or equivalent to the background population risk. However, as discussed below, there has been some change of opinion for some of these conditions, with clarification of risk, since the publication of the ACP consensus document.

ANDI – mastalgia and cyclical nodularity

These are aberrations of normality and therefore should not be labelled as a 'disease'. These clinically diagnosed conditions are not associated with any specific histology and, by definition, they will have the same cancer risk as the normal population, unless a biopsy has been performed which shows an incidental histological marker of risk. The cancer risk of an individual patient suffering from the symptoms must be calculated from the individual risk factors defined in this chapter.

Fibroadenoma

The situation with fibroadenoma is complex and is dealt with in detail in Chapter 7. In general, studies in the past have shown no increase in subsequent cancer. Clinical experience suggests that most fibroadenomas involute by hyalinization if they are not removed. Carcinoma arising in a fibroadenoma is a very rare event and has been estimated

at 1 in 1000 fibroadenomas by Azzopardi.[30] These tumours are usually lobular in type, as would be expected from the lobular origin of fibroadenoma.

Semb[31] failed to find a single case of carcinoma in his series of 142 patients with fibroadenoma followed up from 4 to 27 years postoperation. A second study by Oliver and Major[32] of 175 patients reported one case of carcinoma in a 4–25-year follow-up. In our follow-up of 369 cases of fibroadenoma followed for 1–10 years, only two cases of cancer were detected, both in the opposite breast.

However, recent, more formal studies are slightly less reassuring. Levi et al.[33] showed a slightly increased risk in a follow-up of 1461 cases of fibroadenoma, with a standardized incidence ratio of 1.6 (relative risk, RR = 1.1–2.1). The risk appeared to persist indefinitely, so that the cumulative risk of invasive breast cancer was 0.7% at 5 years and 2.2% at 12 years following the diagnosis of fibroadenoma. Although this is a low incidence, it is not insignificant because of the young age of many patients with fibroadenoma. Another group[34] have found fibroadenoma to be an independent risk factor for subsequent cancer with an odds ratio of 1.7 (95% confidence limits, CL = 1.1–2.5) in a case control study.

A recent study by Dupont and colleagues[35] has helped clarify this situation. They divided fibroadenomas into simple and complex, the latter designation being given to fibroadenomas also showing cysts, sclerosing adenosis, epithelial calcifications or papillary apocrine change. The complex group had an increased subsequent incidence of cancer RR = 3.10 (CL = 1.9–5.1), a similar figure to those with benign proliferative disease in the adjacent breast tissue, and to those with a family history of cancer. The risk in these groups is long term, it does not seem to decrease with time. Two-thirds of the patients were non-complex, and had no family history, so were at no increased risk.

However, because simple fibroadenoma occurs in a young population, lifetime follow-up would be necessary to provide definitive guidance and such long-term data are not available at present. It would seem prudent to follow up those with complex histology and/or a strong family history from the age of 35.

Blunt duct adenosis and sclerosing lesions

Blunt duct adenosis and sclerosing adenosis are both histological appearances of ANDI and do not alone carry an increased cancer risk.[26,36] These lesions are usually found incidentally in a biopsy performed for a dominant lump or radiological finding and of themselves require no follow-up.

However, while sclerosing adenosis itself appears to carry no increase in risk of subsequent cancer, there is some evidence that it may act synergistically with atypical hyperplasia to increase the risk, in much the same way as a family history of breast cancer seems to do. Tavassoli and Norris[37] found the rate of cancer following hyperplasia with atypia to be 17% in those who also had sclerosing adenosis, compared with only 4.2% in those without.

Radial scar was put in a separate category in the ACP consensus document (Table 18.1) – 'insufficient evidence to assign a risk'. This condition and its larger counterpart, complex sclerosing lesion, have received much more attention in the past decade. The associated cancer risk is still controversial, although there is increasing consensus that the cancer risk is that of the individual histological patterns associated with the lesion. The chance of significant associated histology increases with the size of the lesion and with increasing age of the patient. This subject has been dealt with in more detail in Chapter 10.

Microglandular adenosis is another uncommon condition which is not covered by the ACP consensus document. There are no convincing prospective data available, but there are increasing numbers of reports of its association with cancer, or with subsequent cancer.[38] Nevertheless, at present recommended management is by complete excision and long-term follow-up.

Macroscopic breast cysts

The ACP consensus statement places all forms of cysts in the 'no increased risk' group without comment. However, the subject is more controversial than this suggests and requires more detailed discussion. Attention has been focused on gross cystic disease because it is a common benign breast condition which is often found coexisting in cancerous breasts and it appears around the age that cancer becomes common. It is important to specify 'gross cystic disease' as defined by Haagensen et al.[36] to denote macroscopic cysts, which can be felt, aspirated or seen at operation, in contradistinction to microscopic cysts, which are impalpable and only found in association with other pathology in the breast.

Many studies have reported the incidence of cystic disease in cancerous breasts, but most have found that cysts are just as common in non-cancerous breasts studied at autopsy as in cancerous breasts. Thus, gross cysts taken in isolation from hyperplastic lesions do not appear to be commoner in cancerous breasts. Many investigations have also examined the question of subsequent breast cancer development after a diagnosis of cystic disease in 'prospective' studies dating as far back as 1940, but as Azzopardi[30] points out: 'These studies are in reality mostly retrospective observation studies and suffer from a variety of methodological and statistical errors which give rise to varying estimates of increased risk.' Also, many of these studies were carried out before the specific histological subgroups detailed above had been described adequately and so many of the series have failed to identify accurately those histological patterns which would influence subsequent cancer rates.

Davis et al.[39] in 1964 reviewed the results of six studies and found a 2.6 times increase in cancer risk in the published works and a 1.73 times increase in their own material. However, Haagensen et al.[36] and Azzopardi[30] both concluded that none of the earlier studies was valid because of poorly defined pathology or invalid statistics. Nevertheless, Haagensen et al.[36] describe a relative risk of three times for their private patients with gross cystic disease and two times for their public patients. Page et al.,[26] in their study of over 4000 women, found that cysts alone had a risk of only 1.2 times, i.e. not significantly different from normal. A more recent study from this group showed a higher risk (RR 2–4) only for cysts in association with proliferative disease or a family history.[40]

However, the most recent work suggests that Haagensen may be right. The evidence is discussed more fully in Chapter 9. In brief, prospective studies show an increased cancer risk of about 4 times over the general population,[41,42] although there is conflicting evidence regarding the effect of multiplicity or cyst type. A raised blood level of the cyst fluid protein GCDFP-15 seems to have an enhancing effect.

The small increase in cancer risk can be accommodated by reducing the age for screening from 50 to 40 years, since cysts are uncommon before this age. This can be justified at present only in those with multiple or type I cysts, until the uncertainties regarding different cyst parameters are clarified.

There is some evidence of an association between macrocysts and benign duct papilloma, although this association is not seen sufficiently often to be of clinical significance.

Apocrine metaplasia (papillary apocrine change)

Apocrine metaplasia or pink cell change is such a common finding in the breast that it has long been considered to be of no importance in cancer risk. It is very commonly seen in cysts. Studies in the 1980s suggested that apocrine metaplasia in biopsies may be an indicator of increased risk. Page et al. showed a 2.7 times increase in risk for papillary apocrine change[26] and Roberts et al. reported a 6.9 times increase for pink cell metaplasia.[28]

A more recent study from Page's group shows no evidence of increased cancer risk associated with papillary apocrine change alone after a median follow-up of 20 years.[43] Many women with apocrine change had associated proliferative disease, and this accounted for the slightly increased risk; those with apocrine change alone had no increase. These same authors categorized papillary apocrine change on the basis of cytological and histological findings, and a small group whose changes were categorized as highly complex appeared to have a slight increase in cancer risk (RR = 2.4), but this did not reach statistical significance.

Seidman et al. have reported a study of 37 patients with atypical apocrine adenosis, defined as apocrine adenosis with enlarged nucleoli and greater than three-fold variation in nuclear area.[44] They found this carried a relative risk of 14 (CI 4.1–48) in women more than 60 years of age at time of diagnosis. The risk in younger women appeared to be low.

Haagensen's long-term follow-up of his series of gross cystic disease[36] noted increased risk in patients with gross cysts who had apocrine metaplasia on their biopsies in addition to the cyst; patients without apocrine metaplasia had a lower risk. This is in keeping with the finding of Bruzzi et al.[42] that the increased cancer risk in gross cystic disease was associated with type I cysts.

These studies suggest that apocrine metaplasia in association with cystic disease and papillary apocrine change by itself are associated with a small increase in risk which only reaches clinically significant proportions where atypical forms are found on histology.

Duct ectasia/periductal mastitis

There is no evidence that DE or periductal mastitis predisposes to subsequent development of cancer, although we are not aware of any formal follow-up study and some degree of DE is so common in the general population that it will often coexist with other conditions carrying their own risk factors. Despite the stasis of duct content which must occur after total duct excision operations, there is no evidence that this is associated with increased cancer risk. Follow-up data presently available cannot be regarded as definitive, although we have no evidence to suggest that long-term follow-up is necessary.

Solitary duct papilloma

Solitary intraduct papilloma presenting as nipple discharge with or without a subareolar mass is usually considered to be a benign condition which carries no increased risk of breast cancer. A clear distinction must be made between the solitary intraductal papilloma and the much rarer (by a factor of 10) multiple intraduct type, which does carry an increased cancer risk.[36] The differences between these two types are discussed in Chapter 12. Prolonged follow-up is not regarded as necessary if the surgeon and pathologist are happy that the papilloma is indeed a solitary one and has been excised by microdochectomy. However, Table 18.1 shows that the consensus statement from the American College of Pathologists[29] puts papilloma with a fibrovascular core in the moderate risk group (1.5–2 times). Furthermore, a paper by Ciatto et al.[45] puts the RR at 3.3 (CL = 1.6–6.3). They followed 339 patients for a mean period of 6 years. It is difficult to explain this higher incidence than usually found: they noted no difference with solitary and multiple papillomas, and all 10 cancers occurred in the same segment as the papilloma, raising the possibility that some local pathology may have been missed at the original excision.

A conclusion of an increased risk seems surprising in relation to the general clinical view given above, but is perhaps less surprising when we consider the long-running controversy on this subject, as reviewed by Azzopardi.[30] Once again the basic defect is the lack of large series of well-defined cases followed up for life. At present it is reasonable to treat cases as having a risk so little increased that long-term follow-up is unnecessary unless some other risk factor is present.

Mild epithelial hyperplasia

The work of Page and others shows that mild epithelial hyperplasia (defined in the consensus statement as more than two but not more than four epithelial cells in depth) does not carry an increased risk. For notes on the nomenclature and groupings of hyperplasias, see Chapter 5.

Conditions with slightly increased risk (1.5–2 times)

Moderate or florid hyperplasia without atypia is considered to carry this slight increase in risk of later developing cancer. This accurate characterization of risk is crucially dependent on assessment of the pattern of hyperplasia by the histopathologist. Such accuracy of assessment of benign and malignant patterns, and of the gradation between the extremes, as used in the ACP consensus statement, depends heavily on the work of Azzopardi and Page. It is essential that each individual case is discussed by the pathologist and clinician to ensure that the pathologist's interpretation is understood by the clinician. It is important that the pathologist uses standard terminology such as that of Page's group, the criteria for which have been set out explicitly.[46] Recent multicentre studies have shown that histopathologists, after discussion of the problems, can reproduce Page's criteria with a reasonable degree of congruence.[47] Equally, the clinician needs an understanding of the spectrum and patterns of hyperplasia and of modern terminology. This is discussed at the end of this chapter.

It is important to realize that minor degrees of hyperplasia are common and have no increased risk of breast cancer, so that the term 'hyperplasia' does not itself indicate an increase in risk. When the cytology and architecture change to move closer to that of intraduct or lobular carcinoma-in-situ (LCIS) then the risk of subsequent malignancy increases. The description and definition of the limits of each stage of increasing hyperplasia are difficult and a subject of considerable debate. Several grading systems with different names have been

Table 18.2 Classification of hyperplasias

Black and Chabon[48]	Wellings et al.[25]	Dupont and Page[26,27]	Risk
Grade 1	ALA-I	Minimal	None
Grade 2	ALA-II	Mild hyperplasia with atypia	None
Grade 3	ALA-III	Moderate and florid hyperplasia without atypia	Slight increase
Grade 4	ALA-IV	Florid hyperplasia with atypia	Moderate increase
Grade 5	ALA-V	Carcinoma in situ	High

described by different pathologists, but it should be appreciated that the process is a continuum rather than a series of well-defined stages. The principal systems are outlined in Table 18.2 with approximate levels of equivalent severity of change indicated.

The diagnostic features of each grade are outside the scope of this work and lie in the province of detailed pathology textbooks. The interested reader is referred to the works by Azzopardi,[30] Black and Chabon,[48] Wellings *et al.*[25] and Dupont and Page.[26,46] It is particularly important to note that the use of the word atypical (or atypia) differs between Page's group and the other workers, hence the presence of some overlap in the comparability of lesions III and IV (Table 18.2) and Page's hyperplasias with and without atypia. It is inevitable that some borderline cases will be graded differently by different pathologists, hence the importance of understanding the spectrum of appearance.

Intraduct hyperplasia without evidence of atypia (often called epitheliosis (UK) or papillomatosis (USA) in the past) is a lesion which is commonly seen in biopsies undertaken for a dominant lump and was present in 22% of putatively normal breasts in a post-mortem study.[5] It is clear that malignancy is not inevitable even in those patients with a pathological state which carries a high risk. This histological entity has caused endless debate among pathologists and interpretation of published series has been difficult due to imprecise definition of this term. Careful histopathological studies by Page's group[26] have shown an increased risk of subsequent breast cancer if atypia or atypical lobular hyperplasia was present in the biopsy (discussed below), but the risk was not increased where the hyperplasia was cytologically and morphologically bland. Page further showed that a family history of breast cancer in a first-degree relative in a patient showing hyperplasia with atypia increases the relevant risk from 5 to 11 times.[27]

Because the distinction between the degrees of hyperplasia is made on the fine morphological and cytological detail, it is important that the surgeon encourages the pathologist to produce clear descriptive reports that specify the situation of epithelial changes along the spectrum from normal through hyperplasia to atypias, rather than using ill-defined general terms such as 'chronic mastopathy' or 'fibrocystic disease'. Fortunately this has become much more common and accepted over the past decade.

Conditions with moderate increase in cancer risk (5 times)

This group includes lobular and ductal hyperplasias with atypia. The quantitation of risk has been derived particularly from the work of Page's group.[26] The cancer risk following the diagnosis of lobular hyperplasia with atypia has been found to be 6 times in women aged less than 45 and 3 times in older women. This risk estimate has been validated by a further study[28] which set the risk at 6.4 times normal.

Page's group found the risk of ductal hyperplasia with atypia to be 2.6 times, and papillary apocrine change to be 2 times normal, so that ductal hyperplasia lies more in the slightly increased risk group (less than the corresponding patterns with assessment of lobular hyperplasia). This may reflect the greater difficulties associated with ductal hyperplasia: Azzopardi did not consider the case for an increased risk for ductal hyperplasia with atypia to be established.

Two more recent studies looking at different populations have come to similar conclusions, in each case showing a slightly higher risk than in the earlier studies. Dupont and colleagues[40] found that the presence of atypical hyperplasia in a biopsy carried a subsequent cancer risk of 4.3 times that of women without proliferative disease (CL = 1.7–11), while the presence of ductal hyperplasia without atypia had a relative risk of 1.3 (CL = 0.7–2.2). In each case a family history of breast cancer increased the risk 2.4 times (CL = 1.4–4.3).

The second study came from a prospective follow-up of 121,700 US registered nurses.[49] The corresponding figures with and without atypia were RR of 3.7 and 1.6. London *et al* do not comment on family history, but note the atypia-associated risk to be greater in premenopausal women (RR = 5.9) than postmenopausal women (RR = 2.3). The similarities between these studies suggests that the figures arrived at are a valid assessment of the risk.

Page and Simpson have recently reviewed this subject.[50]

An interesting corollary of these studies is whether prophylactic mastectomy reduces the risk of subsequent cancer. It has long been recognized that mastectomy by no means guarantees complete protection, but there have been few hard data to quantify the effect. A recent report from the Mayo Clinic, where 950 women undergoing bilateral prophylactic mastectomy were followed for an average of 17 years, suggests that the women were given a 90% risk reduction.[51]

The same question might be asked about the lesser diminution of glandular tissue achieved by reduction mammoplasty. Attempts to correlate breast size with cancer risk have been confounded by many factors, especially the varying amounts of adipose and glandular tissue. However, a large Danish study followed 7720 women undergoing reduction mammoplasty between 1977 and 1992.[52] Breast cancer was significantly reduced by almost 50% over that expected; cancers of other sites were unaffected. Interestingly, the benefit was only seen in women over 40 years at time of surgery, and particularly those over 50.

Conditions associated with a high risk of invasive cancer

The two entities of LCIS and ductal carcinoma-in-situ (DCIS) are cytologically cancers and not within the remit of benign breast disease. These two lesions were uncommon in the past, and presented rarely as a clinical mass or with nipple discharge. LCIS is normally discovered as an incidental finding on about 0.8% of benign biopsies and DCIS is commonly seen in cancerous breasts as an associated finding.

However, the situation has changed dramatically with the widespread use of screening and improvements in radiological diagnosis. Because the frequency with which it is diagnosed has increased so much, and the controversies regarding management are the subject of many ongoing studies, the subject is of great clinical importance. Full discussions are found in recent textbooks on malignant breast disease.

Non-histological risk factors

Study of the epidemiology of breast cancer has revealed a few personal and familial risk factors which can be elicited on the initial history. The increased risk from each of these factors is relatively weak with only a few reaching a relative risk higher than 4, approximately the risk for a contralateral breast cancer. These factors were summarized by Kalache,[53] who states that only two such factors reach a relative risk of 4: a family history of premenopausal bilateral breast cancer and a previous cancer in the other breast. Three other demographic factors of risk are obvious: female versus male, old versus young and North European/American versus Asian, but clearly these features are of no help in the management of the individual patient.

Thus the effect of the history on the management of patients with benign breast disease is simply that a family history in a mother or a sister (especially if premenopausal) should encourage follow-up and heighten the suspicion of the clinician towards any questionable dominant lump or borderline histology. Family history is a highly significant additive risk factor once atypical hyperplasia has been demonstrated in a biopsy (see above).

Mammographic patterns

Much interest in the last decade has been focused on the role of mammography of the benign breast in determining the cancer risk for individual patients. Wolfe proposed an apparently simple classification of mammograms based on parenchymal patterns which he considered would divide patients into high- and low-risk groups, with the high-risk groups having as much as a 12-fold increase in risk, and the higher risk group (DY pattern) a relative risk as high as 27.[54] However, this concept ran into fierce criticism and, although parenchymal patterns seem to have some interesting correlations with other non-radiological risk factors,[55] many studies failed to confirm Wolfe's original observations.[56]

All of these studies were retrospective and therefore subject to sampling errors, until the report from Verbeek *et al.*[57] which was a prospective case-control study. When the papers on this subject were reviewed it was concluded that there is likely to be some increased risk associated with the DY pattern, but not to the degree reported by Wolfe.[58] A prospective study of a screened population from the island of Guernsey showed that Wolfe's DY pattern was associated with an increased risk of subsequent breast cancer but only at the level of 4 times risk, one-sixth of that proposed by Wolfe.[59] Interest in this work has waned over the past decade, although some studies continue. Wolfe patterns do not at present alter our management policies.

New techniques for estimating risk

It will be clear from the preceding discussions of borderline or premalignant histology that pathological estimations of risk are not easy and depend crucially on the experience and knowledge of the individual pathologist, and require a section of breast tissue, hopefully representative. There is no reason to believe that the clinical presentations that induce a surgeon to perform a biopsy will be associated with high-risk pathology as most of the hyperplastic lesions with atypia are found incidentally at biopsy for a condition such as dominant nodularity. This situation has been summarized succinctly by Sloane[60] when he said: 'Effective screening is the major problem as several clinico-pathological studies suggest that the lesions with the greatest potential for neoplastic change usually produce no premonitory symptoms and are discovered incidentally.' An ideal method of risk estimation should be accurate in its prediction, be able to be performed on readily accessible body constituents – preferably blood or urine – and should not depend on subjective interpretation. No such marker has been discovered to date.

Despite this conclusion there has been much interest in possible biochemical markers, of which the most promising has been Haagensen's work on the breast cyst protein GCDFP-15, discussed above and in Chapter 9.

Khan *et al.* have recently suggested that ER (oestrogen receptor) expression may have a predictive effect in postmenopausal women.[61] They compared the percentage of epithelial cells expressing ER in high-risk (normal epithelium from the contralateral breast in women with breast cancer) and normal risk women. In postmenopausal women ER expression correlated with cancer risk, PR (progesterone receptor) expression was the same in both groups. HRT use confounded the results, since it increased ER expression in low-risk women to the levels seen in the high-risk group. There was a suggestion that increase of the percentage of cells expressing ER in the luteal phase in premenopausal women (when it is normally increased) could also be an indicator of cancer risk, but results were only clear-cut in the postmenopausal, non-HRT group.

Molecular markers and cancer risk

In view of the genetic changes in cancer, the possibility that mutations might occur in benign tissues which would subsequently lead to cancer has raised much interest, as yet without a great deal of progress. A group at the Mayo Clinic analysed benign biopsies for a range of molecular markers, particularly p53.[62] Fourteen of 60 samples showed immunoreactivity to p53, and five to the HER-2/neu protein product, but they were not related to recognized premalignant histological patterns, and no conclusions regarding a relationship to subsequent cancer were drawn.

Similarly, studies of chromosomal changes have detected abnormalities in diffuse proliferative disease, papillomas and fibroadenomas. Some of the changes were the same as have been seen repeatedly in early cancers, suggesting that they may be early neoplasia-relevant changes, but not sufficient in themselves to initiate malignancy.[63]

REFERENCES

1. Hislop TG & Elwood JM. Risk factors for benign breast disease: a 30 year cohort study. *Canadian Medical Association Journal* 1981; **124**: 283–291.

2. Vessey MP, McPherson K & Doll R. Breast cancer and oral contraceptives: findings in the Oxford-FPA contraceptive study. *British Medical Journal* 1981; **282**: 2093–2094.

3. Ader DN & Browne MW. Prevalence and impact of cyclical mastalgia in a United States clinic based sample. *American Journal of Obstetrics and Gynecology* 1997; **177**: 126–132.

4. Cooke MG & Rohan TE. The patho-epidemiology of benign proliferative epithelial disorders of the female breast. *Journal of Pathology* 1985; **146**: 1–15.

5. Sandison AT. An autopsy study of the human breast. *National Cancer Institute Monograph No. 8*, US Dept Health, Education and Welfare, 1962.

6. Aaman TB, Stalsberg H & Thomas DB. Extratumoral breast tissue in breast cancer patients: study of variations with age and country of residence in low- and high-risk countries. *International Journal of Cancer* 1997; **71**: 333–339.

7. Royal College of General Practitioners. Breast cancer and oral contraceptives: findings in Royal College of General Practitioners Study. *British Medical Journal* 1981; **282**: 2089–2093.

8. Pons JY. Medical treatment of mastopathies at risk. [Review] *Revue Française de Gynecologie et d'Obstetrique* 1991; **86**: 29–32.

9. Anderson TJ, Ferguson DJP & Raab GM. Cell turnover in the 'resting' human breast: influence of parity, contraceptive pill, age and laterality. *British Journal of Cancer* 1982; **46**: 376–382.

10. McPherson K, Vessey MP, Neil A *et al.* Early oral contraceptive use and breast cancer: Results of another case control study. *British Journal of Cancer* 1987; **56**: 653–660.

11. Asscher AW. Oral contraceptives and breast cancer. *Lancet* 1987; **ii**: 1267.

12. McGonigle KF & Huggins GR. Oral contraceptives and breast disease. [Review] *Fertility and Sterility* 1991; **56**: 799–819.

13. Stomper PC, Van Voorhis BJ, Ravnikor VA & Meyer JE. Mammographic changes associated with post-menopausal HRT – a longitudinal study. *Radiology* 1990; **174**: 487–490.

14. McNicholas MM, Heneghan JP, Milney MH *et al.* Pain and increased mammographic density in women receiving hormone replacement therapy: a prospective study. *American Journal of Roentgenology* 1994; **163**: 311–315.

15. Litherland JC, Evans AJ & Wilson ARM. The effect of hormone replacement therapy on recall rate in the National Health Service breast screening programme. *Clinical Radiology* 1997; **52**: 276–279.

16. Rickard MT & Selopranoto S. Enlarging and newly appearing fibroadenomas in screening mammography. *The Breast* 1996; **5**: 100–104.

17. Brenner RJ, Bein ME, Sarti DA & Vinstein AL. Spontaneous regression of interval benign cysts of the breast. *Radiology* 1994; **193**: 365–368.

18. Willis DB, Calle EE, Miracle-McMahill HL & Heath CW Jr. Estrogen replacement therapy and risk of fatal breast cancer in a prospective cohort of post-menopausal women in the United States. *Cancer Causes and Control* 1996; **7**: 449–457.

19. Roberts MM, Elton RA, Robinson SE & French K. Consultation for breast disease in general practice and referral patterns. *British Journal of Surgery* 1987; **74**: 1020–1023.

20. Nichols S, Waters WE & Wheeler MJ. Management of female breast disease by Southampton general practitioners. *British Medical Journal* 1980; **281**: 1450–1453.

21. Bywaters JL. The incidence and management of female breast disease in a general practice. *Journal of the Royal College of General Practitioners* 1977; **27**: 353–357.

22. Ernster VL. The epidemiology of benign breast disease. *Epidemiological Review* 1981; **3**: 184–202.

23. Ingram DM, Nottage E & Roberts T. The role of diet in the development of breast cancer: a case control study of patients with breast cancer, benign epithelial hyperplasia and fibrocystic disease of the breast. *British Journal of Cancer* 1991; **64**: 187–191.

24. Lubin F, Wax Y, Ron E *et al.* Nutritional factors associated with benign breast disease etiology: a case-control study. *American Journal of Clinical Nutrition* 1989; **50**: 551–556.

25. Wellings SR, Jensen HM & Marcum RG. An atlas of subgross pathology of the human breast with special reference to possible precancerous lesions. *Journal of the National Cancer Institute* 1975; **55**: 231–273.

26. Page DL, Vander Zwaag R, Rogers LW *et al.* Relation between component parts of fibrocystic disease complex and breast cancer. *Journal of the National Cancer Institute* 1978; **61**: 1055–1063.

27. Dupont WD & Page DL. Risk factors for breast cancer in women with proliferative breast disease. *New England Journal of Medicine* 1985; **312**: 146–151.

28. Roberts MM, Jones V, Elton RA *et al.* Risk of breast cancer in women with a history of benign disease of the breast. *British Medical Journal* 1984; **288**: 275–278.

29. Winchester DP. ACP consensus statement. The relationship of fibrocystic disease to breast cancer. *American College of Surgeons Bulletin* 1986; **71**: 29–31.

30. Azzopardi JG. In: *Major Problems in Pathology*, Vol II, *Problems in Breast Pathology*. London: WB Saunders, 1979.

31. Semb C. Pathologico-anatomical and clinical investigations of fibroadenomatosis cystica mammae and its relation to other pathological conditions in the mamma, especially cancer. *Acta Chirurgica Scandinavica* 1928; **64** (Suppl 10): 1–484.

32. Oliver RL & Major RC. Cyclomastopathy: a physio-pathological conception of some benign breast tumours, with an analysis of four hundred cases. *American Journal of Cancer* 1934; **21**: 1–85.

33. Levi F, Randimbison L, Te VC *et al.* Incidence of breast cancer in women with fibroadenoma. *International Journal of Cancer* 1994; **57**: 681–683.

34. McDivitt RW, Stevens JA, Lee NC *et al.* Histologic types of benign breast disease and the risk of breast cancer. *Cancer* 1992; **69**: 1408–1414.

35. Dupont WD, Page DL, Parl FF *et al.* Long term risk of breast cancer in women with fibroadenoma. *New England Journal of Medicine* 1994; **331**: 10–15.

36. Haagensen CD, Bodian C & Haagensen DE. *Breast Carcinoma, Risk and Detection*, pp 83–105. London: Saunders, 1986.

37. Tavassoli FA & Norris HJ. A comparison of the results of longterm follow up of atypical intraduct hyperplasia and intraductal hyperplasia of the breast. *Cancer* 1990; **65**: 518–529.

38. James BA, Cranor ML & Rosen PP. Carcinoma of the breast arising in microglandular adenosis. *American Journal of Clinical Pathology* 1993; **100**: 507–513.

39. Davis HH, Simons M & Davis JB. Cystic disease of the breast: relationship to carcinoma. *Cancer* 1964; **17**: 957–978.

40. Dupont WD, Parl FF, Hartman WH *et al.* Breast cancer risk associated with proliferative breast disease and atypical hyperplasia. *Cancer* 1993; **71**: 1258–1265.

41. Bundred NJ, West RR, Dowd JO *et al*. Is there an increased risk of breast cancer in women who have had a breast cyst aspirated? *British Journal of Cancer* 1991; **64**: 953–955.

42. Bruzzi P, Dogliotti L, Naldoni C *et al*. Cohort study of risk of breast cancer with cyst type in women with gross cystic disease of the breast. *British Medical Journal* 1997; **314**: 925–928.

43. Page DL, Dupont WD & Jensen RA. Papillary apocrine change of the breast – associations with atypical hyperplasia and risk of breast cancer. *Cancer Epidemiology, Biomarkers and Prevention* 1996; **5**: 29–32.

44. Seidman JD, Ashton M & Lefkowitz M. Atypical apocrine adenosis of the breast: a clinicopathological study of 37 patients with an 8.7 year follow-up. *Cancer* 1996; **77**: 2529–2537.

45. Ciatto S, Andreoli C, Cirillo A *et al*. The risk of breast cancer subsequent to histological diagnosis of benign intraductal papilloma. *Tumori* 1991; **71**: 41–43.

46. Page DL & Rogers RW. Combined histologic and cytologic criteria for the diagnosis of mammary atypical ductal hyperplasia. *Human Pathology* 1992; **23**: 1095.

47. Schnitt SJ, Connolly JL, Tavassoli FA *et al*. Interobserver reproducibility in the diagnosis of ductal proliferative breast lesions using standardised criteria. *American Journal of Surgical Pathology* 1992; **16**: 1133–1143.

48. Black MM & Chabon AB. In situ carcinoma of the breast. In: Sommers SC (ed.) *Pathology Annual*, pp 185–210. New York: Appleton-Century-Crofts, 1969.

49. London SJ, Connolly JL, Schnitt SJ & Colditz GA. A prospective study of benign breast disease and the risk of breast cancer. *Journal of the American Medical Association* 1992; **267**: 941–944.

50. Page DL & Simpson JF. Pathology of pre-invasive and excellent-prognosis breast cancer. [Review] *Current Opinion in Oncology* 1996; **8**: 462–467.

51. Comment. *Journal of the National Cancer Institute* 1997; **89**: 762.

52. Boice JD Jr, Friis S, McLaughlin JK *et al*. Cancer following breast reduction surgery in Denmark. *Cancer Causes and Control* 1997; **8**: 253–258.

53. Kalache A. Risk factors for breast cancer: a tabular summary of the epidemiological literature. *British Journal of Surgery* 1981; **68**: 797–799.

54. Wolfe JN. Risk for breast cancer development determined by mammographic parenchymal pattern. *Cancer* 1976; **37**: 2486–2492.

55. De Waard F, Rombach JJ, Collette HJA & Slotboom B. Breast cancer risk associated with reproductive factors and breast parenchymal patterns. *Journal of the National Cancer Institute* 1984; **72**: 1277–1282.

56. Egan RL & Mosteller RC. Breast cancer mammography patterns. *Cancer* 1977; **40**: 2087–2090.

57. Verbeek ALM, Hendricks JHC, Peters PHM & Sturmans F. Mammographic breast pattern and the risk of breast cancer. *Lancet* 1984; **i**: 591–593.

58. Boyd NF, O'Sullivan B, Fishell E, Simor I & Cooke E. Mammographic patterns and breast cancer risk. Methodologic standards and contradictory results. *Journal of the National Cancer Institute* 1984; **72**: 1258–1259.

59. Gravelle IH, Bulstrode JC, Bulbrook RD *et al*. A prospective study of mammographic parenchymal patterns and risk of breast cancer. *British Journal of Radiology* 1986; **59**(701): 487–491.

60. Sloane JP. Precancerous changes in the breast. In: Carter RC (ed.) *Precancerous States*. London: Oxford University Press, 1984.

61. Khan SA, Rogers MAM, Khuurana KK *et al*. Estrogen receptor expression in benign breast epithelium and breast cancer risk. *Journal of the National Cancer Institute* 1998; **90**: 37–42.

62. Millikan R, Hulka B, Thor A *et al*. P53 mutations in benign breast tissue. *Journal of Clinical Oncology* 1995; **13**: 2293–2300.

63. Dietrich CU, Pandis N, Teixeira MR *et al*. Chromosome-abnormalities in benign hyperproliferative disorders of epithelial and stromal breast tissue. *International Journal of Cancer* 1995; **60**: 49–53.

Chapter 19

Geographical variations – benign breast disorders in non-Western populations

KEY POINTS AND NEW DEVELOPMENTS

1. There is a widely held perception that major differences in various entities of benign breast disorder are found in different populations. There is much less hard evidence to support this than is generally supposed.
2. Some of the apparent differences may be due to low rates of presentation of painful nodularity and other elements of ANDI in non-Western countries. Whether this low incidence of ANDI is due to absence, or merely failure to consult, is unclear. The incidence of painful nodularity has increased dramatically in one centre in India in recent years.
3. While the proportion of fibroadenoma within benign breast disorders is much higher in Africa and India than among white women, the absolute incidence may be as high, or higher, in white women.
4. There appear to be true and unexplained variations in the incidence of phyllodes tumours, even within the same country.
5. Histological evidence of 'fibrocystic disease' in Africa and India is consistently seen in an earlier age group than in Western countries.
6. Many developing countries show a high incidence of chronic abscess associated with inadequate primary treatment of lactational abscess. Abscesses associated with duct ectasia/periductal mastitis (DE/PDM) appear to be rare, but they could be underdiagnosed.
7. There is a great need for well-designed studies comparing benign breast disorders in various countries, particularly longitudinal studies as developing countries take on Western customs and habits.

It is not surprising that benign breast disorders in non-Western countries or non-white populations have evoked little interest when they have been neglected until recently in Western countries. Only in the last 20 years have papers dealing with non-Western populations begun to appear.

Against this paucity of hard data, there has been a general perception that the spectrum of benign breast disorders is different in these countries, with a predominance of pregnancy-related disorders, especially lactational abscess, and with the various manifestations of 'fibrocystic disease' notable by their absence.

In the past, reports of disease incidence (of all kinds) from Third World countries have often come from teaching centres which deal with only a fraction of the population, presenting a biased view from an unrepresentative sample. Patients with non-life threatening conditions may not travel long distances to an overburdened teaching hospital, so these conditions may be perceived to be rare.

Recent experience suggests that these considerations may apply to benign breast disorders, for when surgeons who have worked in centres with special interest and expertise in this area return to their home country, the spectrum appears to be remarkably similar in Western and developing countries,[1,2] although some notable proportional differences are still seen. While we have no practical experience of management of benign conditions in these countries, discussion and correspondence with many colleagues suggests that these similarities may be as significant as the disparities.

Apart from the obvious occurrence of tropical diseases such as tuberculosis and filariasis, the two differences that are reported repeatedly are a higher incidence of fibroadenoma (and possibly giant and multiple fibroadenoma) among black populations (and to a lesser extent among Indian and Chinese women), especially in South Africa and the West Indies; and a corresponding lower incidence of painful nodularity and other elements of ANDI. Even here, the absence of detailed population-based studies means that aberrant referral patterns cannot be excluded.

ASIA

Alagaratnam and Wong reviewed 2065 Chinese women with benign breast disorders seen in a specialist breast clinic in Hong Kong over a 16-year period,[3] during which 939 patients with breast cancer were also seen. The spectrum of benign conditions differed markedly from Indian and African women in that 'fibroadenosis' was twice as common as fibroadenoma. These two formed 53% and 29% of cases respectively, with bacterial infections and duct papilloma making 8% and 4% respectively. Lipomas were surprisingly common at almost 4%, with DE/PDM at 2%, and six benign phyllodes tumours (0.5%). Tuberculosis and paraffinoma (a Hong Kong specialty) each constituted about 1%.

More recently, a series of giant fibroadenomas has been reported from the same unit,[4] 26 patients being seen over a period of 20 years. The lesions behaved in similar fashion to those seen in the UK, all were enucleated without recurrence, and in all cases the defect filled spontaneously without need for reconstruction. The lesions tended to present earlier, probably related to the small breast size of Chinese women, and the sudden rapid growth typical in adolescent white girls was not seen. The incidence in this series is not greatly different to that seen in Western countries, considering the large population covered by this one specialist unit. Thus the perception of a high incidence in Chinese women may not be valid. It has arisen from the report of Nambiar and Kannan-Kutty[5] who reported 15 cases in Chinese women over a 9-year period. These patients were collected over a wide area of Malaysia and Singapore, so again the perceived high incidence may be an artefact of referral pattern.

Cheung and Alagaratnam have also reviewed the cases of nipple discharge seen in Chinese women attending their Hong Kong breast clinic.[6] They constituted 1.5% of women seen, and all aspects were similar to experience in Western countries.

The incidence of high-risk radiological Wolfe patterns in Asian women undergoing mammographic screening has been compared to that in white women,[7] to see if it correlates with the lower incidence of cancer. This was found to be so, with a highly significant excess of Asians in the low-risk N1/P1 categories.

An increase in the incidence of breast cancer in Japan in recent decades has been well recognized, with much speculation as to whether this is related to westernization of diet or other aspects of Japanese life. Whether there has been a parallel increase in benign proliferative lesions has been studied by Schnitt et al.[8] They compared a consecutive series of benign breast biopsies from 1974 to 1975, classified according to the criteria of Dupont and Page (see Chapter 18), with a similar series a decade later. Over the 10-year period there was a highly significant increase in the number of cases showing proliferative lesions, with and without atypia, but this was confined to the younger women, with incidence of 18% versus 6% in women younger than 40, but only 17% versus 13% (NS) in women older than 40.

INDIA

India clearly reflects the lack of published work on benign breast conditions until recently; no publication has been found devoted to this subject prior to 1983.

Rangabashyam and colleagues reported a series of 215 benign breast lesions seen in a single unit in Madras,[9] which showed a similar pattern to many other non-Western countries, with a marked predominance of fibroadenoma (57%), together with chronic pyogenic abscess (8%) and a high incidence of galactocele (also 8%). The range of less common conditions was unremarkable, but there was a 17% incidence of 'fibroadenosis', seen at a young age (70% before the age of 30) similar to that seen in other non-Western countries, but differing by about a decade from rates in Western women.

In 1989, Shukla and Kumar[1] reported a dual study of benign breast disorders, a prospective study of patients seen in two large teaching centres during 1985–1987 and a 10-year retrospective study of histological reports. Once again fibroadenoma was the commonest single lesion, and patients presented at an early age, with a peak in the 20–30 age group and more than 90% presenting before the age of 40. Only 2% of the patients had taken the oral contraceptive pill for a year, and it is interesting to speculate whether this may play a role in the high incidence of fibroadenoma, since the oral contraceptives seem to be protective for fibroadenoma, as well as nodularity in general.

In both series, fibroadenoma predominated, comprising over 40% of all presentations excluding mastalgia. (Thus in four studies in India,[1,2,9,10] the incidence of fibroadenoma was 38%, 46%, 40% and 57%. The incidence of 'fibroadenosis'-related conditions was also similar in the four series, at 20%, 16%, 20% and 16%. Surprisingly, the incidence of phyllodes tumour varied considerably, at 11%, 1%, 14% and 2%.)

Chronic abscess and tuberculosis were seen in the two studies by Rangabashyam et al.[9] and Shukla and Kumar[1] in about 10% and 5% respectively. A total of four cases of filariasis (0.3% of all benign breast disorders) were seen in the two studies. Mastalgia was quite common; the incidence was twice that of cancer and about one quarter that of all benign breast disorders.

A recent paper from India[2] is of interest because it shows considerable changes from earlier papers towards statistics more in keeping with those in the West. Analysing 234 cases over a 2-year period (acute abscess was excluded) from the same hospital as Shukla and Kumar,[1] breast pain and nodularity has become the most common presentation (70%) with fibroadenoma now down to 17.5%. It is not possible to tell whether this represents an absolute decrease in fibroadenoma, or an increase in pain and nodularity. The latter seems the more likely, and may be due either to increased awareness on the part of women, or to a true increase in manifestations of ANDI. Only population-based studies will be able to tell which is the most important, but such information is of prime importance in understanding benign breast disorders. Mastalgia showed a ratio between cyclical and non-cyclical patterns similar to that seen in the West.

AFRICA

There has been a considerable amount of material published on benign breast conditions from various countries of Africa, but it suffers in general with the limitations of ill-defined referral patterns described above.

One study from Kenya avoided these biases by evaluating a population of healthy nurses in Nairobi to assess the importance of the premenstrual syndrome (PMS) in these patients,[11] providing some insight into the problem of mastalgia. A sample of 400 nurses were interviewed with an investigator-administered questionnaire. A surprisingly high percentage of patients (95.5%) reported PMS, with mastalgia the symptom in 80%. However, most women regarded the symptom as a normal part of their feminity, with the result that only 6% changed their activities, and only 3% took medication.

Bjerregaard and Kung'u have reviewed the histological diagnoses of a large series (1084 cases) of benign breast disorders from the same hospital.[12] Benign biopsies were more than twice as common as cancer, partly due to the high incidence of fibroadenoma, which exceeded that of cancer by 25%. Fifteen per cent of the biopsies were for 'mastopathy', and these fell readily into the three main groups of cysts, fibrosis and hyperplastic mastopathy.

Onukak and Cederquist reviewed 306 histologically diagnosed benign conditions from northern Nigeria.[13] Two benign biopsies were performed for each cancer, and fibroadenoma was the dominant condition, comprising 44% of all benign biopsies. Twenty-nine per cent of the masses were more than 6 cm in diameter, suggesting a high incidence of giant fibroadenoma, and similar to the figure of 30% reported in Ugandan Africans.[14] Although there was one malignant phyllodes tumour in the series, benign phyllodes tumour was notably absent, confirming the marked regional variations found with this condition. Virginal hypertrophy was also not seen, suggesting that there may be regional differencs in this condition as well among black women.

One-third of the patients were diagnosed as 'mammary dysplasia', with fibrosis, adenosis and sclerosing adenosis. Two-thirds of these patients were nulliparous, despite the high level of parity in this population. Most conditions seen in Western populations were present, such as lactating adenoma, tubular adenoma, duct papilloma and DE/PDM. The ratio of tubular and lactating adenomas to fibroadenomas of 1:20 was high, but again similar to the figure reported for Uganda.[14] As expected, lactation-related infections were high, with frequent chronicity. Only two cases of tuberculosis of the breast were found, in spite of a high incidence of tuberculosis in the region.

Even within a country such as Nigeria, there are notable differences in benign disorders, which may be related to differences in lifestyle. Otu reported from the rainforest of south-east Nigeria,[15] where fibroadenoma accounted for 70% of masses, infective conditions for 25%, with 'fibrocystic disease' only 3%, compared with tuberculosis at 7%. The incidence of tuberculosis differs from that reported by Onukak discussed above. The mean age for all conditions was only 24 years, although this is not surprising with the dominance of fibroadenoma, and almost all the infective conditions were lactation related.

A report of 657 patients from the urban area of Ibadan is in marked contrast.[16] Here media pressure for breast self-examination was responsible for some (although only a minority of 15%) of the presentations. Simple abscesses were not included in the study. 'Mammary dysplasia' accounted for 29% of the benign disorders, and fibroadenoma was still responsible for 55%. Furthermore, an additional 8% were diagnosed as sclerosing adenosis, and 65% of these presented with pain. Pain was complained of in only 10% of mammary dysplasia. Thirteen phyllodes tumours (2%) were seen, again contrasting with the figures from the north. There were twice as many cancers as benign masses, and the overall incidence of benign disorders was computed as 15/100,000 women years, compared to an incidence of 122 reported from Boston.[17] The figure for fibroadenoma in Boston was 33, compared with about 8 for Ibadan. While there may be many fibroadenomas which go untreated in Ibadan, the figures do not support the widely held view of a very much higher incidence among black populations.

Thus the incidence of fibroadenoma seems similar throughout Nigeria, but the incidence of 'fibrocystic disease' varies greatly, as does that of phyllodes tumour.

It is interesting to compare these African series with a study of black patients in the USA.[18] There 48% of 282 benign lesions were again fibroadenoma, with 'fibrocystic disease' the second largest group at 24%. Intraductal papilloma and sclerosing adenosis were each about 5%, the rest made up of a wide variety of less common conditions. Only one phyllodes tumour was seen (0.5%). The peak age incidence of 15–25 for fibroadenoma is similar to that seen in Africa, and 'fibrocystic disease' is seen at an earlier age than in white Americans, although in the black women it was seen over a wider age range with less of a peak, from 20 to 70.

MIDDLE EAST

Amr and colleagues reported a study of 915 patients with breast disease,[19] of which 15% were cases of cancer. When these were excluded, the pattern of benign disease is similar to that seen in other non-Western populations, with fibroadenoma predominating at 36%. Conditions associated with pregnancy accounted for 32% and 'fibrocystic condition' for 25%. The incidence of breast disease is noted to have increased markedly in the last 5 years.

MELANESIA

Murthy *et al.* have reported a study of 302 biopsy-confirmed benign breast lesions among the native population of New Guinea.[20] Pregnancy-related inflammatory breast diseases were much the most important group, and they attribute this to the high frequency of pregnancy, together with poor general hygiene and lack of antibiotic therapy. There was a high incidence of tuberculous mastitis. Once again 'fibrocystic' disease was found to present in a younger age group than generally reported in Western populations.

INDIVIDUAL CONDITIONS

Fibroadenoma and phyllodes tumour
Fibroadenoma makes up such a large proportion of benign breast disorders in India and Africa that an excess in these populations could be considered likely. However, there are no population-based figures to support this. As discussed above, one study from Africa[16] (fibroadenoma comprised 55% of all benign breast disorders) computed an absolute rate only one-quarter of that reported for white patients in Boston.[17] The reported incidences in Chinese women seem lower than those in African women, and the fibroadenoma proportion of benign breast disorders in India is falling dramatically as painful nodularity becomes more obtrusive.

Giant fibroadenoma
Onukak and Cederquist[13] found that 29% of fibroadenomas exceeded 6 cm in diameter, similar to the 30% reported from Uganda, and qualifying for designation as giant fibroadenoma. In contrast, only 4% of fibroadenomas exceeded 5 cm (and that included pregnancy, lactating adenomas, etc.) in an Indian/African population in South Africa. Although this latter figure is probably higher than in the UK, it is not markedly so. The high figures in Nigeria and Uganda are dramatically different to those reported in Western series, so probably represent a true excess, and a similar pattern is reported anecdotally from the West Indies. Giant fibroadenoma seems to be much less common among Chinese women (3%[10]) and the incidence is probably similar to that seen in UK series.

Phyllodes tumour is particularly interesting, with evidence that the incidence varies considerably, and without obvious reason. There are considerable differences between different areas in Nigeria and India, which are probably significant, even allowing for variation among pathologists regarding diagnostic criteria. Perhaps the absence of virginal hypertrophy (usually seen particularly in black girls) in the series from northern Nigeria where phyllodes tumour was also absent reflects a lack in this area of some agent stimulatory to breast tissue.

Tubular and lactating adenomas
The incidence of these 'pure' adenomas seems to be high in relation to that of fibroadenomas in Africa, as reported from Nigeria,[13] while this has also been reported from Jamaica.[21]

Inflammatory conditions
As would be expected, lactation-related infections and abscesses are seen frequently in countries where very high pregnancy rates are the norm. Less expected is the high incidence of chronic abscess formation in developing countries. This is attributed to poor hygiene, the lack of effective surgery and restricted access to antibiotics, or use of inappropriate antibiotics. The possibility that some of these may be subareolar and due to unrecognized DE/PDM cannot be

excluded, although this is unlikely since in one series where 96% of abscesses, and most of the chronic ones, occurred in relation to lactation only 4% occurred in young women with inverted nipples.

It is not surprising that tuberculosis is relatively common in countries where the disease is still widespread, although the incidence varies and in some cases appears to be inappropriately low.[7] Filariasis also affects the breast where it is endemic.

ANDI

Painful nodularity and histological evidence of 'fibrocystic disease' are much less common in non-Western than in Western countries, typically comprising 3–30% of benign breast disorders in Africa, in contrast to rates of 70% and 55% fibroadenoma in the same two centres. However, for 'fibrocystic disease' the figures from the second centre, which was an urban population in Nigeria subjected to breast awareness campaigns, were remarkably similar to those reported among black women in the USA. A recent study from Hongkong shows cyclical mastalgia to have similar features and response to treatment to those reported from western countries.[22]

It is clear that much more data are required to learn the extent of any geographical variations in benign breast disorders, and equally clear that such studies could provide important insights into these conditions. The collection of such data will become more meaningful as the use of the term 'fibrocystic disease' disappears, to be replaced by specific clinical and histological terms that can be compared from one country to another.

REFERENCES

1. Shukla HS & Kumar S. Benign breast disorders in non-western populations: Part 11–Benign Breast Disorders in India. *World Journal of Surgery* 1989; **13**: 746–749.
2. Khanna AJ, Tapodar J & Misra MK. Spectrum of benign breast disorders in a university hospital. *Journal of the Indian Medical Association* 1997; **95**: 5–8.
3. Alagaratnam TT & Wong J. Benign breast disorders in Chinese women. *World Journal of Surgery* 1989; **13**: 743–745.
4. Alagaratnam TT, Ng WF & Leung EYF. Giant fibroadenoma of the breast in an oriental community. *Journal of the Royal College of Surgeons of Edinburgh* 1995; **40**: 161–162.
5. Nambiar R & Kannan-Kutty M. Giant Fibro-adenoma (cystosarcoma phyllodes) in adolescent females – a clinicopathological study. *British Journal of Surgery* 1974; **61**: 113–117.
6. Cheung KL & Alagaratnam TT. A review of nipple discharge in Chinese women. *Journal of Royal College of Surgeons of Edinburgh* 1997; **42**: 179–181.
7. Turnbull AE, Kapera L & Cohen ME. Mammographic parenchymal patterns in Asian and Caucasian women attending for breast screening. *Clinical Radiology* 1993; **48**: 38–40.
8. Schnitt SJ, Jimi A & Kojiro M. The increasing prevalence of benign proliferative breast lesions in Japanese women. *Cancer* 1993; **71**: 2528–2531.
9. Rangabashyam N, Gnanaprakasam D, Krishnaraj B *et al.* Spectrum of benign breast lesions in Madras. *Journal of the Royal College of Surgeons of Edinburgh* 1983; **28**: 369–373.
10. Khanna S, Arrya NC & Khanna NN. Spectrum of benign breast disease. *Indian Journal of Surgery* 1988; **50**: 169.
11. Rupani NP & Lema VM. Premenstrual tension among nurses in Nairobi, Kenya. *East African Medical Journal* 1993; **70**: 310–313.
12. Bjerregaard B & Kung'u A. Benign breast lesions in Kenya: a histological study. *East African Medical Journal* 1992; **69**: 231–235.
13. Onukak EE & Cederquist RA. Benign breast disorders in Northern Nigeria. *World Journal of Surgery* 1989; **13**: 750–752.
14. Templeton AC. Tumors of the breast. In: *Tumors in a Tropical Country, a Survey of Uganda 1964–1968*, pp 94–100. London: Heinemann, 1973.
15. Otu AA. Benign breast tumours in an African population. *Journal of the Royal College of Surgeons of Edinburgh* 1990; **35**: 373–375.
16. Ihekwaba FN. Benign breast disease in Nigerian women: a study of 657 patients. *Journal of the Royal College of Surgeons of Edinburgh* 1994; **39**: 280–283.
17. Cole P, Elwood JM & Kaplan SD. Incidence rates and risk factors of benign breast neoplasms. *American Journal of Epidemiology* 1978; **108**: 112–120.
18. Oluwole SF & Freeman HP. Analysis of benign breast lesions in blacks. *American Journal of Surgery* 1979; **137**: 786–789.
19. Amr SS, Sadi ARM, Ilahi F & Sheikh SS. The spectrum of breast diseases in Saudi Arab females – a 26 year pathological survey at Dharhran Health Centre. *Annals of Saudi Medicine* 1995; **15**: 125–132.
20. Murthy DP, SenGupta SK & Muthaiah AC. Benign breast disease in Papua New Guinea. *Papua New Guinea Medical Journal* 1992; **35**: 101–105.
21. Persaud V, Talerman A & Jordan R. Pure adenoma of the breast. *Archives of Pathology* 1968;**86**:481–485
22. Cheung KL. Management of cyclical mastalgia in Oriental women. *Australian and New Zealand Journal of Surgery* 1999;**69**:492–494.

Operations

CONTENTS

The detailed indications for various operations have been outlined in previous chapters dealing with individual conditions. The general indications, detailed technique and complications of each operation are gathered together in this chapter.

TISSUE DIAGNOSIS IN THE CLINIC

It is now clear that the majority of breast abnormalities can and should be diagnosed in the clinic, in most cases all diagnostic modalities except open biopsy being used at the first visit. In our own practice diagnostic open biopsy is now an unusual event in symptomatic patients but is still sometimes necessary in the screening clinic. The two important techniques are cytological examination and core needle biopsy for histology. Sampling may be clinically or image guided.

Breast samples for cytological examination may be obtained either by aspiration cytology or by exfoliative cytology of nipple discharge or by imprint cytology of ulcerated lesions of the breast or nipple.

Two forms of needle biopsy need to be differentiated: fine needle aspiration for cytology and core needle biopsy for definitive histology.

Fine needle aspiration (FNA) cytology is simple, causes little discomfort and can be used to sample lesions of all sizes. It is unlikely to spread tumour cells or lead to implantation along the needle track. Accurate interpretation is critically dependent on the availability of a skilled experienced cytologist.

Core needle biopsy is easily performed under local anaesthesia, and with newer spring-loaded techniques, need cause no more pain than FNA. The coarser instrument is efficient in obtaining satisfactory specimens from carcinomas of 2 cm diameter or more but it is more difficult to locate small lesions than is the case with FNA, unless with the aid of image guidance. The rubbery fibrotic tissue typical of benign breast conditions rarely gives a good tissue core with a hand-held needle, but better results are obtained with the newer spring-loaded instruments. An adequate core can provide definitive histology equivalent to that from an open biopsy. There is a small risk of needle track implantation from carcinoma.

With both techniques, the benefit lies only in obtaining a positive diagnosis and little credence should be placed on a negative result unless sampling error can be excluded with certainty.

Some authorities avoid core biopsy for very small lesions (e.g. <5 mm) for fear that a small cancer may be removed completely, leaving no indication of its location for re-excision. With such small lesions, usually of excellent prognosis and with follow-up available, this may be a more theoretical than practical problem.

Fine needle aspiration
The first description of aspiration cytology was that of Martin and Ellis,[1] who described the technique and the results in 65 patients (six breast) with cancer. Stewart[2] described the results

in 500 breast lumps and gave clear descriptions of both benign and malignant breast lesions. He recognized many of the pitfalls of this technique and showed how they might be avoided. In spite of the advantages of the technique described by these authors it was little taken up until popularized in Europe at the Karolinska Institute in Sweden.[3] Webb was the first to report a series in Britain in 1970, and did much to establish the value of this approach.[4] Bates *et al.* [5] have shown that introduction of aspiration cytology leads to a reduced open biopsy rate. The benign/malignant ratio dropped from 1.9 to 0.7 without increase in the number of patients who subsequently developed cancer.

Indications
This technique is used with advantage in every discrete lump in the breast whether this is demonstrated by palpation, on ultrasound or on mammography. It may also be used for more diffuse lesions where there is some suspicion of underlying malignancy, e.g. inflammatory carcinoma masquerading as infection. The use of aspiration cytology in diffuse nodularity of ANDI is problematic. The usual result in this situation is a few specks of clear fluid reported as acellular.

Aspiration cytology may also be used to obtain tissue in screen-detected lesions. If there is no palpable lump then two techniques for obtaining tissues may be considered: ultrasound and stereotactic-guided aspiration cytology. Ultrasound-guided biopsy is obviously suitable for those mass lesions which can be identified sonographically. As it is unusual to be able to detect microcalcification on ultrasound; stereotactic-guided techniques are appropriate for microcalcification, and those masses not visible on ultrasound. (However, the development of high-frequency ultrasound is increasing the likelihood of detecting microcalcifications by ultrasound.) These two techniques are described below.

Important principles
- Ensure that the patient does not have any form of internal mammary prosthesis.
- Use a fine needle without local anaesthetic.
- Make sure the technique used is that approved by your cytologist.
- Interpret the result in the light of the other components of triple assessment (see Chapter 6).

Technique
The equipment necessary for making satisfactory smears should be available (Figure 20.1, Table 20.1).

No anaesthetic is required. The skin is cleansed with a spirit-based antiseptic and a 21-gauge needle attached to a syringe is inserted into the lump which is steadied between two fingers of the second hand. The syringe should be large enough to aspirate the total volume if it proves to be a cyst. A special syringe holder (CAMECO) is available to facilitate one-handed manipulation but many prefer the more direct feel obtained by holding the syringe. Considerable information can be acquired in this way, as the consistency of the breast tissue, and of the lump in particular, is 'sensed' with the needle point: the lack of resistance of fat, the toughness of fibrous tissue, the characteristic gritty sensation of cancer, and the firmness followed by a sudden 'give' as the needle enters a cyst.

If the lesion proves to be a cyst, a record should be made of the site, colour and quantity of the aspirate. Unless the fluid is blood stained, cytology is not indicated. Measurement of electrolyte content[6] may give some indication of likelihood of recurrence, but is not used routinely. Cysts may be deeper than suggested by palpation, so if no cyst is located on the first needle pass, it is worthwhile exploring a little deeper. After withdrawing the needle, the area is palpated to ensure that the lump has disappeared completely. The use of ultrasound in the clinic allows precise localization of cysts and eliminates most of these uncertainties.

If the lesion proves to be solid, the needle should be moved in and out of the mass in several directions while maintaining modest negative pressure until material appears in the hub of the needle. Fifteen or 20 passes may be necessary. Accurate placement of the needle is confirmed by moving the lesion while observing the needle and syringe. Care is taken to enter the lesion in a plane parallel to the chest wall to reduce risk of penetrating the underlying pleura. The negative pressure is released before removing the needle from the lump; failure to do this results in the sample becoming splattered around the barrel of the syringe rather than being retained in the needle. The needle is disconnected, the syringe filled with air and the needle replaced to expel the contents onto a labelled microscope slide. Expulsion should be repeated several times before it is assumed that no specimen is present; a completely dry aspirate is rare.

Gross blood contamination interferes with cytology so that, if a blood vessel is hit, it is usually best to repeat the procedure later. Some authorities pass the needle without using suction, maintaining that this gives specimens just as satisfactory and with a much reduced incidence of bleeding. A cottonwool ball is then held firmly over the entry point to reduce the chances of a haematoma, more common in the relatively vascular cancers, before covering it with an adhesive dressing.

The exact technique and the method of fixing the specimen need to be discussed with the cytologist. The specimens may be fixed immediately in alcohol as for cervical smears or air-dried prior to fixation. An alternative technique, that is claimed to be more reliable in inexperienced hands, is to flush out the needle and syringe with Cytofix. This fluid suspension is sent to the laboratory where it is spun down before being mounted on the slide by the cytologist.[7,8] Some cytologists prefer a small amount of heparinized saline in the syringe. The results of cytological assessment are graded as shown in Table 20.2.

Contraindications and complications

There are no real contraindications to performing aspiration cytology, although it is better avoided in very uncooperative and restless patients. Occasional patients will not give consent to this procedure.

Table 20.1 Equipment for aspiration cytology
21-gauge needle
10-mL syringe
Mediswab
Slides with ground glass end
Fixative
Pencil
Cottonwool ball
Adhesive dressing (Airfix)
+/- Syringe holder

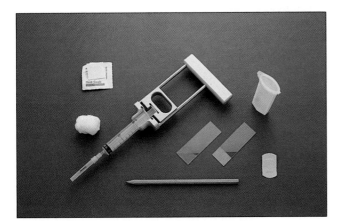

20.1 The instruments and equipment needed for FNA.

Table 20.2 Grading of cytological reports	
Cytological grading	Interpretation
C1	Inadequate[a]
C2	Benign
C3	Probably benign
C4	Probably malignant
C5	Malignant

[a]Inadequate = no epithelial cells. If the aspirate contains inflammatory cells such as macrophages or lymphocytes appropriate deductions may be made in the clinical context.

Pneumothorax is a well-recognized complication of FNA (and the most important), and it is important that doctors using the technique be aware of it. There have been a number of reports since Gateley *et al.* first described seven cases in 1991.[9] They estimated the frequency of this complication to be 1 per 1000 FNA procedures. The clinical picture is similar in most cases, although varying in severity. The patient typically complains of some pain at the time of the procedure, and further pain in the chest after a period of a few minutes to a few hours. There is frequently mild distress, but shock or other severe symptoms are not usually seen. The patient rapidly recovers. The suggested mechanism is a valsalva manoeuvre by an apprehensive patient at the time of needle insertion, with the lung expanded under pressure against the parietal pleura.

A second paper from Italy[10] reported 19 cases from 201,000 aspirations carried out in 48 institutions. This gives an incidence of 0.01%, but as it is a retrospective survey, it probably underestimates the frequency. Kaufman *et al.*[11] also found an incidence of 1:417; all procedures were carried out by experienced personnel. It is now clear that this complication can occur with the most experienced operators, and is seen more commonly in thin women and in peripheral or axillary needlings, where the thickness of the breast is least, although it has been seen with lumps in all sites and breasts of all configurations. If suspected, a chest X-ray will show a small to moderate pneumothorax, which resolves spontaneously over 7–10 days.

While some patients have been treated aggressively by insertion of a chest drain, especially when admitted on a thoracic service, most cases resolve quickly without active interference. If suspected, the patient should be observed for a few hours (or occasionally overnight) to ensure stabilization. If the pneumothorax is large enough to cause respiratory distress, simple aspiration of the air should be sufficient.

No serious complications have been reported, and would be very unlikely because of the fine needle used. Diagnosis is dependent on awareness of the complication and knowledge of those situations where it is most likely to occur: thin, restless patients and a needle passed directly into a peripherally sited lump, at right angles to the chest wall.

Other complications

The most common, but still rare, complication of aspiration cytology is haematoma. This is undesirable for a number of reasons: it is uncomfortable for the patient; if the lesion proves to be malignant there is the theoretical risk of spreading cancer cells further in the breast; it may become infected; and it may make further evaluation of the lesion, clinically or by imaging, more difficult. Sometimes a cyst will become painful after aspiration, either from infection, or more often when cyst contents leak into the surrounding breast.

Horobin *et al.*[12] have examined the effect of fine needle biopsy on subsequent mammograms. Fifty-two women had mammograms before and 3–4 days after fine needle biopsy.

In ten cases there were differences in the mammographic appearance but none were sufficient to lead to a change in radiological diagnosis. In seven of these, cystic lesions became less obvious; in three cases an increased density was noted and the authors expressed concern that a malignant lesion might have been overlooked or that haematoma around a benign lesion might be misread as having features of malignancy; in consequence they recommend performing mammography before aspiration cytology or waiting for 1 week afterwards. Provided the radiologist has the information that aspiration has been performed these rules need not be absolute.

One further situation in which caution should be urged is the patient with augmentation mammoplasty. The silicone prosthesis may be close to the lump and perforation of the envelope must be avoided. In this situation ultrasound or stereotactic-guided aspiration may reduce the chance of inadvertent damage to the prosthesis.[13]

Core needle biopsy

Core needle biopsy is easily performed under local anaesthesia, but can cause some discomfort. The facility with which this procedure may be performed has been greatly enhanced by the development of an automated spring-loaded firing device which is also less painful for the patient. It permits biopsy of subclinical lesions visualized on ultrasonography and mammography. An adequate core can provide definitive histology equivalent to that from an open biopsy.

Indications

An attempt should be made to obtain a core biopsy in any solid mass more than 1 cm in diameter,[14] and with imaging control even smaller lesions. Needle biopsy can cause sufficient tissue oedema to obscure mammographic detail so mammography should precede core biopsy in triple assessment, hence biopsy should be deferred until after mammography, or mammography deferred for 1 week after biopsy. (If the purpose of mammography is to screen the rest of the breast after a dominant mass has been assessed by image-guided biopsy, there is no need to defer mammography.)

While most patients readily tolerate needle biopsy, some find that it causes considerable pain, so it should be used with discretion for tender masses or those deep to the areola. We generally use it together with and following FNA cytology.

Important principles

- Ensure that the patient does not have any form of internal mammary prosthesis.
- Use local anaesthetic but avoid this form of biopsy if the lump is particularly painful.
- Develop a one-hand technique for needle manipulation so the other hand can stabilize the lump.
- Insert the closed needle up to, but not into, the lump as the spring-loading mechanism carries both trocar and sheath into the lump.

- Ensure that the direction of the instrument allows for a 2-cm throw without encountering any vital structure.
- Apply pressure after biopsy for at least 3 minutes, to minimize early and late bleeding.

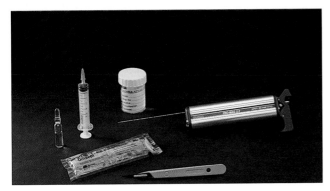

20.2 The instruments and equipment needed for core needle biopsy using a spring-loaded needle carrier.

Technique

The equipment necessary for the procedure (Figure 20.2) should be available and a no-touch technique used, although gloves are not absolutely necessary.

A number of biopsy needles are available. Our preference for breast biopsy is a spring-loaded instrument with a short (3 inch; 7.6 cm) needle because short needles are easier to control. An instrument with a 2-cm throw will give the best biopsy specimens (Figure 20.3).

Our impression accords with that of McMahon *et al.*[15] that the spring-loaded device for automatic sampling is less painful than the hand-held procedure. After cleansing the skin, a small intradermal weal of local anaesthetic (1% lignocaine) is raised at the biopsy site (Figure 20.4).

The proposed line of the needle should also be infiltrated down to the lesion to be biopsied, but excessive infiltration is to be avoided because it will obscure the position of the underlying mass. Using a sterile technique, a small nick is made in the skin and through to the subcutaneous fat with a pointed disposable scalpel blade (No. 11 or 15; Figure 20.5), and the closed needle, held in the spring-loaded gun,

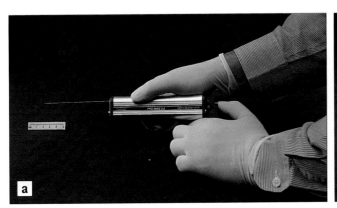

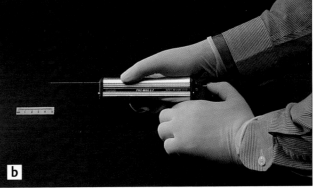

20.3 An instrument with a 2-cm throw will provide optimal specimens.

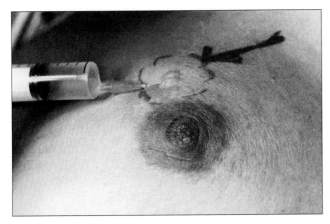

20.4 Infiltration of skin and underlying tissues with local anaesthetic.

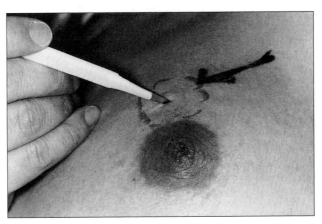

20.5 A small stab incision is made through the skin and subcutaneous tissue with a fine pointed scalpel.

is inserted through this until it abuts against the lesion (Figure 20.6).

The gun allows the needle to be manipulated with one hand, leaving the second hand free to steady and manipulate the mass or hold the ultrasound probe. The safety catch on the gun is then released and the gun fired. The needle is withdrawn in the closed position and the core of tissue placed straight into formalin. If necessary, further cores of tissue can be taken until a satisfactory specimen is obtained (Figure 20.7).

A general guide to the nature of the specimens can be obtained by examining the cores. If these float on the formalin they are likely to be fat only. If they sink, they are likely to be breast tissue (Figure 20.8).

Bleeding is not uncommon, so haemostasis is secured by firm digital pressure over the area for several minutes. The small skin incision is then covered with an occlusive dressing. (Note that when using a Trucut needle alone, the trocar must be advanced into the mass, and the sheath advanced over it. With the spring-loaded device, the needle is inserted to the mass because both needle and sheath are advanced together. Inserting the needle into the mass might result in it moving through the mass into tissues behind it.)

Complications
The contraindications and complications of needle biopsy are similar to those of aspiration cytology but bruising is noticeably commoner. Roberts et al.[14] reported a 37% incidence of bruising, although none of these were described as a haematoma. Haematoma may occur when a vascular lesion has been biopsied or a subcutaneous vein punctured and moderate bruising is common, hence the need for local pressure for at least 3 or 4 minutes. Extensive bruising is more common in patients on anticoagulants such as warfarin (Figure 20.9), when special precautions should be taken.

Image-guided needle biopsy
Ultrasound-guided biopsy
This technique is used for impalpable lesions that can be defined ultrasonically. A 7.5–13-Mhz linear probe is used. The technique is similar to the method used for palpable lumps except that the operator holds the ultrasound head with one hand while guiding the needle with the other. The lesion and the needle are both apparent to the operator so very accurate localization can be achieved. The major advantages of this method are that it is quick and without radiation exposure.

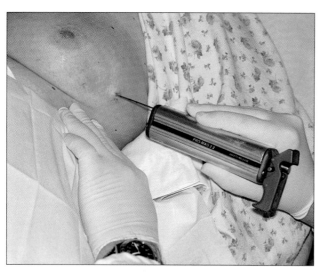

20.6 The needle is inserted up to, but not into, the mass.

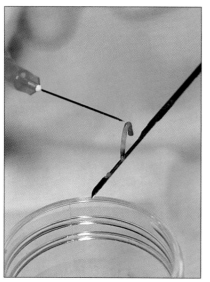

20.7 A satisfactory specimen.

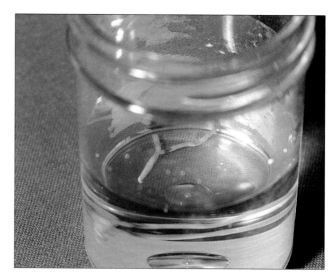

20.8 Breast tissue (in contrast to fat) usually sinks to the bottom of the fluid.

Stereotactic biopsy

Stereotactic biopsy can be used where a lesion is not visible on ultrasound. It is useful in performing both localized aspiration cytology and core needle biopsy, and provides very accurate localization of microcalcifications.

This technique has the disadvantage of requiring specialized equipment and radiation exposure. Some earlier reports were not favourable: Evans and Cade[16] found that stereotactic localization did not improve the yield of positive aspirates when compared to those obtained during a standard localization technique. However, Parker et al.[17] and Donkers[18] have successfully adapted this approach to obtain core needle biopsies that are particularly useful in obtaining definitive histology in marginal conditions such as complex sclerosing lesions. Using both imaging techniques for guiding needle biopsy has greatly reduced the need for open biopsy in our practice. Clinics should monitor their use of open biopsy to ensure that unnecessary operations are eliminated.

Open biopsy procedures

Open biopsy covers a number of procedures, including excision biopsy, incision biopsy, removal of a fibroadenoma and biopsy under radiological control. Each procedure carries different indications and requires a special technique.

Local anaesthesia

Many breast lumps can be satisfactorily removed under local anaesthesia. Lignocaine 1% without adrenaline is infiltrated along the line of the proposed incision. Usually the procedure is painless but there is some discomfort if too much traction is placed on the breast tissue during mobilization of the lump. A further injection of local anaesthetic deep to the lump will usually solve this problem. Diathermy

haemostasis is safe. The use of a long-acting local anaesthetic such as bupivacaine in combination with lignocaine can assist pain control with outpatient procedures. Many women prefer the discomfort of local anaesthesia to the experience of recovery from a general anaesthetic.

The theoretical danger of disseminating tumour cells by the local anaesthetic has not been fully evaluated; provided the spread of the anaesthetic fluid is confined to an area that will be encompassed by subsequent treatment fields, surgical or radiotherapeutic, this concern is more apparent than real. The relative vascularity of many cancers also makes local anaesthesia a less attractive option for these patients. This technique is particularly applicable in the removal of small fibroadenomas.

A further problem of local anaesthesia for small lumps is that occasionally the lesion is less readily palpable after the anaesthetic has been introduced. Walker et al.[19] have established the general advantages of local anaesthetic removal of breast lumps. The biopsy rate under local anaesthetic in 997 consecutive patients increased from 15% to 60% over a 5-year period.

General anaesthesia

This is an elective procedure, but in general can be carried out on an outpatient (daycase) basis. The patient is starved and as muscle relaxation is not required endotracheal intubation is unnecessary. A laryngeal mask technique is safe and satisfactory.

Indications

Open biopsy is indicated for removal of any persistent undiagnosed discrete lump in the breast or for removal of previously diagnosed benign lumps at the patient's request, as outlined in Chapter 4.

Wounds in young girls may be complicated by hypertrophic scars and this is particularly frequent and noticeable in the upper inner quadrant of the breast, and close to the sternum. Account should be taken of this before recommending removal of lumps in young girls.

Important principles

- Think carefully before excising breast lumps under local anaesthetic, especially in young girls, where breast tissue is dense and deep lumps may feel superficial.
- Never remove a lump before triple assessment.
- Define the lump carefully before operation. Avoid the temptation to keep removing fibrotic breast tissue which looks and feels 'abnormal' at operation – this can lead to inadvertent subcutaneous mastectomy.
- Be careful with haemostasis; vessels in fibrotic breast tissue are difficult to control.
- Mark the site of the lump before operation with the patient in the position in which she will be placed on the operating table.

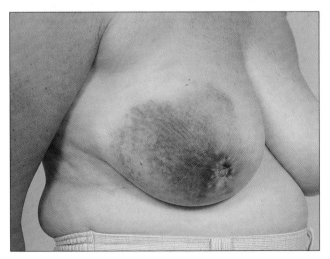

20.9 Extensive haematoma of the breast following core needle biopsy in a woman on warfarin.

Benign Disorders and Diseases of the Breast

Technique

It is customary to lie the patient supine but occasionally it is helpful to rotate the patient a little if the breast is large and the planned incision lies laterally. Diathermy is a useful but not essential adjunct to the procedure. Care needs to be exercised if it is intended to send tissue for oestrogen receptor analysis. Receptors are heat labile and the use of diathermy near the lesion may lead to misleading assays.[20] Rosenthal[20] reported that 53% of tumours were ER-positive when a scalpel was used and 27% when the lesion was excised with diathermy. More recent reports[21,22] suggest that provided a cuff of normal breast tissue is retained around the tumour then this problem can be avoided. It seems simpler to wait until the lesion has been removed before using diathermy haemostasis. The development of immunocytochemical assays for oestrogen receptors perhaps makes the concerns about the handling of specimens less critical but it is important to ascertain from the laboratory how best to present the specimens to them.

Periareolar incisions are preferred for all masses within 5 cm of the areola and curved incisions parallel to, the circumference for more peripheral masses (Figure 20.10).

Incisions close to, but parallel to the areolar margin are to be avoided, as the double line can give an unsightly appearance (Figure 20.11).

In general, the blood supply to the breast is so profuse that ischaemia need not cause concern except in extensive periareolar incisions. The blood supply of the breast and its implications for biopsy are discussed by Robertson.[23] Where cancer is suspected, the incision should be planned to take into account subsequent treatment. In re-excising a biopsy wound for malignancy, the whole of the wound and contaminated tissue should be removed without re-entering the original wound, so a badly orientated biopsy wound may necessitate excessive sacrifice of skin at the second procedure (Figure 20.12).

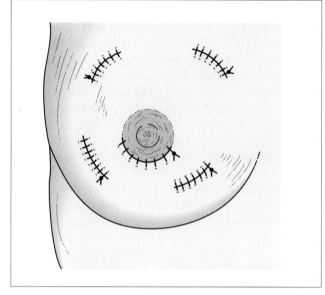

20.10 Incisions for breast biopsy for benign conditions. Where the mass lies within 5 cm of the areola, a periareolar incision is used. For more distant masses, a curved incision parallel to the areola is used.

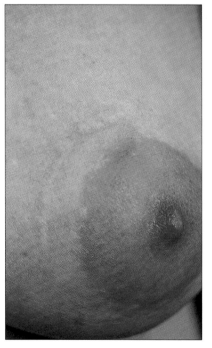

20.11 Scar resulting from an excision through a close para-areolar incision, giving an unnecessarily obvious scar.

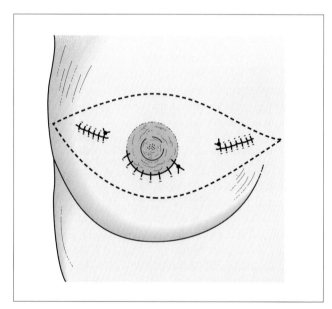

20.12 In patients of cancer age group, biopsy incisions should be sited in such a way as to be readily re-excised within the skin island of a mastectomy wound, should this be necessary.

The skin at the selected site of incision is held under slight tension by the assistant and a slightly curved incision made with a number 10 blade. The incision is deepened throughout its length into the subcutaneous fat and veins divided and ligated. A self-retaining retractor will allow good exposure of the lesion while giving excellent haemostasis from the sometimes troublesome superficial vessels.

The incision is deepened until the breast disc is encountered. In young patients this is easily identified; in the postmenopausal involuted breast it may be represented by a few strands of fibrous tissue. The lesion should now be palpated and the decision to perform either excision or incision biopsy confirmed or occasionally revised. Many discrete lumps will prove to be a prominent area of fibrotic nodularity. This is a diffuse process and the lump palpated can rarely be defined visually. It must be carefully defined by palpation – both preoperatively and through the wound. The further one goes into the breast, the more difficult it is to define the mass precisely. It is sometimes useful to insert a needle into the mass at an early stage to ensure that the area which was felt preoperatively is the area that will be excised. The mass is grasped with an Allis forceps and excised with a scalpel, suppressing any impulse to continue excising the surrounding breast tissue which may look the same as the palpable nodule. Pursuit of all apparently abnormal tissue will lead to an inadvertent subcutaneous mastectomy.

Bleeding is often troublesome because the small vessels lie embedded in the dense fibrous tissue. This can be tedious as tumours are often vascular and the vessels bleed easily; meticulous haemostasis now will be rewarded by a low incidence of subsequent bleeding and haematoma formation. A combination of diathermy and suture transfixion of vessels in fibrous tissue is used, and the wound carefully inspected for bleeding prior to closure.

The use of drains is controversial but if one is to be used a suction drain is appropriate. One randomized trial reported no difference in haematoma rate between wounds drained or not drained.[24] The increasing use of daycase surgery in patients undergoing removal of breast lumps also militates against the use of drainage. Our practice is to obtain adequate haemostasis and reserve drainage with a size 14 exudrain for large wounds or where there is doubt as to the adequacy of haemostasis. The exit site of the drain must remain within the planned treatment areas if the lesion proves to be a cancer. For practical purposes this means the drain should be brought out between the incision and the nipple.

There is also a difference of opinion as to whether the defect in the breast tissue should be closed. This will require an absorbable suture on a heavy cutting needle because of the fibrous nature of the breast tissue. Such suturing may lead to further haematoma formation and distortion of the breast. On the other hand, large defects may persist and leave a palpable ridge which is prone to be mistaken for a further lump, especially in the central breast

area. Neither situation is satisfactory but our preference is to leave the defect in most cases. The skin should be closed with a fine intracuticular suture: 4/0 prolene is satisfactory or 5/0 polydioxanone (PDS) which obviates the need for suture removal.

Complications

The common complications of breast biopsy are confined to persistent bleeding from the wound and haematoma formation. Johnson et al.[25] recorded marked bruising in 35/119 breast biopsies done under local anaesthesia but in only one was this considered a haematoma. The incidence of bruising was not affected by the use of a pressure pad; haemostasis at the time of surgery is the most important preventive. Wound infection is rare except as a complication of a haematoma.

Painful haematomas occurring in the first 48 hours are best managed by opening the wound and evacuating the clot rather than allowing spontaneous resolution. After ensuring haemostasis, the wound should be closed with suction drainage and antibiotic cover. Allowing natural resolution may take some time, may cause considerable pain both early and late and may make subsequent assessment of the breast more difficult. Haematomas presenting late after liquefaction may be managed by repeated aspiration through a wide bore needle.

One situation where special care needs to be taken is in the irradiated breast. The use of breast-conserving treatments for early breast cancer makes the need to evaluate such patients important. Pezner et al.[26] reported that 30% of patients having open biopsies had wound-healing problems with significant deterioration in the cosmetic appearance of the biopsied breast. Complications were more common in women with large breasts. They reported no complications in a small number of women who had needle biopsies of irradiated breasts, so image-guided biopsy should be used as much as possible.

Postoperative care

Most patients will be able to go home on the same day, with adequate provision of analgesia. For those who have required drainage the drain may be removed the following day (at home or after overnight stay) provided drainage is minimal and there is no haematoma formation. If nonabsorbable, the subcuticular sutures are removed at 7 days. At this time a check should be made that the pathology has been reviewed and arrangements made for further management and follow-up depending on the diagnosis.

Incision biopsy

Since incision biopsy is used mainly to confirm the diagnosis of large carcinomas and to obtain material for oestrogen receptor analysis, it is largely outside the scope of this book. However, it is an important rule that a diagnosis should be made before definitive treatment is planned for large masses of obscure aetiology, benign or malignant. This will prevent unsatisfactory procedures such as a poorly planned excision of a large phyllodes tumour, which may make it impossible to ensure an adequate excision margin at a secondary procedure. This can usually be achieved by cytology or core needle biopsy. In the rare instances where neither technique has been satisfactory, it is better to perform an incision biopsy than to do a wide excision for a lump which may prove to be no more than fibrous tissue. Details of the technique are given above under excision biopsy.

Removal of a fibroadenoma

The early stages of the operation are the same as those described under open biopsy. However, fibroadenoma in young women usually lies within a well-defined capsule and can be enucleated easily. The pedicle may require ligation or diathermy (Figure 20.13) and the base of the pedicle may require excision if this is broad because there may be some extension of fibroadenomatous tissue into the area of the capsule (Figure 20.14).

Bleeding is minimal and there should be no need to insert a drain into the cavity if haemostasis of the vascular pedicle has been obtained. Because the parenchyma of the breast is hardly disturbed, there is no need to close the defect in the breast tissue which will soon disappear.

In older women, a fibroadenoma usually presents as a dominant mass in an involuting breast. These fibroadenomas often do not enucleate satisfactorily and are best removed by the technique of excision biopsy described earlier.

Image-controlled biopsy
Indications

This procedure is indicated to remove a lesion seen on mammography but which cannot be felt clinically. The commonest indication is a small area of microcalcification or trabecular distortion for which the differential diagnosis usually lies between early carcinoma (in situ or invasive), radial scar and sclerosing adenosis. Because these conditions cannot be safely differentiated radiologically, excision biopsy is usually indicated (see Chapter 10).

Important principles

- Close cooperation is required between surgeon, radiologist and pathologist.
- The radiological abnormality is localized by the radiologist in the radiology department (Figure 20.15).
- Excision biopsy is performed by the surgeon under general anaesthetic.
- Immediate specimen radiology is carried out by the radiologist to confirm that the area in question has been removed.
- Further tissue excision is performed if the abnormal area was not located in this specimen.
- The specimen is dissected by the radiologist to isolate the radiological abnormality.
- Rapid paraffin section is taken.

Techniques – wire localization

This technique is the most widely practised in localizing non-palpable breast lesions. A hooked wire enclosed within a needle is placed in the breast where the radiologist judges the lesion to be. Further views are taken and the relationship of the tip of the needle to the lesion ascertained. Multiple wires may be used to delineate large or multiple lesions, such as extensive areas of microcalcification. The needle is removed, leaving the wire *in situ*, which is then taped to the skin while the patient is transferred to the operating theatre.

Fixation of the wire is usually secure, but migration may occur, especially in large and fatty breasts. Although some surgeons report that the subsequent search of the breast can

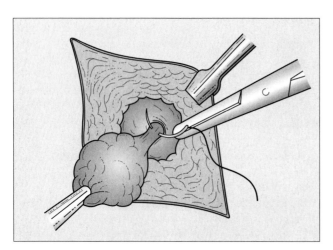

20.13 Removing a fibroadenoma. The blood supply comes only through the pedicle so this should be ligated if it is substantial.

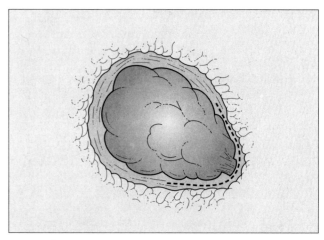

20.14 There is sometimes extension of fibroadenomatous tissue in the pedicle so that, where this is broad, an area adjacent to the base should be removed to minimize recurrence.

be satisfactorily done under a local anaesthetic most patients prefer this under general anaesthetic. There are a number of different wires available. The one selected is unimportant but our current preference is for the Reidy needle.

The general conduct of the operation is as for an open biopsy, with either a periareolar incision or one related to the wire exit. After the incision has been made the wire is found under the skin. It is divided with wire cutters and brought into the wound; the external part is discarded. A mosquito forceps is placed on the wire to allow the assistant to keep the wire steady while its track is followed through the fat into the breast tissue. A pair of Allis forceps is placed on either side of the wire in a plane opposite to the side of the lesion, so that if the wire lies inferior and lateral to the lesion the forceps are placed in this quarter. The Allis forceps are then lifted to bring the breast tissue to the incision, the breast tissue is divided along the wire in this plane for a short distance and haemostasis secured.

The Allis forceps are now repositioned adjacent to the place where the wire disappears into the tissue and the process is repeated. Gentle palpation will eventually reveal the recurved hook on the wire. When this is found the suspicious area can be defined and excised; a palpable abnormality may or may not be apparent. Gentle handling of the wire is required at this stage so as not to dislodge it.

The tissue is excised and sent for specimen radiology to confirm that the correct area has been removed (Figures 20.16 and 20.17). The remainder of the operation proceeds as for biopsy of a palpable lump.

Careless excision can result in large defects with unnecessary cosmetic deformity from benign lesions, so emphasis should be placed on accurate localization. The document entitled 'Guidelines for surgeons in the management of symptomatic breast disease in the United Kingdom' (1995), endorsed by the Senate of the Royal Surgical Colleges, recommends

that as a quality outcome measure, >90% of diagnostic biopsies which subsequently prove to be benign should weigh less than 20 g and that the surgeon should ensure that the biopsy is weighed in the theatre and by the pathologist.

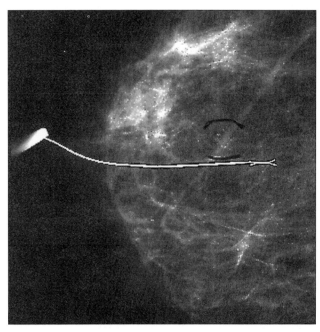

20.15 A subclinical radiological lesion has been localized with a wire inserted into the breast.

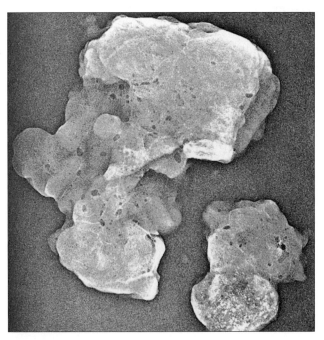

20.17 Where a small lesion is present in a relatively large specimen, excision of the lesion on the basis of specimen radiology may help the pathologist.

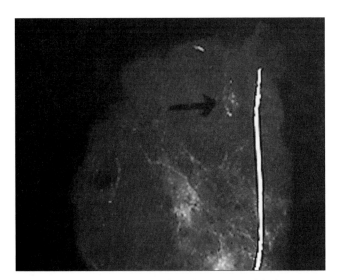

20.16 The specimen radiology confirms the presence of the lesion.

Technique – double dye localization (Figure 20.18)

In this technique the radiologist injects a mixture of hypaque and a vital blue dye into an area adjacent to the radiographic lesion.[27] The area of interest is then related to the dye and the surgeon given clear instructions as to the relationship of the two. At operation the surgeon identifies the dye and removes the indicated area. This technique has been replaced by wire-insertion procedures.

A variation on this theme is the Svane technique.[28,29] The lesion is identified stereotactically and then marked with carbon; a tract is then led to the surface so that the lesion can be identified. The carbon remains in place so that this approach has an advantage over the double dye technique in that the marker will not diffuse and there is no urgency in carrying out the biopsy procedure. It has the advantage over wire methods in that there is nothing to disturb during transportation of the patient to the operating theatre. Although we have no experience of this technique in Cardiff it would seem appropriate where stereotactic aspiration cytology is performed when the tattoo could be used to localize the lesion during subsequent definitive surgery.

Complications of localization biopsy

Helvie et al.[30] have reported the immediate complications of localization and needle aspiration in 370 cases while still in the radiology department. Vasovagal attacks occurred in 7%, four patients developed syncope. They also recorded prolonged bleeding in three patients and severe pain in two. Rappaport et al.[31] have examined the complications following localization biopsy in 144 consecutive patients. They reported an infection rate of 1.2% and cases of diathermy burns of the skin.

Problems may occur with the wire, including total migration into the breast, possibly requiring a second localization to remove it, migration outside the breast (into the pleural cavity has been recorded), and accidental transection of the wire during dissection, with loss of the deep portion.

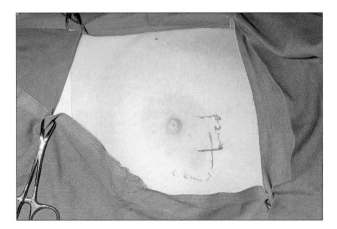

20.18 The double dye technique may still be used but has been largely replaced by hooked wires.

REMOVAL OF GIANT FIBROADENOMA AND PHYLLODES TUMOUR

In a young patient (<20 years)

A giant fibroadenoma is usually defined as a lesion more than 5 cm in diameter. These lesions may lie close to the surface of the breast and may then be removed in the same way as a smaller fibroadenoma. Larger lesions tend to lie deeper in the breast and are best approached from behind through a submammary incision which will give a better cosmetic result than one located on the breast.

Technique

A submammary incision (Figure 20.19) is taken down to the fascia over the serratus anterior and pectoralis major muscles and dissection is carried upwards in this largely avascular retromammary plane (Figure 20.20).

The fibroadenoma is then pushed through the posterior aspect into the wound, the capsule incised (Figure 20.21) and the tumour shelled out in the usual way.

A suction drain is inserted into the retromammary space and the wound closed with subcuticular prolene. This approach to the back of the breast through the submammary fold was described by Gaillard–Thomas in 1882.[32]

It is important that more radical procedures are avoided in young girls and that no attempt is made to close the cavity, and even more important that no complex reconstructive procedures are used, for reasons given in Chapter 7.

In an older patient

Giant fibroadenoma and phyllodes tumour in older patients differ from those in young girls in a number of ways. They vary in the degree of malignancy and may not shell out from surrounding involuting breast tissue. Hence, they are best managed by core needle or incision biopsy to provide definitive histological assessment before planning management, which is usually by a measured wide local excision or by simple mastectomy.

Where a 1-cm clearance is required, as is usually the case with phyllodes tumour, this should be measured around the whole surface. This is done most satisfactorily by the surgeon placing the fingers of his left hand on the tumour, and cutting outside his finger. The details of the technique do not differ from those of the operations described above; the all-important principles are considered in Chapter 7.

MICRODOCHECTOMY

Indications

This operation is indicated for blood-stained or serous discharge from a solitary duct when the opening of the affected duct on to the nipple can be identified. We use this operation for patients under the age of 40, preferring the operation of major duct excision for blood-stained nipple discharge in patients over this age (see Chapters 11 and 12). No attempt

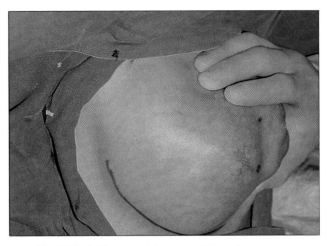

20.19 The Gaillard–Thomas incision for giant fibroadenoma.

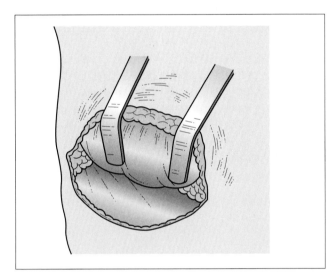

20.20 The dissection is carried upwards in the submammary plane at the level of the pectoral fascia.

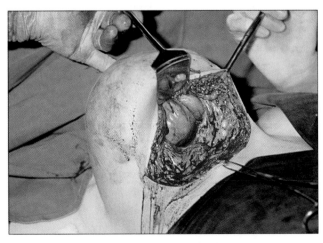

20.21 The fascial layer on the posterior aspect of the breast is incised and the fibroadenoma enucleated and delivered through the wound.

should be made to express discharge from the nipple for several days prior to operation so that some discharge is present to identify the duct at operation. Alternatively, the nipple may be sprayed with a plastic dressing such as Nobecutane® 2 or 3 days before operation to ensure retention of secretion.

Important principles
- Avoid expressing fluid for a few days before operation.
- Radial or periareolar incisions are both satisfactory, the latter preferable in younger women.
- Identify the duct with a lacrimal probe.
- Excise all dilated parts of the duct system if operating for blood-related discharge.

Operative technique
The orifice of the affected duct is identified by squeezing the nipple to express a drop of discharge. A lacrimal probe is inserted into the duct and passed as far into the breast tissue as possible (Figure 20.22).

This should be done gently to avoid creating a false passage. The probe will frequently pass only 1–2 cm because passage along the duct may be blocked by little pockets which tend to occur as the duct dilates around a papilloma. This distance is sufficient to demonstrate the direction of the duct and, after making the incision, the dark fluid in the dilated duct is usually visible. Some authorities recommend injecting dye into the duct to facilitate localization, but there is a

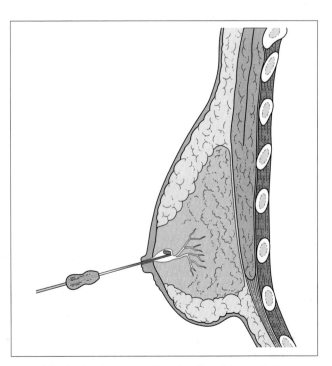

20.22 A lacrimal probe is passed into the affected duct to find its direction within the breast. It often will not go very far because it catches in small pockets of the dilated duct.

tendency for the dye to leak from the ducts into the tissues, precluding precise dissection.

Using the direction of the lacrimal probe as a guide, a racquet-shaped incision is made to enclose the immediate termination of the duct with a minimal amount of surrounding nipple tissue and carried radially across the areola and on to the breast skin for a total distance of 5 cm (Figure 20.23).

The skin flaps are raised over a short distance and the whole of the affected duct and its branching system dissected out in segmental fashion for a distance of at least 5 cm from its orifice (Figure 20.24).

The main portion of the duct can usually be identified for about 2.5 cm. It is dissected carefully to interfere as little as possible with surrounding ducts, although if a central duct is affected, some damage to the adjacent ducts may be inevitable. A further segmental area of breast tissue about 2.5 cm long is removed in continuity with the duct (Figure 20.25).

A length of 5–6 cm of the duct system will usually remove any papillomas present because these are lesions of the large ducts.

However, if the duct remains dilated beyond 5 cm, it should be followed further towards the periphery of the breast. Normally a duct is only dilated between the papilloma and the nipple. So, if peripheral ducts are dilated, peripheral papillomas – benign or malignant – should be anticipated and a segmental resection of the breast carried out to encompass all dilated, blood-filled ducts.

Peripheral dilatation of ducts is particularly seen in older patients with multiple 'discrete' papillomas occupying a single ductolobular system. Such papillomas tend to be benign or of very low-grade malignancy, and complete excision of that system should be curative.

Haemostasis is secured and the specimen removed. The terminal portion of the duct is marked with a silk suture to help the pathologist orientate the tissue. Having done this, the duct system may be opened and inspected for the presence of a papilloma. However, macroscopic papilloma is found in only about half the cases, others being due to duct ectasia (DE). A suction drain is inserted and the skin closed with fine sutures, subcuticular or interrupted.

Variations of technique

Several variations have been described for this procedure. The tissues around the duct may be infiltrated with saline containing 1:300,000 adrenaline solution to help maintain haemostasis and allow more exact dissection. The use of binocular magnifying loupes will also help precise dissection.

Some surgeons (e.g. Haagensen[33]) prefer to use a peri-areolar incision, dissecting the flap upwards in the same manner as described under major duct excision. The dilated duct is then dissected to its entry on to the nipple. The peripheral flap is raised to allow segmental excision of the duct drainage area. Haagensen advocates this incision on cosmetic grounds, although we find a radial incision usually gives a satisfactory cosmetic result. The radial incision has the advantage that it can more readily be extended where this is necessary, so is particularly appropriate in the older patient. In contrast, a periareolar incision is to be preferred in younger women since a hypertrophic scar, although rare, is more likely with radial incisions (Figure 20.26).

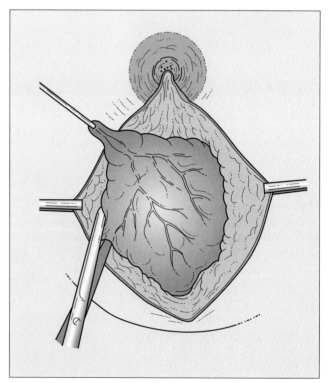

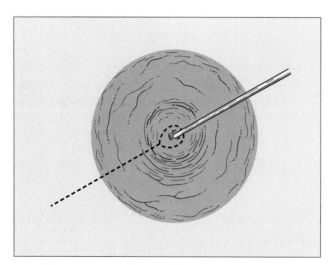

20.23 The racquet incision for microdochectomy. The skin surrounding the terminal duct is removed in continuity within the duct.

20.24 The segment drained by the duct is dissected back into the breast for a distance of 2–3 cm, but further if the ducts remain dilated at this level.

EXCISION OF MAMMARY DUCT FISTULA

Indications
- Established duct fistula with a single opening.
- A localized abscess which always presents at the same spot.
- In a patient who does not seek correction of an inverted nipple.

Important principles
- Conservative drainage of periareolar abscess as an acute procedure if the fistula is not established.
- The central (nipple) opening of the duct must be excised.
- Healing by granulation has proved a reliable method of obtaining a satisfactory result but the wound must be well shaped and managed correctly.
- Recently there has been a strong move towards primary closure under antibiotic cover.

Fistulotomy or fistulectomy?
In his original description, Atkins[34] simply laid the fistula open and allowed it to granulate (fistulotomy). This is probably a satisfactory procedure, but we have preferred fistulectomy because it ensures that the central portion of the duct is excised (important in minimizing recurrence), removes some of the ductal system and leaves healthy tissue to granulate. This operation is described, but similar principles apply to fistulotomy. A probe is passed into the external opening of the fistula and passes easily out of the duct opening on to the nipple (Figure 20.27).

The skin incision encompasses the fistula and an ellipse of skin is removed which need be only about 1 cm wide at its maximum (Figure 20.28).

More important is that the incision includes the whole of the affected lactiferous sinus and the opening on to the nipple; this is the portion of terminal duct lined by squamous epithelium. The ellipse and underlying tissue also include a centimetre or two of the duct system distal to the fistula. The incision is deepened through subcutaneous fat into the breast tissue just below the affected duct (Figure 20.29).

If the wound is allowed to granulate, healing will be rapid and certain, provided the wound is well shaped (Figure 20.30) and does not close prematurely.

This is ensured by sewing in a loose pack of gauze soaked in proflavine/paraffin emulsion for 2–3 days to maintain an

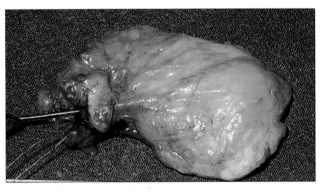

20.25 A typical specimen following microdochectomy from a large breast.

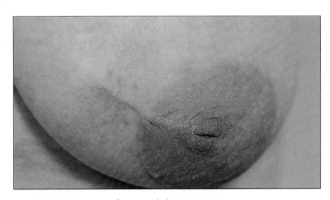

20.26 An obvious scar from a radial incision in a young woman.

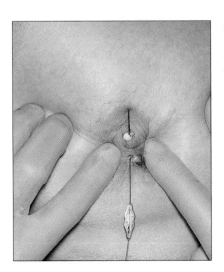

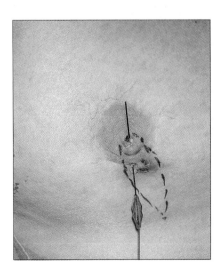

20.27 A probe is passed through the duct fistula and out through the nipple.

20.28 The skin excision for mammary duct fistula.

open cavity while the walls of the wound stiffen (Figure 20.31).

The disadvantage of granulation lies in the pain associated with wounds in the nipple region with conventional gauze dressings, and the longer period of hospitalization associated with this technique. Both these disadvantages can be avoided by using one of the many non-adherent cavity dressings, such as Silastic Foam® (Figure 20.32) or Kaltostat.

These cause no pain on dressing change and can be managed by the patient at home, allowing a shorter period of hospitalization than with primary wound closure. An alternative is to close the wound primarily under antibiotic cover.[35]

MAJOR DUCT EXCISION (ADAIR/URBAN/HADFIELD)

This important procedure has an interesting history. It was first reported in 1960 by Hadfield,[36] based on 31 cases, and in the UK the operation is commonly referred to as Hadfield's procedure. In his paper he paid tribute to Adair and Urban of the Memorial Hospital, New York, for having taught him the operation. Three years later, Urban described his technique,[37] reporting 167 operations. Hence, the operation is also frequently known as Urban's duct excision, although in his own paper, Urban assigns his own precedence to Adair, whose first operation preceded Urban's by 2 years, although Adair published no account of his technique.

Indications (see Chapter 11 for details)
- Blood-related discharge in a patient over the age of 40 years. Here it is preferred to microdochectomy because of the more generous pathological material provided in a patient with a significant risk of cancer. Urban[37] found 41 unsuspected cancers in 434 duct excision operations mainly in the older age groups. Major duct excision gives more certain control of symptoms should the symptoms prove to be due to DE.
- Non-blood-related discharge sufficiently copious to be an embarrassment to the patient. If the discharge is milky, prolactinoma should first be excluded.
- Subareolar abscess, selected according to the criteria discussed in Chapter 11, or a peripheral mass or abscess with central major DE, when the mass and major ducts can be excised in continuity.

The operation is not necessary for biopsy for small areas of periductal mastitis (PDM) with moderate DE. These are satisfactorily managed by core needle or local excision biopsy.

Important principles
The areolar flap, confined to one-third of the circumference, is dissected in a plane deep to the venous plexus to avoid ischaemia. The under surface of the nipple is bared completely:
- to remove all terminal duct tissue;
- to ensure that no ducts are missed at the back of the duct cone.
- Remove the central portion of the nipple if the nipple does not evert easily.
- Ignore peripheral dilated ducts.
- Submit all excised tissue to histology.

Technique – incision
The ducts are approached through a periareolar incision extending for 30–40%, and no further than 50% around

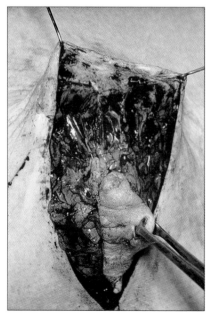

20.29 The underlying tissue is excised conservatively.

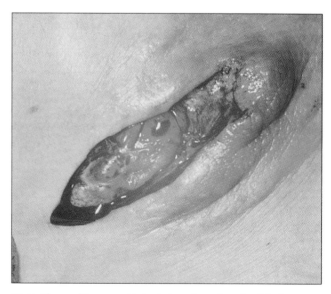

20.30 The resulting wound is boat shaped – as broad as it is deep – so that it will heal from below.

the circumference. It is usually based inferiorly but may be centred anywhere towards localized pathology. It should be placed accurately at the areolar margin to obtain maximum cosmetic benefit (Figure 20.33).

Urban[37] recommended a radial incision removing an ellipse of skin stopping short of the nipple. He found it easier to repair the oval-shaped defect in the breast tissue (Figure 20.34).

We advise this approach where there is severe scarring from periareolar sepsis, because it allows easy entry to the subareolar plane through relatively normal tissue, instead of through dense scar tissue. It has the disadvantage that it may encourage the surgeon to leave small amounts of terminal duct on the undersurface of the nipple.

A 'Z'-shaped incision transecting the nipple has been recommended. We quickly abandoned this approach because it proved tedious, was more destructive and presented no advantages.

Technique – dissection

The incision is deepened until the prominent radially running subcutaneous veins are reached. These are divided and ligated with fine absorbable suture material and the plane of dissection developed immediately deep to these veins (Figure 20.35).

By preserving the vascular plexus of the areola, the viability of nipple and areola is assured. The penalty for neglecting this careful definition of tissue planes is shown in Figure 20.36.

The areolar flap is dissected in this plane until about one-third of the areola has been elevated and the cone of fibroductal tissue passing to the nipple is reached. A subareolar tunnel is then developed behind the ductal cone by blunt dissection with a haemostat working from each side (at 3 o'clock and 9 o'clock, respectively) to meet in the middle behind the ducts (Figure 20.37).

This can be done in the correct plane without great difficulty because both the ductal tissue and the skin of the

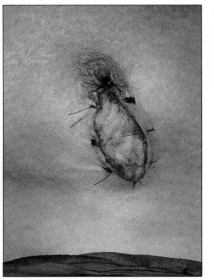

20.31 A satisfactory shape of the wound is ensured by sewing in a loose pack for 2–3 days (see text for details).

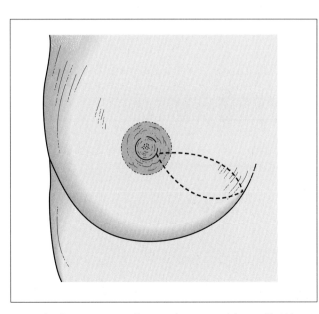

20.32 Non-adherent dressings such as Silastic Foam® allow painless management as an outpatient.

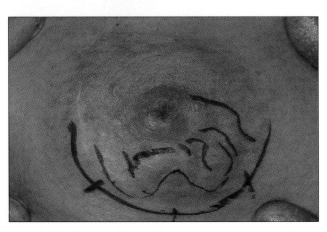

20.33 Incision for major duct excision, exactly at the areolar margin.

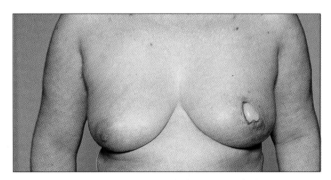

20.34 The alternative incision for major duct excision advocated by Urban.[37]

areola are tough structures and the subcutaneous fat represents the path of least resistance.

The core of ductal tissue is grasped by a Kocher forceps passed through the subareolar tunnel. The ducts are divided on the forceps to ensure that an inverted nipple is not damaged by this manoeuvre (Figure 20.38).

With retraction on the Kocher forceps, the ductal mass is dissected back into the breast for a distance of 3 cm or so and then transected. During this process, any bleeding vessels should be caught and ligated before they retract back into the breast substance.

It is not uncommon for ducts to remain dilated at the site of transection. Hadfield recommends that they be ligated with fine catgut, but this is not easy because they are embedded in fibrous tissue. Urban recommended that dissection be extended into the breast until the ducts are of normal size, but this will sometimes result in a major defect, little short of subtotal mastectomy. There seems to be no disadvantage in ignoring the transected dilated ducts, as recommended by Haagensen, and wounds without overt sepsis

can be expected to heal in spite of some continuing leakage of duct contents. (Total duct excision for blood-related discharge requires a different approach to peripheral dilated ducts as described under microdochectomy.)

Attention is drawn to the under-surface of the nipple to ensure that the terminal ducts are removed completely. The nipple is fully inverted and stretched over the tip of the index finger and the remaining duct tissue excised with scissors (Figure 20.39).

This manoeuvre also ensures that no ducts are missed as can happen if the tunnelling traverses the duct mass rather than the subcutaneous plane, leaving some ducts at the far side of the incision.

If dissection is complete, the nipple will usually resume the everted position. If there is any tendency to reinvert, a further examination should be made to ensure that all ductal tissue has been excised and a loose purse-string suture of fine PDS may be placed around its base (a tight purse-string suture may produce nipple ischaemia).

Sometimes the centre of a deeply inverted nipple is

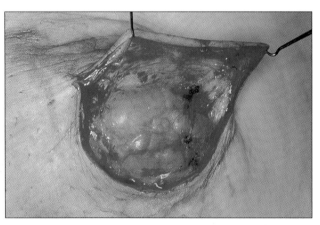

20.35 The areolar flap is elevated in the subvenous plane.

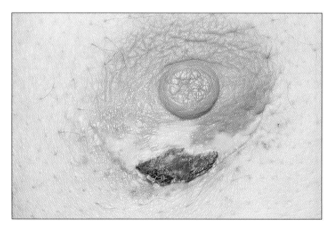

20.36 Partial nipple necrosis due to dissection of the flap in too superficial a plane.

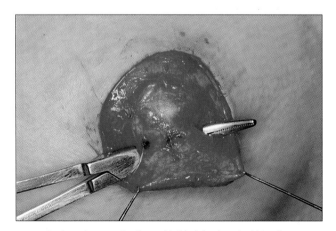

20.37 A subareolar tunnel is formed behind the ducts by blunt dissection, and a Kocher forceps passed through the tunnel to grasp the ducts.

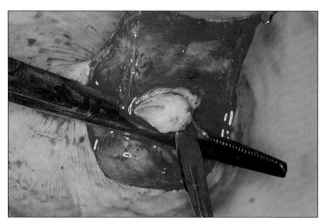

20.38 The ducts are divided immediately below the nipple by cutting on to the Kocher forceps.

thickened, keratotic and contains dilated terminal ducts, and cannot be inverted satisfactorily after duct division. It may then be best to excise, in conservative fashion, the central portion of the nipple and close the defect with one or two fine sutures. This central portion needs to be only 5 mm or so in diameter; the tough fibromuscular layer of the nipple with overlying skin maintains the shape of the nipple and gives a satisfactory result (see Core nipple duct excision below).

Drainage and closure

In the absence of infection a small suction drain should be inserted and the wound closed with fine interrupted or subcuticular suture. Some authors recommend obliteration of the subareolar cavity by a series of approximating purse-string sutures. We omit this step and have not found it to be a disadvantage. The cosmetic result of this operation is excellent when there has been little or no tissue destruction before surgery (see Figure 11.21). When the operation is performed after extensive sepsis the cosmetic result is likely to be less satisfactory.

In the presence of overt or recent infection, the wound should not be closed primarily because of a considerable risk of postoperative infection (Figure 20.40).

This predisposes to nipple necrosis or chronic infection leading to sinus formation. It is best to pack the wound with gauze soaked in proflavine and paraffin emulsion and subsequently allow the wound to granulate using a Silastic Foam® or similar non-adherent dressing. In some situations, where extensive sepsis extends into the breast, it may be satisfactory to close the periareolar portion of the incision and leave a radial portion of the incision open for counter-drainage (Figure 20.41).

The increasing evidence for a role for bacterial infection in some of these abscesses, particularly recurrent ones, raises the question of whether they may be safely closed primarily in the presence of adequate antibiotic therapy. If this is done, the minimum spectrum of cover should be that of anaerobic organisms and Gram-positive cocci. Metronidazole and flucloxacillin or Augmentin® seem to be satisfactory regimens.

On balance, our experience leads us to prefer continuation of our policy of open granulation. However, where the infection has been well controlled by antibiotics and prior drainage so that only a track remains, we close the wound after excision of this tract under antibiotic cover. Hence our preference for two-stage management of abscesses where possible: preliminary conservative drainage, followed by major duct excision 6–8 weeks later with primary closure under antibiotic cover.

There does not seem to be any carcinogenic risk from leaving the peripheral ducts *in situ*. Urban found only seven cancers developing in his 434 patients having duct excision and followed for 2–14 years. Three were *in situ* and and four infiltrating.

CORE NIPPLE DUCT EXCISION

The terminal centimetre of breast ducts, together with apex of the nipple containing the duct orifices, may readily be removed in continuity with the underlying ductoglandular

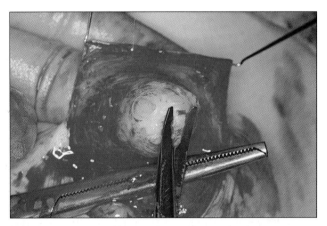

20.39 Any residual terminal duct tissue is removed after inverting the nipple over the index finger.

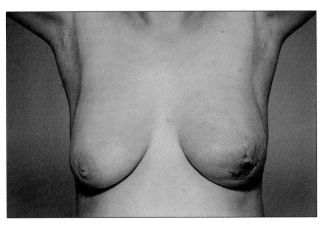

20.40 Severe wound infection resulting from ill-advised closure following major duct excision in the presence of active infection.

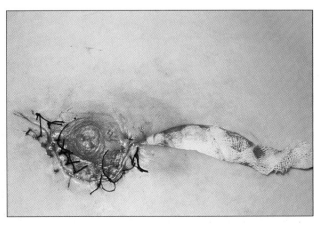

20.41 In cases with extensive incision for recurrent sepsis, partial closure may be appropriate.

cone. This is a simple and effective procedure, which we have not seen used elsewhere or described previously.

Indications

It is particularly useful in two situations: severe PDM to facilitate nipple eversion, and as an extension of subcutaneous mastectomy to ensure total duct removal without sacrificing the cosmetic contribution of the nipple–areolar complex.

In longstanding cases of PDM with much sepsis the nipple remains inverted even after conventional duct excision. If left, epithelial debris collects in the inverted nipple where it is malodorous and acts as a focus of persisting infection. For this reason we believe that total nipple eversion should be achieved in all such cases, and that this removes the need for excision of the nipple and areola sometimes recommended in this situation.

When subcutaneous mastectomy is carried out as a prophylactic measure, or for intraduct cancer extending to within about 2 cm of the nipple, core nipple duct excision should be added to avoid the late risk of Paget's disease in the nipple. Where intraduct cancer extends closer to the nipple (or where invasive cancer approaches the nipple), we would prefer the more conventional subcutaneous mastectomy with removal of nipple and areola.

Technique

The ductoglandular cone is dissected towards the nipple as in a standard subcutaneous mastectomy or major duct excision procedure. As the nipple is approached, the ducts are isolated from the areola, but instead of dividing them just below the nipple in an Urban's procedure, or including the nipple and areola in a mastectomy, dissection around the ducts is continued into the nipple in a plane between the duct cone and the fibromusculo-cutaneous outer tissues of the nipple until the surface is reached (Figure 20.42).

The plane is well defined, because of the robust nature of both inner duct cone and the outer tissues, although some sharp dissection is required. The apical skin of the nipple containing the duct orifices is excised in continuity with the ducts, leaving a stiff hollow cylinder to maintain much of the nipple's shape and bulk. The apex of the nipple is refashioned with a couple of loose sutures (Figure 20.43).

DRAINAGE OF A LACTATIONAL BREAST ABSCESS

This is indicated when percutaneous drainage has not given rapid resolution, or when the overlying skin is compromised. It should be performed under general anaesthetic. Antibiotic cover is given if there is surrounding widespread cellulitis, otherwise it is unnecessary. In the vast majority of cases, a curvilinear incision parallel to the areola should be made over the area of maximum tenderness after confirmation of the presence of pus by ultrasound or needle aspiration (Figure 20.44).

The abscess is usually multilocular and these loculi will need to be broken down with the finger but without unnecessary disturbance of the uninvolved breast tissue (Figure 20.45).

The skin incision should be adequate – at least three-quarters of the diameter of the abscess (Figure 20.46). The cavity is then lightly packed with gauze soaked in proflavine/paraffin emulsion and the wound left open (see Figure 20.31). Tight packing must be avoided as it interferes with drainage. After a day or two, the pack should be replaced with a non-adherent absorbent dressing. These

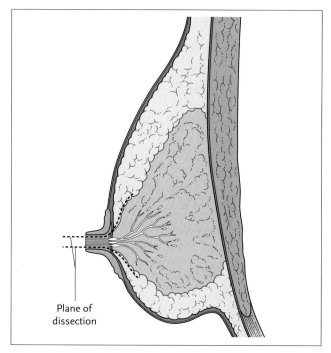

20.42 Core nipple duct excision. The plane of dissection is between the ductoglandular cone and the outer nipple.

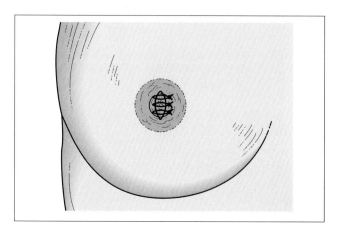

20.43 The outer layer is loosely approximated by a few interrupted sutures.

materials eliminate pain from wound dressing, give excellent drainage and allow the patient to manage her own wound at home. The cavity rapidly fills and healing is usually complete by 2–3 weeks provided the incision is generous and the wound is pyramidal shaped (Figures 20.47 and 20.48).

Treated in this way there is surprisingly little deformity of the breast.

An alternative approach to the drainage of breast abscess is that of Benson and Goodman[38]: curettage and primary closure under antibiotic cover. The abscess cavity is opened as before, and emptied, and the lining of granulation tissue curetted out. The cavity is then closed primarily with interrupted vertical mattress sutures which pass deep to the cavity. These authors recommend removing the sutures on the fourth day. This approach lies midway between needle aspiration and formal drainage, and may be less applicable with the advent of ultrasound-guided drainage.

SUBCUTANEOUS MASTECTOMY IN MALE PATIENTS

This is indicated in a minority of patients with gynaecomastia, where gross degrees of breast enlargement are causing cosmetic and psychological trauma, and in cases where

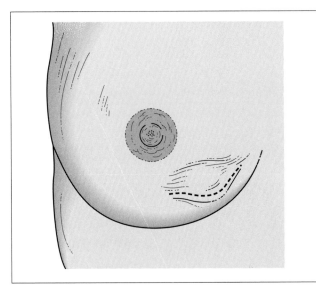

20.44 The presence of pus should always be confirmed by needle aspiration before proceeding to open drainage of an abscess.

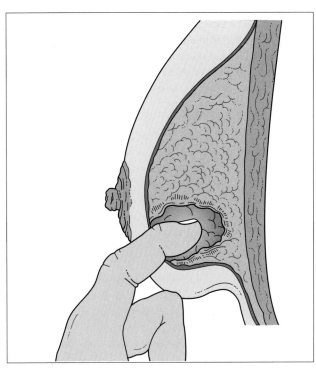

20.45 All loculi must be broken down with an exploring finger.

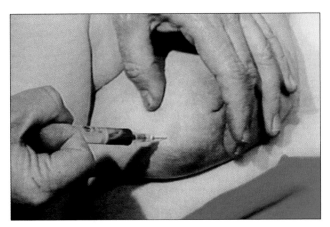

20.46 The incision for abscess drainage. It should be of generous proportion.

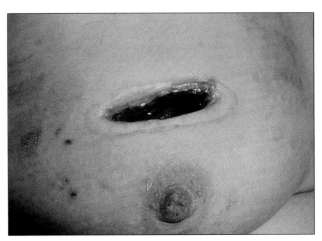

20.47 A satisfactory, well-shaped wound following removal of a proflavine emulsion pack from a very large abscess.

there is no underlying correctable cause and which have not responded to hormone therapy (see Chapter 16).

Important principles

1. Submammary incision should be used for very large volumes of breast tissue.
2. Periareolar incisions are preferred for moderate gynaecomastia.
3. Splitting the breast tissue down to the pectoral fascia gives mobility which facilitates dissection.
4. Leave a modest amount of subcutaneous fat and breast tissue adherent to the areola with closure as a separate layer beneath the nipple.
5. It is not as easy to obtain a good cosmetic result as might be imagined, especially with grosser and dependent examples of gynaecomastia. For this reason, adjuvant liposuction and more complex plastic procedures are being used in such cases as discussed in Chapter 16.

Technique

A periareolar incision is made around the lower half of the circumference. It is often necessary to extend this laterally for a short distance to achieve adequate haemostasis. Alternatively, an inframammary incision may be used, although this is cosmetically less satisfactory, especially in young patients who have a greater tendency to keloid formation. In practice the periareolar incision is best in young patients and a submammary incision in elderly obese patients with dependent breast tissue.

The nipple is elevated with much greater difficulty than is the case in the female breast because the fibroglandular tissue of gynaecomastia is adherent to the areola. A small amount of subcutaneous fat and adherent breast tissue is left behind the nipple, both to avoid damage to the nipple (much more easily done than might be thought) and to improve the cosmetic result by preserving normal nipple protrusion. The amount of tissue left behind the nipple is a matter of judgement and experience.

The flaps are dissected only a small distance upwards and downwards in a deep subcutaneous plane, so that a considerable thickness of subcutaneous fat is retained. The breast cone is then grasped and split tranversely down to the pectoral fascia (Figure 20.49).

Upper and lower halves are dissected from the pectoral fascia upwards and downwards, respectively, so that the flap dissection is completed with a much more mobile breast cone.[39] With very marked gynaecomastia, the breast cone can be quartered rather than halved and this further facilitates dissection through a small periareolar incision. It is important to dissect superficial to the pectoral fascia, as its preservation ensures that the skin retains its mobility. Haemostasis is obtained as the dissection proceeds because it is difficult to obtain adequate access to the periphery of the depth of the wound once the tissues have retracted after the breast has been removed.

Haematomas are a common complication of this procedure when done through a subareolar incision and, in cases where haemostasis is excessively difficult, a lateral extension of the wound should be made to give adequate access (Figure 20.50) and lighted retractors used.

Suction drains (two) are then inserted and the wound closed either with subcuticular prolene or with interrupted sutures. Saline should be instilled into the wound while it is being closed to prevent clot formation with blockage of the suction drains.

The drains can be removed as soon as drainage is reduced to a small quantity, usually on the first postoperative day.

SUBCUTANEOUS MASTECTOMY IN WOMEN

Important principles

1. Think carefully, twice or even three times, about the validity of the indication for the operation.
2. Accept the risk of skin or nipple necrosis where many previous biopsy scars are present.

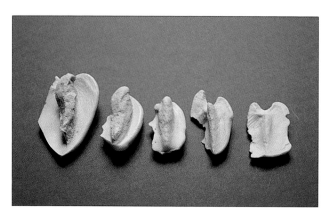

20.48 Sequential Silastic Foam® dressings as a large abscess cavity heals uneventfully – a convenient and painless method.

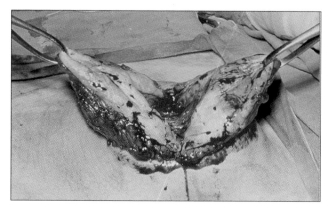

20.49 Excision of gynaecomastia through a periareolar incision is facilitated by splitting the breast tissue cone into two (or four) pieces.

3. Use an incision which will allow removal of all breast tissue, including the axillary tail and central nipple ducts.
4. Warn the patient that silicone prosthesis reconstruction is associated with considerable long-term problems.

Technique

This operation is very rarely indicated for non-malignant conditions (see Chapter 4) and should not be undertaken lightly. It is a difficult procedure to perform if complete removal of breast tissue is to be achieved with minimal complications. Only a basic account of operative detail can be given here.

There are many possible complications, especially in the breast scarred by numerous previous biopsies. Incision needs to be planned to take account of these scars which may predispose to skin necrosis. A submammary incision is used most commonly. However, it should be recognized that total excision of the breast tissue (especially the axillary tail) is not achieved through a small submammary incision. For this reason, we prefer a periareolar incision with a lateral extension because it is important that all breast tissue be excised, particularly when the operation is being carried out for preneoplastic states.

The procedure differs from the operation in the male in that all the tissue behind the nipple needs to be removed, and preferably the central core of the nipple should be taken as well to eliminate the terminal ducts. Fortunately, the areola can be elevated without difficulty in the female and this part of the procedure does not differ from major duct excision combined with central nipple duct excision. This is achieved by continuing the excision of the ductal core right through the nipple, taken in continuity with the central nipple skin containing the duct orifices. This central core is only about 5–8 mm in diameter (see Figure 20.42). The plane between the subcutaneous tissue and the breast tissue is more easily found with scissors than with a scalpel. It is important that all breast tissue be removed and this extends further medially, superiorly and laterally than may be anticipated.

The most troublesome part of the dissection is the axillary tail and breast tissue is very often left in this region.

The axillary tail is best defined by blunt dissection and its limit defined by palpation. A curved haemostat should be placed around the axillary tissue at its upper level and tied after the pedicle has been divided. Meticulous haemostasis is especially important to avoid haematoma; lighted retractors help in achieving this. It is advisable to insert at least two suction drains at the completion of this procedure. In appropriate cases, a silicone gel prosthesis or a Becker type tissue expander may be inserted into a subpectoral pocket. The skin is closed with subcuticular or interrupted sutures.

Complications

The main complication of subcutaneous mastectomy is haematoma formation, resulting from inadequate haemostasis associated with the use of small incisions. Skin flap or nipple necrosis is not uncommon, particularly in patients who have had multiple previous biopsies.

The inevitable consequence of leaving ductal tissue under the nipple is the risk of cancer developing in the major ducts, a risk which is not just theoretical.[40] Similarly, the development of late cancer due to residual breast tissue left in the periphery of the breast is a significant problem. Where the operation is being done for putative prophylaxis against the development of cancer, this possibility should be considered carefully at the time of surgery, for total removal of breast tissue is necessary but not easily achieved through conventional cosmetic incisions, and should be combined with central duct excision.

There are many complications of silicone gel reconstruction; these are dealt with in plastic surgery textbooks.

In spite of these problems, a modest result is often satisfactory to the patient (Figure 20.51), although individual patients will react very differently to similar cosmetic results.

Operations for inverted nipples

A surgeon setting out to correct congenital inverted nipples, or secondarily inverted nipples, has a wide variety of procedures from which to choose, and new approaches continue

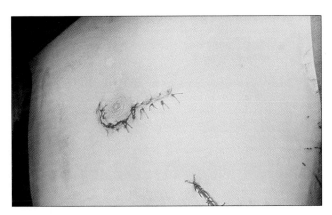

20.50 A lateral extension to a periareolar wound impairs cosmesis, but may be necessary to give adequate access.

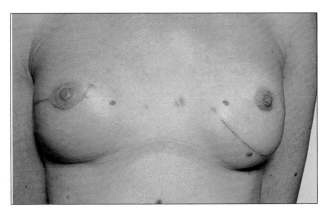

20.51 Result of insertion of bilateral subpectoral prostheses following subcutaneous mastectomy. Previous biopsy incisions have been utilized and extended to ensure that all breast tissue has been removed.

to appear in the literature in large numbers. So wide a choice makes it difficult to choose any individual technique and also suggests that no particular method is satisfactory. This is confirmed by the paucity of papers reporting large series of cases with long-term follow-up.

On general principles, one would expect that a successful procedure would need to deal with the underlying pathology, which is poor development or fibrotic shortening of the major ducts. This can only be corrected by transecting the ducts completely.

Reported techniques fall into two main groups:

1. Those which correct by pulling on the ducts and attempt to hold them out, by sutures or by providing an underlying buttress of tissue.
2. Those that divide the ducts completely and then use one of the methods in (1) to hold the nipple everted.[41,42] Although these reports are of small numbers with little follow-up, they at least meet the basic principles.

In our experience, major duct excision, combined if necessary with excision of the central core of the nipple, will cure inverted nipples without any additional buttressing procedures. Hence our recommendation is that this operation, performed as described earlier in this chapter, is the procedure of choice, provided the patient is aware that she will be unable to breastfeed following this procedure.

It is possible that simple division of the ducts by transfixion may be satisfactory,[43] but we have no experience of this technique. We prefer to do a conservative major duct excision.

In the absence of long-term follow-up, those procedures which do not divide the ducts must be considered unproven. It is also possible that some conservative procedures divide the ducts without recognizing it, so details of subsequent breastfeeding should accompany long-term results of operation for nipple inversion.

REFERENCES

1. Martin HE & Ellis EB. Biopsy by needle puncture and aspiration. *Annals of Surgery* 1930; **92**: 169–181.
2. Stewart FW. The diagnosis of tumours by aspiration. *American Journal of Pathology* 1933; **9**: 801–808.
3. Franzen S & Zajicek D. Aspiration biopsy in diagnosis of palpable lesions of the breast: critical review of 3479 consecutive biopsies. *Acta Radiologica* (Therapy) 1968; **7**: 41–262.
4. Webb AJ. The diagnostic cytology of breast carcinoma. *British Journal of Surgery* 1970; **57**: 259–264.
5. Bates AT, Bates T, Hastrich DJ *et al*. Delay in the diagnosis of breast cancer. The effect of the introduction of fine needle aspiration cytology to the breast clinic. *European Journal of Surgical Oncology* 1992; **18**: 433–437.
6. Dixon JM, Scott WN & Miller RW. Natural history of cystic disease: the importance of cyst type. **British Journal of Surgery** 1985; **72**: 190–192.
7. Ross DA, Cunningham S, Vincenti A & Rainsbury RM. Breast cytology made simple with a cell suspension medium. *European Journal of Surgical Oncology* 1992; **18**: 404–405.
8. Howat AJ, Armstrong GR, Briggs WA *et al*. Fine needle aspiration of palpable breast lumps: a 1 year audit using the cytospin method. *Cytopathology* 1992; **3**: 17–22.
9. Gateley CA, Maddox PR & Mansel RE. Pneumothorax: a complication of fine needle aspiration of the Breast. *British Medical Journal* 1991; **303**: 627–628.
10. Catania S, Veronesi P, Marassi A *et al*. Risk of pneumothorax after FNA of the breast: Italian experience of more than 200,000 aspirations. *The Breast* 1993; **2**: 246–247.
11. Kaufman Z, Shpitz B, Shapiro M *et al*. Pneumothorax: A complication of FNA of breast tumours. *Acta Cytologica* 1994; **38**: 737–738.
12. Horobin JM, Matthew BM, Preece PE & Thompson A. Effects of fine needle aspiration on subsequent mammograms. *British Journal of Surgery* 1992; **79**: 52–54.
13. Mitnick JS, Vazquez MF, Roses DF *et al*. Stereotactic localization for fine needle aspiration biopsy in patients with augmentation prostheses. *Annals of Plastic Surgery* 1992; **29**: 31–35.
14. Roberts JG, Preece PE, Bolton PM *et al*. The Trucut biopsy in breast cancer. *Clinical Oncology* 1975; **1**: 287–303.
15. McMahon AJ, Lufty AM, Matthew A *et al*. Needle core biopsy of the breast with a spring loaded device. *British Journal of Surgery* 1992; **79**: 1042–1045.
16. Evans WP & Cade SH. Needle localization and fine needle aspiration biopsy of nonpalpable breast lesions with the use of standard and stereotactic equipment. *Radiology* 1989; **173**: 53–56.
17. Parker SH, Lovin JD, Jobe WE *et al*. Stereotactic breast biopsy with a biopsy gun. *Radiology* 1990; **176**: 741–747.
18. Donkers DJ. Stereotactic core biopsy of breast lesions. *Radiology* 1992; **183**: 631–634.
19. Walker GM, Foster RS, McKegny CP & McKegny FP. Breast biopsy. A comparison of outpatient and inpatient experience. *Archives of Surgery* 1978; **113**: 942–946.
20. Rosenthal LJ. Discrepant estrogen receptor protein levels according to surgical technique. *American Journal of Surgery* 1979; **138**: 6801–6811.
21. Pilnik S & Steicher F. The use of haemostatic scalpel in operations upon the breast. *Surgery, Gynecology and Obstetrics* 1986; **162**: 589–591.
22. Glen PM & Margulies D. Electrocautery and hormone receptors in breast biopsy. *American Journal of Surgery* 1989; **158**: 6–7.
23. Robertson JLA. The choice of incision for biopsy in large breasted women. *South African Journal of Surgery* 1980; **18**: 9–12.
24. Wheeler MH & Lakhany Z. Breast biopsy – A trial of wound drainage. *American Journal of Surgery* 1976; **31**: 581–582.
25. Johnson AJ, Thompson AM, John TG *et al*. Wound compression pads are of no value after local anaesthetic breast biopsy. *Annals of the Royal College of Surgeons of England* 1991; **73**: 303–304.
26. Pezner RD, Lorant JA, Terz J *et al*. Wound healing

complications following biopsy of the irradiated breast. *Archives of Surgery* 1992; **127**: 321–324.

27. Preece PE, Gravelle IH, Hughes LE *et al.* The operative management of subclinical breast cancer. *Clinical Oncology* 1977; **3**: 165–169.

28. Svane G. A stereotactic technique for preoperative marking of impalpable breast lesions. *Acta Radiologica* 1983; **24**: 145–151.

29. Potchen EJ, Sierra A, MacKenzie C & Osuch J. Svane localisation of non-palpable breast lesions. *Lancet* 1991; **338**: 816.

30. Helvie MA, Ikeda DM & Adler DD. Localization and needle aspiration of breast lesions: complications in 370 cases. *American Journal of Roentgenology* 1991; **157**: 711–714.

31. Rappaport W, Thompson S, Wong R *et al.* Complications associated with needle localization biopsy of the breast. *Surgery, Gynecology and Obstetrics* 1991; **172**: 303–306.

32. Thomas JG. *New York Medical Journal* 1882; **xxv**: 337.

33. Haagensen CD. *Diseases of the Breast*, 3rd edn. Philadelphia: WB Saunders, 1986.

34. Atkins HJB. Mammillary fistula. *British Medical Journal* 1955; **2**: 1473–1474.

35. Bundred NJ, Dixon JM, Chetty U & Forrest APM. Mammillary fistula. *British Journal of Surgery* 1987; **74**: 466–468.

36. Hadfield GJ. Excision of the major duct system for benign disease of the breast. *British Journal of Surgery* 1960; **47**: 472–477.

37. Urban JA. Excision of the major duct system of the breast. *Cancer* 1963; **16**: 516–520.

38. Benson EA & Goodman MA. Incision with primary suture in the treatment of acute puerperal breast abscess. *British Journal of Surgery* 1970; **57**: 55–58.

39. Von Kessel F, Pickrell KL, Huger WE & Matton G. Surgical treatment of gynaecomastia: an analysis of 275 cases. *Annals of Surgery* 1963; **157**: 142–151.

40. Srivastava A & Webster DJT. Isolated nipple recurrence 17 years after subcutaneous mastectomy for breast cancer – a case report. *European Journal of Surgical Oncology* 1987; **13**: 459–461.

41. Hartrampf CR & Schneider WJ. A simple direct method for correction of inversion of the nipple. *Plastic and Reconstructive Surgery* 1976; **58**: 678–679.

42. Broadbent TR & Woolf RM. Benign inverted nipple. Trans nipple areola correction. *Plastic and Reconstructive Surgery* 1976; **58**: 673–677.

43. Crestinu JM. The inverted nipple – a blind method of correction. *Plastic and Reconstructive Surgery* 1987; **79**: 127–130.

Chapter 21

Cosmetic aspects of benign breast disorders

CONTENTS

KEY POINTS AND NEW DEVELOPMENTS

1. Careful assessment of a patient's concerns and motivations is essential to maximize patient satisfaction after cosmetic procedures, with psychological assessment added in cases of uncertainty.
2. Reduction mammoplasty is a complex procedure with many possible complications. Both the surgeon and the patient should be fully aware of these. The most important technical preoperative assessment is the new position of the nipple-areolar complex.
3. Of many possible procedures, transposition of the nipple-areolar complex on an inferior glandular pedicle is a well-proven technique.
4. Claims of systemic complications from silicone prostheses have affected the popularity of augmentation mammoplasty, although the balance of evidence at present is convincingly against any causal relationship.
5. The legal position regarding implants varies from country to country.
6. Simple augmentation is not appropriate where the nipple lies below the inframammary groove. This situation requires some form of mastopexy, with or without augmentation.
7. Uncommon congenital abnormalities, such as Poland's syndrome and tubular breasts, are difficult to correct completely, leading to a variety of procedures being recommended.
8. The increasingly sought after gender reassignment surgery should only be considered on the recommendation of a psychiatrist experienced in this field.

PSYCHOLOGICAL ASPECTS

Society places great demands on our appearance and our ability to conform to stereotypes. Nowhere is this more evident than with the female breast. As a generality most people like to think that their body appearance is normal. This normality is presented to us through daily experiences and in particular through modern advertising. Most people like to conform to the dictates of fashion and if they fall outside of the bands of 'normality' they feel self-conscious. This self-consciousness may be reinforced by friendly teasing and results in a small number of people becoming so concerned about their body image that they resort to either alteration in behaviour or disguise. A few patients cannot cope psychologically and seek surgical alteration of the abnormality. Research by Harris[1] using psychometric testing has shown that in the female, perceived abnormality of the breasts causes more psychological distress and greater satisfaction when surgically corrected than abnormalities of the face or abdomen.

Cosmetic surgery of the breast also has a functional basis. Large-breasted women may be unable to take part in sports, they may suffer with shoulder and neck pain and they may have an abnormal posture. What is less often realized is that small-breasted women may be equally disadvantaged in that they find it difficult to buy clothing that fits, the garments available having been designed for 'average' proportioned women.

It has been shown that in correctly selected, motivated patients cosmetic breast surgery is of great therapeutic value.[2] However, breast surgeons should be cautioned that if they undertake cosmetic surgery they should be properly trained in the latest techniques and be capable of producing results that fall consistently within accepted surgical standards. Breast surgery is becoming a minefield for the inexperienced surgeon, not only from the pressure of the dissatisfied patient but also from the escalating litigation associated with it.

HYPERTROPHY OF THE BREAST

The normal breast has a variety of shapes, sizes and levels of firmness. Some breasts continue to grow following normal puberty, resulting in either physical or psychological morbidity. Patients requesting a breast reduction can be divided into two groups: first, those with so-called virginal hypertrophy present before pregnancy, including the sometimes difficult to assess teenagers, and secondly, a group consisting mainly of postmenopausal women presenting with advancing breast hypertrophy in middle age, often associated with an increasing body mass index.

Frequently the patient with large breasts will complain of interference with daily activity such as sport and an inability to run, or abnormal posture associated with a varying degree of shoulder and upper back pain. Sometimes the patient will complain of intertrigo under the breasts or mastalgia.

In the younger group there is undoubtedly often a body image distortion. Patients will frequently feel that their breasts are a source of sexual signal to the opposite sex and that it is their breasts that are being visualized and not their person.

Patient selection

It is important to establish the fitness of the patient for such surgery as undoubtedly complications are higher in patients who are smokers or those with chronic respiratory or cardiovascular disease and obesity. A psychological assessment must be made of the patient's motivation for surgery. In breast reduction this is usually straightforward in older patients provided they are aware of the necessary scars and possible complications. The help of a clinical psychologist or breast counsellor may prove invaluable.

Patients in the younger group, however, can be more difficult to advise. In those where at least 500 g are going to be excised then the decision is usually straightforward. However, in the moderately large-breasted patient, in whom perhaps only 200 g of breast tissue will be excised and where self-consciousness is as much a factor as the practical problems of a large breast, caution needs to be exercised. In this sort of patient it is important to advise them that they will certainly be self-conscious about their breasts once scars are visible. Scars in young patients are frequently red, hypertrophic and spread and this outcome should be reinforced by showing postoperative photographs of appropriate results. It should be explained to such patients that cosmetic surgery is a balance between the benefits of surgery and the possible complications of poor scarring through to nipple necrosis. Most patients will reluctantly accept the advice for delay and if there is any cause for anxiety then the patient should be referred on for more appropriate detailed psychological counselling.

The examination should include a body mass index assessment by measuring the height and weight, a measurement of the nipple height measured from the suprasternal notch, an assessment of asymmetry both in breast size and the thoracic wall curvature and the noting of any excess adiposity in the axillae. Photographs should be taken as a record. The patient is then advised on the common complications of breast reduction which should include the position and quality of scars, the inability to breastfeed, loss of nipple sensation through to nipple necrosis, haematoma formation and fat necrosis with their various managements. Patients are frequently offered a second consultation closer to the time of planned surgery.

Surgical techniques

There are a multiplicity of surgical procedures. Essentially the nipple is either resited as a free graft which is indicated in very large reductions and in older medically compromised patients, or the nipple-areolar complex is transposed on the underlying breast tissue, thus retaining the potential for breastfeeding and sensation postoperatively.

Nipple size and position

The most important preoperative decision is the new position of the nipple-areolar complex. Frequently it is placed too high. The result of this is that with gradual reptosis of the breast the nipple retains its new position and ends up lying on top of the breast. In most women the nipple should be positioned about 23 cm from the suprasternal notch, which is about the level of the inframammary groove. Traditionally the areolar diameter varies between 38 and 45 mm in diameter and the nipple lies along a line dropped vertically from the midclavicular line to the inframammary crease.

The safest technique to move the nipple-areolar complex (in my opinion) is on the underlying breast tissue on an inferior glandular pedicle as described by Hester *et al.*[3] Once the reduction has been effected the skin is tailored and this results in an inverted T scar with the vertical element running down from the newly positioned nipple-areolar complex to the inframammary groove and the transverse scar lying in the inframammary groove.

A further point in the design of this operation is how much skin is excised. A Wise keyhole pattern has been used by many to design the skin excision.[4] However, the angle of the Wise keyhole pattern does require to be varied depending upon the preoperative size and shape. Reduction mammoplasty is an operation in which the fine technical details of planning and execution are the most important variables in determining the outcome of surgery.

Liposuction can be used as an isolated procedure in elderly women with heavy breasts who want a fast and safe operation without too much consideration for aesthetics. However, Lejour[5] has shown that liposuction as part of a breast reduction surgery can be beneficial allowing limitation of the extent of the scars and in particular the reduction of lateral/axillary tail prominence.

Newer surgical procedures have concentrated on limiting the extent of scarring and in particular many small to moderate breast reductions can be undertaken using only a vertical scar together with the scar around the nipple-areolar complex as opposed to the inverted T scar described above. The vertical scar breast reduction has been popularized by Lejour[5] and Asplund and Davies[6] (Figures 21.1 and 21.2).

Such techniques depend upon reducing the breast size with elevation of the nipple-areolar complex and then shaping the remaining breast tissue with sutures (glanduloplasty). Following some skin reduction the remaining skin is draped over the breast mound. Over the ensuing 12 weeks the skin will contract down to the shape and size of the underlying gland. This is in direct comparison with the inverted T scar where the skin reduction and resuturing tend to produce the shape of a new breast.

Surgery is routinely undertaken with the patient semirecumbant. It has been shown that infiltrating the breast preoperatively with a dilute solution of adrenaline and bupivacaine[7] decreases intraoperative bleeding and helps the postoperative pain. Subcuticular sutures should always be used to close the skin.

Complications

Aesthetics

The most common complication for the inexperienced surgeon is a lack of planning and placing the nipple-areolar complex too high.

Fat necrosis

Fat necrosis is probably the second most common complication and in most cases is a self-limiting condition. The breast frequently becomes red, indurated and hard but the patient has no systemic symptoms. The patient is frequently

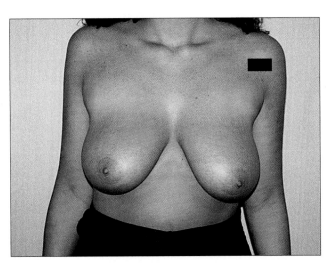

21.1 Vertical scar reduction mammoplasty. Preoperative photograph.

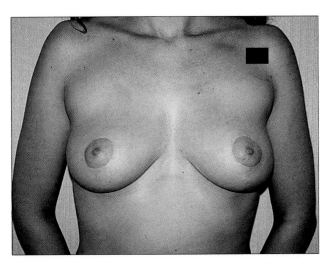

21.2 Vertical scar reduction mammoplasty. Postoperative photograph showing the cosmetic result that should be sought.

placed on antibiotics and over a period of 3-4 weeks this induration settles. Unfortunately, the resulting fibrosis around fat necrosis takes many months to resolve and some patients may be left with a marked palpable tumour within the breast. It is probably safer for this tumour to be excised as (a) it will interfere with future mammograms and (b) patients are often disturbed by having a palpable lump. This may affect the overall breast size.

Haematoma

Haematoma is less common but more important as if undiagnosed it may lead to compromise of the vascular supply to the nipple-areolar complex. In my opinion drains should always be used postoperatively.

Nipple sensation

Loss of sensation in the nipple is a well-known complication of reduction mammoplasty. The extent will depend on what type of breast reduction is undertaken and the amount of breast tissue excised. Gonzalez et al.[8] reported in a study of 84 breasts an overall loss of sensation in the nipple in 10% of cases.

Breastfeeding

In a retrospective analysis of 292 patients who underwent breast reduction by six different procedures Sandsmark et al.[9] found that of 49 women who gave birth during the follow-up period 32 could nurse their babies although milk production varied widely and in no case was sufficient for complete infant feeding. Harris et al.[10] found that 50% of patients who became pregnant after breast reduction were able to breastfeed for 2 weeks but then failed to continue for a variety of reasons. One-third succcessfully breastfed for at least 2 months.

Patient satisfaction

Strombeck[11] and most recently Klassen et al.[12] have shown the great physical and psychological benefits of breast reduction.

Free nipple grafting

Women who have gigantomastia or severe hypertrophy or medical conditions likely to compromise surgery are probably better served by reduction with free nipple transplantation. The skin reduction is the same as for the inverted T procedure using the Wise keyhole pattern and usually the whole of the gland lying below the inframammary groove is amputated. The conical shape of the breasts is restored by reapproximating the vertical limbs of the keyhole and the nipple is grafted on to its new position. Nipple-areolar projection and survival is improved by grafting on to a dermal bed rather than fat and usually there is a good take of graft. There is always mild to moderate hypopigmentation of the areolar. Romano et al.[13] reported a series in which the average resection was 1838 g of breast tissue per

breast. One-year follow-up showed that there were minimal complications and excellent aesthetic results with shorter operating time, reduced blood loss and less risk of wound-healing complications.

HYPOPLASIA OF THE BREAST

Augmentation of the small breast is a common cosmetic procedure recently drawn to everyone's attention by the controversy surrounding the use of silicone gel implants. In the past a variety of substances have been used to make the breast larger. These have included the injection of free paraffin and silicone and more recently fat, with occasional good short-term results which have been far outweighed by the long-term complications. Dermal fat grafts have also been tried but these frequently result in both atrophy and calcification of the graft and have now been abandoned.

Silicone gel implants were introduced 35 years ago for breast augmentation and until recently this was one of the most commonly performed cosmetic operations. All breast implants available today consist of a silicone bag and in the UK there are three commonly used fillers: saline, Hydrogel and silicone. The indications for breast augmentation are usually for breast hypoplasia. This can result in either self-consciousness and a poor self-image leading to psychosexual disturbances or a more practical problem of the difficulty of finding clothes that fit. Again there are usually two groups of patients: younger nulliparous patients who require careful counselling and selection and older patients who have completed their families and their breasts have become smaller with successive pregnancies. The latter group is a much easier group to advise provided their motivation is for personal confidence and self-motivation.

Preoperative evaluation

Accurate preoperative evaluation of the patient is required and in particular any asymmetry of the breasts in position and size should be noted and measured and asymmetries of the shape of the thorax should also be identified. The patient should be photographed preoperatively. One of the difficult problems is sizing the patient for an implant; the simplest approach is to advise the patient to bring a sports bra with a full cup to the size which she aspires to fill then use sizers to fill the bra cup so that an estimation can be made. Nowhere is it more important to discuss with the patient the complications of such surgery. This can include loss of nipple sensation, hardening around the prosthesis due to scarring or encapsulation and a palpable edge to the prosthesis. The type of prosthesis which may be used, with its pros and cons, should also be discussed. Access to the surgical plane, which is either in front of or behind the pectoralis major muscle, is through an inframammary, a periareolar or a transaxillary incision. The principal contraindication to simple breast augmentation is if the patient has a degree of ptosis of the breast such that the nipple-areolar complex lies below the inframammary groove. If simple breast augmentation is undertaken in this situation then the nipple-areolar complex will lie low compared to a higher breast mound. This group of patients will always require a mastopexy, elevating the nipple-alveolar complex with or without breast augmentation.

A full discussion of the necessary scars for this latter procedure is obviously required and many patients decide against surgery at this point.

Prostheses

In the USA saline is the most commonly used filler for breast prostheses. However, it has two drawbacks: first, the prosthesis cannot be overfilled and therefore wrinkling of the silastic shell of the prosthesis is common and is frequently obvious through normal breast tissue. Secondly, where there is a fold in the prosthesis this leads to weakness and then rupture. Implant failure rates of 20% have been reported, although newer prostheses introduced in the mid-1980s report a much lower failure rate.[14] Saline prostheses may have a slightly lower instance of capsule formation and can also be inserted through smaller incisions.

Recently in the UK prostheses filled with soyabean extract (Triluscent) have been banned.

In the UK silicone gel-filled implants have not been removed from clinical use. In the US, lawyers have claimed that silicone gel-filled mammary prostheses have been implicated in cases of breast cancer, in congenital abnormalities in children born to mothers who had had a breast augmentation and in a range of diseases from arthritis to autoimmune disorders grouped together under a label of connective tissue disease.

Carcinogenicity

Deapen et al.[15] studied 3111 women after augmentation mammoplasty for a mean 6.2 years. In that group 15.7 cases of breast cancer would have been expected but only nine were observed. Statistically this was a non-significant difference. In a further study by Berkel et al.[16] in Alberta the records of women who had undergone breast augmentation between 1973 and 1986 were checked against those of a group of women who had had primary breast cancer diagnosed between 1973 and 1991. The expected incidence of breast cancer in the implant cohort was calculated to be 86.2 cases. In fact 41 cases were observed and the authors concluded there was no increased risk of breast cancer. There has been one reported case of squamous cell carcinoma arising from the capsule around the implant 15 years after breast augmentation,[17] with a further two cases of synovial metaplasia of the periprosthetic capsule. To date there is no evidence to support a cause-and-effect relationship between silicone breast implants and breast cancer in humans.

Teratogenicity

Similarly there is no evidence to support a cause and effect between silicone breast implants and congenital abnormalities in children born to mothers with breast implants.

Autoimmune disorders

The term human adjuvant disease was introduced by Miyoshi et al.[18] in 1964 upon noticing connective tissue-like illness in two patients whose breasts had been injected with paraffin for augmentation. Van Nunen et al.[19] published the first report linking mammary implants used for augmentation with symptoms of collagen disease. There has been much conjecture as to which autoimmune diseases have been caused and how they are caused. This has been summarized in an article by the Counsel on Scientific Affairs of the American Medical Association.[20] Subsequently there have been 23 retrospective studies comparing groups of women who have had breast augmentation using silicone gel implants with controlled groups who have not. The conclusion of all these studies involving nearly 30,000 patients is that there is no positive proof of silicone gel being implicated in the cause of any disease, i.e. there is no difference in disease patterns between the augmented and the non-augmented groups.[21,22]

Apart from the controversy surrounding the use of silastic gel the operation of breast augmentation has other complications. The most common is scarring around the prosthesis: so-called capsule formation. Some patients will make a thick scar, some patients will make a thin scar. If the patient makes a thick scar with capsular contraction the prosthesis will feel hard and will assume a more rounded shape. If the patient makes a thin scar the prosthesis will remain soft and flat. The prosthesis itself in all cases remains unchanged.

It has now been shown that a rough-coated or textured surface to the prosthesis interferes with the alignment of collagen myofibroblast matrix in the scarring and this results in the degree of encapsulation being greatly reduced. Malata et al.[23] reported an encapsulation rate interfering with the results of surgery of only 7% if the prosthesis was textured and placed behind the pectoralis major muscle. The introduction of textured prostheses has radically altered the outcome of breast augmentation to the benefit of many women.

Polyurethane-coated prostheses working on the same principle are generally no longer available as there have been concerns about the degradation products from the polyurethane.

Surgical technique

The patient should be marked out preoperatively as to the extent of dissection of the pocket and the position of the incision. In general, surgery is undertaken under general anaesthetic either as a day case, or as a one-night stay in hospital when excessive pain in anticipated, especially if the prosthesis is to be placed behind the pectoralis major muscle.

The patient's breast may be infiltrated with a mixture of adrenaline and bupivacaine to help with haemostasis and postoperative pain control. Depending upon the incision and plane of dissection, either sharp dissection aided by a lighted retractor or blunt dissection can be used to develop a pocket. Perioperative antibiotics may or may not be used, Redivac drains may or may not be used and the implants may or may not be washed in an antiseptic agent.

Wounds should be closed using a subcuticular stitch and the breast prosthesis should be checked for symmetry by sitting the patient up on the table and maintaining their posture with a brassière or adhesive stretch bandage (Figures 21.3 and 21.4).

Postoperative complications
The following complications have been reported.

Haematoma
Williams[24] reported an incidence of haematoma of 3% in breast augmentation, and significant haematomas are associated with both infection and capsular firmness and should therefore be evacuated.

Wound infections
An incidence of 2% in 899 cases was reported by Courtiss et al.[25] Le Roy and Given[26] studied the role of prophylactic antibiotics in breast augmentation surgery and concluded that the routine use of antibiotics to prevent wound infection after augmentation mammoplasty is beneficial.

Nipple sensation
The incidence of diminished nipple sensation after augmentation ranges from negligible to almost 50% and probably the average is about 15%. As common are areas of hypoaesthesia in the skin surrounding the nipple-areolar complex and in some cases patients complain of hyperaesthesia after breast augmentation.

Pain
Pain after augmentation can be either in the immediate postoperative period, especially where the pectoralis major muscle has been manipulated, or late and associated with severe capsular contraction.

Capsule formation
Severe capsular contraction is reported in one series at 7% at 3 years.[23] Capsular contraction can either be accepted, the prosthesis removed, with or without replacement, with or without capulotomy or capulectomy. Obviously it cannot be guaranteed that open capsulectomy, which can only be performed through a submammary incision and replacement of the prosthesis, will not result in a further significant capsule.

Misplacement
Displacement or incorrect position of the implant can occur in the immediate postoperative period. It is important therefore to point out to the patient any asymmetries in breast shape and size preoperatively.

Rupture
All prosthesis will 'bleed' to a certain extent and there will be a small leak of silicone gel from the prosthesis. Of more concern is rupture in which there is a major tear or disruption of the shell, which becomes evident clinically when the patient complains of pain and deformity in the previously augmented breast. Many ruptures of implants are silent, however, and this has been recently highlighted by the paper of Brown et al.[26] who reported a rupture rate of 72% in prostheses that had been implanted up to 25 years previously. In this alarming paper the vast majority of patients had implants inserted at least 10 years previously which were of a type with very thin capsules. The modern implant has a very different type of laminated construction and it is hoped that the rupture rate of these prostheses will be much lower. The most sensitive way of telling whether the prosthesis is ruptured or not is by magnetic resonance

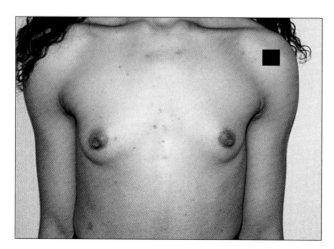

21.3 Augmentation mammoplasty. Preoperative photograph.

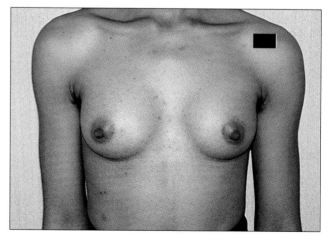

21.4 Augmentation mammoplasty. Postoperative photograph showing a satisfactory result.

imaging, but ultrasound does not have a place in the routine screening of these prostheses.

Again routine mammography is not contraindicated with silastic gel prostheses *in situ*. All that is required is for the radiographer to be informed and alternative views can usually be obtained of the breast tissue.[27]

MASTOPEXY (CORRECTION OF BREAST PTOSIS)

Some women present with a reasonable breast volume but with a loss of breast shape, either as a result of weight loss or following pregnancy. In these cases the breast becomes ptosed with the nipple-areolar complex lying well below the inframammary groove. The patient may request either a simple mastopexy procedure to elevate the nipple and reshape the gland with no increase in volume, or a mastopexy with breast augmentation.

Most mastopexies can be achieved by repositioning the nipple-areolar complex and tailoring the skin, leaving a single vertical scar down to the submammary groove. In severe cases where there has been marked volume loss from the breast or the skin and breast tissues have extremely poor tone, more skin will require excision and a transverse scar lying in the inframammary groove will also be required with a skin excision based on the Wise keyhole pattern.

The surgical technique is as for a breast reduction in most cases. The operation itself carries the same possible complications but the incidence of these is greatly reduced.

Undertaking augmentation at the same operation can be extremely difficult and it is usually best to place the prosthesis in a submuscular pocket.

AMASTIA AND POLAND'S SYNDROME

Amastia is a rare condition and is probably due to failure of the milk gland to develop to its complete evolution. It is not surprising that such an obvious abnormality was recorded in Biblical times (Song of Solomon, VIII). Congenitally, amastia may be part of Poland's syndrome, which consists of varying degrees of absence of the pectoralis major muscle and overlying breast associated with a small nipple which is usually higher than the normal contralateral side and a hypoplastic arm and hand, with or without abnormalities of the fingers (Figure 21.5). In spite of its popular eponym, this condition was apparently first described in 1839 by Floriep and the terminology has been challenged by Ravitch.[28] The condition occurs in both male and females.

In the male, treatment of the more severe presentations can be undertaken using customized silastic inserts. A better alternative is to transpose a latissimus dorsi muscle flap. This can provide bulk, provided it has not denervated, and it requires detachment of its humeral head to reconstruct the anterior axillary fold with the insertion of the body of the latissimus muscle into the pocket on the anterior aspect of the chest wall.[29]

In the female, reconstruction is more difficult in that usually one is asked to see and advise a girl in adolescence and definitive reconstruction should be avoided. The easiest and most satisfactory temporization is to insert a tissue expander through a submammary crease incision, placing the prosthesis under any pectoral muscle that may be present. The prosthesis should be placed low, allowing for developing ptosis in the normal contralateral side. As the adolescent grows then the tissue expander can be adjusted appropriately and a definitive augmentation undertaken when growth is complete. Frequently there is a contour deformity at the upper pole of the breast where the pectoralis major is rudimentary, and in many cases the nipple on the affected side will remain too high and too small.

Trauma is another cause of amastia, mainly as a result of thermal injury. Often there is a shortage of skin and the breast bud is damaged. Simple augmentation with an implant may be possible but resurfacing with a latissimus dorsi flap prior to augmentation may be required. Other causes of amastia include radiotherapy in childhood.

TUBULAR BREASTS

This is where there is a marked degree of ptosis of the breast associated with a very large areola and narrow breast base. Correction is difficult and involves overexpanding the breast base together with dividing some of the subcutaneous bands that lie circumferentially around the breast tissue, then at a later date augmenting the breast by placing the prosthesis into the overexpanded pocket (Figures 21.6 and 21.7).

SYMAZIA

This is a very rare deformity in which the breasts are fused in the midline. It can cause difficulty and discomfort with clothing but more often self-consciousness because of the

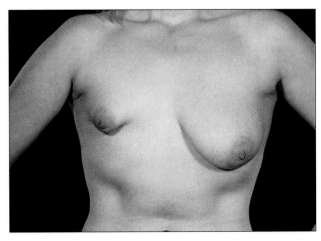

21.5 Right-sided Poland's syndrome.

lack of cleavage. It is probably not correctable surgically. There are reports of correction by undertaking breast reduction and separating the breasts by removing the subcutaneous tissues overlying the sternum and then suturing the skin down on to the sternum itself, but these results are not always reproducible.

GYNAECOMASTIA

This is defined as an asymptomatic palpable discrete button of firm subareolar tissue measuring at least 2 cm in diameter. It has a high incidence in the normal population, increasing with advancing age. It is important to differentiate clinically between breast tissue, fat and well-developed pectoral muscle. The latter is particularly important to establish as weightlifters frequently take hormones and have a very high critical appearance of their body image. In these cases usually by tensing the underlying pectoral muscle it can be shown that there is virtually no degree of gynaecomastia. In my opinion breast tissue cannot be aspirated down a liposuction instrument. It can only be removed surgically and the best approach is through a Webster's periareolar incision.[30] Where there is a significant degree of fat then liposuction or, more recently, ultrasonic-assisted liposuction (UAL) may be indicated, especially to chamfer the edges of a surgical excision.

The object is to restore a healthy body image. The most common complication is over-resection of the gland, producing a very flat-lying nipple-areolar complex. Other complications include haematoma and seroma, nipple-areolar necrosis or partial necrosis, loss of sensation, conspicuous scars or residual skin redundancy.

GENDER REASSIGNMENT SURGERY

Patients should only be operated on for gender reassignment if they have been referred by a psychiatrist experienced in gender dysphoria and with two psychiatrists agreeing that surgery is in the best interest of the patient.

Male to female: breast augmentation

The initial assessment and informed consent are exactly the same as for a female undergoing breast augmentation. Most males have a wide torso and require a larger augmentation. Scars are probably best situated in the axilla but there is a size limitation and my personal preferred plane of pocket is submuscular. Patients should be warned about loss of nipple sensation and the fact that a cleavage is difficult to produce in view of the fact that the chest is wide and the breast prosthesis manufactured for women tends to have a relatively narrow base.

Female to male: breast mastectomy

Mastectomy in this situation is based upon two operations. First, if there is marked skin excess with nipple ptosis then the best operation is to undertake a mastectomy, leaving the incision as close to the submammary groove as possible, and repositioning the nipples as a composite graft. Smaller breasts with good skin and breast tone can be reduced through a periareolar incision with or without a medial and lateral extension which, in my experience, is not often necessary. The complications are as for a gynaecomastia reduction and, or course, patients need to be warned that this is frequently an incomplete mastectomy and that a significant amount of breast tissue may be left behind. The main complication of this surgery is an over-reduction of the tissues, resulting in an extremely flat or uneven looking chest wall, sometimes with no adipose tissue between the skin and the underlying pectoralis muscle. This should be avoided as it is impossible to correct as a secondary procedure.

SUBCUTANEOUS MASTECTOMY

This is best done as a two-operator procedure with an ablative surgeon and a reconstructive surgeon. Unfortunately

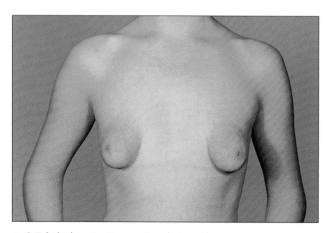

21.6 Tubular breasts. Preoperative photograph.

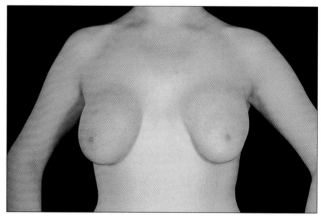

21.7 The patient shown in Figure 21.6, after surgery to correct tubular breasts.

there are two diametrically opposing factors involved. First, subcutaneous mastectomy in order to be prophylactic against cancer should remove as much of the underlying glandular tissue as possible. This frequently leaves an extremely thin skin envelope which has a precarious blood supply, certainly not sufficient to allow any transposition of the nipple-areolar complex to a newer position. Secondly, as much tissue as possible should be left behind in order to disguise the underlying breast prosthesis and to preserve a safe blood supply to the skin.

In smaller-breasted women where there is no ptosis of the nipple-areolar complex, subcutaneous mastectomy can be undertaken through a submammary groove incision with immediate reconstruction placing a prosthesis into a submuscular pocket, frequently involving not only the pectoralis major muscle but serratus anterior . Ablative surgeons should be reminded that the female breast stops at the inframammary groove and, where possible, this landmark should not be disturbed.

The problem case of subcutaneous mastectomy is where the nipple-areolar complex needs to be elevated to a new position. If this is to be done safely at the time of a mastectomy then there has to be compromise on the amount of glandular tissue removed. Sometimes a two-stage procedure can be undertaken, whereby the nipple-areolar complex is first raised as it would be in a breast reduction with the necessary periareolar scars and inframammary scars, and then at a later date a subcutaneous mastectomy can be performed more safely. On the other hand, a skin reduction with a free nipple-areolar graft can be undertaken, but this always results in some loss of the nipple-areolar sensation.

Subcutaneous mastectomy is a very difficult operation, producing very variable results and patients are frequently dissatisfied with the outcome of their surgery, either from an aesthetic point of view or because the breast prosthesis is easily palpable with contour deformities or deformity because of capsular contracture.

REFERENCES

1. Harris DL. Self consciousness of disproportionate breast size: A primary psychological reaction to abnormal appearance. *British Journal of Plastic Surgery* 1983; **36**: 191–195.

2. Shakespeare V & Cole RP. Measuring patient based outcomes in a plastic surgery service: Breast reduction surgical patients. *British Journal of Plastic Surgery* 1997; **50**: 242–248.

3. Hester TR, Bostwick J, Miller L & Cunningham SJ. Breast reduction utilizing the maximally vascularised central breast pedicle. *Plastic and Reconstructive Surgery* 1985; **76**: 890–898.

4. Wise RJ. A preliminary report on a method of planning the mammoplasty. *Plastic and Reconstructive Surgery* 1956; **17**: 367.

5. Lejour M. Vertical mammoplasty and liposuction of the breast. *Plastic and Reconstructive Surgery* 1994; **94**: 100.

6. Asplund OA & Davies DM. Vertical scar reduction with medial flap or glandular transposition of nipple areolar. *British Journal of Plastic Surgery* 1996; **49**: 507.

7. Metaxitos N, Asplund O & Hayes M. Bipuvacaine with adrenaline in breast reduction: A control study about peri- and post-operative bleeding and post-operative pain control. *British Journal of Plastic Surgery* 1999 (in press).

8. Gonzalez F, Brown FE, Gold ME *et al.* Pre-operative and post operative nipple areolar sensibility in patients undergoing reduction mammoplasty. *Plastic and Reconstructive Surgery* 1993; **92**: 809–814.

9. Sandsmark M, Amland PF, Abyholm *et al.* Reduction mammoplasty. A comparative study of the Orlando & Robbins method in 292 patients. *Scandanavian Journal of Plastic and Reconstructive Hand Surgery* 1992; **26**: 203–209.

10. Harris L, Morris SF & Frieberg A. Is breast feeding possible after reduction mammoplasty? *Plastic and Reconstructive Surgery* 1992; **89**: 836.

11. Strombeck JO. Macromastia in women and its surgical treatment. A clinical study based on 1042 cases. *Acta Chirurgica Scandinavica* 1964; **341** (Suppl 1): 128.

12. Klassen A, Jenkinson C, Fitzpatrick R & Goodacre T. Patient's health related quality of life before and after aesthetic surgery. *British Journal of Plastic Surgery* 1996; **49**: 433.

13. Romano JJ, Francel JJ & Hoopes JE. Free nipple graft reduction mammoplasty. *Annals of Plastic Surgery* 1992; **28**: 271.

14. Gutowski KA, Mesna GT & Cunningham BL. Saline filled breast implants. *Plastic and Reconstructive Surgery* 1997; **100**: 1019.

15. Deapen DM, Bernstein L & Brody GS. Are breast implants anti-carcinogenic? A 14 year follow up of the Los Angeles study. *Plastic and Reconstructive Surgery* 1997; **99**: 1346.

16. Berkel H, Birdsell DC & Jenkins H. Breast augmentation: A risk factor for breast cancer. *New England Journal of Medicine* 1992; **326**(25): 1649.

17. Paletta C, Paletta Fx Jr & Paletta Fx Sr. Squamous cell carcinoma following breast augmentation. *Annals of Plastic Surgery* 1992; **29**: 425.

18. Miyoshi K, Miyamura T, Kobayashi Y *et al.* Hypergammaglobulinaemia by prolonged adjuvanticity in men. Disorders developed after augmentation mammoplasty. *Journal of the Keio Medical Society* 1964; **2122**: 9–14.

19. Van Nunen SA, Gatenby PA & Basten A. Post mammoplasty connective tissue disease. *Arthritis and Rheumatism* 1982; **25**: 694.

20. Counsel on Scientific Affairs, American Medical Association. Silicone gel breast implants. *Journal of the American Medical Association* 1993; **270** (21): 2602.

21. Gabriel SE, O'Fallon WM, Kurland LT *et al.* Risk of connective tissue diseases and other disorders after breast implantation. *New England Journal of Medicine* 1994; **330** (24): 1697–1708.

22. Sanchez-Guerrero J, Colditz GA, Karlson EW *et al.* Silicone breast implants and the risk of connective tissue diseases and symptoms. *New England Journal of Medicine* 1995; **332** (25): 1666.

23. Malata CM, Feldberg L, Coleman DJ, Foo ITH & Sharpe DT.

Textured or smooth implants for breast augmentation? Three year follow up of a prospective randomized controlled trial. *British Journal of Plastic Surgery* 1997; **50**: 99–105.

24. Williams JE. Experiences with a large series of silastic breast implants. *Plastic and Reconstructive Surgery* 1972; **49**: 253.

25. Courtiss EH, Goldwyn RM & Anastasia GW. The fate of breast implants with infections around them. *Plastic and Reconstructive Surgery* 1979; **63**: 812.

26. Le Roy J & Given KS. Wound infection in breast augmentation: The role of prophylactic perioperative antibiotics. *Aesthetic and Plastic Surgery* 1991; **15**: 303.

27. Samuels JB, Rohrich RJ, Weatherall PT, Ho AMN & Goldberg KL. Radiographic diagnosis of breast implant rupture: Current status and comparison of techniques. *Plastic and Reconstructive Surgery* 1995; **96**: 865–877.

28. Ravitch MM. Poland's syndrome – a study of an eponym. *Plastic and Reconstructive Surgery* 1997; **59**: 508–512.

29. Bostwick J. Correction of breast asymmetries. In: *Aesthetic and Reconstructive Breast Surgery*, p103. St Louis: CV Mosby, 1983.

30. Webster JP. Mastectomy for gynaecomastia through a semicircular intra-areolar incision. *Annals of Surgery* 1946; **124**: 556.

Psychological aspects of BBD

CONTENTS

KEY POINTS AND NEW DEVELOPMENTS

1. Patients presenting to breast clinics have a high degree of anxiety. This is related mainly to fear of cancer and resolves when a benign diagnosis is found.
2. However, some women exhibit permanent behaviour change following benign biopsy, possibly related to continued anxiety generated by their physician.
3. Patients presenting with moderate to severe mastalgia fall into two broad groups: those accepting reassurance and those requesting treatment.
4. The first group have scores for anxiety and depression similar to controls.
5. The second group have cyclical variation in anxiety and depression scores, reaching pathological levels in the luteal period.
6. It is not clear whether these luteal phase changes are the result of the pain or the cause.
7. Dermatitis artefacta of the breast is an uncommon expression of an underlying psychological problem.

Following the recognition in the 1970s that breast cancer treatment was associated with significant psychosocial morbidity, an extensive body of literature has developed on a variety of aspects of the psychological correlates of breast cancer. In contrast, the literature on the psychological aspects of benign breast disease is scanty. Often cases of benign breast disease (BBD) are studied purely to act as 'normal' controls for the cancer cases.

A complex relationship exists between an individual's psychological state, physical well-being and underlying personality. Presented with an anxious patient complaining of breast symptoms, it can be difficult to decide whether the primary problem is somatic or psychological. The problem is compounded by a lack of clarity among breast clinicians on what is meant by 'psychological' problems. Three areas have been regarded as contributing to the psychological dimensions of benign breast disease: personality, stress and mood.

Personality is a poorly defined concept which is, as a result, difficult to quantify. There tends to be a certain circularity about definitions of personality. A questionnaire will be designed to determine personality type. The personality type is then defined by a certain score on that questionnaire which is determined because people of that personality type achieve that score. As a result attempts to associate breast disease with personality are unconvincing.

The earliest suggestion that a breast condition could result from psychological causes came from Sir Astley Cooper, who described women who suffered from cyclical breast pain as being 'of an irritable and suggestive nature'.[1] Atkins considered that 'chronic mastitis' was the result of endocrine factors, neuralgic factors and psychological factors.[2] He felt that endocrine factors were the least important and postulated that the 'seed of psychological pain' lay in the woman's awareness of the breast as a common site for cancer. In 1949 Patey rejected the concept of chronic mastitis and classified benign breast disease as 'cystic diseases of the breast' and the 'pain syndrome'.[3] The latter he felt to be a 'subjective disorder' resulting from an exaggeration of the normal premenstrual feeling of engorgement and sensitivities of the breast. He, too, thought that the fear of cancer played a major role in the aetiology of the disorder but felt that a small proportion might be purely psychological in origin and might result from the patient being 'sexually maladjusted with her husband'. The view that breast pain had a psychological origin was commonly held until 1978 when Preece et al.[4] measured the neuroticism scores in women presenting with cyclical mastalgia using the Middlesex Hospital Questionnaire (MHQ). They found no difference between women with cyclical mastalgia and women presenting at the varicose veins clinic, although both were significantly different from female psychiatric outpatients. They concluded that there was no evidence of psychological abnormality in women with breast pain.

More recent studies have examined the patient's mood or the external stress which she is experiencing. These latter studies have the advantage of examining clearly definable parameters. Studies on the inter-relationship of psychological factors and breast disease should use well-accepted, independently validated measurement instruments.[5] When this is done, it is clear that there are definite patterns of psychological morbidity associated with benign breast disease.

PSYCHOLOGICAL PROBLEMS RESULTING FROM BENIGN BREAST DISEASE

The commonest interaction between benign breast disease and the psyche is the development of anxiety as a result of breast symptoms.

Patients presenting to breast clinics have a high level of anxiety irrespective of their subsequent diagnosis.[6] While most studies do not specifically explore the reasons for that anxiety, it is apparent that most patients are worried that they might have breast cancer. The anxiety levels of women who undergo surgical biopsy for benign breast disease remain high until the results of the biopsy are known, at which time they fall to the expected levels for the general population.[7] In one study, women waiting for breast biopsy were compared with a group of women waiting for cholecystectomy. The highest levels of anxiety were found in women who subsequently were found to have benign breast disease. The women with breast cancer had the same levels of anxiety as the cholecystectomy group. The authors interpret this as indicating that women with benign breast disease might have a predisposition to psychological morbidity.[8]

Women recalled for further assessment from breast screening programmes who are subsequently found not to have breast cancer have high levels of anxiety at the time of their clinical attendance.[9] Clearly, in these cases the anxiety is generated by concerns about cancer and not by any underlying psychological problem and it does not give rise to long-term morbidity. It can be argued that short-term morbidity which resolves rapidly after the confirmation of a benign diagnosis is of little importance, but such patients do have a persistent increased awareness of the possibility of developing breast cancer.[10]

A similar finding was noted in a retrospective study of women who had had a breast biopsy for benign disease up to 2 years previously.[11] Fifty-eight per cent recalled severe amounts of anxiety during the period between discovery of an abnormality and the final diagnosis. The mean length of time for discovery to diagnosis was 35 days. Curiously, there was no relationship between the length of delay from discovery to diagnosis and the level of anxiety experienced. The long-term effects of this period of anxiety are unknown and it seems reasonable to try to shorten this period of uncertainty as much as possible. This is the main justification for the introduction of Rapid Diagnosis Clinics, but so far no studies of the psychological effects of such clinics have been published.

There is some evidence of a permanent behaviour change following benign breast biopsy.[12] Women who have undergone benign biopsies are more likely to carry out regular breast self-examination than the general population, suggesting a higher level of specific anxiety. The study is contaminated in that those women also undergo more frequent mammography and physical examination and their anxieties about their breasts may be generated by their medical advisors and be a reflection of the physician's anxieties. The anxiety may become self-reinforcing as women who had had a previous breast biopsy reported greater levels of fear about the outcome of subsequent mammograms, although they were more likely to undergo them than the general population.

PSYCHOLOGICAL ABNORMALITY AS A CAUSE OF BENIGN BREAST DISEASE

Cyclical mastalgia

Cyclical breast pain is common. In population surveys more than 60% of women report that they have experienced cyclical mastalgia which they grade as severe.[13,14]

Despite the findings of Preece et al.,[4] there are difficulties in accepting the organic explanation as the entire explanation for the syndrome. Only 3–10% present for treatment, which raises the question of what precipitates that presentation. Some are concerned that the symptom is a sign of underlying disease. Such women can be reassured by clinical assessment and an explanation of the reason for their symptoms. Other women remain adamant that they need treatment. No difference between the two groups can be detected in the severity of the pain and an alternative explanation must be sought.

The MHQ measures neuroticism, which is a difficult concept to define. More recent instruments measure mood, which is a definite concept that can be defined independently of the results of the psychological instrument, so that the results of the instruments can be validated. In addition, the MHQ contains some ambiguous questions in which a positive response could be the result of physical disease rather than psychological disorder. More recent studies have assessed mood (anxiety and depression) using well-validated instruments.

We examined two groups of women presenting to the breast pain clinic complaining of cyclical mastalgia.[15] Both groups had moderate to severe mastalgia. One group were reassured by their examination at the clinic and did not require any treatment but the other group requested treatment despite being told they had no serious condition affecting their breasts. We compared both groups with a control group of similar age who did not have any breast symptoms.

All the women completed a series of questionnaires in the follicular and luteal phases of the menstrual cycle. The women who had cyclical mastalgia but did not want treatment had results for anxiety and depression similar to those for the control group of women. Their results for state anxiety, trait anxiety and depression were within the limits expected for the general population and did not alter significantly with their cycle. In contrast, the women who requested treatment had a marked cyclical variation in their levels of anxiety and depression and in the luteal phase these levels were in the pathological range. Similar levels of anxiety were found by Ramirez et al. in their study but they did not look for cyclical variation.[16] They did examine the patients' psychosocial adjustment using the Psychosocial Adjustment to Illness Scale (PAIS). This showed a marked impairment of social functioning which improved in those women responding to therapy, suggesting that at least some of the distress is a result of the pain rather than a cause. However, both Downey and Ramirez found that effective pain relief (using goserelin) did not result in elimination of anxiety.

It is not clear, therefore, whether the mood disturbance is the primary problem or whether it is secondary to an underlying hormonal disorder. It appears that the majority of women regard cyclical mastalgia as normal and it only becomes a disease when it is associated with mood disturbance.

Dermatitis artefacta

Occasionally, patients present with persistent ulceration of the breast which defies diagnosis. Biopsy reveals chronic inflammation without any specific features and local measures fail to alleviate the problem. Even excision of the lesion with primary closure is followed by further breakdown. In these circumstances a diagnosis of dermatitis artefacta should be considered.[17] The ulcer often has a bizarre and atypical shape but there is no specific diagnostic feature other than the failure to respond to therapy. Total occlusion may result in temporary healing but recurrence is common.

When there are grounds for suspecting a diagnosis of dermatitis artefacta the opinion of a clinical psychologist or psychiatrist should be sought. The condition can often be cured by directly challenging the patient with the possibility that she is producing the injury herself. Almost always, she will deny this but will stop aggravating the lesion which will rapidly heal. Unfortunately, if it proves impossible to deal satisfactorily with the underlying psychological problem, she is likely to re-present with other psychosomatic problems.

REFERENCES

1. Cooper, Sir Astley. Part 1, pp 3, 78–79. In: *Illustrations of Diseases of the Breast*. London: Longmans, 1823.

2. Atkins HJB. Chronic mastitis. *Lancet* 1938; 707–712.

3. Patey DH. Two common non-malignant conditions of the breast. The clinical features of cystic disease and the pain syndrome. *British Medical Journal* 1949; 1: 96–99.

4. Preece PE, Mansel RE & Hughes LE. Mastalgia: Psychoneurosis or organic disease? *British Medical Journal* 1978; 1: 29–30.

5. Leinster SJ. How to measure psychological morbidity in women with benign breast disease. In: *Proceedings of the 4th International Symposium of Benign Breast Disease*, pp 191–195. Casterton: Parthenon Publishing, 1991.

6. Heim E, Augustiny KF, Blaser A *et al.* Coping with breast cancer – a longitudinal prospective study. *Psychotherapy and Psychosomatics* 1987; 48: 44–59.

7. Ashcroft JJ, Slade PD & Leinster SJ. Psychological aspects of breast cancer treatment. In: Karras E (ed.) *Current Issues in Clinical Psychology*, Vol 3. New York: Plenum, 1986.

8. Hughson AV, Cooper AF, McArdle CS & Smith DC. Psychosocial morbidity in patients awaiting breast biopsy. *Journal of Psychomatic Research* 1988; 32: 173–180.

9. Gram IT, Lund E & Slenker SE. Quality of life following a false positive mammogram. *British Journal of Cancer* 1990; 62: 1018–1022.

10. Bull AR & Campbell MJ. Assessment of the psychological impact of a breast screening programme. *British Journal of Radiology* 1991; 64: 510–515.

11. Benedict S, Williams RD & Baron PL. Recalled anxiety: from discovered to diagnosis of a benign breast mass. *Oncology Nursing Forum* 1994; 21: 1723–1727.

12. Benedict S, Williams RD & Baron PL. The effect of benign breast biopsy on subsequent breast cancer detection practices. *Oncology Nursing Forum* 1994; 21: 1467–1475.

13. Leinster SJ, Whitehouse GH & Walsh PV. Clinical mastalgia: clinical and mammographic observations in a screened population. *British Journal of Surgery* 1987; 74: 220–222.

14. Maddox P & Mansel R. The treatment of mastalgia. *Breast News* 1988; 2: 4–6.

15. Downey HM & Leinster SJ. Mood changes – an explanation why women request treatment for clinical mastalgia. In: Mansel RE (ed.) *Recent Developments in the Study of Benign Breast Disease*, pp 117–132. London: Parthenon, 1993.

16. Ramirez AJ, Jarrett SR, Hamed H, Smith P & Fentiman IS. Psychosocial distress associated with severe mastalgia. In: Mansel RE (ed.) *Recent Developments in the Study of Benign Breast Disease*, pp 109–116. London: Parthenon, 1993.

17. Puig L, Perez M, Llaurado A, Esquius J, Moreno A & de Morgas JM. Factitial dermatosis of the breast: a possible dermatologic manifestation of Munchausen's syndrome. *Cutis* 1989; 44: 292–294.

Index